# Best Practices in Midwifery

Barbara A. Anderson, DrPH, CNM, FACNM, FAAN, was lead editor of the first edition of *Best Practices in Midwifery: Using the Evidence to Implement Change* and now has led the initiative to broaden the scope of this work in the second edition. She currently serves on the board of directors of the American College of Nurse-Midwives. She has had a long career in nursing and public health, field-based teaching, mentorship, program planning, curriculum development, and academic administration. She is lead editor of *DNP Capstone Projects: Exemplars of Excellence in Practice* (2015) and is co-editor of the award-winning text *Caring for the Vulnerable: Perspectives in Nursing Theory, Research, and Practice* (2008, 2012, 2016). Dr. Anderson currently serves as a journal referee for *Social Science & Medicine*. She has served as chair of the Population, Reproductive, and Sexual Health section of the American Public Health Association and led the urban initiative in California that won the Safe Motherhood Initiative—USA Model Program award. She has been a program consultant in midwifery, public health, and nursing in Africa, Asia, and Latin America and has prepared nurses, midwives, and physicians in public health and the midwifery model of care in more than 100 countries. She began her career as a Peace Corps volunteer in Ethiopia, writing a textbook on maternal health for Ethiopian nursing students.

Judith P. Rooks, MPH, MS, CNM, FACNM, is past president of the American College of Nurse-Midwives. As a nurse-midwife and epidemiologist, she has had many years of service with the Centers for Disease Control and Prevention. She was the principal investigator of major studies published in professional journals, including the *New England Journal of Medicine* and the *Journal of the American Medical Association*. She has been a consultant to family planning and midwifery programs globally and served in the Office of the U.S. Surgeon General. She has authored more than 100 published papers and is the author of *Midwifery & Childbirth in America* (2007). In 1993, she received the American Public Health Association's award for outstanding service to the health of mothers and babies. She is currently involved in work related to the safety and risks of home births in the United States. Although retired, she continues to work on behalf of mothers, babies, and midwives.

Rebeca Barroso, DNP, MSN, CNM, FACNM, is an assistant professor of midwifery at Frontier Nursing University and practices full-scope midwifery at HealthEast Care, Saint Paul, Minnesota, serving low-income national and international clientele at Seton Catholic Charities Clinic. She has an extensive background in clinical midwifery and women's health, working with vulnerable women experiencing health disparities from multiple cultural backgrounds. She has been in continuous full-scope certified nurse-midwife (CNM) practice for more than 20 years. She is a preceptor and coordinates clinical education for CNM, women's health nurse practitioner, and family nurse practitioner students, chairing the Education Committee of HealthEast Care. She is a faculty member and mentors midwifery and doctor of nursing practice students at Frontier Nursing University. She is co-editor of *DNP Capstone Projects: Exemplars of Excellence in Practice* (2015). Dr. Barroso won the 2011 W. Newton Award from the American College of Nurse-Midwives and is active in the American College of Nurse-Midwives and the Minnesota Advance Practice Nurses Coalition.

# Best Practices in Midwifery

Using the Evidence to Implement Change

**Second Edition**

Barbara A. Anderson, DrPH, CNM, FACNM, FAAN

Judith P. Rooks, MPH, MS, CNM, FACNM

Rebeca Barroso, DNP, MSN, CNM, FACNM

*Editors*

L.C.C.C. LIBRARY  DISCARD

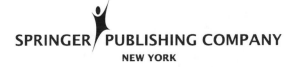

SPRINGER PUBLISHING COMPANY
NEW YORK

Copyright © 2017 Springer Publishing Company, LLC

All rights reserved.

No part of this publication may be reproduced, stored in a retrieval system, or transmitted in any form or by any means, electronic, mechanical, photocopying, recording, or otherwise, without the prior permission of Springer Publishing Company, LLC, or authorization through payment of the appropriate fees to the Copyright Clearance Center, Inc., 222 Rosewood Drive, Danvers, MA 01923, 978-750-8400, fax 978-646-8600, info@copyright.com or on the Web at www.copyright.com.

Springer Publishing Company, LLC
11 West 42nd Street
New York, NY 10036
www.springerpub.com

*Acquisitions Editor*: Margaret Zuccarini
*Composition*: Westchester Publishing Services

*ISBN*: 978-0-8261-3178-2
*e-book ISBN*: 978-0-8261-3179-9
*Instructor's PowerPoints*: 978-0-8261-3213-0

*Instructor's Materials: Qualified instructors may request supplements by e-mailing textbook@springerpub.com*

16 17 18 19 20 / 5 4 3 2 1

The author and the publisher of this Work have made every effort to use sources believed to be reliable to provide information that is accurate and compatible with the standards generally accepted at the time of publication. Because medical science is continually advancing, our knowledge base continues to expand. Therefore, as new information becomes available, changes in procedures become necessary. We recommend that the reader always consult current research and specific institutional policies before performing any clinical procedure. The author and publisher shall not be liable for any special, consequential, or exemplary damages resulting, in whole or in part, from the reader's use of, or reliance on, the information contained in this book. The publisher has no responsibility for the persistence or accuracy of URLs for external or third-party Internet websites referred to in this publication and does not guarantee that any content on such websites is, or will remain, accurate or appropriate.

**Library of Congress Cataloging-in-Publication Data**

Names: Anderson, Barbara A. (Barbara Alice), 1944– , editor. | Rooks, Judith, editor. | Barroso, Rebeca, editor.
Title: Best practices in midwifery : using the evidence to implement change / Barbara A. Anderson, Judith P. Rooks, Rebeca Barroso, editors.
Description: Second edition. | New York, NY : Springer Publishing Company, LLC, [2017] | Includes bibliographical references and index.
Identifiers: LCCN 2016010822 | ISBN 9780826131782 (hardcopy : alk. paper) | ISBN 9780826131799 (ebook) | ISBN 9780826132130 (instructors powerpoints)
Subjects: | MESH: Midwifery—methods | Nurse Midwives | Evidence-Based Nursing | Labor, Obstetric | Obstetric Labor Complications | United States
Classification: LCC RG950 | NLM WY 157 | DDC 618.2—dc23
LC record available at http://lccn.loc.gov/2016010822

Special discounts on bulk quantities of our books are available to corporations, professional associations, pharmaceutical companies, health care organizations, and other qualifying groups. If you are interested in a custom book, including chapters from more than one of our titles, we can provide that service as well.
**For details, please contact:**
Special Sales Department, Springer Publishing Company, LLC
11 West 42nd Street, 15th Floor, New York, NY 10036-8002
Phone: 877-687-7476 or 212-431-4370; Fax: 212-941-7842
E-mail: sales@springerpub.com

Printed in the United States of America by Bradford & Bigelow.

*To all midwives, whose vision, voice, scholarship, and astute clinical observation and practice have forged the path of evidence-based practice*

# CONTENTS

# CONTRIBUTORS

**Barbara A. Anderson, DrPH, CNM, FACNM, FAAN** Independent Consultant in Midwifery and DNP Education; Formerly Professor and University Administrator in Nursing and Public Health (Tenured, Retired); Member of Board of Directors, American College of Nurse-Midwives, Silver Spring, Maryland

**Laura A. Aughinbaugh, DNP, CRNP, CNM, LC** Midwife Clinician in Women's Health, Women's Pelvic Medicine Center, University of California, San Diego, California; Adjunct Instructor, Hahn School of Nursing and Health Science, University of San Diego, San Diego, California

**Mary Paul Backman, MN, CNM** Full Scope Midwife and Educator, Department of Obstetrics and Gynecology, Madigan Army Medical Center, Tacoma, Washington

**Mary K. Barger, PhD, MPH, CNM, FACNM** Associate Professor, Hahn School of Nursing and Health Science, Betty and Bob Beyster Institute of Nursing Research, University of San Diego, San Diego, California; Associate Editor, *Journal of Midwifery and Women's Health*

**Rebeca Barroso, DNP, MSN, CNM, FACNM** Assistant Professor, Midwifery & Women's Health, Frontier Nursing University, Hyden, Kentucky; Full Scope Midwife, Preceptor, and Clinical Educator, HealthEast Care, St. Paul, Minnesota

**Cheryl Tatano Beck, DNSc, CNM, FAAN** Distinguished Professor, School of Nursing, University of Connecticut, Storrs, Connecticut; Member of Board of Trustees, University of Connecticut, Storrs, Connecticut

**Heather M. Bradford, MSN, ARNP, CNM, FACNM** Full Scope Midwife and Preceptor, Evergreen Health Midwifery Care, Kirkland, Washington; Adjunct

Faculty, Nurse-Midwifery/Women's Health Nurse Practitioner Program, School of Nursing and Health Studies, Georgetown University, Washington, DC

**Ginger K. Breedlove, PhD, APRN, CNM, FACNM**    Professor, Graduate Programs, The Eleanor Wade Custer School of Nursing, Shenandoah University, Winchester, Virginia; Immediate Past President, American College of Nurse-Midwives, Silver Spring, Maryland

**Deborah M. Brickner, DNP, FNP-BC, CNM**    Founder and Director, Kaleidocope Family Health, Inc., Madisonville, Tennessee

**Jesse S. Bushman, MA, MALA**    Director, Department of Advocacy and Government Affairs, American College of Nurse-Midwives, Silver Spring, Maryland

**Nicole S. Carlson, PhD, CNM**    Midwife Clinician, Northside Women's Specialists, Atlanta, Georgia; Assistant Professor, School of Nursing, Emory University, Atlanta, Georgia; President, Georgia Affiliate, American College of Nurse-Midwives

**Melody J. Castillo, MSN, CNM, FNP-BC**    Midwife Clinician, Sunset Women's Medical Group, Sunset Community Health Center, Yuma, Arizona

**Michelle R. Collins, PhD, CNM, FACNM**    Professor and Director, Nurse-Midwifery Program, School of Nursing, Vanderbilt University, Nashville, Tennessee

**Jane M. Dyer, PhD, MBA, CNM, FACNM**    Assistant Professor, College of Nursing and Clinical and Translational Scholar, University of Utah, Salt Lake City, Utah; Member of Board of Directors, American College of Nurse-Midwives, Silver Spring, Maryland

**Eunice K. M. Ernst, MPH, CNM, DSc (Hon), FACNM**    Professor and Mary Breckinridge Endowed Chair of Midwifery, Frontier Nursing University, Hyden, Kentucky

**Judith T. Fullerton, PhD, CNM, FACNM**    Independent Consultant in Midwifery and Women's Health Evaluation and Research; Consultant to International Confederation of Midwives; formerly Professor, School of Medicine, University of California, San Diego, California (tenured, retired)

**Meghan Garland, MSN, CNM**    Instructor and Regional Clinical Coordinator, Midwifery & Women's Health, Frontier Nursing University, Hyden, Kentucky

**Billie Anne Gebb, MSLS**    Director of Library Services and Faculty, Frontier Nursing University, Hyden, Kentucky

**Margaret S. Hutchison, MSN, CNM**   Director, CenteringPregnancy® Program, San Francisco General Hospital; Clinical Professor, Department of Obstetrics and Gynecology, University of California, San Francisco, California

**John C. Jennings, MD**   Professor of Obstetrics and Gynecology, Texas Tech University Health Science Center, Permian Basin, Texas; Immediate Past President, American College of Obstetrics and Gynecology, Washington, DC

**Cecilia M. Jevitt, PhD, CNM, FACNM**   Associate Professor, Midwifery and Women's Health Nurse Practitioner Specialties Coordinator, Yale University School of Nursing, West Haven, Connecticut

**Robin G. Jordan, PhD, CNM, FACNM**   Adjunct Instructor, Nurse-Midwifery/ Women's Health Nursing Practitioner Program, School of Nursing & Health Studies, Georgetown University, Washington, DC

**Mayri Sagady Leslie, EdD, MSN, CNM**   Assistant Professor and Director, MSN Concentration in Nurse-Midwifery Program, School of Nursing, The George Washington University, Washington, DC

**Patricia O. Loftman, MS, LM, CNM**   Co-Chair and Leader, Midwives of Color Committee, American College of Nurse-Midwives, Silver Spring, Maryland; formerly Midwife Clinician at The Special Prenatal Clinic, Harlem, New York

**Jody R. Lori, PhD, CNM, FACNM, FAAN**   Associate Professor, Department of Health Behavior and Biological Sciences; Associate Dean of Global Affairs and Director, PAHO/SHO Collaborating Center, University of Michigan, Ann Arbor, Michigan

**Amy Marowitz, DNP, CNM**   Associate Professor, Midwifery & Women's Health, Frontier Nursing University, Hyden, Kentucky

**Kathleen A. Moriarty, PhD, CAFCI, CNM, FACNM**   Instructor, Midwifery & Women's Health, Frontier Nursing University, Hyden, Kentucky; Clinician Midwife, Hutzel Women's Hospital, Detroit, Michigan; Member of Board of Directors, American College of Nurse-Midwives, Silver Spring, Maryland

**Elizabeth Nutter, DNP, CNM**   Deputy Director, U.S. Army Obstetric-Gynecology Course, Fort Hood, Texas

**Julia C. Phillippi, PhD, CNM, FACNM**   Assistant Professor, School of Nursing, Vanderbilt University, Nashville, Tennessee

**Judith P. Rooks, MPH, MS, CNM, FACNM**   Past President of the American College of Nurse-Midwives, Silver Spring, Maryland; Consultant to the American College of Nurse-Midwives Home Birth Task Force; Principal Investigator of National Birth Center Study

**Mavis N. Schorn, PhD, CNM, FACNM** Professor and Senior Associate Dean for Academics, School of Nursing, Vanderbilt University, Nashville, Tennessee

**Kathryn Schrag, MSN, FNP, CNM** Founder, Birth and Women's Health, Tucson, Arizona; Faculty, American Association of Birth Centers, How to Start a Birth Center; Instructor, Midwifery & Women's Health, Frontier Nursing University, Hyden, Kentucky

**Kerri D. Schuiling, PhD, NP, CNM, FACNM, FAAN** Provost and Vice President of Academic Affairs, Northern Michigan University, Marquette, Michigan

**Jenna Shaw-Battista, PhD, CNM** Associate Health Sciences Clinical Professor and Associate Education Director, CNM, WHNP Specialty Program, Department of Family Health Care Nursing, University of California, San Francisco, California

**Joan K. Slager, DNP, CNM, CPC, FACNM** Director, Nurse-Midwifery Program, Bronson Women's Service, Kalamazoo, Michigan; Treasurer, Member of Board of Directors, American College of Nurse-Midwives, Silver Spring, Maryland

**Denise Colter Smith, PhD, CNM** Staff Midwife and Clinical Instructor for Family Medicine Residency Program, Fort Belvoir Community Hospital, Fort Belvoir, Virginia

**Susan R. Stapleton, DNP, CNM, FACNM** Data Coordinator, American Association of Birth Centers, Perkiomenville, Pennsylvania

**Susan E. Stone, DNSc, CNM, FACNM, FAAN** Professor and President, Frontier Nursing University, Hyden, Kentucky

**Lisa Summers, DrPH, CNM, FACNM** Senior Policy Advisor, APRN Issues, Department of Health Policy, American Nurses Association, Silver Spring, Maryland

**Melanie R. Thomas, MS, MD** Assistant Adjunct Professor, Department of Psychiatry, University of California, San Francisco, California

**Suzan Ulrich, DrPH, CNM, FACNM** Assistant Dean for Graduate Nursing Programs, St. Catherine University, St. Paul, Minnesota; Robert Wood Johnson Executive Nurse Fellow

**Zach G. Young, MSLS** Information Services Librarian and Faculty, Frontier Nursing University, Hyden, Kentucky

**Susan M. Yount, PhD, CNM, WHNP-BC, FACNM** Associate Professor, DNP and Midwifery & Women's Health, Frontier Nursing University, Hyden, Kentucky

# FOREWORD

Evidence-based practice (EBP) was established to contest clinical decision making based on tradition rather than science. The original visionary formula for EBP comprised three pillars: (a) the best available evidence; (b) professionals' skills, expertise, and judgment; and (c) the needs and preferences of patients and families (Evidence-Based Medicine Working Group, 1992; National Health Service Executive, 1999). The goal is to use evidence to arrive at best clinical decisions in partnership with women and colleagues of the health care team.

A recent series on midwifery evidence published in *The Lancet* reflects the original three pillars of EBP (Homer et al., 2014; Renfrew et al., 2014; ten Hoope-Bender et al., 2014; Van Lerberghe et al., 2014). The authors' evaluation of evidence to date revealed that 80% of maternal and newborn deaths, including stillbirths, could be averted globally if midwifery were accessible to all women and newborns. Unique to this series was the development of an evidence-informed Quality Maternal and Newborn Care (QMNC) Framework (Renfrew et al., 2014). The framework is presented as a matrix encompassing clinical services founded on philosophy and values, including respect, communication, community knowledge and understanding, and care tailored to a woman's circumstances and needs. Although first-line management of complications and referral services are part of the framework, there is marked attention to optimizing biological, psychological, social, and cultural processes, as well as strengthening a woman's capabilities. Management is expectant and interventions are used only when indicated. "The services provided by midwives are best delivered not only in hospital settings but also in communities—midwifery is not a vertical service offered as a narrow segment of the health system. Midwifery services are a core part of universal health coverage" (Horton & Austudillo, 2014, p. 1).

Every chapter in this second edition of *Best Practices in Midwifery: Using the Evidence to Implement Change* captures the evidence for midwifery as presented in the QMNC Framework. Issues on the organization of care—both globally and locally—are examined, including the midwifery workforce, facilitating access, challenges of advocating for women, migration, and creating a collaborative workplace. Evidence is presented to facilitate best practices in caring for women across the continuum of prenatal, intrapartum, and postpartum care such as therapeutic presence in labor, nutrition and weight management, mental health, and vaccination. The evidence on place of birth describes birth center and home birth data and practicalities. There is innovation and excitement throughout the chapters, creating a culture of change based on best evidence.

This book is intended to assist midwives, nurses, physicians, and administrators to design safe care of the highest quality during pregnancy, birth, and postpartum. It will facilitate changes in institutional policies that work with women to make informed decisions for themselves and their babies. It will help us to reduce health disparities and improve outcomes across populations through the systematic application of the data presented in these pages.

*Holly Powell Kennedy, PhD, CNM, FACNM, FAAN*
*Helen Varney Professor of Midwifery*
*Yale University*
*New Haven, Connecticut*
*Past President, American College of Nurse-Midwives*
*Silver Spring, Maryland*

## REFERENCES

Evidence-Based Medicine Working Group. (1992). Evidence-based medicine: A new approach to teaching the practice of medicine. *Journal of the American Medical Association, 268*(17), 2420–2425.

Homer, C. S., Friberg, I. K., Dias, M. A., ten Hoope-Bender, P., Sandall, J., Speciale, A. M., & Bartlett, L. A. (2014). The projected effect of scaling up midwifery. *Lancet , 384*, 1146–1157. doi:10.1016/S0140-6736(14)60790-X

Horton, R., & Astudillo, O. (2014). The power of midwifery. *Lancet, 384*, 1075–1076. doi:10.1016/S0140-6736(14)60855-2

National Health Service Executive. (1999). *What is evidence-based health care?* Unit 1. *Critical Appraisal Skills Programme and Health Care Libraries Unit*. Oxford, UK: Oxford University Press.

Renfrew, M. J., McFadden, A., Bastos, M. H., Campbell, J., Channon, A. A., Cheung, N. F., . . . Declercq, E. (2014). Midwifery and quality care: Findings from a new evidence-informed framework for maternal and newborn care. *Lancet, 384*, 1129–1145. doi:10.1016/S0140-6736(14)60789-3

ten Hoope-Bender, P., de Bernis, L., Campbell, J., Downe, S., Fauveau, V., Fogstad, H., . . . Van Lerberghe, W. (2014). Improvement of maternal and newborn health through midwifery. *Lancet, 384*, 1226–1235. doi:10.1016/S0140-6736(14)60930-2

Van Lerberghe, W., Matthews, Z., Achadi, E., Ancona, C., Campbell, J., Channon, A., . . . Turkmani, S. (2014). Country experience with strengthening of health systems and deployment of midwives in countries with high maternal mortality. *Lancet, 384*, 1215–1225. doi:10.1016/S0140-6736(14)60919-3

# PREFACE

*The greatest joy is to become a mother; the second greatest is to be a midwife.*
—Norwegian Proverb

The landscape in health care and midwifery has changed considerably since the first edition of *Best Practices in Midwifery: Using the Evidence to Implement Change* was released in 2013. Global and domestic events have highlighted the critical role that midwives play in improving the odds for survival and enhancing the health of mothers and infants. As the first decade of this century closed, the United Nations (UN) Millennium Development Goals (MDGs) merged into the next global initiative, the UN Sustainable Development Goals (SDGs). Many of the MDGs had considerable success. Globally, between 1990 and 2015, the maternal mortality ratio declined by 45% and the under-5-year-old mortality rate declined by more than 50% (UN, 2015). By 2014, more than 71% of births were assisted by a skilled provider, an increase from 59% in 1990 (UN, 2015). Frequently, that skilled provider was a midwife.

In 2014, *The Lancet* published the Series on Midwifery, a critical analysis of the impact and potential for high-quality midwifery care in saving lives and improving the health of women and children (Frenk, Gómez-Dantés, & Moon, 2014). The National Institute for Health and Care Excellence (NICE) guidelines demonstrated the efficacy of physiologic birth in low-technology settings, with midwives as key players (NICE, 2014).

Yet, the world, including the United States, continues to face a critical short-age and maldistribution of midwives and other health professionals. Building capacity across the globe for a skilled midwifery workforce, educated to the Standards of the International Confederation of Midwives (ICM), is an essential component in combatting this deficiency in the global workforce (ICM, 2013; *Lancet* Series, 2014).

The health care landscape in the United States faces enormous challenges. The United States ranked 22 out of 180 nations in a global ranking of maternal deaths in 1990, but fell to 60 of 180 in 2013; the United States has seen a sharp rise in maternal deaths (Kassebaum et al., 2014). As maternal mortality has risen (currently 18.5/100,000 live births) so has morbidity—with many near misses; unplanned events that did not result in death but easily could have (Kassebaum et al., 2014). Women of color, especially those in poverty, continue to bear the burden of mortality and morbidity in childbearing, reflecting higher numbers than the published amalgamated figures of mortality and morbidity (Brown, Small, Taylor, Chireau, & Howard, 2011).

Midwives are central to many of the efforts to combat these appalling statistics. In this book, we examine efforts involving midwifery to improve the health of women and children in the United States, including Strong Start, US MERA, CenteringPregnancy®, and focus on physiologic birth. We also look at excellent endeavors on the global front.

The second edition of this book picks up where the first edition ended. With colleagues Susan Stone, Kitty Ernst, and the faculty at Frontier Nursing University (FNU), the first edition sought to reflect the vision of Mary Breckinridge, founder of the Frontier Nursing Service and the Frontier Graduate School of Midwifery in Hyden, Kentucky (Breckinridge, 1952). The second edition seeks to bring together the voices and knowledge of midwifery experts from across the nation.

This second edition examines updated evidence on a range of topics affecting midwifery, including evidence-based clinical practice, the impact of institutional and national policies, and the effects of diversity and globalization. With contributions from 44 authors, clinicians, scholars, and leaders, the book reflects a vision and voice of best practices grounded in the evidence. Section I examines the external environment that impacts the profession. Section II drills down into the evidence for optimal outcomes. Section III explores the evidence for major midwifery contributions to physiologic birth, and Section IV reminds us that we do not live in a silo but need to work collaboratively with our colleagues across the globe.

Qualified instructors may request PowerPoint supplements to this text from Springer Publishing Company by e-mailing textbook@springerpub.com.

The editors are grateful to the many persons who have supported our efforts to present current evidence and best practices, especially the 43 authors who took time away from their busy practices, positions, and responsibilities to share their knowledge. We are grateful to our reviewers: American Association of Birth Centers past president and current director of Strong Start, Jill Alliman; American College of Nurse-Midwives (ACNM) past president, Katherine Camacho Carr; and external reviewer, E. N. Anderson, professor emeritus of anthropology. It is an honor to have Holly Powell Kennedy sharing her wisdom in the Foreword. Dr. Kennedy is an inspiration to all. We wish to acknowledge Susan Stone, president of FNU, for her visionary ideas in the first edition, and Kitty Ernst, Mary Breckinridge Chair of Midwifery, FNU, who is truly a force of nature in promoting the vision of midwifery. We wish to acknowledge the expertise of co-editor Rebeca Barroso and copy editor Prudence Hull, in editing the manuscript. As always, the Springer Publishing Company editors have given timely and knowledgeable support. Thank you to assistant editor Amanda Devine and to long-time nurse and friend of nursing and midwifery, acquisition editor and Springer Nursing publisher Margaret Zuccarini, for creating a climate of collegiality. As the lead editor, Barbara A. Anderson is indebted to the co-editors of this work, ACNM past president Judith P. Rooks, and clinician par excellence, Rebeca Barroso.

Lastly, to our midwife colleagues, certified nurse-midwives, certified midwives, certified professional midwives, registered midwives, and all those around the world who hold the professional and honorable title of "midwife," we share with you the vision of "a midwife for every woman" (ACNM, 2015, para. 1). That vision has never been more achievable.

*Barbara A. Anderson*
*Judith P. Rooks*
*Rebeca Barroso*

# REFERENCES

American College of Nurse-Midwives (ACNM). (2015). Forging our future: ACNM Strategic Plan 2015-2020. Retrieved from www.midwife.org/ACNM/files/ccLibraryFiles/FILENAME/000000005401/2015-20-strategicplanexecsummary-final-070915.pdf

Breckinridge, M. (1952). *Wide neighborhoods: A story of the Frontier Nursing Service.* Lexington, KY: University Press of Kentucky.

Brown, H. L., Small, M., Taylor, Y. S., Chireau, M., & Howard, D. L. (2011). Near miss maternal mortality in a multiethnic population. *Annals of Epidemiology, 21*(2), 73–77. doi:10.1016/j.annepidem.2010.10.009

Frenk, J., Gómez-Dantés, O., & Moon, S. (2014). From sovereignty to solidarity: A renewed concept of global health for an era of complex interdependence. *Lancet, 383*(9911), 94–97. doi:10.1016/S0140-6736(13)62561-1

International Confederation of Midwives (ICM). (2013). Global standards for midwifery education, with companion guidelines (ICM Core Document 2010, amended 2013). Retrieved from www.internationalmidwives.org

Kassebaum, N. J., Bertozzi-Villa, A., Coggeshall, M. S., Shackelford, K. A., Steiner, C., Heuton, K. R., . . . Lozano, R. (2014). Global, regional, and national levels and causes of maternal mortality during 1990–2013: A systematic analysis for the Global Burden of Disease Study. *Lancet, 384*(9947), 980–1004. doi:10.1016/S0140-6736(14)60696-6

National Institute for Health and Care Excellence (NICE). (2014). Intrapartum care for healthy women and babies. Retrieved from https://www.nice.org.uk/guidance/CG190/chapter/About-this-guideline#copyright

United Nations (UN). (2015). The Millennium Development Goals report. Retrieved from http://www.un.org/millenniumgoals/2015_MDG_Report/pdf/MDG%202015%20rev%20(July%201).pdf

# ADVANCING MIDWIFERY CARE

Barbara A. Anderson

*Section I, "Advancing Midwifery Care," examines the wider context of the profession, with emphasis on the global and domestic midwifery workforce issues. Chapter 1 discusses deficiencies and maldistribution in the global workforce and examines the role of midwifery in meeting global health goals as well as the crucial need to scale up midwifery education and services. Chapter 2 focuses on current initiatives in the United States that seek to address the serious disparities in maternal and child health and the role of midwifery in meeting these needs. This chapter presents current data from the American College of Nurse-Midwives on the challenges facing the scaling up of the midwifery workforce in the United States, offering practical approaches for the individual midwife for involvement in advocacy and the legislative process. Chapter 3, from the field of library science, describes how to obtain and interpret the scientific evidence that is essential for implementing change in practice and advocacy. The authors make a strong argument that best practices in midwifery include excellent skills in searching for evidence-based information. In order to advance the profession and provide optimal care for women, infants, and families, midwives need to understand the external environment affecting practice and use scientific library tools to communicate, practice, and advocate.*

# CHAPTER ONE

# THE MIDWIFERY WORKFORCE: ISSUES GLOBALLY AND IN THE UNITED STATES

Judith T. Fullerton and Barbara A. Anderson

## THE GLOBAL MIDWIFERY WORKFORCE IN CONTEXT

This chapter describes the current definition and state of the global midwifery workforce. We discuss definitions, trends, issues, and best practices in the provision of an adequate midwifery workforce. In the recent decade, the role and contribution of midwives received particular attention as progress toward the United Nation (UN) Millennium Development Goals (MDGs) 4 and 5 was reviewed (Lomazzi, Borisch, & Lasser, 2014; UN, 2015) and the post-2015 agenda was deliberated (Hill, Buse, Brolan, & Ooms, 2014; World Health Organization [WHO], 2015a). These deliberations included addressing the impact of scaling up global midwifery services (Homer et al., 2014).

### Health Statistics and Health Disparities

Health disparities and poor health statistics for women and infants result in the need for a skilled midwifery workforce, with backgrounds, language, and social attributes accessible to diverse populations. The annual number of maternal deaths worldwide declined by 45% between 1990 and 2013, from approximately 546,000 to 289,000 deaths (WHO, 2014). The majority of the global burden of maternal deaths shifted from Asia to sub-Saharan Africa, in large part because of differential trends in fertility, the HIV/AIDS epidemic, and access to reproductive health (Zureick-Brown et al., 2013). Between 2003 and 2009, hemorrhage, hypertensive disorders, and sepsis were responsible for more than half of the maternal deaths worldwide (Say et al., 2014).

In 2013 in the United States, 18.5 mothers died for every 100,000 births, a total of almost 800 deaths. That figure was more than double the maternal mortality rate in countries at complementary levels of economic development, such as Canada, and more than triple the rate in the United Kingdom (Kassebaum et al., 2014). This statistic represents a steep rise in pregnancy-related deaths in

3

the United States since at least 1987, when the mortality rate was 7.2 per 100,000 births. This increase is in stark contrast to most other countries, which have had notable decreases, including many nations in East Asia and Latin America. The United States now ranks 60th for maternal deaths on a list of 180 countries, down markedly from its rank of 22nd in 1990 (Kassebaum et al., 2014). Three major factors are identified as contributing causes: (a) inconsistent obstetric practice (lack of standardization in guidelines for managing obstetric emergencies and complications); (b) an increasing number of women who present for antenatal care with chronic conditions and diseases, which contribute to pregnancy-related conditions; and (c) a general lack of good data about maternal health outcomes (e.g., maternal mortality reviews; Agrawal, 2015).

Mortality statistics mask the additional impact of maternal morbidity that arises from near-miss, unplanned events that did not result in maternal death, but had the clear potential to do so (Pattinson et al., 2009; WHO, 2011a). Timely access to appropriately skilled providers is clearly a variable in near-miss events. This finding has been validated in studies conducted in a multitude of settings both in the United States and across the world (Haddad et al., 2014; Hankins et al., 2012; Kaye, Kakaire, & Osinde, 2011; Nelissen et al., 2013; Tunçalp, Hindin, Souza, Chou, & Say, 2012). A study of near-miss maternal mortality in a U.S. multiethnic population indicated greater risk for Hispanic women, attributed to interaction among health status, socioeconomic level, and ethnicity (Brown, Small, Taylor, Chireau, & Howard, 2011).

Infant and newborn statistics are also compelling. In 2013, 4.6 million (74% of all deaths among those younger than age five) occurred within the first year of life. The risk of a child dying before completing the first year of age was highest in the WHO African region (60 per 1,000 live births), about five times higher than that in the WHO European region (11 per 1,000 live births). Globally, however, the infant mortality rate has decreased from an estimated rate of 63 deaths per 1,000 live births in 1990 to 34 deaths per 1,000 live births in 2013. Annual infant deaths have declined from 8.9 million in 1990 to 4.6 million in 2013 (WHO, 2015b).

Infant mortality declined in the United States between 2005 and 2011 (MacDorman, Hoyert, & Mathews, 2013), although this finding represents a higher infant mortality than 27 other wealthy countries (Ingraham, 2014). Neonatal mortality levels decreased from 4.6 million in 1990 to 3.3 million in 2009 (Oestergaard et al., 2011). The U.S. neonatal mortality rate was 4.01 in 2011. The rate of late fetal deaths (still births $\geq$ 100 g and/or $\geq$ 28 weeks gestation) was 17.7 per 1,000 births. The rate of early neonatal deaths was 8.4 per 1,000 live births, with 67.1% of these occurring by day 3 of life (Vogel et al., 2014).

The goal of achieving health equity is the effort to attain the highest level of health for all people (Ruano, Friedman, & Hill, 2014). Global disparities in mortality statistics are, to some degree, a reflection of very real biological predispositions and propensities (risk factors and indicators) that influence health status of both mothers and infants (Awasogba et al., 2013; Ravelli et al., 2013; Schaaf, Liem, Mol, Abu-Hanna, & Ravelli, 2013).

However, observed differences are also, to some undefined but impactful degree, a difference in health status that results from social disadvantage associated, by region or geography, with race or ethnicity, social, financial, and cultural differences. These characteristics create disparities in access to appropriate and high-quality health care services (Beal, 2011; Kruk, Prescott, & Galea, 2008; Louis, Menard, & Gee, 2015; Vanderbilt et al., 2013). This disparity becomes even more evident in countries, such as the United States, in which the population shows great heterogeneity. Racial/ethnic minority groups in the United States are at disproportionate risk of being uninsured, lacking access to care, and experiencing worse health outcomes from preventable and treatable conditions (Jackson & Gracia, 2014). In a population-based analysis, it was determined that U.S. women who were poor and unemployed, lacked health insurance, and educational attainment were far less likely to utilize reproductive health care services (Hall, Dalton, & Johnson, 2014).

The global action agenda in the post-2015 millennium era is for political will, partnerships, social development, and equity—a rights-based framework for reproductive health care (George, Branchini, & Portela, 2015). These strategies, coupled with health systems strengthening, improvements in quality of care, and expansion of a qualified reproductive health workforce, can bring evidence-based life-saving services to scale (Bhutta, Cabral, Chan, & Keenan, 2012; Pyone, Sorensen, & Tellier, 2012; Sakala, 2012; Souza et al., 2014; Yakoob et al., 2011).

## THE MIDWIFERY WORKFORCE: DEFINITIONS, SCOPE OF PRACTICE, AND GLOBAL CONCEPTS

The profession of midwifery and the titled designation of *midwife* are deeply embedded in history, culture, and tradition. This chapter emphasizes the role and scope of practice of the fully qualified (professional) midwife within the global health workforce. The contributions of other health workers in countries that include the designation of midwife within the regulatory title (auxiliary midwife, community midwife, for example) and those who self-identify as a midwife are acknowledged.

### Definition of the Fully Qualified Midwife

The distinctions in definition and scope of practice are of great importance as countries develop their road maps for achieving sustainable development goals and targets for maternal and newborn health (WHO, 2015c). The distinctions are clearly important to those who are charged with crafting educational policy based on evidence that links provider competency to health outcomes and impact. The International Confederation of Midwives (ICM) definition of the midwife was written in 2011. The definition is a clear mandate for adherence to educational standards:

> A midwife is a person who has successfully completed a midwifery education program that is duly recognized in the country where it is located and that is based on the ICM *Essential Competencies for Basic Midwifery*

*Practice* and the framework of the ICM *Global Standards for Midwifery Education*. (ICM, 2011a, para. 1)

Further, according to the ICM, a midwife is a person who demonstrates competency in the practice of midwifery and has met the qualifications to be registered and/or legally licensed to practice midwifery and use the title "midwife" (ICM, 2011a, para. 1).

There are, in general, two cadres of midwives globally: those educated first as nurses, followed by additional preparation in midwifery, and *direct-entry* midwives who are not prepared initially as nurses. Some countries combine nursing and midwifery in a single program of study. These education programs are not endorsed by the ICM, as the period of education is typically too short to acquire competency in the full scope of practice of either profession.

There are also various pathways within nurse-midwifery and direct-entry midwifery programs of study that offer options and opportunities for advanced degrees and other specializations. Some countries, notably the United States, advocate for or require the minimum of a bachelor's degree for entry into the profession (Phillips, 2015).

## Scope of Midwifery Practice

ICM defines the scope of midwifery practice as follows:

> The midwife is recognized as a responsible and accountable professional who works in partnership with women to give the necessary support, care and advice during pregnancy, labor and the postpartum period, to conduct births on the midwife's own responsibility and to provide care for the newborn and the infant. (ICM, 2011a, para. 1)

This definition further states that the midwife may practice in any setting, including the community, clinics and health units, hospitals, and the home. Qualities of midwifery care include:

- Employing prevention measures
- Promoting normal birth
- Detecting maternal or infant complications
- Accessing appropriate assistance and medical care
- Providing emergency care
- Offering health counseling to the woman, family, and community
- Offering antenatal education and preparation for becoming a parent
- Offering sexual and reproductive health education
- Educating about care of the child (ICM, 2011a)

The scope of midwifery practice overlaps several other cadres that also make a contribution to reproductive and newborn health. The greatest degree of overlap occurs across the perinatal continuum, and may be reflected in the role of the skilled birth attendant (SBA). A 2004 joint statement by WHO, ICM, and the International Federation of Gynecology and Obstetrics (FIGO) defines the SBA as:

> [A]n accredited health professional—such as a midwife, doctor or nurse—who has been educated and trained to proficiency in the skills needed to manage normal (uncomplicated) pregnancies, childbirth and the immediate postnatal period, and in the identification, management and referral of complications in women and newborns. (WHO, 2004, p. 1)

However, the concept of being trained to proficiency requires consideration of the concept of competence (Fullerton, Ghéressi, Johnson, & Thompson, 2011). Research has demonstrated difficulties inherent in measurement and wide variation among countries in the application of the concept of competence (Adegoke, Utz, Msuya, & van den Broek, 2012; Cragin, DeMaria, Campero, & Walker, 2007; Harvey et al., 2007).

## The Global Midwifery Workforce

The basic premise that underpins effective workforce planning is that there must be sufficient quantity and variety of health workers appropriately distributed and competent in the skills needed to meet current and evolving demands of the population. The basic challenges encountered in the effort to conduct effective workforce planning are that many countries are already in a state of workforce deficit and imbalance while epidemiological transformations and the aging of the population continue to modify workforce priorities (WHO, 2015d).

WHO (2006) conducted the most recent study of the global health workforce almost a decade ago. The density of the total health workforce per 1,000 population indicated a range of 2.3 (Africa) to 24.8 (the Americas). The report estimated that a total of 57 (of 192) countries would experience critical shortages of doctors, nurses, and midwives (WHO, 2006). Periodic updates have estimated that the current density of the nursing and midwifery health workforce per 10,000 population ranges from a low of 1.4 to 172.7 (over the period 2007–2013; WHO, 2015b). By WHO region, this ranges from a low of 12.4 per 10,000 population for Africa to 44.9 per 10,000 in the Americas, and a high of 80.2 per 10,000 for the European region. The density also ranges from 5.3 per 10,000 for low-income groups to 88.2 per 10,000 for high-income groups. Current data indicate that about 43% of WHO member states report having fewer than two nursing and midwifery personnel per 1,000 population and 28% report less than one (WHO, 2015b).

The *State of the World's Midwifery, 2014* (UN Population Fund [UNFPA], 2014) provides details concerning the midwifery workforce in 73 low- and middle-income countries. The report generally uses the term *midwife* to include those health professionals who are educated to undertake the roles and responsibilities of a midwife, regardless of their educational pathway to midwifery, whether direct entry, integrated within, or following basic nursing. The report does not link country-based use or definition of the title midwife either to the set of competencies defined by WHO/ICM/FIGO for the SBA or those referenced within the ICM definition of the midwife. Further, *The Lancet's* Series on Midwifery, published in 2014, although providing a full description of core characteristics of practice, nonetheless limits midwifery scope of practice to reproductive health, childbirth, and newborn care:

> [T]he skilled, knowledgeable, and compassionate care for childbearing women, newborn infants, and families across the continuum throughout pre-pregnancy, pregnancy, birth, postpartum, and the early weeks of life. (Renfrew et al., 2014, p. 16)

## The U.S. Midwifery Workforce

A recent estimate indicates that certified nurse-midwives (CNMs) and certified midwives (CMs; direct entry) delivered 7.8% of all hospital births in 2013 (the most current data available; Martin, Hamilton, Osterman, Curtin, & Mathews, 2015), and an additional small proportion of births that occurred in out-of-hospital settings. This figure is based on the U.S. Standard Certificate of Live Birth (Centers for Disease Control and Prevention [CDC], 2003), which specifically captures data for CNM/CM and "other midwife" cadres within the U.S. midwifery workforce. The number of births attended by midwives, other than CNMs/CMs, cannot be subcategorized by title, certification, or licensure. Birth data are a small proportion of the scope of services rendered by the midwifery workforce in the United States, but are the only indicator available within national databases.

Information about the actual size of the midwifery workforce is also elusive, given that titling varies among each of the 50 U.S. states and territories. The American Midwifery Certification Board (AMCB), which maintains a registry of CNMs and CMs, reports that 11,291 persons held active certificates as of May 2015. The North American Registry of Midwives (NARM), which maintains similar information for certified professional midwives (CPMs; of whom the majority are direct-entry midwives), reports that 1,921 credentials had been issued as of June 2015. The additional number of midwives who practice under state-issued authority, but without national certification status, cannot be estimated.

U.S. government reports about the health workforce offer additional information about the midwifery workforce. However, these data focus on CNMs, who also hold the credential of an advanced practice registered nurse (APRN), thus excluding CMs and CPMs (and others) from consideration (U.S. Department of Health and Human Services, Health Resources and Services Administration [HRSA], 2013a, 2015).

## THE POTENTIAL IMPACT OF THE MIDWIFERY WORKFORCE

These differences and distinctions have important implications for educational and health policy. Countries are placing great focus on development of a health human resource policy for sexual, reproductive, maternal, neonatal, child, and adolescent health services. Research emphasis is placed on estimates of workforce needs (Crowe, Utley, Costello, & Pagel, 2012) and affirmation of the impact of skilled birth attendance (Högberg, 2010; Singh, Brodish, & Suchindran, 2014). Policy research focuses on both short- and long-term strategic responses (Prata et al., 2011).

For example, a recent systematic review of studies addresses human resources prepared and positioned to contribute to the improvement of maternal health outcomes (Bhutta, Lassi, & Mansoor, 2010). The review included 83 studies involving SBAs. The authors acknowledge that the positive outcomes demonstrated in that systematic review cannot be disaggregated or attributed to the contribution made by any single cadre of health workers that practices under the umbrella designation of SBA, and certainly not to the cadre of professional midwives. Similarly, targeted research, and a recent critical review of the methods used for the global Demographic and Health Surveys, concluded that the methods used to classify providers of maternal and reproductive care are inconsistent in definitions used across the various countries and even inconsistent with the WHO definition of an SBA. These variations limit cross-country comparisons of the impact of skilled attendance on reproductive health outcomes (Footman et al., 2015; Garenne, 2011).

In September 2013, a review of progress toward meeting MDGs was conducted under the leadership of the UN Secretary-General. A strategy document, "The Midwifery Services Framework," was developed to assist countries in their considerations about development of the role of midwives in advancing an agenda for reproductive, maternal, neonatal, child, and adolescent health services. The guiding framework lays a foundation of pragmatic steps and supporting tools for global use to initiate, develop, strengthen, monitor, and evaluate midwifery services (ICM, 2014). The definitions of a midwife and the practice of midwifery are central in this document.

Taking the MDGs for maternal and child health forward into the post-2015 agenda requires an assessment of the factors that have limited some countries from making sufficient progress and/or meeting the MDG targets for maternal and child health. The going-forward strategy recognizes the need for universal access to reproductive health services and supportive legal, regulatory, and financial frameworks surrounding reproductive health services (WHO, 2015a).

Bergevin, Faveau, and McKinnon (2015) hypothesize that an end to preventable maternal deaths could be achieved by 2035 in nearly all countries if a package of strategically integrated actions would be adopted. These actions include emphasizing universal health coverage, scaling up of human resources, and improving skills. The governance, management, and targeting of appropriate skills of the health workforce is central to any country's response to the challenges of achieving universal coverage and health equity (Campbell et al., 2014; Germain, Sen, Garcia-Moreno, & Shankar, 2015; Grady et al., 2011; Hammonds & Ooms, 2014).

The recent global analysis conducted by the UNFPA (2014) concluded that midwives, when educated and regulated to international standards (ICM, 2011b, 2013a, 2013b), have the competencies to deliver 87% of the 46 essential reproductive maternal and newborn health services needed by women and newborns. The analysis indicated, however, that professional midwives made up only 36% of the reported midwifery workforce.

The potential impact of midwifery services (Renfrew et al., 2014) and the effect of scaling up midwifery globally (Homer et al., 2014) were discussed in *The Lancet's* Series on Midwifery in 2014. Additional analysis indicates that midwives alone can achieve remarkable mortality reductions and that this impact is further enhanced by collaborative services provided by midwives and obstetricians (Bartlett, Weissman, Gubin, Patton-Molitors, & Friberg, 2014; Waldman, Kennedy, & Kendig, 2012).

The WHO's *Strategic Directions for Strengthening Nursing & Midwifery Services—2011–2015* (WHO, 2011b) defines policy actions that must be taken to advance the professions. Key Result Area 3 calls for enhancement of institutional capacity for the intake and production of suitably skilled practitioners to provide comprehensive people-centered services (WHO, 2011b).

## BEST POLICIES AND PRACTICES IN EXPANSION OF THE MIDWIFERY WORKFORCE

The response of governments has frequently been to focus on shorter term solutions that aim to increase the numbers of providers (Mumtaz, Levay, Bhatti, & Salway, 2015) or task shifting/task sharing combined with community-based interventions to address regional shortages (Ni Bhuinneain & McCarthy, 2015), rather than a focus on competencies (Frenk et al., 2010). Strong political will and substantial financial commitment are fundamental to scaling up access to a skilled midwifery workforce (Frenk, Gómez-Dantés, & Moon, 2014; Rosskam, Pariyo, Hounton, & Aiga, 2014).

### Education of the Professional Midwifery Workforce

The guidelines that accompany the ICM global standards for midwifery education (ICM, 2013b) provide support for educators in designing midwifery education programs and curricula that focus on health workforce needs and their country's burden of disease while still adhering to the ICM global standards for education of the professional midwife. Countries are free to design these programs of study in accordance with any of the several evidence-based theories of best practices in education. Transformative and constructivist program approaches hold current prominence. These and other theoretical frameworks share a common theme of competency-based teaching and learning (Fullerton, Johnson, Thompson, & Vivio, 2010; Fullerton, Thompson, & Johnson, 2013; Johnson, Fogarty, Fullerton, Bluestone, & Drake, 2013).

Countries need to focus on the development of the professional midwifery workforce. Shorter term solutions that focus on greater numbers of workers (e.g., the trained traditional birth attendants or the community or auxiliary midwife) have diverted human and financial resources. Demonstrated improvements in quality outcomes of care provided by these health workers are limited (Chary, Diaz, Henderson, & Rohloff, 2013; Pyone, Adaji, Madaj, Woldetsadik, & van den Broek, 2014; Sibley, Sipe, & Barry, 2012; Thompson, Land, Camacho-Hubner, & Fullerton, 2015). Several major investments aimed at short-term improvements in access to care have proven to be unsustainable (Mansoor et al., 2013; Mansoor, Hill, & Barss, 2012; Turkmani et al., 2013).

In the United States, expansion of the midwifery workforce is challenged, in part by reliance on the pipeline of nursing students who elect to enter programs of nurse-midwifery education. This pipeline shortage is exacerbated by current and projected shortages in the nursing workforce (American Association of Colleges of Nursing [AACN], 2014; HRSA, 2013b; Jurascheck, Zhang, Ranganathan, & Lin, 2012). Additional challenges arise from the variation among the U.S. states and territories in licensure of CNMs (Phillips, 2015). Direct-entry midwives are also recognized in many states within the United States. Those who qualify as CMs or CPMs via licensure, certification, registry, or permit also contribute to the U.S. professional midwifery workforce.

The various professional associations, certification agencies, and accreditation authorities that represent the interests of professional and other categories of state-licensed or unregulated midwives are engaged in efforts to achieve uniformity and harmony in the U.S. midwifery workforce. The U.S. Midwifery, Education, Regulation and Association (US MERA) workgroup have identified ICM standards and guidelines as a common goal (Camacho Carr, Collins-Fulea, Krulewitch, & Breedlove, 2015).

## Appropriate Task Shifting/Task Sharing

Task shifting is defined as either (a) developing a new provider cadre with competencies to perform tasks normally performed by health professionals with more education and higher qualifications or (b) expanding the scope of practice of an existing health professional cadre to accept additional tasks and functions (Deller et al., 2015). Appropriate task sharing is a type of collaborative practice in which the higher order/higher impact skills are reserved for the most appropriately skilled professional and delegation of remaining tasks to other health providers trained to proficiency in their performance. It is a reflection of the overarching scopes of practice among various health workers across the perinatal continuum.

Task shifting, also known as task sharing, has become an identified global strategy for remediation of health worker shortages. The WHO published global recommendations and guidelines with an initial focus on response to the HIV/ AIDS epidemic (WHO, 2008). In 2012, this focus was expanded to maternal and newborn health (WHO, 2012). Task sharing is an effort to expand the reach of lifesaving services to women, newborns, and their families. It is a strategy for maximizing the quality and performance of existing cadres of health workers (WHO, 2015d).

Renfrew et al. (2014) conducted an exhaustive analysis of the broad range of practices within the domain of maternal and newborn care that could or should be within the scope of midwifery practice. The review also identified the effectiveness of interventions delivered by midwives and other workforce groups that provided some or all of the components of midwifery care. A final extension of the review identified components of midwifery care delivered by community and traditional health workers. The outcome of these reviews underpinned an evidence-based framework that describes a system for high-quality maternal and newborn care. This system is most effective when integrated into a collaborative approach to care (task sharing) and referral (Renfrew et al., 2014).

Dawson, Buchan, Duffield, Homer, and Wijewardena (2014) conducted a similar synthesis of the literature, which indicated that task sharing may increase access, availability, and cost-effectiveness of maternal and reproductive health services without compromising performance or patient outcomes. The issues and barriers to task sharing necessitate the need for appropriate education of the cadre to whom any task is shifted, and a supportive, effective health system that enables prompt and responsive referrals among care partners (Dawson et al., 2014). These findings were congruent with the findings of Renfrew et al. (2014).

## Appropriate Recruitment, Migration, and Licensure Across Nations

The movement of health professionals among countries of origin (source) and other countries (destination) for purposes of employment has benefits and limitations for individual midwives and the global community (Aluttis, Bishaw, & Frank, 2014). Economic conditions in both source and target countries are a key factor in stimulating workforce migration (Anderson, 2012; Anderson & Isaacs, 2007). A WHO analysis indicates that there is considerable variation in midwifery-to-personnel ratios within countries, which is consistent with the variation in the level of economic development of the region. Africa and Southeast Asia report the lowest average ratios and Europe the highest (Buchan, O'May, & Dussault, 2013). Nair and Webster (2013) estimates that about one third of the countries affected by shortage of human resources for health are the emerging market economies. These are some of the same countries that see out-migration of their workforce, which is seeking to improve personal employment opportunities and economic status (Brock, 2013; Marcus, Quimson, & Short, 2014).

The experience of midwives who obtained employment in target countries was the subject of a systematic review (Moyce, Lash, & de Leon Siantz, 2015), which concluded that licensing barriers, language challenges, racism, marginalization, and discrimination were common, a finding consistent with a number of similar single-country studies (Bourgeault, Neiterman, & Lebrun, 2011; Pittman, 2013), including the United States (Chen, Auerbach, Muench, Curry, & Bradley, 2013; Sherwood & Shaffer, 2014). Reliance on international recruitment is a short-term solution to health workforce planning (Anderson & Isaacs, 2007; Buchan, Twigg, Dussault, Duffield, & Stone, 2015; Humphries, Brugha, & McGee, 2012).

It is the responsibility of individual governments to develop solutions to retain their own health professionals so as to mitigate the adverse effects of workforce maldistribution and shortages. It is also the responsibility of each destination country to be aware of the fact that its gain may generate risk and impact within source countries, and to adhere to principles of accountability and social justice in recruitment of the workforce from source countries.

The WHO has developed a code of practice that speaks to the responsibilities of governments in the recruitment of health personnel (WHO, 2010). A set of guidelines for career moves and migration that incorporates an ethical framework for nurse recruitment has been developed by the International Council of Nurses (2010). A voluntary code of conduct for ethical recruitment of foreign-educated health professionals has been distributed within the United States ("Alliance," 2011).

There has been at least one larger scale study of the effect of compliance with codes of conduct (Young, 2013). A major finding of that inquiry was that adherence to these policies slowed international recruitment. More importantly, it placed emphasis on acknowledging the value of those professionals who have been recruited to a target country as contributing members of the target country workforce. In turn, this places responsibility on source countries for continued professional development of the individual midwife already in practice, and for development of their national workforce, as a contribution to quality of the global midwifery workforce.

Internationally educated midwives face significant challenges in obtaining licensure to practice in the United States. Those wishing to quality as CNMs must meet eligibility for the AMCB national certification examination. At present, this is not available outside of re-enrollment in a basic midwifery education program (AMCB, 2015). There are mechanisms leading to eligibility for the NARM certification and the CPM credential (NARM, 2015). Further work of the US MERA workgroup may, in the future, expand these options and opportunities.

International migration also involves migration of faculty among countries, which can adversely affect the ability of source countries to build the capacity of their health workforce (Anderson & Isaacs, 2007). A recent systematic review of the literature addressing nurse faculty migration (Benton, González-Jurado, & Beneit-Montesinos, 2013) concluded that this topic has not been adequately addressed in the policy debate. A global summit was convened to generate a relevant sub-Saharan regional policy agenda (Thompson et al., 2014). That body of work has not been implemented to date.

## CONCLUSION

The landmark document, *The Lancet's* Series on Midwifery, identifies midwifery as key to promoting the health and well-being of women and newborns globally and in the United States. Stability and scaling up of the midwifery workforce are critical issues in the provision of services (Renfrew et al., 2014). Although maternal mortality has declined in many areas of the world, it has risen steeply in the United States (Kassebaum, 2014). This demographic shift places an increased burden on the United States to plan effectively for both midwifery education and expansion of services.

The basic premise of effective workforce planning is sufficient quantity and variety of appropriately distributed competent health workers. Many countries, including the United States, are in a state of workforce deficit and imbalance (WHO, 2015b). The going-forward strategy of the post-2015 MDGs agenda recognizes the need for universal access to reproductive health services and legal, regulatory, and financial frameworks to support those services (WHO, 2015a). Key to this agenda is the scaling up of the midwifery workforce.

Best practices in the expansion of the midwifery workforce include education in line with the ICM standards, task shifting as appropriate, and equitable distribution of the workforce. The latter requires special attention to the global issues of workforce recruitment and migration. Unregulated recruitment and migration place a huge burden upon source nations and can have a profound impact on the health of women and newborns globally. The issues of ethical conduct and social justice are central to the resolution of the global midwifery workforce shortage.

## REFERENCES

Adegoke, A., Utz, B., Msuya, S. E., & van den Broek, N. (2012). Skilled birth attendants: Who is who? A descriptive study of definitions and roles from nine Sub Saharan African Countries. *PLoS One*, 7(7), e40220. doi:10.1371/journal.pone.0040220

Agrawal, P. (2015). Maternal mortality and morbidity in the United States of America. *Bulletin of the World Health Organization*, 93(3), 135. doi:10.2471/BLT.14.148627

Alliance for Ethical International Recruitment Practices. (2011). Voluntary code of conduct for the recruitment of foreign-educated health professionals to the United States. Retrieved from http://www.nursingworld.org/MainMenuCategories/ThePracticeofProfessionalNursing/workforce/ForeignNurses/CodeofConductforRecruitmentofForeignEducatedNurses.pdf

Aluttis, C., Bishaw, T., & Frank, M. W. (2014). The workforce for health in a globalized context—Global shortages and international migration. *Global Health Action*, 7, 23611. doi:10.3402/gha.v7

American Association of Colleges of Nursing (AACN). (2014). Nursing shortage fact sheet. Retrieved from http://www.aacn.nche.edu/media-relations/NrsgShortageFS.pdf

American Midwifery Certification Board (AMCB). (2015, May). AMCB report of CNM/CM by state. Retrieved from http://www.amcbmidwife.org/docs/default-document-library/number -of-cnm-cm-by-state—may-2015.pdf?sfvrsn=2

Anderson, B. A. (2012). The nursing workforce shortage: The vulnerability of the health care system. In M. de Chesnay & B. A. Anderson (Eds.), *Caring for the vulnerable: Perspectives in nursing theory, research, and practice* (3rd ed., pp. 557–563). Boston, MA: Jones & Bartlett.

Anderson, B. A., & Isaacs, A. A. (2007). Simply not there: The impact of international migration of nurses and midwives—Perspectives from Guyana. *Journal of Midwifery and Women's Health*, 52(4), 392–397. doi:10.1016/j.jmwh.2007.02.021

Awasogba, T., Betancourt, J. R., Conyers, F. G., Estapé, E. S., Francois, F., Gard, S. J., . . . Yeung, H. (2013). Prioritizing health disparities in medical education to improve care. *Annals of the New York Academy of Sciences*, 1287(1), 17–30. doi:10.1111/nyas.12117

Bartlett, L., Weissman, E., Gubin, R., Patton-Molitors, R., & Friberg, I. K. (2014). The impact and cost of scaling up midwifery and obstetrics in 58 low- and middle-income countries. *PLoS One*, 9(6), e98550. doi:10.1371/journal.pone.0098550

Beal, A. C. (2011). High-quality health care: The essential route to eliminating disparities and achieving health equity. *Health Affairs, 30*(10), 1868–1871. doi:10.1377/hlthaff.2011.0976

Benton, D. C., González-Jurado, M. A., & Beneit-Montesinos, J. V. (2013). Nurse faculty migration: A systematic review of the literature. *International Nursing Review, 60*(2), 157–166. doi:10.1111/inr.12008

Bergevin, Y., Faveau, V., & McKinnon, B. (2015). Towards ending preventable maternal deaths by 2035. *Seminars in Reproductive Medicine, 33*(1), 23–29. doi:10.1055/s-0034-1395275

Bhutta, Z. A., Cabral, S., Chan., C. W., & Keenan, W. J. (2012). Reducing maternal, newborn, and infant mortality globally: An integrated action agenda. *International Journal of Gynaecology and Obstetrics, 119*(Suppl. 1), S13–S17. doi:10.1016/j.ijgo.2012.04.001

Bhutta, Z. A., Lassi, Z. S., & Mansoor, N. (2010). Systematic review on human resources for health interventions to improve maternal health outcomes: Evidence from developing countries. Retrieved from http://www.who.int/pmnch/activities/human_resources/hrh_maternal_health_2010.pdf

Bourgeault, I. L., Neiterman, E., & Lebrun, J. (2011). Midwives on the move: Comparing the requirements for practice and integration contexts for internationally educated midwives in Canada with the U.S., U.K., and Australia. *Midwifery, 27*(3), 368–375. doi:10.1016/j.midw.2011.03.010

Brock, G. (2013). Is active recruitment of health workers really not guilty of enabling harm or facilitating wrongdoing? *Journal of Medical Ethics, 39*(10), 612–614. doi:10.1136/medethics-2012-101136

Brown, H. L., Small, M., Taylor, Y. S., Chireau, M., & Howard, D. L. (2011). Near miss maternal mortality in a multiethnic population. *Annals of Epidemiology, 21*(2), 73–77. doi:10.1016/j.annepidem.2010.10.009

Buchan, J., O'May, F., & Dussault, G. (2013). Nursing workforce policy and the economic crisis: A global overview. *Journal of Nursing Scholarship, 45*(3), 298–307. doi:10.1111/jnu.12028

Buchan, J., Twigg, D., Dussault, G., Duffield, C., & Stone, P. W. (2015). Policies to sustain the nursing workforce: An international perspective. *International Nursing Review, 62*(2), 162–170. doi:10.1111/inr.12169

Camacho Carr, K., Collins-Fulea, C., Krulewitch, C., & Breedlove, G. (2015). The United States midwifery education, regulation and association work group: What is it and what does it hope to accomplish? *Journal of Midwifery & Women's Health, 60*(2), 125–127. doi:10.1111/jmwh.12306

Campbell, J., Buchan, J., Cometto, G., David, B., Dussault, G., Fogstad, H., . . . Tangcharoensathien, V. (2014). Human resources for health and universal health coverage: Fostering equity and effective coverage. *Bulletin of the World Health Organization, 91*(11), 853–863. doi:10.2471/BLT.13.118729

Centers for Disease Control and Prevention (CDC). (2003). U.S. standard certificate of live birth. Retrieved from http://www.cdc.gov/nchs/data/dvs/birth11-03final-ACC.pdf

Chary, A., Diaz, A. K., Henderson, B., & Rohloff, P. (2013). The changing role of indigenous lay midwives in Guatemala: New frameworks for analysis. *Midwifery, 29*(8), 852–858. doi:10.1016/j.midw.2012.08.011

Chen, P. G., Auerbach, D. I., Muench, U., Curry, L. A., & Bradley, E. H. (2013). Policy solutions to address the foreign-educated and foreign-born health care workforce in the United States. *Health Affairs, 32*(11), 1906–1913. doi:10.1377/hlthaff.2013.0576

Cragin, L., DeMaria, L. M., Campero, L., & Walker, D. M. (2007). Educating skilled birth attendants in Mexico: Do the curricula meet International Confederation of Midwives standards? *Reproductive Health Matters, 15*(30), 50–60. doi:10.1016/S0968-8080(07)30332-7

Crowe, S., Utley, M., Costello, A., & Pagel, C. (2012). How many births in sub-Saharan Africa
and South Asia will not be attended by a skilled birth attendant between 2011 and 2015?
*BMC Pregnancy and Childbirth, 12*(1), 4. doi:10.1186/1471-2393-12-4

Dawson, A. J., Buchan, J., Duffield, C., Homer, C. S., & Wijewardena, K. (2014). Task shifting
and sharing in maternal and reproductive health in low-income countries: A narrative
synthesis of current evidence. *Health Policy and Planning, 29*(3), 396–408. doi:10.1093/
heapol/czt026

Deller, B., Tripathi, V., Stender, S., Otolorin, E., Johnson, P., & Carr, C. (2015). Task shifting
in maternal and newborn health care: Key components from policy to implementation.
*International Journal of Gynecology and Obstetrics, 130*(Suppl. 2), S25–S31. doi:10.1016/j
.ijgo.2015.03.005

Footman, K., Benova, L., Goodman, C., Macleod, D., Lynch, C. A., Penn-Kekana, L., &
Campbell, O. M. (2015). Using multi-country household surveys to understand who pro-
vides reproductive and maternal health services in low-and middle-income countries:
A critical appraisal of the Demographic and Health Surveys. *Tropical Medicine &
International Health, 20*(5), 589–606. doi:10.1111/tmi.12471

Frenk, J., Chen, L., Bhutta, Z. A., Cohen, J., Crisp, N., Evants, T., . . . Zurayk, H. (2010).
Health professionals for a new century: Transforming education to strengthen health
systems in an interdependent world. *Lancet, 376*(9756), 1923–1958. doi:10.1016/S0140
-6736(10)61854-5

Frenk, J., Gómez-Dantés, O., & Moon, S. (2014). From sovereignty to solidarity: A renewed
concept of global health for an era of complex interdependence. *Lancet, 383*(9911), 94–97.
doi:10.1016/S0140-6736(13)62561-1

Fullerton, J. T., Ghérissi, A., Johnson, P. G., & Thompson, J. B. (2011). Competence and
competency: Core concepts for international midwifery practice. *International Journal of
Childbirth, 1*(1), 4–12. doi:10.1891/215652811795481140

Fullerton, J. T., Johnson, P. J., Thompson, J. B., & Vivio, D. (2010). Quality considerations
in midwifery pre-service education: Exemplars from Africa. *Midwifery, 27*(3), 308–315.
doi:10.1016/j.midw.2010.10.011

Fullerton, J. T., Thompson, J. B., & Johnson, P. (2013). Competency-based education: The essential basis of pre-service education for the professional midwifery workforce. *Midwifery,
29*(10), 1129–1136. doi:10.1016/j.midw.2013.07.006

Garenne, M. (2011). Estimating obstetric mortality from pregnancy-related deaths recorded
in demographic censuses and surveys. *Studies in Family Planning, 42*(4), 237–246. doi:
10.1111/j.1728-4465.2011.00287.x

George, A. S., Branchini, C., & Portela, A. (2015). Do interventions that promote awareness
of rights increase use of maternity care services? A systematic review. *PLoS One, 10*(10),
e0138116. doi:10.1371/journal.pone.0138116

Germain, A., Sen, G., Garcia-Moreno, C., & Shankar, M. (2015). Advancing sexual and
reproductive health and rights in low- and middle-income countries: Implications for the
post-2015 global development agenda. *Global Public Health, 10*(2), 137–148. doi:10.1080/
17441692.2014.986177

Grady, K., Ameh, C., Adegoke, A., Kongnyuy, E., Dornan, J., Falconer, T., . . . van den Broek, N. (2011). Improving essential obstetric and newborn care in resource-poor countries. *Journal of Obstetrics and Gynaecology, 31*(1), 18–23. doi:10.3109/01443615.2010.533218

Haddad, S. M., Cecatti, J. G., Souza, J.P., Sousa, M. H., Parpinelli, M. A., Costa, M. L., . . . Mattar, R. (2014). Applying the maternal near miss approach for the evaluation of quality of obstetric care: A worked example from a multicenter surveillance study. *BioMed Research International,* 1. doi:10.1155/2014/989815

Hall, K. S., Dalton, V., & Johnson, T. R. (2014). Social disparities in women's health service use in the United States: A population-based analysis. *Annals of Epidemiology, 24*(2), 135–143. doi:10.1016/j.annepidem.2013.10.018

Hammonds, R., & Ooms, G. (2014). The emergence of a global right to health norm—The unresolved case of universal access to quality emergency obstetric care. *BMC International Health and Human Rights, 14*(1), 4. doi:10.1186/1472-698X-14-4

Hankins, G. D., Clark, S. L., Pacheco, L. D., O'Keefe, D., D'Alton, M., & Saade, G. R., (2012). Maternal mortality, near misses, and severe morbidity: Lowering rates through designated levels of maternity care. *Obstetrics & Gynecology, 120*(4), 929–934. doi:10.1097/AOG .0b013e31826af878

Harvey, S. A., Blandón, Y. C., McCaw-Binns, A., Sandino, I., Urbina, L., Rodriguez, C., . . . Djibrina, S. (2007). Are skilled birth attendants really skilled? A measurement method, some disturbing results and a potential way forward. *Bulletin of the World Health Organization,* 85(10), 783–790. doi:10.2471/BLT.06.038455

Hill, P. S., Buse, K., Brolan, C. E., & Ooms, G. (2014). How can health remain central post-2015 in a sustainable development paradigm? *Globalization and Health, 10*(1), 1–5. doi:10 .1186/1744-8603-10-18

Högberg, U. (2010). Midlevel providers and the fifth millennium goal of reducing maternal mortality. *Sexual & Reproductive Healthcare, 1*(1), 3–5. doi:10.1016/j.srhc.2009.11.002

Homer, C. S., Friberg, I. K., Dias, M. A., ten Hoope-Bender, P., Sandall, J., Speciale, A. M., & Bartlett, L. A. (2014). The projected effect of scaling up midwifery. *Lancet, 384*(9948), 1146–1157. doi:10.1016/S0140-6736(14)60790-X

Humphries, N., Brugha, R., & McGee, H. (2012). Nurse migration and health workforce planning: Ireland as illustrative of international challenges. *Health Policy, 107*(1), 44–53. doi:10.1016/j.healthpol.2012.06.007

Ingraham, C. (2014, September 29). Our infant mortality rate is a national embarrassment. *Washington Post.* Retrieved from http://www.washingtonpost.com/blogs/wonkblog/wp/ 2014/09/29/our-infant-mortality-rate-is-a-national-embarrassment

International Confederation of Midwives (ICM). (2011a). ICM international definition of the midwife. Retrieved from http://www.internationalmidwives.org/assets/uploads/documents/ Definition%20of%20the%20Midwife%20-%202011.pdf

International Confederation of Midwives (ICM). (2011b). Global standards for midwifery regulation. Retrieved from http://www.internationalmidwives.org/assets/uploads/documents/ Global%20Standards%20Competencies%20Tools/English/GLOBAL%20STANDARDS%20 FOR%20MIDWIFERY%20REGULATION%20ENG.pdf

International Confederation of Midwives (ICM). (2013a). Essential competencies for basic midwifery practice (ICM Core Document 2010, amended 2013). Retrieved from http://www .internationalmidwives.org/assets/uploads/documents/CoreDocuments/ICM%20Essential

%20Competencies%20for%20Basic%20Midwifery%20Practice%202010,%20revised%20 2013.pdf

International Confederation of Midwives (ICM). (2013b). Global standards for midwifery education, with companion guidelines (ICM Core Document 2010, amended 2013). Retrieved from http://www.internationalmidwives.org/assets/uploads/documents/CoreDocuments/ ICM%20Standards%20Guidelines_ammended2013.pdf

International Confederation of Midwives (ICM). (2014). The ICM Midwifery Services Framework for reproductive, maternal, neonatal, child health services. Retrieved from http://www.internationalmidwives.org/projects-programmes/icm-msf-page1

International Council of Nurses. (2010). Guidelines. Career moves and migration: Critical questions. Retrieved from http://www.icn.ch/images/stories/documents/publications/ guidelines/guideline_career_moves_migration_eng.pdf

Jackson, C. S., & Gracia, J. N. (2014). Addressing health and health-care disparities: The role of a diverse workforce and the social determinants of health. *Public Health Reports, 129*(Suppl. 2), 57–61.

Johnson, P., Fogarty, L., Fullerton, J., Bluestone, J., & Drake, M. (2013). An integrative review and evidence-based conceptual model of the essential components of pre-service education. *Human Resources for Health, 11*(1), 42. doi:10.1186/1478-4491-11-42

Jurascheck, S. P., Zhang, X., Ranganathan, V., & Lin, V. W. (2012). United States registered nurse workforce report card and shortage forecast. *American Journal of Medical Quality, 27*(3), 241–249. doi:10.1177/1062860611416634

Kassebaum, N. J., Bertozzi-Villa, A., Coggeshall, M. S., Shackelford, K. A., Steiner, C., Heuton, K. R., . . . Lozano, R. (2014). Global, regional, and national levels and causes of maternal mortality during 1990–2013: A systematic analysis for the Global Burden of Disease Study. *Lancet, 384*(9947), 980–1004. doi:10.1016/S0140-6736(14)60696-6

Kaye, D. K., Kakaire, O., & Osinde, M. O. (2011). Systematic review of the magnitude and case fatality ratio for severe maternal morbidity in sub-Saharan Africa between 1995 and 2010. *BMC Pregnancy and Childbirth, 11*(1), 65. doi:10.1186/1471-2393-11-65

Kruk, M. E., Prescott, M. R., & Galea, S. (2008). Equity of skilled birth attendant utilization in developing countries: Financing and policy determinants. *American Journal of Public Health, 98*(1), 142–147. doi:10.2105/AJPH.2006.104265

Lomazzi, M., Borisch, B., & Lasser, U. (2014). The Millennium Development Goals: Experiences, achievements and what's next. *Global Health Action, 7.* doi:10.3402/gha.v7.23695

Louis, J. M., Menard, M. K., & Gee, R. E. (2015). Racial and ethnic disparities in maternal morbidity and mortality. *Obstetrics & Gynecology, 125*(3), 690–694. doi:10.1097/AOG .0000000000000704

MacDorman, M. F., Hoyert, D. L., & Mathews, T. J. (2013). Recent declines in infant mortality in the United States, 2005—2011. *NCHS Data Brief, No. 120.* Retrieved from http://www .cdc.gov/nchs/data/databriefs/db120.pdf

Mansoor, G. F., Hashemy, P., Gohar, F., Wood, M. E., Ayoubi, S. F., & Todd, C. S. (2013). Midwifery retention and coverage and impact on service utilization in Afghanistan. *Midwifery, 29*(10), 1088–1094. doi:10.1016/j.midw.2013.07.021

Mansoor, G. F., Hill, P. S., & Barss, P. (2012). Midwifery training in post-conflict Afghanistan: Tensions between educational standards and rural community needs. *Health Policy and Planning, 27*(1), 60–68. doi:10.1093/heapol/czr005

Marcus, K., Quimson, G., & Short, S. D. (2014). Source country perceptions, experiences, and recommendations regarding health workforce migration: A case study from the Philippines. *Human Resources for Health, 12*(1), 62. doi:10.1186/1478-4491-12-62

Martin, J. A., Hamilton, B. E., Osterman, M. J., Curtin, S. C., & Mathews, T. J. (2015). Births: Final data for 2013. *National Vital Statistics Report, 64*(1). Retrieved from http://www.cdc.gov/nchs/data/nvsr/nvsr64/nvsr64_01.pdf

Moyce, S., Lash, R., & de Leon Siantz, M. L. (2015). Migration experiences of foreign educated nurses: A systematic review of the literature. *Journal of Transcultural Nursing* [E-pub ahead of print]. doi:10.1177/1043659615569538

Mumtaz, Z., Levay, A., Bhatti, A., & Salway, S. (2015). Good on paper: The gap between programme theory and real-world context in Pakistan's Community Midwife programme. *British Journal of Obstetrics and Gynaecology, 122*(2), 249–258. doi:10.1111/1471-0528.13112

Nair, M., & Webster, P. (2013). Health professionals' migration in emerging market economies: Patterns, causes and possible solutions. *Journal of Public Health, 35*(1), 157–163. doi:10.1093/pubmed/fds087

Nelissen, E., Mduma, E., Broerse, J., Ersdal, H., Evjen-Olsen, B., van Roosmalen, J., & Stekelenburg, J. (2013). Applicability of the WHO maternal near miss criteria in a low-resource setting. *PLoS One, 8*(4), e61248. doi:10.1371/journal.pone.0061248

Ni Bhuinneain, G. M., & McCarthy, F. P. (2015). A systematic review of essential obstetric and newborn care capacity building in rural sub-Saharan Africa. *British Journal of Obstetrics and Gynaecology, 122*(2), 174–182. doi:10.1111/1471-0528.13218

North American Registry of Midwives (NARM). (2015). Current status. Retrieved from http://narm.org/certification/current-status

Oestergaard, M. Z., Inoue, M., Yoshida, S., Manhanani, W. R., Gore, F. M., Counsens, S., . . . Mathers, C. D. (2011). Neonatal mortality levels for 193 countries in 2009 with trends since 1990: A systematic analysis of progress, projections, and priorities. *PLoS Medicine, 8*(8), e1001080. doi:10.1371/journal.pmed.1001080

Pattinson, R., Say, L., Souza, J., van den Brooek, N., Rooney, C. I., & the WHO Working Group on Maternal Mortality and Morbidity Classifications. (2009). WHO maternal deaths and near-miss classifications. *Bulletin of the World Health Organization, 87*(10), 734–734A. doi:10.2471/BLT.09.071001

Phillips, S. J. (2015). 27th annual APRN legislative update: Advancements continue for APRN practice. *Nurse Practitioner, 40*(1), 16–42. doi:10.1097/01.NPR.0000457433.04789.ec

Pittman, P. (2013). Nursing workforce education, migration and the quality of health care: A global challenge. *International Journal of Quality in Health Care, 25*(4), 349–351. doi:10.1093/intqhc/mzt048

Prata, N., Passano, P., Rowen, T., Bell, S., Walsh, J., & Potts, M. (2011). Where there are (few) skilled birth attendants. *Journal of Health Population and Nutrition, 29*(2), 81–91. doi:10.3329/jhpn.v29i2.7812

Pyone, T., Adaji, S., Madaj, B., Woldetsadik, T., & van den Broek, N. (2014). Changing the role of the traditional birth attendant in Somaliland. *International Journal of Gynecology and Obstetrics, 127*(1), 41–46. doi:10.1016/j.ijgo.2014.04.009

Pyone, T., Sorensen, B. L., & Tellier, S. (2012). Childbirth attendance strategies and their impact on maternal mortality and morbidity in low-income settings: A systematic review.

*Acta Obstetricia et Gynecologica Scandinavica, 91*(9), 1029–1037. doi:10.1111/j.1600-0412 .2012.01460.x

Ravelli, A. C., Schaff, J. M., Eskes, M., Abu-Hanna, A., de Miranda, E., & Mol, B. W. (2013). Ethnic disparities in perinatal mortality at 40 and 41 weeks of gestation. *Journal of Perinatal Medicine, 41*(4), 381–388. doi:10.1515/jpm-2012-0228

Renfrew, M. J., McFadden, A., Bastos, M. H., Campbell, J., Channon, A. A., Cheung, N. F., . . . Declercq, E. (2014). Midwifery and quality care: Findings from a new evidence-based informed framework for maternal and newborn care. *Lancet, 384*(9948), 1129–1145. doi:10 .1016/S0140-6736(14)60789-3

Rosskam, E., Pariyo, G., Hounton, S., & Aiga, H. (2014). Increasing skilled birth attendance through midwifery workforce management. *International Journal of Health Planning and Management, 28*(1), e62–e71. doi:10.1002/hpm.2131

Ruano, A. L., Friedman, E. A., & Hill, P. S. (2014). Health, equity and the post-2015 agenda: Raising the voices of marginalized communities. *International Journal for Equity in Health, 13*(1), 1–3. doi:10.1186/s12939-014-0082-6

Sakala, C. (2012). Letter from North America: Rapidly evolving national maternity care landscape in the United States. *Birth, 39*(3), 263–265. doi:10.1111/j.1523-536X.2012.00556.x

Say, L., Chou, D., Gemmill, A., Tunçalp, O., Moller, A. B., Daniels, J., . . . Aikema, L. (2014). Global causes of maternal death: A WHO systematic review. *Lancet, 2*(6), e323–e333. doi: 10.1016/S2214-109X(14)70227-X

Schaaf, J. M., Liem, S. M., Mol, B. W., Abu-Hanna, A., & Ravelli, A. C. (2013). Ethnic and racial disparities in the risk of preterm birth: A systematic review and meta-analysis. *American Journal of Perinatology, 30*(6), 433–450. doi:10.1055/s-0032-1326988

Sherwood, G. D., & Shaffer, F. A. (2014). The role of internationally educated nurses in a quality, safe workforce. *Nursing Outlook, 62*(1), 46–52. doi:10.1016/j.outlook.2013.11.001

Sibley, L. M., Sipe, T. A., & Barry, D. (2012). Traditional birth attendant training for improving health behaviours and pregnancy outcomes. *Cochrane Database of Systematic Reviews, 2012*(8). doi:10.1002/14651858.CD005460.pub3

Singh, K., Brodish, P., & Suchindran, C. (2014). A regional multilevel analysis: Can skilled birth attendants uniformly decrease neonatal mortality? *Maternal and Child Health Journal, 18*(1), 242–249. doi:10.1007/s10995-013-1260-7

Souza, J. P., Tunçcalp, Ö., Vogel, J. P., Bohren, M., Widmer, M., Oladapo, O. T., . . . Temmerman, M. (2014). Obstetric transition: The pathway towards ending preventable maternal deaths. *British Journal of Obstetrics and Gynaecology, 121*(Suppl. 1), 1–4. doi:10.1111/1471-0528 .12735

Thompson, J. E., Land, S., Camacho-Hubner, A. V., & Fullerton, J. T. (2015). Assessment of provider competence and quality of maternal/newborn care in selected Latin American and Caribbean countries. *Pan American Journal of Public Health, 37*(4–5), 343–350.

Thompson, P. E., Benton, D. C., Adams, E., Morin, K. H., Barry, J., Prevost, S. S., . . . Oywer, E. (2014). The global summit on nurse faculty migration. *Nursing Outlook, 62*(1), 16–21. doi:10 .1016/j.outlook.2013.05.004

Tunçalp, O., Hindin, M. J., Souza, J. P., Chou, D., & Say, L. (2012). The prevalence of maternal near miss: A systematic review. *British Journal of Obstetrics & Gynaecology, 119*(6), 653–661. doi:10.1111/j.1471-0528.2012.03294.x

Turkmani, S., Currie, S., Mungia, J., Assefi, N., Rahmanzai, A. J., Azfar, P., & Bartlett, L. (2013). "Midwives are the backbone of our health system": Lessons from Afghanistan to guide expansion of midwifery in challenging settings. *Midwifery, 29*(10), 1166–1172. doi: 10.1016/j.midw.2013.06.015

UN Population Fund (UNFPA). (2014). The State of the World's Midwifery 2014: A universal pathway. A woman's right to health. New York, NY: Author. Retrieved from http://www .unfpa.org/sowmy

United Nations (UN). (2015). The Millennium Development Goals report 2015. Retrieved from http://www.un.org/millenniumgoals/2015_MDG_Report/pdf/MDG%202015%20rev%20 (July%201).pdf

United States Department of Health and Human Services, Health Resources and Services Administration (HRSA). (2013a). The U.S. health workforce chartbook. Retrieved from http://bhpr.hrsa.gov/healthworkforce/supplydemand/usworkforce/chartbook/index.html

United States Department of Health and Human Services, Health Resources and Services Administration (HRSA). (2013b). The U.S. nursing workforce: Trends in supply and education. Retrieved from http://bhpr.hrsa.gov/healthworkforce/reports/nursingworkforce/ nursingworkforcefullreport.pdf

United States Department of Health and Human Services, Health Resources and Services Administration (HRSA). (2015). Sex, race, and ethnic diversity of U.S. health occupations (2010-2012). Retrieved from http://bhpr.hrsa.gov/healthworkforce/supplydemand/ usworkforce/diversityushealthoccupations.pdf

Vanderbilt, A. A., Isringhausen, K. T., VanderWielen, L. M., Wright, M. S., Slashcheva, L. D., & Madden, M. A. (2013). Health disparities among highly vulnerable populations in the United States: A call for action for medical and oral health care. *Medical Education Online, 18.* doi:10.3402/meo.v18i0.20644.

Vogel, J. P., Souza, J. P., Mori, R., Morisaki, N., Lumbiganon, P., Laopaiboon, M., . . . Gülmezoglu, A. M. (2014). Maternal complications and perinatal mortality: Findings of the World Health Organization Multicountry Survey on Maternal and Newborn Health. *British Journal of Obstetrics and Gynaecology, 121*(Suppl. 1), 76–88. doi:10.1111/1471-0528.12633

Waldman, R., Kennedy, H. P., & Kendig, S. (2012). Collaboration in maternity care: Possibilities and challenges. *Obstetrics and Gynecology Clinics of North America, 39*(3), 435–444. doi:10 .1016/j.ogc.2012.05.011

World Health Organization (WHO). (2004). Making pregnancy safer: The critical role of the skilled attendant. A joint statement of WHO, ICM and FIGO. Retrieved from http://www .who.int/maternal_child_adolescent/documents/9241591692/en

World Health Organization (WHO). (2006). The World Health Report 2006—Working together for health. Retrieved from http://www.who.int/whr/2006/en

World Health Organization (WHO). (2008). Task shifting: Global recommendations and guidelines. Retrieved from http://www.who.int/workforcealliance/knowledge/resources/ taskshifting_guidelines/en

World Health Organization (WHO). (2010). WHO Global Code of Practice on the International Recruitment of Health Personnel. Retrieved from http://www.who.int/hrh/migration/code/ practice/en

World Health Organization (WHO). (2011a). The WHO near-miss approach. Evaluating the quality of care for severe pregnancy complications. Retrieved from http://www.who.int/ reproductivehealth/topics/maternal_perinatal/nmconcept/en

World Health Organization (WHO). (2011b). Strategic directions for strengthening nursing and midwifery services—2011–2015. Retrieved from http://www.who.int/hrh/resources/nmsd/en

World Health Organization (WHO). (2012). Optimizing health worker roles to improve access to key maternal and newborn health interventions through task shifting. Retrieved from http://www.who.int/reproductivehealth/publications/maternal_perinatal_health/978924504843/en

World Health Organization (WHO). (2014). Trends in maternal mortality: 1990 to 2013. Retrieved from http://www.who.int/reproductivehealth/publications/monitoring/maternal-mortality-2013/en

World Health Organization (WHO). (2015a). Strategies toward ending preventable maternal mortality (EPMM). Retrieved from http://www.who.int/reproductivehealth/topics/maternal_perinatal/epmm/en

World Health Organization (WHO). (2015b). World health statistics. Retrieved from http://www.who.int/gho/publications/world_health_statistics/EN_WHS2015_Part2.pdf?ua=1

World Health Organization (WHO). (2015c). Global strategy for women's, children's and adolescents' health, 2016–2030. Retrieved from http://www.who.int/life-course/partners/global-strategy/global-strategy-2016-2030/en/?utm_source=MHTF+Subscribers&utm_campaign=97a8a8fb80-MH_Buzz_Sept_29_2015&utm_medium=email&utm_term=0_8ac9c53ad4-97a8a8fb80-183740093

World Health Organization (WHO). (2015d). Health workforce 2030: Towards a global strategy on human resources for health. Retrieved from http://www.who.int/hrh/documents/15-295Strategy_Report-04_24_2015.pdf?ua=1

Yakoob, M. Y., Ali, M. A., Ali, M. U., Imdad, A, Lawn, J. E., Van Den Broek, N., & Bhutta, Z. A. (2011). The effect of providing skilled birth attendance and emergency obstetric care in preventing stillbirths. *BMC Public Health*, *11*(Suppl. 3), S7. doi:10.1186/1471-2458-11-S3-S7

Young, R. (2013). How effective is an ethical international recruitment policy? Reflections on a decade of experience in England. *Health Policy*, *111*(2), 184–192. doi:10.1016/j.healthpol.2013.03.008

Zureick-Brown, S., Newby, H., Chou, D., Mizoguchi, N. M., Say, L., Suzuki, E., & Wilmoth, J. (2013). Understanding global trends in maternal mortality. *International Perspectives on Sexual and Reproductive Health*, *39*(1), 32–41. doi:10.1363/3903213

# ADVOCATING FOR CHILDBEARING WOMEN: CURRENT INITIATIVES AND WORKFORCE CHALLENGES

Heather M. Bradford and Jesse S. Bushman

## MATERNITY CARE DEFICITS IN THE UNITED STATES

Over the past decade, the United States has averaged nearly 4.1 million births per year (Hamilton, Martin, Osterman, Curtin, & Matthews, 2015). Childbirth is the most common reason for a hospital stay (Weiss & Elixhauser, 2014). However, achieving quality maternity care has been challenging. Although childbirth costs more in the United States than any other developed country, babies continue to be born prematurely and at a low birth weight (Hamilton et al., 2015). The United States ranks behind 26 other countries with respect to neonatal mortality and exclusive breastfeeding rates (MacDorman, Mathews, Mohangoo, & Zeitlin, 2014; World Health Organization [WHO], 2015a, 2015b). Racial, socioeconomic, and ethnic disparities exist with regard to infant and maternal morbidity and mortality (Lu et al., 2010).

African American women are more than three times as likely to die as a result of pregnancy and childbirth when compared to Caucasian women (Centers for Disease Control and Prevention [CDC], 2015). Maternal mortality rates are high; the United States now ranks last among developed nations in maternal mortality, with a continued *rising* rate of maternal morbidity and mortality (Kilpatrick et al., 2014; Lu, 2015). More than 600 women die each year in the United States from pregnancy and childbirth, with more than 50,000 suffering a life-threatening complication (Lu, 2015). The most common preventable conditions that result in severe maternal morbidity and mortality are obstetric hemorrhage, severe hypertension, infection, and venous thromboembolism (Creanga et al., 2015; Main, McCain, Morton, Holtby, & Lawton 2015).

### Unnecessary Interventions

Given the high costs of birth in addition to these troubling statistics, many unnecessary and unwanted interventions in labor and birth continue to occur.

In terms of U.S. health care, the culture reflects the adage "the more technology, the better"; a cascade of interventions often interrupts the normal birth process (Buckley, 2015). Although the American College of Obstetricians and Gynecologists (ACOG) and the American Academy of Pediatrics have published standards for more than 30 years recommending waiting until the 39th week of gestation before considering an elective induction, this policy has often not been practiced. Between 1990 and 2006, the labor induction rates increased from 9.5% to 22.5%; and one meta-analysis of births between 2003 and 2006 found 44% of nulliparous women underwent induction, of which 40% were done electively (Signore, 2010). A recent study of the use of episiotomy found that for the 10% of hospitals where episiotomy was most frequently performed, the average rate of use was 34.1%. In contrast, in the 10% of hospitals where the procedure was least performed, the average rate of use was 2.5% (Friedman, Ananth, Prendergast, D'Alton, & Wright, 2015).

## High Cesarean Rates

Although cesarean sections can be life saving for both mother and/or baby, 60% more cesarean sections were performed in 2009 (reaching 32.9%) as compared to 1996. Cesarean section is the most common operating room procedure in the United States (Main et al., 2011; Weiss, Elixhauser, & Andrews, 2011). However, the rise in the cesarean section has not been associated with a concurrent decrease in maternal or neonatal morbidity or mortality (ACOG & the Society for Maternal–Fetal Medicine [SFMFM], 2014). In fact, for low-risk women, cesarean birth poses a greater risk of maternal morbidity and mortality compared to vaginal birth (Curtin, Gregory, Korst, & Uddin, 2013).

The current stagnant cesarean section rate of 32.2% exceeds the Healthy People 2020 national target rate of 24% (Hamilton et al., 2015; Office of Disease Prevention and Health Promotion, 2015). A 2015 Leapfrog Hospital Survey of 1,122 voluntary hospitals revealed that more than 60% had rates of cesarean section that exceeded the target rate of 24%, with some hospital rates ranging between 26% and 40% (Leapfrog Group, 2015). A 2015 review of hospital rates within California varied from 18% to 56% (Gorman, 2015). In 2014, ACOG and SFMFM issued a landmark joint consensus statement, arguing the procedure is overused. Both organizations speculated the varied rate can only be explained by differing clinical practice patterns among providers and hospitals, despite similar patient populations (ACOG & SFMFM, 2014).

## INITIATIVES FOR CHANGE

With staggering deficits in the U.S. maternity care system, many opportunities for improving maternal and child health outcomes exist. For decades, public and professional organizations have striven to address these issues and improve the quality, cost, and clinical outcomes of maternity care. However, in the past 5 years, these initiatives have dramatically increased, with a confluence of public awareness campaigns, quality-improvement programs, and new laws aimed at improving maternal and child outcomes.

## Transforming Maternity Care: Childbirth Connection's Blueprint for Action

In 2009, Childbirth Connection hosted a national policy symposium, Transforming Maternity Care: A High-Value Proposition, to address the poor outcomes in our maternity care system. More than 100 national leaders actively engaged in the symposium, with a focus on answering the question, "Who needs to do what, to, for, and with whom to improve the quality of maternity care over the next 5 years?" (Angood et al., 2010). As a result, a Symposium Vision Team developed and published the "2020 Vision for a High-Quality, High-Value Maternity Care System," which continues to inform approaches to an optimal maternity care system. The companion direction-setting consensus report "Blueprint for Action: Steps Toward a High-Quality, High-Value Maternity Care System," published in 2010, identified many actionable strategies for broad-based maternity care system reform (Angood et al., 2010; National Partnership for Women and Families, 2015).

Given the rapidly evolving health care environment and the growing body of research findings on labor and birth interventions that disturb the normal hormonal process but are commonly used in the United States, a revised action plan was released in 2016. This plan focused on addressing the aim of creating a high-quality, high-value maternity care system that consistently facilitates physiologic childbearing for women and babies, whenever safely possible, and judiciously provides indicators for interventions based upon robust evidence. Utilizing the recently published evidence-based report "The Hormonal Physiology of Childbearing: Evidence and Implications for Women, Babies, and Maternity Care" (Buckley, 2015), Childbirth Connection convened a multistakeholder, multidisciplinary National Advisory Council with recommendations for effective and efficient ways to use the seven improvement levers over the next 5 years (M. Corry, personal communication, December 2, 2015). The levers are:

- Innovative payment and delivery systems, and quality-improvement initiatives
- Performance measurement and leveraging results for improvement
- Engaging women in their care, including making informed choices among quality care options
- Health information technology, including use of electronic health records, patient portals, care plans, and mobile health
- Health professions education, across all levels and relevant disciplines
- Workforce composition and distribution
- Filling in crucial research gaps, from reproductive biology to clinical epidemiology to health services research (M. Corry, personal communication, December 2, 2015)

Further information on how to participate in this quality-improvement process is available through the Childbirth Connection's "Reports" (Childbirth Connection, 2016; see transform.childbirthconnection.org/reports).

## Perinatal Quality Measures

There has been an increase in the evaluation of quality measures capable of improving maternity care. In 2010, The Joint Commission discarded the previously used pregnancy-and-related-condition set, and replaced these documents with an expanded measure set that was more evidence based. This perinatal care measure set (consisting of five core measures) was endorsed by the National Quality Forum in 2012 and includes:

- Cesarean rates (nulliparous, term, singleton, vertex [NTSV])
- Elective delivery before 39 weeks gestation
- Antenatal steroids
- Health care–associated bloodstream infections in newborns
- Exclusive breast-milk feeding during the hospital stay (The Joint Commission, 2015)

In 2013, as a result of pressure from perinatal care organizations, The Joint Commission began requiring hospitals to submit these accountability performance measures in order to be accredited. Beginning in 2014, hospitals with more than 1,100 births per year were required to submit these core measures (The Joint Commission, 2013). Effective 2016, the threshold for mandatory reporting of the perinatal care performance measure set changed from a minimum of 1,100 births annually to 300 births per year, encompassing more than 80% of accredited hospitals with birthing units (The Joint Commission, 2015).

In addition to the above five perinatal core measures determined by The Joint Commission, the National Quality Forum has also refined its endorsed measures related to perinatal care. Previously, its 33 perinatal and reproductive health measures were focused on ambulatory care, emergency care, and patient outcomes. In 2012, through a rigorous endorsement process, the National Quality Forum limited the list to 14 perinatal core measures focused on reproductive health, pregnancy, childbirth, postpartum, and newborn care. The intent was to measure data sets more suitable for accountability and quality improvement (National Quality Forum, 2012).

After these core data sets were endorsed by The Joint Commission and the National Quality Forum, the Leapfrog Group became the first to publish rates of early elective deliveries (EED) by a hospital in 2012 (Leapfrog Group, 2014). In 2015, Leapfrog published the NTSV cesarean section rates by hospital, becoming the first organization to release this single, standardized validated measure publicly. These data were voluntarily provided by 1,122 hospitals in the United States (Leapfrog Group, 2015).

## Reducing Early Elective Inductions

Although ACOG has been recommending against elective deliveries prior to 39 weeks gestation since 1979, and March of Dimes initiated its premature birth report card in 2008, it was not until 2010 that an unprecedented number of stake-holders, public awareness campaigns, and resources emerged to endorse reduc-ing the rate of EED (Perelman, Delbanco, & Vargas-Johnson, 2013). Organizations from varied perspectives, including patients, health care professionals, hospitals, health systems, the business community, public health agencies, and public and private payers, have called jointly for the reduction of EED. Specific patient and provider-focused tools and resources include:

- American College of Nurse-Midwives (ACNM): *Normal Healthy Childbirth for Women and Families: What You Need to Know*
- March of Dimes: *Why the Last Weeks of Pregnancy Count*
- ACOG: *Five Things Physicians and Patients Should Question*
- Association of Women's Health, Obstetric and Neonatal Nurses (AWHONN): *40 Reasons to Go the Full 40*
- Childbirth Connection: *Quick Facts About Induction of Labor* (National Quality Forum Maternity Action Team, 2014)

The Association of Maternal and Child Health Programs created provider-focused and consumer-based campaigns to support the effort (Centers for Medicare & Medicaid Services [CMS], 2012). Within the Health Resources and Services Administration (HRSA), the Maternal and Child Health Bureau and its partners are continuing to work together to support HRSA's Collaborative Improvement & Innovation Network (CoIIN) to Reduce Infant Mortality, with a focus on reducing EED (as one of five broad strategies to improve outcomes in 13 southern states; HRSA, 2015).

Through the implementation of a multistakeholder Birth Outcomes Initiative, South Carolina used a policy of nonpayment for EED to underscore a multistake-holder commitment to improving birth outcomes. South Carolina was the first state to have its Medicaid program partner with the largest local commercial insurer, BlueCross BlueShield of South Carolina, to adopt a nonpayment policy. Many other state Medicaid agencies have followed suit, and have adopted edu-cational and payment strategies to reduce EED (CMS, 2012).

The reduction in state and hospital-wide EED efforts has been remarkable, and many stakeholders have lauded these efforts as one of the greatest quality-improvement successes in health care history (National Quality Forum, 2014). According to Leapfrog Group data, EED rates decreased to 4.6% in 2013, repre-senting a 73% decrease in 3 years (Leapfrog Group, 2014).

## Reducing EED

National efforts to reduce EED rates have been led by three initiatives:

- National Priorities Partnership Maternity Action Team (NPPMAT; 2014)
- Strong Start's Mother and Newborn Initiative (Conway, 2015)
- California Maternal Quality Care Collaborative (CMQCC; 2011)

### Partnership for Patients Initiative

In 2011, the Department of Health and Human Services (HHS) launched the Partnership for Patients Initiative, with an overall goal of reducing harm. This group consists of more than 7,200 partners, including over 3,200 hospitals. Upon the request of HHS, in conjunction with the Partnership for Patients and the National Quality Forum, the NPPMAT convened in 2012 and spearheaded a specialized initiative on reducing EED among low-risk women to less than 5% nationwide, and reducing cesarean section rates among low-risk women to 15% or less (NPP, 2012).

Established in 2007, the NPP is a partnership of more than 50 organizations from across the health care spectrum that provides consultation to the U.S. government on achieving national improvement priorities. The NPPMAT established a multiprong strategy to achieve this goal, including:

● Encouraging widespread collection and reporting of The Joint Commission's set of perinatal measures as described previously
● Helping providers implement *hard-stop* policies and patient-safety checklists to prevent nonmedically indicated inductions and cesarean sections
● Improving and aligning consumer and provider messaging around normal healthy birth and the harms of EED (NPP, 2012)

Through this quality-improvement program, many states and payers began drastically reducing their EED rates. For example, in 2012, the Michigan Health and Hospital Association encouraged their board of directors to promote the elimination of all EED. Among 39 reporting hospitals, EED rates fell to under 2% (NPP, 2012).

Despite the dramatic decrease in EED rates across the country over 2 years, and a national rate of 5% or less in 2013, some hospitals continued to experience EED rates higher than 20% to 30% (Leapfrog Group, 2014). HHS requested that the National Quality Forum reconvene the NPPMAT in 2014 with the goal to reduce EEDs to 5% or less in every state. This team of 20 private and public stakeholders, including ACNM, developed a *Playbook for the Successful Reduction of Early Elective Deliveries* (NPPMAT, 2014). The primary objective of this resource was to provide specific guidance and strategies to those hospitals facing barriers in their quality-improvement efforts to reduce their EED rates. The ACNM led efforts in promoting aligned messaging around spontaneous birth through a public education campaign, a normal birth toolkit (ACNM, 2015a), and an interprofessional joint clinician statement supporting physiologic birth (Camacho Carr, Collins-Fulea, Krulewitch, & Breedlove, 2015; United States Midwifery Education, Regulation, and Association [US MERA], 2015). In addition, the *Playbook* incorporated the March of Dimes *Late Preterm Brain Development Card* (National Quality Forum, 2014).

### Strong Start Initiative

In 2012, under the Affordable Care Act (ACA), HHS announced the Strong Start Initiative to address two goals: reduce EED and reduce the rate of preterm births for at-risk women covered by Medicaid. Their work related to reducing preterm births will be discussed later in this chapter.

In conjunction with the activities of many public and private stakeholders, Strong Start aimed to encourage best practices for reducing the number of EED that lack medical indication across all payer types. Using a broad-based multimedia and educational outreach campaign focused on providers and pregnant women, in conjunction with professional organizations, such as ACOG and the March of Dimes, the project leveraged the existing infrastructure of the NPPMAT. The initiative funded 26 national, state, and regional hospital system organizations to serve as Hospital Engagement Networks. These networks were selected to identify solutions to adverse outcomes, develop collaborative initiatives, and provide technical support to individual hospitals with the goal of facilitating the adoption of evidence-based clinical practices, including the reduction in EED (CMS, 2012; NPP, 2012).

### California Maternal Quality Care Collaborative

In 2010, the CMQCC, in conjunction with the March of Dimes and the California Department of Health, Maternal, Child and Adolescent Health Division, created an EED task force, which led the development of a maternal quality toolkit. The goals of the toolkit were focused on reducing EED in California, determining, and disseminating best practices for the prevention of EED, and outlining the most effective strategies for supporting California health care providers in implementing those practices (CMQCC, 2011). March of Dimes used the toolkit to pilot a demonstration project with 25 hospitals in the five states with the highest number of births (California, New York, Texas, Illinois, and Florida), successfully reducing the rate of EED by 83% (Oshiro et al., 2013). This toolkit quickly became the national model, an initiative that demonstrated that provider education, coupled with consumer education and hospital quality-improvement efforts, can yield dramatic results.

Since 2014, CMQCC has joined forces with the NPP, enabling widespread dissemination and implementation of the *Playbook*, which has subsequently been widely adopted across the United States (Perelman et al., 2013).

## Reducing Primary Cesarean Rates in Low-Risk Women

On the heels of tremendous success to reduce rates of EED through multistakeholder collaboration, some members of the medical community and maternity health care leaders have addressed the United States stagnant cesarean section rates. As of 2016, few initiatives have been implemented on the national level, but traction is growing, initially generated by two landmark documents. These include ACOG and the SFMFM's 2014 consensus document, which suggested opportunities for improvement related to redefining latent and active phases of labor (ACOG & SFMFM, 2014) as well as the CMQCC's 2011 white paper, which called for the implementation of statewide quality-improvement toolkits (Main et al., 2011).

### CMQCC's Toolkit: Reduce Cesarean Sections

With proven success in reducing EED, a multidisciplinary task force of the CMQCC plans to release a toolkit in 2016 focusing on reducing unnecessary cesarean section births among nulliparous women at term with a singleton pregnancy in vertex position. Mirroring other CMQCC bundles, the comprehensive toolkit provides a guide for clinicians and health care teams focusing on evidence-based care for those women with an intended vaginal birth. This work uses the Alliance for Innovation on Maternal Health's (AIM) Safe Reduction of Primary Cesarean Birth Bundle as the main blueprint for the project (Council on Patient Safety in Women's Health Care, 2015a). AIM's work will also capitalize on the work of ACNM's Birth Toolkit, referencing its bundles as well (H. Smith, personal communication, December 7, 2015).

This innovative approach to reducing cesarean section rates was tested in several pilot hospitals in California, including Hoag Memorial Hospital Presbyterian, during a 3-year period. The cesarean section rate decreased from 38% to 25% among low-risk women. The initiative also increased rates of vaginal births in women who had a cesarean previously (Gorman, 2015). The toolkit strategies used to improve these outcomes at Hoag Memorial Hospital Presbyterian included:

- Transparency among maternity care providers regarding their individual cesarean rates
- Educating patients about the value of waiting for labor to start, as well as greater scrutiny for providers when scheduling an induction
- Developing and implementing an obstetric emergency department and laborist model
- Educating obstetric nurses about supporting laboring women in a manner that promotes physiologic birth, providing financial incentives if the rates decreased
- Enlisting local employers/insurers to adjust payments regarding birth type (Gorman, 2015)

### ACNM Project: Reducing Primary Cesarean

In 2015, as part of the Birth Toolkit, ACNM launched the Reducing Primary Cesarean Project (ACNM, 2015b). This project, funded by the Transforming Birth Fund, is focused on the development of hospital-based perinatal collaboratives through the implementation of one of three bundles (including intermittent auscultation, promoting spontaneous labor progress, and promoting comfort in labor). This multistate, multihospital project will create opportunities for maternity care professionals and health systems to initiate action steps and prompt system change aimed at reducing the incidence of primary cesarean births (ACNM, 2015b).

## Improving Access, Outcomes, and Safety

### The Affordable Care Act

The 2012 ACA advanced the health of women and children by improving access to care and expanding coverage with no cost sharing, including maternity-related preventive services and programs to achieve better maternal and child health outcomes (Simmons, Warren, & McClain, 2015). The primary focus of the ACA was to expand coverage and reduce the number of uninsured persons. Before the ACA was enacted, Medicaid eligibility was limited to women with dependent children, pregnant women, and the disabled. The coverage expansion in the ACA was designed to broaden Medicaid to many more low-income individuals and offer a new coverage pathway to economically disadvantaged adults without children who were largely ineligible before the law was passed. Two years into the passage of the ACA, 56% of new enrollees are women (9% are children; CMS, 2015; Salganicoff, Ranji, Beamesderfer, & Kurani, 2014). Also, 8.7 million women have gained coverage, which includes specific maternity-related preventive services with no cost sharing (Simmons et al., 2015).

### Maternal, Infant, and Early Childhood Home Visiting

The goal of the Maternal, Infant, and Early Childhood Home Visiting (MIECHV) program is improving health and development outcomes for at-risk children through evidence-based home-visiting programs. This program has provided more than 670,000 visits to parents and children with services now available in 75% of urban areas. In addition, under the ACA, employers must provide a reasonable break time for a woman to express milk for her nursing child up to 1 year of age; and a place, other than a bathroom, for an employee to express breast milk (Simmons et al., 2015).

### ACA Strong Start Initiative to Reduce Preterm Deliveries

The Strong Start for Mothers and Newborns Initiative developed a two-strategy approach geared toward testing innovative practices to improve maternal and infant health outcomes and reducing costs in the care of low-income families. The first awareness campaign (2010–2013) focused on reducing EED. The second strategy sought innovative approaches to prenatal care for Medicaid and Children's Health Insurance Program (CHIP) participants with the ultimate goal of reducing preterm birth and low-birth-weight infants. The program partnered with 27 organizations with 213 provider sites in 30 states, Washington, DC, and Puerto Rico. The 3-year program tests evidence-based approaches to reducing the rate of preterm births (Conway, 2015). Four approaches included:

- Group prenatal care, incorporating peer-to-peer support in a facilitated setting for three components: health assessment, education, and support
- Birth centers with comprehensive care

- Prenatal care facilitated by midwives and teams of health professionals, including peer counselors and doulas
- Maternity care homes, that is, enhanced prenatal care at traditional prenatal sites with expanded access to care coordination, education, and other services (Conway, 2015)

Results to date indicate that Strong Start participants have lower rates of cesarean, higher rates of breastfeeding, and overall lower rates of preterm birth when compared to national averages (Conway, 2015).

### National Partnership for Maternal Safety Initiative

The Council on Patient Safety in Women's Health Care (i.e., "The Council") is a coalition of more than 16 national provider and health organizations, including ACOG and ACNM. In 2012, under The Council, the National Partnership for Maternal Safety initiative was formed to address maternal morbidity, mortality, and safety. The group consisted of representatives from 15 organizations in women's health care (including ACNM and ACOG) and other provider, state, federal, and regulatory bodies. The primary work of this initiative was the development of *patient safety bundles*—small, straightforward sets of evidence-based practices proven to improve patient outcomes (Institute for Healthcare Improvement, 2016; Main & Menard, 2013). The three bundles of primary focus include obstetric hemorrhage, severe hypertension in pregnancy, and venous thromboembolism prevention in pregnancy (Council on Patient Safety in Women's Health Care, 2015b; Main, Goffman, et al., 2015). These bundles were chosen because they are the leading causes of maternal morbidity and mortality.

The goal of the initiative is to implement all three bundles in every U.S. birthing facility within 3 years. The purpose of the bundles was not to introduce new guidelines but rather to organize existing, evidence-based materials, confirming guidelines that each hospital should have in place and providing examples if modifications are needed (Council on Patient Safety in Women's Health Care, 2015b). The safety bundles also call on hospital teams to debrief after obstetric emergencies occur and monitor their outcomes to improve their response (Schneider, 2015).

### The National Improvement Challenge

One of the other programs of The Council is the National Improvement Challenge, which is aimed at improving maternal morbidity through the education of medical residents, midwives, and nurses. Launched in 2014, this innovative program solicits applications from individuals or teams who are affiliated with a nursing, midwifery, or medical residency program; have used The Council's tools; and have documented improved structures, processes, and/or outcomes through multidisciplinary collaborative engagement targeting a specific bundle (e.g., obstetric hemorrhage). A monetary award is given to the winners, as well as the opportunity to share the project with the larger national audience. The focus areas are the three obstetric bundles, as well as reducing cesarean section rates, reducing surgical site infections with gynecological patients, and improving perinatal mood disorders (Council on Patient Safety in Women's Health Care, 2015c, 2015d).

*AIM Program to Reduce Maternal Morbidity and Mortality*
The Council also partnered with the HHS Maternal and Child Health Bureau (MCHB) to form the AIM program, a coalition of eight professional and public organizations. The goal of AIM is to:

- Prevent 1,000 maternal deaths and 100,000 cases of severe maternal morbidity nationally by 2018
- Improve uptake and content of postpartum care
- Provide guidance and implementation strategies on the consistent content and delivery of well-woman care (AIM, n.d.).

Over a 4-year period starting in 2016, AIM is partnering with states, perinatal quality collaboratives, maternity care providers, birth facilities, and major hospital systems to implement and provide technical assistance regarding the three evidence-based maternal safety bundles in all birth settings, as well as additional bundles focused on reducing low-risk primary cesarean deliveries and improving postpartum care to enhance interconception care (AIM, 2015). In addition, the AIM program is providing intensive assistance and implementation support to eight states with the highest rates of maternal morbidity and mortality in our nation, chosen based on high acuity and need for improved infrastructure, capacity building, and leadership engagement (ACNM, 2015c).

# THE WORKFORCE SHORTAGE IN U.S. MATERNITY CARE

## OB/GYN Workforce Shortage

A 2011 study by ACOG examined several factors impacting the obstetrician/gynecologist (OB/GYN) workforce and concluded that the United States is facing a very serious shortage of maternity care providers (Congress of OB/GYN, 2011). The meaning of this shortage is being driven by several significant trends. The Census Bureau estimates that the number of births between 2014 and 2060 will increase by 14% (U.S. Census Bureau, 2014). The number of medical school graduates entering an OB/GYN residency has remained almost flat for three decades (Accreditation Council for Graduate Medical Education, 2015; Congress of OB/GYN, 2011).

In addition, the OB/GYN workforce is undergoing a dramatic shift from a mostly male profession to a mostly female profession. Women balance their lives differently than their male counterparts, working fewer hours per week, working part time more often, and retiring from obstetric practice several years earlier. A much larger percentage of OB/GYN residents are choosing to subspecialize into fields where they may not attend births at all. For example, in 2000, only 7% of OB/GYN residents chose subspecialization. In 2012, that figure had grown to 19.5% (Congress of OB/GYN, 2011; Rayburn, Gant, Gilstrap, Elwell, & Williams, 2012). Using a measure of demand that accounts for population increase, prevalence and incidence of conditions and disease, rates of insurance coverage, the available supply of providers, and utilization of care, this organization has projected a shortage of between 15,723 and 21,723 OB/GYN providers by 2050 (Congress of OB/GYN, 2011).

## Workforce Maldistribution

Compounding the problem of OB/GYN provider shortage is the issue of maldistribution. Across the United States, there are significant areas of the country without access to a skilled maternity care provider. Data from the Area Resource File maintained by the HRSA clearly shows that 40% of counties have neither an OB/GYN nor a certified nurse-midwife (CNM) or certified midwife (CM) provider (E. DeClercq, personal communication, May 29, 2014; see Figure 2.1).

## Structure of the Maternal Care Provider Workforce

In 2014, CNMs/CMs collectively attended 8% of U.S. births (Hamilton et al., 2015). However, as specialists in normal physiologic birth, CNMs/CMs are in fact capable of attending a much larger portion of births. For example, in several states CNMs/CMs attend 20% or more of all births (Hamilton et al., 2015). Most

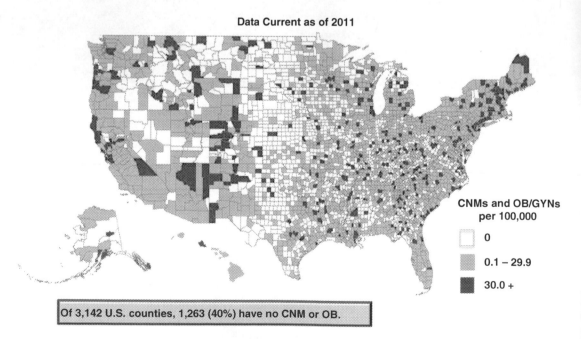

**Data Current as of 2011**

CNMs and OB/GYNs per 100,000

☐ 0

▨ 0.1 – 29.9

▦ 30.0 +

Of 3,142 U.S. counties, 1,263 (40%) have no CNM or OB.

**Figure 2.1** CNMs and OB/GYNs per 100,000 population.

*Source:* American College of Nurse-Midwives (2015d). Reprinted by permission of Jesse Bushman, Director of Advocacy and Government Affairs, American College of Nurse-Midwives.

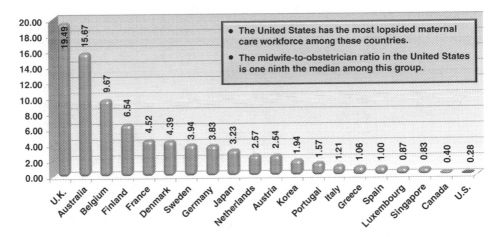

**Figure 2.2**  Maternal care workforce structure in several developed countries: Midwives per obstetrician.
*Source:* American College of Nurse-Midwives (2015d). Reprinted by permission of Jesse Bushman, Director of Advocacy and Government Affairs, American College of Nurse-Midwives.

high-resource countries have reached the conclusion that midwives are the appropriate providers for a significant portion of pregnant women, and have structured their maternal care workforces to more closely reflect the acuity needs of the patient population. For example, among 20 different high-resource countries, the median midwife-to-obstetrician ratio is 2.5 to 1. For a number of complex reasons, within the United States this ratio is inverted, with 0.28 CNMs/CMs per obstetrician. Including certified professional midwives (CPMs), a group not certified by the American Midwifery Certification Board (AMCB), that ratio is 0.32 midwives per obstetrician (AMCB, 2015; Association of American Medical Colleges [AAMC], 2014; Eguchi, 2009; Emons & Luiten, 2001; Rowland, McLeod, & Froese-Burns, 2012; see Figure 2.2).

In several of these countries, midwives attend a significant majority of births (Emons & Luiten, 2001; WHO, 2014a, 2014b; H. Kristjánsdóttir, Iceland midwife leader, personal communication, April 30, 2015; see Figure 2.3). Studies in these same countries have concluded that midwifery care is, in fact, appropriate for most women (Emons & Luiten, 2001; Shah, 2015; ten Hoope-Bender et al., 2014).

It is notable that the model of maternal care in Europe is not analogous to that of the United States. In those countries, midwives are frequently the default maternal care providers, with care being transferred to an obstetrician if and when complications arise (Emons & Luiten, 2001; Shah, 2015; ten Hoope-Bender et al., 2014). In the United States, obstetricians are the most common attendants at births with and without complications. Further, guidelines for transfer of care between midwives practicing in a home environment in the United States are variable around the country, whereas in several European countries there are clear guidelines and mechanisms to accomplish the needed transfer (Shah, 2015). Finally, as noted previously, the midwifery workforce in the United States is made up of two major categories of midwives (CNMs/CMs and CPMs). In the United States, a subset of CPM educational pathways does not meet standards of the International

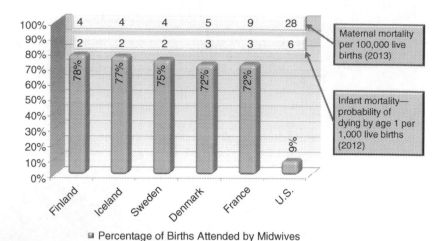

Figure 2.3 Maximizing midwifery: What is possible.

*Source:* American College of Nurse-Midwives (2015d). Reprinted by permission of Jesse Bushman, Director of Advocacy and Government Affairs, American College of Nurse-Midwives.

Confederation of Midwives (ICM), which may lead to variations in practice. In contrast, in many European countries there is typically a single type of midwife, whose education, certification, licensure, and scope of practice are uniform and reflect the ICM standards (ICM, 2014). Concerted efforts are currently underway in the United States to ensure that all midwives, regardless of credential, meet ICM (2014) standards (Camacho Carr et al., 2015; US MERA, 2015). Many other high-resource countries have aligned the structure of their maternal care provider workforces with the structure of their populations (see Figure 2.4), with a larger number of well-prepared midwives managing normal births and a smaller number of highly skilled obstetricians caring for women whose needs rise to that level.

Statements about the value and comparative prominence of midwifery in other high-resource countries have captured the attention of providers and health policy experts in the United States, some of whom have asked whether the United States should seek to modify the structure of its maternal care workforce more along those lines (Shah, 2015; ten Hoope-Bender et al., 2014).

## Interprofessional Practice—The Ideal

The ideal workforce structure involves a mix of providers who are trained to address the normal processes while also being able to recognize complications and transfer care to another group of providers skilled in addressing complications. An argument might be made that a single set of providers, skilled in both normal birth and interventions, would suffice, but there are two important results that arise from such a situation.

First, when human beings are trained to use a specific set of tools, they will tend to use those tools to address problems placed before them. If education and training emphasize the use of intervention, they will naturally gravitate toward

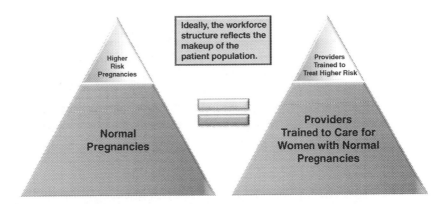

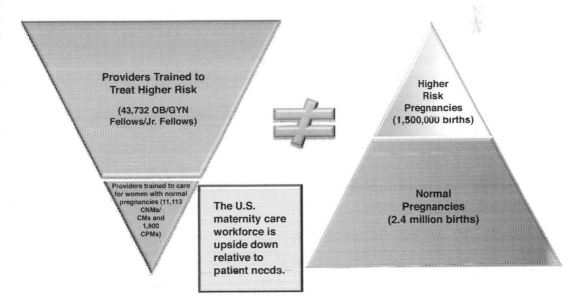

**Figure 2.4**   Ideal maternal care workforce structure.

*Source:* American College of Nurse-Midwives (2015d). Reprinted by permission of Jesse Bushman, Director of Advocacy and Government Affairs, American College of Nurse-Midwives.

**Figure 2.5**   Current U.S. maternal care workforce structure.

CM, certified midwife; CNM, certified nurse-midwife; CPM, certified professional midwife.

*Source:* American College of Nurse-Midwives (2015d). Reprinted by permission of Jesse Bushman, Director of Advocacy and Government Affairs, American College of Nurse-Midwives.

that course of action. As discussed earlier and as will be demonstrated later in a review of the evidence, individuals who have extensive training in intervention to address complications find it difficult to abstain from using those interventions. This difficulty arises even when situations before them do not necessarily call for intervention and the better course of action would be to support the body's normal processes (Buckley, 2015; Cragin & Kennedy, 2006). Interventions bring with them their own sets of complications and costs and should not be used unnecessarily. A person whose training and experience focuses on supporting normal physiologic birth will naturally gravitate toward using those approaches. Because birth is primarily a normal event, it is critical that our maternal care workforce include a substantial body of providers who specialize in supporting normal birth (Fagerlund & Germano, 2009).

The second reason to question the single-provider approach is an economic one. Obstetricians must necessarily understand what is normal before they begin to specialize in caring for patients with complications. With a foundational understanding of what is normal, obstetricians subsequently spend years developing skills for treating complications. Obstetricians also develop skills in gynecologic care and surgery, as well as primary care services other than those focused on obstetric care. As a result, obstetricians' training is much more lengthy and expensive than that of midwives (AAMC, 2015; College Board, 2016; Fagerlund & Germano, 2009; see Figure 2.6).

Because of the time and cost entailed in physician education and training, Congress has chosen to make an investment of public money into this process, to ensure that appropriately skilled physicians are available to the citizenry. According to the Institute of Medicine (IOM), payments made to teaching institutions to support physicians' training and education amount to some $15 billion per year (IOM, 2014). In 2014, there were 117,427 medical interns and residents in the United States (Brotherton & Etzel, 2014). On average, in 2014 the U.S. taxpayers invested $127,000 per resident into the development of the physician workforce (ACNM, 2015d).

Because of the complexity of the methodology used to determine graduate medical education (GME) payments to any given hospital, actual payments vary widely. The past president of the ACOG recently stated in a presentation at ACNM's annual conference that GME funding for OB/GYN residents amounted to approximately $100,000 per resident per year. Given the 4-year length of an OB/GYN residency, taxpayers are investing some $400,000 in the training and education of each OB/GYN resident (Jennings, 2015).

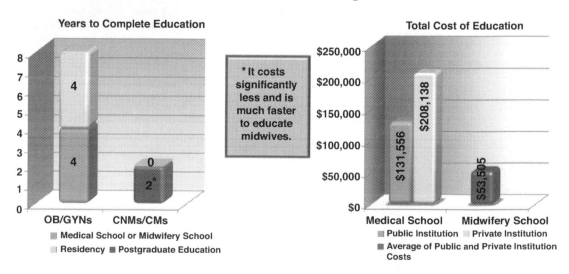

**Figure 2.6**  Cost and length of education—OB/GYNs and CNMs/CMs.

CM, certified midwife; CNM, certified nurse-midwife.

*Source:* American College of Nurse-Midwives (2015d). Reprinted by permission of Jesse Bushman, Director of Advocacy and Government Affairs, American College of Nurse-Midwives.

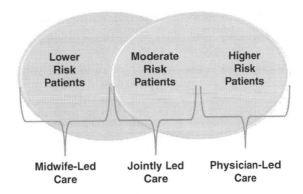

**Figure 2.7**   Interprofessional collaboration—the Ideal.
*Source:* American College of Nurse-Midwives (2015d). Reprinted by permission of Jesse Bushman, Director of Advocacy and Government Affairs, American College of Nurse-Midwives.

From an economic standpoint, using a provider (an obstetrician) who needs 8 years and hundreds of thousands of dollars to complete training to address a health care need that can be fully met by a different provider (a midwife) whose graduate training takes 2 to 3 years and entails far less cost is not an optimal use of resources. These years of education only account for the specialty education, not the basic medical school or basic nursing school plus the master's degree earned by CNMs. Furthermore, because payment methodologies more highly reward complex, difficult, and resource-intensive services, physicians generate more revenue when they recognize the economic value of their own training and focus it on situations in which the depth of that training is fully utilized.

The Medical Group Management Association (MGMA) noted in a recent report that the use of nonphysician providers in physician practices serves more patients and enables physicians to practice to the full extent of their skills. Furthermore, MGMA data over many years show that practices with nonphysician providers usually perform better financially, generating more physician income (MGMA, 2014).

For purposes of ensuring not just safe but optimal outcomes, and to best utilize the economic resource represented by the billions of taxpayer dollars invested in the development of the OB/GYN workforce, the most rational approach is to ensure that the number of maternal care providers specializing in support of normal physiologic birth and those specializing in care for women who develop complications during pregnancy or labor be proportionate to the number of women falling into each of these categories. Both provider types are necessary and they are not interchangeable (see Figure 2.7).

## The Midwifery Return on Investment

As noted previously, educating a midwife is more rapid and less costly than educating on OB/GYN. Because midwives are capable of attending a large portion of births, it makes sense for policy makers to consider an investment in their education.

Midwifery education programs consistently have reported to ACNM Office of Advocacy and Government Affairs that the primary challenge they face in educating more midwives is their ability to secure a sufficient number of clinical sites for their students (Germano, Schorn, Phillippi, & Schuiling, 2014). There are several reasons for this situation. First, hundreds of millions of taxpayer dollars are being invested into the training of obstetricians every year, strongly encouraging hospitals to prioritize OB/GYN training. Public investment in midwifery education comes primarily through two sources:

- Graduate Nurse Education (GNE) demonstration program that was created under the ACA
- National Health Service Corps, which provides loans and scholarships directly to midwifery students, but does not support the clinical sites (ACNM, 2015d)

The second reason, according to Jesse Bushman, director of advocacy and government affairs at the ACNM, is that the difficulty in securing training sites for midwifery students arises from how CNMs are treated under the Medicare program. Teaching physicians can supervise interns and residents, and then bill for the supervised services under their own billing numbers. Although CNMs often instruct interns and residents, and are largely responsible for the instruction of student midwives, the Medicare statute and regulations are completely silent on how supervising CNMs can bill for services. As a result, cautious compliance officers may preclude the CNM from billing for these services at all, unless the CNM can completely repeat the procedure and document it as such (ACNM, 2015d).

The GNE demonstration under the ACA was established to explore methods of increasing the number of advanced practice registered nurses (APRNs), including CNMs, in the United States. Under this demonstration, five hospitals received funding over 4 years to be used for APRN education programs in an effort to increase the number of available precepting clinical sites. During this demonstration, only one of the five sites has included a midwifery education program in its operations and the amount given to preceptors was a few thousand dollars. Some midwifery education programs independently pay the midwives who precept their students. However, a 2014 study found that 62% of preceptors are not financially compensated for their work (Germano et al., 2014).

According to Bushman, the enormous disparity in public funding for OB/GYN and CNM/CM education, coupled with billing issues for midwifery-supervised services, poses significant barriers to finding stable clinical sites for midwifery students. Hospitals recognize the strong financial drivers and are likely to prioritize the education of OB/GYNs. From a public policy standpoint, however, investment in midwifery education is cost-effective. As noted, taxpayer investment into each OB/GYN resident is $400,000, whereas the GNE demonstration is providing approximately $24,000 per student to support precepting costs.

From numerous studies of risk-adjusted populations, it is known that the rate of cesarean births for women attended by midwives is lower than that for women attended by physicians (Altman, 2015; Cragin & Kennedy, 2006; Jackson et al., 2003). Given that Medicaid funding covers nearly half of all births, if a state or the federal government were to invest $24,000 to secure precepting for a midwife, the Medicaid programs would expect to realize savings arising from that midwife's caring for patients covered by that program within a short period of time (Markus, Andres, West, Garro, & Pellegrini, 2013). ACNM (2015d) estimates that the 1-year return on investment for the average Medicaid program, for a state investment of $24,000 into midwifery education, is $8,705. During that same period, commercial payers would save $23,988. These savings would accrue from reductions in cesarean births alone. Further savings from the midwifery model would accrue based on other aspects of their practice (e.g., reduced use of epidurals). Clearly, an investment in midwifery education will not only help with provider shortages, but will also result in cost savings (ACNM, 2015d).

A public investment in midwifery education would have a very significant impact in terms of the number of births that could be attended. Given the shortage and maldistribution of maternal care providers in this country, midwifery care is an excellent answer. There is a continuing need for OB/GYNs, and support for their education is essential. However, with a shift in providers focusing their care on those who need it most, coupled with a public investment in midwifery education, a balanced workforce would emerge. This balanced workforce would expand the role of midwifery while concurrently addressing the workforce shortage. With the growth of the midwifery profession and its focus on physiologic birth, childbearing women would be better served.

## BEST PRACTICES IN SHAPING POLICY

There are steps that policy makers can take to invest in the development of the midwifery workforce. The needed steps must address the shortages of providers and ensure an appropriately structured maternity care workforce. At the time of this writing, significant steps are being undertaken toward that end.

## Policy for Workforce Development

### Legislative Changes to Identify Shortage Areas

ACNM and ACOG have been closely cooperating during 2014 and 2015 to advocate for legislation that would require HRSA to identify areas of the country experiencing a shortage of full-scope maternity care providers. These newly identified data would give insight into the exact nature of the shortage.

### Expanding the GNE Program

The GNE program is currently a demonstration that is limited to five sites. If this program were expanded nationwide, it would greatly facilitate efforts to increase access to clinical sites for midwifery students. The ACA requires that the GNE program report its results to Congress by October 2017, so it is unlikely that any significant legislative efforts will be underway until that report has been finalized. However, preliminary information from participating organizations are positive and Bushman anticipates that this report will demonstrate the value of the program.

### Preceptor Reimbursement

As Bushman has described, ACNM has been working with legislators in the U.S. House of Representatives to develop legislation modifying the Medicare statute to provide reimbursement to CNMs for the services of medical interns, residents, and student midwives under their supervision, just as teaching physicians are paid for such supervised services. Certified registered nurse anesthetists (CRNAs) can currently be paid for the supervised services of student CRNAs, which creates a precedent for such a legislative provision (ACNM, 2015d).

### State Tax Credits for Preceptors

The state of Georgia has developed an innovative solution to the shortage of primary care providers in their state. Under their preceptor tax incentive program, a clinical preceptor invites certain students into his or her clinic to provide training. If these students are present for an aggregate of at least 480 hours (as reported to the state by their educational programs), the preceptor can receive a tax credit equal to $1,000 for every 160 hours of precepting, up to a total of $10,000. This tax credit goes directly to the individual preceptor, which helps offset losses that might occur if he or she is slowed down by the need to work with the students (ACNM, 2015d).

## Advocating for Midwifery

In order to address the obstetric provider workforce shortage and grow the midwifery workforce, midwives must be involved in the legislative process. In asking a midwife why he or she entered the profession of midwifery, the response might be to care for women or attend births. Few midwives would respond that they wanted to engage in the politics of the profession. However, because midwifery has historically been relatively invisible in the larger health care arena, and most of the laws and regulations regarding the profession are defined through political activity, it is imperative that every student midwife and midwife engage in the legislative process and advocate for the profession.

There are many opportunities to do so. The simplest method is to contact state and federal legislators about important issues. For example, with respect to the legislation mentioned previously, which requires HRSA to identify areas of the country experiencing a shortage of full-scope maternity care providers, all students and midwives can play an important role in helping to move this bill forward.

Once a bill has been introduced by a specific member of Congress (preferably from the political party who holds control of the chamber), it is given a bill number and assigned to the appropriate committee. HR 1209, the Improving

Access to Maternity Care Act, was introduced in March 2015 by Congressman Michael Burgess (R-TX) and referred to the House Energy and Commerce Subcommittee on Health (Library of Congress, 2016). Each year, thousands of bills are sent to committees and only several hundred actually make it out of committee. Therefore, federal legislators need to hear from their constituents regarding the bills in order to influence their opinion. The goal with any bill is to gain support from all members of Congress through cosponsorship. If a bill has gathered strong bipartisan support with a significant number of cosponsors, it has a much better chance of moving out of committee toward a vote. ACNM maintains an updated page addressing professional advocacy concerns (ACNM, 2016). There are many ways to contact a legislator to ask for cosponsorship of a specific bill:

- Ask to meet with staff at the federal legislators' local office to discuss the bill and educate them about midwifery, or watch for the scheduling of town hall meetings
- E-mail, fax, or call federal legislators' health aides in their Washington, DC office. Handwritten letters are no longer recommended because of the length of time it takes to process them
- Sign a letter prewritten by ACNM regarding the bill (ACNM, n.d.)
- Ask patients, colleagues, family members, and neighbors to advocate

Legislative aides are often inexperienced and have a high turnover rate. However, legislative aides advise the legislators about health care issues and are helpful in the lobbying process. The most important aspect of lobbying is the relationship established with the legislators and their staff. There are many ways to build that relationship. Some suggestions for the caller or visitor are as follows:

- Always self-identify as a constituent
- Connect with legislators at least once a year
- Visits or e-mails do not have to be issue related: messages can focus on educating about the midwifery profession; the population served; scope of practice; and/or the education, licensing requirements, and certification of midwives
- Business cards and information about the profession of midwifery should be shared (available on the ACNM website)
- Legislators need to be thanked for voting on a bill in a manner that supports midwifery
- Exchanges with the staff and/or legislator should be made memorable by providing examples
- Requests should be simple and one-issue focused
- Business attire is essential

A second key action step for students and midwives is to advocate for the profession of midwifery by providing financial support as possible to the ACNM PAC (political action committee) and other organizations supporting the practice of licensed, certified midwifery. The ACNM PAC solicits voluntary contributions from ACNM members to distribute strategically as campaign contributions to federal legislators. PAC contributions create a relationship between legislators and midwives. These contributions also allow ACNM to support legislators who have a proven record on the federal issues that matter to the profession. PAC contributions can be made online at the ACNM website.

## REFERENCES

Accreditation Council for Graduate Medical Education. (2015). Graduate medical education data resource book 2011–2014. Retrieved from http://www.acgme.org/acgmeweb/tabid/259/GraduateMedicalEducation/GraduateMedicalEducationDataResourceBook.aspx

Alliance for Innovation on Maternal Health (AIM). (n.d.). AIM program description. Retrieved from http://www.safehealthcareforeverywoman.org/downloads/AIM/AIM-Program-Description.pdf

Altman, M. R. (2015). *Exploration of nurse-midwifery care for childbirth* (Unpublished doctoral dissertation). Washington State University College of Nursing, Spokane, WA.

American College of Nurse-Midwives (ACNM). (n.d.). Action center: Active issues. Retrieved from https://www.votervoice.net/ACNM/Campaigns

American College of Nurse-Midwives (ACNM). (2015a). BirthTOOls.org: Tools for optimizing the outcome of labor safely. Retrieved from http://birthtools.org/Get-Involved

American College of Nurse-Midwives (ACNM). (2015b). Reducing primary cesareans. Retrieved from http://birthtools.org/HBI-Reducing-Primary-Cesareans

American College of Nurse-Midwives (ACNM). (2015c). Alliance for innovation on maternal health (AIM). Retrieved from http://www.midwife.org/Alliance-for-Innovation-on-Maternal-Health-AIM

American College of Nurse-Midwives (ACNM). (2015d). *The midwifery model of care: A value proposition. Unpublished material from the Department of Advocacy and Government Affairs.*

American College of Nurse-Midwives (ACNM). (2016). Advocacy. Retrieved from http://www.midwife.org/Advocacy

American College of Obstetricians and Gynecologists (ACOG), & Society for Maternal–Fetal Medicine (SFMFM). (2014). Safe prevention of the primary Cesarean section (ACOG/SMFM Consensus). *American Journal of Obstetrics and Gynecology, 210*(3), 179–193. doi:10.1016/j.ajog.2014.01.026

American Congress of Obstetricians and Gynecologists (Congress of OB/GYN). (2011). The obstetrician gynecologist workforce in the US: Facts, figures, and implications. Retrieved from http://www.acog.org/Resources-And-Publications/The-Ob-Gyn-Workforce

American Midwifery Certification Board (AMCB). (2015, May). Number of certified nurse-midwives/certified midwives by state. Retrieved from http://www.amcbmidwife.org/docs/default-document-library/number-of-cnm-cm-by-state—may-2015.pdf?sfvrsn=2

Angood, P. B., Armstrong, E. M., Ashton, D., Burstin, H., Corry, M. P., Delblanco, S. F., . . . Salganifoff, A. (2010). Blueprint for action: Steps toward a high-quality, high-value maternity care system. *Women's Health Issues, 20*(Suppl. 1), S18–S49. doi:10.1016/j.whi.2009.11.007

Association of American Medical Colleges (AAMC). (2014). Physician specialty data book 2014. Retrieved from https://members.aamc.org/eweb/DynamicPage.aspx?Action=Add&Object KeyFrom=1A83491A-9853-4C87-86A4-F7D95601C2E2&WebCode=PubDetailAdd&Do NotSave=yes&ParentObject=CentralizedOrderEntry&ParentDataObject=Invoice%20De tail&ivd_formkey=69202792-63d7-4ba2-bf4e-a0da41270555&ivd_prc_prd_key=41FE F42C-6D95-4E8D-AC8A-1173945902A4

Association of American Medical Colleges (AAMC). (2015). Tuition and student fees, first year medical school students 2014–2015. Retrieved from https://services.aamc.org/tsfreports/ select.cfm?year_of_study=2015

Brotherton, S. E., & Etzel, S. I. (2014). Graduate medical education, 2013–2014. *Journal of the American Medical Association, 312*(22), 2427–2445. doi:10.1001/jama.2014.12575

Buckley, S. J. (2015). *Hormonal physiology of childbirth: Evidence and implications for women, babies, and maternity care.* Washington, DC: Childbirth Connections.

California Maternal Quality Care Collaborative (CMQCC). (2011). Early elective deliveries toolkit. Retrieved from https://www.cmqcc.org/resource/errata-2-83111-elimination-non -medically-indicated-elective-deliveries-39-weeks-gestational

Camacho Carr, K., Collins-Fulea, C., Krulewitch, C., & Breedlove, G. (2015). The United States Midwifery Education, Regulation and Association Work Group: What is it and what does it hope to accomplish? *Journal of Midwifery & Women's Health, 60*(2), 125–127. doi:10.1111/jmwh.12306

Centers for Disease Control and Prevention (CDC). (2015). Pregnancy mortality surveillance system. Retrieved from http://www.cdc.gov/reproductivehealth/maternalinfanthealth/ pmss.html

Centers for Medicare & Medicaid Services. (2012). Reducing early elective deliveries in Medicaid and CHIP. Retrieved from http://www.medicaid.gov/medicaid-chip-program -information/by-topics/quality-of-care/downloads/eed-brief.pdf

Centers for Medicare & Medicaid Services. (2015, July 28). Medicaid & CHIP: May 2015 monthly applications, eligibility determinations and enrollment report. Retrieved from http://www.medicaid.gov/medicaid-chip-program-information/program-information/ downloads/may-2015-enrollment-report.pdf

Childbirth Connection. (2016). Reports. Retrieved from http://transform.childbirthconnec tion.org/reports

College Board. (2016). Average rates of growth of published charges by decade. Retrieved from http://trends.collegeboard.org/content/average-rates-growth-published-charges-decade-0

Conway, P. (2015, May 5). Strong start for mothers and newborns II. First annual evaluation report. The CMS blog: Centers for Medicare and Medicaid Services. Retrieved from http:// blog.cms.gov

Council on Patient Safety in Women's Health Care. (2015a). Alliance for Innovation on Maternal Health (AIM). Retrieved from http://www.safehealthcareforeverywoman.org/aim.php

Council on Patient Safety in Women's Health Care. (2015b). National partnership for maternal safety. Retrieved from http://www.safehealthcareforeverywoman.org/national-partnership .php

Council on Patient Safety in Women's Health Care. (2015c). National improvement challenge. Retrieved from http://www.safehealthcareforeverywoman.org/national-improvement -challenge.php

Council on Patient Safety in Women's Health Care. (2015d). National improvement challenge on obstetric hemorrhage award winners [Press release]. Retrieved from http://www .safehealthcareforeverywoman.org/downloads/National-Improvement-Challenge/Press -Release-Winners-Cycle-1.pdf

Cragin, L., & Kennedy, H. P. (2006). Linking obstetric and midwifery practice with optimal outcomes. *Journal of Obstetric, Gynecologic, & Neonatal Nursing, 35*(6), 779–785. doi:10.1111/ j.1552-6909.2006.00106.x

Creanga, A. A., Berg, C. J., Syverson, C., Seed, K., Bruce, F. C., & Callaghan, W. (2015). Pregnancy-related mortality in the US, 2006–2010. *Obstetrics & Gynecology, 125*(1), 5–12. doi:10.1097/AOG.0000000000000564

Curtin, S. C., Gregory, K. D., Korst, L. M., & Uddin, S. F. (2015). Maternal morbidity for vaginal and cesarean deliveries, according to previous cesarean history: New data from the birth certificate, 2013. *National Vital Statistics Reports, 64*(4), 1–14. Retrieved from http:// www.cdc.gov/nchs/data/nvsr/nvsr64/nvsr64_04.pdf

Eguchi, N. (2009). Do we have enough obstetricians? A survey of the Japan Medical Association in 15 countries. *Japan Medical Association Journal, 52*(3), 150–157.

Emons, J. K., & Luiten, M. I.. (2001). Midwifery in Europe: An inventory in fifteen EU-member states. Retrieved from http://www.deloitte.nl/downloads/documents/website_deloitte/ GZpublVerloskundeinEuropaRapport.pdf

Fagerlund, K., & Germano, E. (2009). The costs and benefits of nurse-midwifery education: Model and application. *Journal of Midwifery and Women's Health, 54*(5), 341–350. doi: 10.1016/j.jmwh.2009.04.008

Friedman, A. M., Ananth, C. V., Prendergast, E., D'Alton, M. E., & Wright, J. D. (2015). Variation in and factors associated with use of episiotomy. *Journal of the American Medical Association, 313*(2), 197–199. doi:10.1001/jama.2014.14774

Germano, E., Schorn, M. N., Phillippi, J. C., & Schuiling, K. (2014). Factors that influence midwives to serve as preceptors: An American College of Nurse-Midwives survey. *Journal of Midwifery & Women's Health, 59*(2), 167–175. doi:10.1111/jmwh.12175

Gorman, A. (2015, May 9). How one hospital brought its C-section rate down fast. *Kaiser Health News*. Retrieved from http://health.usnews.com/health-news/hospital-of-tomorrow/ articles/2015/05/09/how-one-hospital-brought-its-c-section-rate-down-fast

Hamilton, B., Martin, J., Osterman, M., Curtin, S., & Mathews, T. J. (2015). Births: Final data for 2014. *National Vital Statistics Report, 64*(12), 1–64. Retrieved from http://www.cdc.gov/ nchs/data/nvsr/nvsr64/nvsr64_12.pdf

Health Resources and Services Administration (HRSA). (2015). Collaborative improvement and innovation network to reduce infant mortality. HRSA Maternal and Child Health. Retrieved from http://mchb.hrsa.gov/infantmortality/coiin

Institute for Healthcare Improvement. (2016). What is a bundle? Retrieved from http://www .ihi.org/resources/Pages/ImprovementStories/WhatIsaBundle.aspx

Institute of Medicine (IOM). (2014). Graduate medical education that meets the nation's health needs. Retrieved from https://iom.nationalacademies.org/~/media/Files/Report%20Files/ 2014/GME/GME-RB.pdf

International Confederation of Midwives (ICM). (2014). ICM global standards, competencies, and tools. Retrieved from http://www.internationalmidwives.org/what-we-do/global-stan dards-competencies-and-tools.html

Jackson, D. J., Lang, J. M., Swartz, W. H., Ganiats, T. G., Fullerton, J., Ecker, J., & Nguyen, U. (2003). Outcomes, safety, and resource utilization in a collaborative care birth center program compared with traditional physician-based perinatal care. *American Journal of Public Health, 93*(6), 999–1006.

Jennings, J. C. (2015, July). Women's health care workforce issues and collaborative practice. Paper presented at the meeting of the American College of Nurse-Midwives, National Harbor, MD.

Kilpatrick, S. J., Berg, C., Bernstein, P., Bingham, D., Delgado, A., Callaghan, W. M., . . . Harper, M. (2014). Standardized severe maternal morbidity review. *Obstetrics & Gynecology, 124*(2, Part 1), 361–366. doi:10.1097/AOG.0000000000000397

Leapfrog Group. (2014, March 3). Dramatic decline in dangerous early elective deliveries; The Leapfrog Group cautions against babies being born too soon, hits national target. Retrieved from http://www.leapfroggroup.org/policy_leadership/leapfrog_news/5164214

Leapfrog Group. (2015). C-section rates by hospital. Retrieved from http://www.leapfroggroup.org/patients/c-section

Library of Congress. (2016). Current legislative activities. Retrieved from http://www.congress.gov

Lu, M. C. (2015, May 21). Call to action: Saving 100,000 U.S. mothers in 5 years. *Ob.Gyn. News.* Retrieved from http://www.obgynnews.com/home/article/call-to-action-saving-100000-us-mothers-in-5-years/5c2a222691ff139b391ff263242c28ed.html

Lu, M. C., Kotelchuck, M., Hogan, V., Jones, L., Wright, K., & Halfon, N. (2010). Closing the black-white gap in birth outcomes: A life-course approach. *Ethnicity and Disease, 20*(1, Suppl. 2), 62–76.

MacDorman, M. F., Mathews, T. J., Mohangoo, A. D., & Zeitlin, J. (2014). International comparisons of infant mortality and related factors: United States and Europe, 2010. *National Vital Statistics Reports, 63*(5), 1–6. Retrieved from http://www.cdc.gov/nchs/data/nvsr/nvsr63/nvsr63_05.pdf

Main, E. K., Goffman, D., Scavone, B. M., Low, L. K., Bingham, D., Fontaine, P. L., . . . Levy, B. S. (2015). National partnership for maternal safety: Consensus bundle on obstetric hemorrhage. *Obstetrics & Gynecology, 126*(1), 155–162. doi:10.1097/AOG.0000000000000869

Main, E. K., McCain, C. L., Morton, C. H., Holtby, S., & Lawton, E. S. (2015). Pregnancy-related mortality in California: Causes, characteristics, and improvement opportunities. *Obstetrics & Gynecology, 125*(4), 938–947. doi:10.1097/AOG.0000000000000746

Main, E. K., & Menard, M. K. (2013). Maternal mortality: Time for national action. *Obstetrics & Gynecology, 122*(4), 735–736. doi:10.1097/AOG.0b013e3182a7dc8c

Main, E. K., Morton, C. H., Hopkins, D., Giuliani, G., Melsop, K., & Gould, J. B. (2011). *Cesarean deliveries, outcomes, and opportunities for change in California: Toward a public agenda for maternity care safety and quality.* Retrieved from https://www.cmqcc.org/resource/cesarean-deliveries-outcomes-and-opportunities-change-california-toward-public-agenda

Markus, A. R., Andres, E., West, K. D., Garro, N., & Pellegrini, C. (2013). Medicaid covered births, 2008 through 2010, in the context of the implementation of health reform. *Women's Health Issues, 23*(5), e273–e280. doi:10.1016/j.whi.2013.06.006

Medical Group Management Association (MGMA). (2014). NPP utilization in the future of US healthcare: An MGMA research and analysis report. Retrieved from https://www.mgma.com/Libraries/Assets/Practice%20Resources/NPPsFutureHealthcare-final.pdf

National Partnership for Women and Families. (2015). Transforming maternity care: Improvement tools. Retrieved from http://transform.childbirthconnection.org/resources

National Priorities Partnership (NPP). (2012, August). Report from the National Quality Forum: National priorities partnership quarterly synthesis of action in support of the partnership for patients. Retrieved from http://public.qualityforum.org/actionregistry/Documents/report_quarterly%20PfP_August%202012_final.pdf

National Quality Forum. (2012, April). Endorsement summary: Perinatal and reproductive health measures. Retrieved from https://www.qualityforum.org/.../Perinatal_Endorsement_Summary

National Quality Forum Maternity Action Team. (2014). Playbook for the successful elimination of early elective deliveries. Retrieved from http://www.39weeksfl.com/wp-content/uploads/2014/08/NQF-Maternity-Action-Team-Playbook-2014.pdf

Office of Disease Prevention and Health Promotion. (2015). Healthy People 2020. Maternal, infant and child health: Morbidity and mortality. Retrieved from http://www.healthy people.gov/2020/topics-objectives/topic/maternal-infant-and-child-health/objectives

Oshiro, B. T., Kowalewski, L., Sappenfield, W., Alter, C. C., Bettegowda, V. R., Russell, R., . . . Berns, S. D. (2013). A multistate quality improvement program to decrease elective deliveries before 39 weeks of gestation. *Obstetrics &-Gynecology*, *121*(5), 1025–1031. doi:10.1097/AOG.0b013e31828ca096

Perelman, N., Delbanco, S., & Vargas-Johnson, A. (2013). Using education, collaboration, and payment reform to reduce early elective deliveries: A case study of South Carolina's birth outcomes initiative. Retrieved from http://www.milbank.org/uploads/documents/reports/South_Carolina_Birth_Outcomes_Case_Study.pdf

Rayburn, W. F., Gant, N. F., Gilstrap, L. C., Elwell, E. C., & Williams, S. B. (2012). Pursuit of accredited subspecialties by graduating residents in obstetrics and gynecology, 2000–2012. *Obstetrics & Gynecology*, *120*(3), 619–625. doi:10.1097/AOG.0b013e318265ab0a

Rowland, T., McLeod, D., & Froese-Burns, N. (2012). Comparative study of maternity systems. Retrieved from http://www.health.govt.nz/publication/comparative-study-maternity-systems

Salganicoff, A., Ranji, U., Beamesderfer, A., & Kurani, N. (2014). Women and health care in the early years of the ACA: Key findings from the 2013 Kaiser Women's Health Survey. Retrieved from https://kaiserfamilyfoundation.files.wordpress.com/2014/05/8590-women-and-health-care-in-the-early-years-of-the-affordable-care-act.pdf

Schneider, M. E. (2015, June 19). Multidisciplinary group unveils OB hemorrhage safety bundle. *Ob.Gyn. News Digital Network*. Retrieved from http://www.obgynnews.com/specialty-focus/obstetrics/single-article-page/multidisciplinary-group-unveils-ob-hem orrhage-safety-bundle/3b12ff98234c53e514cd4971a0edc2de.html

Shah, N. (2015). A NICE delivery—The cross-Atlantic divide over treatment intensity in childbirth. *New England Journal of Medicine*, *372*(23), 2181–2183. doi:10.1056/NEJMp1501461

Signore, C. (2010). No time for complacency: Labor inductions, cesarean deliveries and the definition of "term." *Obstetrics & Gynecology*, *116*(1), 4–6. doi:10.1097/AOG.0b013 e3181e598d4

Simmons, A., Warren, K., & McClain, K. (2015). The Affordable Care Act: Advancing the health of women and children. Department of Health and Human Services, Office of the Assistant Secretary for Planning and Evaluation (ASPE Issue Brief). Retrieved from https://aspe.hhs.gov/sites/default/files/pdf/77191/ib_mch.pdf

ten Hoope-Bender, P., de Bernis, L., Campbell, J., Downe, S., Fauveau, V., Fogstad, H., . . . Van Lerberghe, W. (2014). Improvement of maternal and newborn health through midwifery. *Lancet, 384*(9949), 1226–1235. doi:10.1016/S0140-6736(14)60930-2

The Joint Commission. (2013). Improving performance on perinatal care measures. *Source, 11*(7), 16–19. Retrieved from http://www.jointcommission.org/assets/1/6/S7_TS_V11_N7.pdf

The Joint Commission. (2015). Expanded threshold for reporting perinatal care measure set. Retrieved from http://www.jointcommission.org/issues/article.aspx?Article=A9Im9xfNb Bo97ZcgWQAj/SE+KRiZJsPtdFLyHUR1bZU=

United States Midwifery Education, Regulation, and Association (US MERA). (2015). Creating the future of midwifery in the US. Retrieved from http://www.usmera.org

U.S. Census Bureau. (2014). 2014 National population projections. Retrieved from https://www.census.gov/population/projections/data/national/2014/downloadablefiles.html

Weiss, A. J., & Elixhauser, A. (2014). *Overview of hospital stays in the United States, 2012* (Healthcare Cost and Utilization Project Statistical Brief #180). Retrieved from http://www.hcup-us.ahrq.gov/reports/statbriefs/sb180-Hospitalizations-United-States-2012.pdf

Weiss, A. J., Elixhauser, A., & Andrews, R. M. (2014). *Characteristics of operating room procedures in U.S. hospitals, 2011* (Healthcare Cost and Utilization Project Statistical Brief #170). Retrieved from http://www.hcup-us.ahrq.gov/reports/statbriefs/sb170-Operating-Room-Procedures-United-States-2011.jsp

World Health Organization (WHO). (2014a). Trends in maternal mortality: 1990 to 2013. Estimates by WHO, UNICEF, UNFPA, The World Bank and the United Nations Population Division. Retrieved from http://apps.who.int/iris/bitstream/10665/112682/2/97892415 07226_eng.pdf

World Health Organization (WHO). (2014b). World Health Statistics, 2014. Retrieved from http://apps.who.int/iris/bitstream/10665/112738/1/9789240692671_eng.pdf

World Health Organization (WHO). (2015a). Global Health Observatory (GHO) data: Neonatal mortality. Retrieved from http://www.who.int/gho/child_health/mortality/neonatal/en

World Health Organization (WHO). (2015b). Global Health Observatory (GHO) data: Exclusive breastfeeding under 6 months: Data by country. Retrieved from http://apps.who.int/gho/data/node.main.1100?lang=en

# CHAPTER THREE

# EVALUATING AND USING SCIENTIFIC EVIDENCE: FOUNDATION FOR IMPLEMENTING CHANGE

Billie Anne Gebb, Zach G. Young, and Barbara A. Anderson

## THE HIERARCHY OF EVIDENCE

In their seminal 1996 article, published in the *British Medical Journal*, Sackett, Rosenberg, Gray, Haynes, and Richardson defined *evidence-based medicine* (EBM) as "the conscientious, explicit, and judicious use of current best evidence in making decisions about the care of individual patients" (para. 2). Sackett, Straus, Richardson, Rosenberg, and Haynes (2000) proposed a simpler definition "Evidence based medicine is the integration of best research evidence with clinical expertise and patient values" (p. 1). The concept of EBM was introduced "to provide a framework, methodological approach, and set of skills to enable clinicians to more effectively access clinically relevant research" (Perry & Kronenfeld, 2005, p. 3).

The theory has since evolved into evidence-based health care (EBHC) because other health care fields, including midwifery, have adopted the model (Perry & Kronenfeld, 2005). The methodology relies upon a series of steps to improve health care delivery and outcomes:

- Identifying a clinical problem
- Formulating a focused, answerable question
- Locating relevant and appropriate resources
- Searching for information
- Critically appraising the information
- Implementing a clinical practice model (Perry & Kronenfeld, 2005)

Performing these steps and implementing the theory of EBM can be considered evidence-based practice (EBP; Perry & Kronenfeld, 2005; Scott & McSherry, 2008). EBM, EBHC, and EBP are often used interchangeably, although many argue that these concepts are not exactly the same (Scott & McSherry, 2008). Likewise, many specialty areas of health care have adopted the evidence-based model to refer to their specialty, such as evidence-based health promotion (Scott & McSherry, 2008). Midwifery is one of several health care fields that have embraced the use of evidence in clinical decision making.

In an editorial in *Women and Birth*, Fahy (2008) calls for a more expansive definition of evidence and EBP for midwives. She advocates that EBP should include evidence of *appropriateness, meaningfulness*, and *feasibility*, mirroring the approach of the Joanna Briggs Institute (JBI; 2014a), an international collaboration that provides reliable evidence for nursing, allied health, and medical professionals.

Kronenfeld et al. (2007) point out that midwives and other advanced practice nurses, in their role as direct care providers, may approach EBP in a manner more similar to physicians. However, midwives bring elements of direct patient care to their practice and may elect to forge their own definition of evidence-based midwifery.

Although there may not be a clear agreement on terminology relating to EBP, all definitions include some form of research and utilization of evidence (Scott & McSherry, 2008). EBP is predicated on finding and evaluating evidence. So, what is considered evidence? It most often refers to research studies but can also include anecdotes and personal experience. Generally, evidence is organized into a hierarchy with the highest quality evidence at the top and less reliable types of information on the bottom. The highest quality evidence comes from studies that are least prone to threats to internal validity. Studies at the bottom of the hierarchy are more susceptible to those threats (Ho, Peterson, & Masoudi, 2008; Trustees of Dartmouth College and Yale University, 2006).

## Systematic Reviews

Systematic reviews are at the top of the evidence hierarchy (Figure 3.1). Many articles may be called review articles, but a systematic review is an overview of all primary studies on a given topic. A systematic review contains a statement of objectives, materials, and methods, and must be conducted in a transparent fashion that is explicitly explained and can be reproduced (Greenhalgh, 2010). The Center for Outcomes Research and Education (CORE) describes a systematic review as "a thorough, comprehensive, and explicit way of interrogating the medical literature" (2015, para. 2). Performing a systematic review is a multistep process. The author begins with a stated objective of answering a clinical question, searches for studies, selects the studies to be included based on inclusion and exclusion criteria, and summarizes the data in a standardized format (CORE, 2015; Greenhalgh, 2010).

## Meta-Analyses

Meta-analyses are at the same level as systematic reviews on the evidence hierarchy. Meta-analyses combine the statistical data from the individual studies into a systematic review and recalculate the statistical tests to provide further evaluation of the topic. Meta-analyses are based on systematic reviews, but not all systematic reviews become meta-analyses (CORE, 2015; Greenhalgh, 2010).

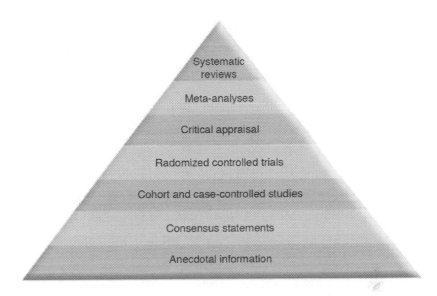

**Figure 3.1**   The hierarchy of evidence.

## Critical Appraisal

Next on the evidence hierarchy are critically appraised topics and articles. These critical appraisals are short summaries created to answer a specific clinical question (Law & Howick, 2014). Critically appraised topics can be found in a number of evidence-based, point-of-care research tools and may also be published in journals.

## Randomized Controlled Trials

Another high-quality evidence type is the randomized controlled trial (RCT). In the RCT, patients or research subjects are randomly assigned to either intervention or control groups. Because the subjects are assigned randomly, other variables do not come into play. Any difference in outcomes between the two groups can be attributed to the intervention (Ho et al., 2008).

## Cohort and Case–Controlled Studies

Below RCTs in the hierarchy of evidence are cohort and case–controlled studies. These studies follow particular groups of people over time. A cohort study follows two groups of patients: one group with a certain condition or intervention and the second group without the condition or intervention. Outcomes from the two groups are compared (SUNY Downstate Medical Center, 2002a). Case–controlled studies are similar in that they also compare a group with a certain condition or intervention to a group without that condition or intervention, but the groups are not followed over time. Comparisons are derived from the histories of the study participants (SUNY Downstate Medical Center, 2002b).

## Consensus Statements

Consensus statements often provide guidelines issued by professional organizations. The main purpose of these guidelines is to make evidence-based standards both clear and accessible and to facilitate clinical decision making (Greenhalgh, 2010). For instance, the American College of Obstetricians and Gynecologists (ACOG) issues practice bulletins, which are subtitled as "Clinical Management Guidelines for Obstetrician-Gynecologists." The American College of Nurse-Midwives (ACNM) produces clinical bulletins. Midwives may also be interested in the clinical practice guidelines from the American Academy of Pediatrics (AAP). Derived from consensus statements, these guidelines are verified data that may be published in textbooks, journals, or online.

## Anecdotal Information

Anecdotal information is the least reliable source because it cannot be verified. However, it does provide a rich description of experience. It builds on the bank of experiences that clinicians have and often corroborates best practices. However, a higher level of evidence must verify these practices.

## DATABASES FOR EVIDENCE-BASED MIDWIFERY PRACTICE

Large-scale bibliographic databases house most evidence-based information. For midwifery, the most relevant databases are MEDLINE and the Cumulative Index to Nursing and Allied Health Literature (CINAHL).

## MEDLINE

Consisting of more than 22 million journal article and book citations, MEDLINE is the largest index of biomedical literature in the world (U.S. National Library of Medicine [U.S. NLM], 2015a). Items indexed in MEDLINE are assigned medical subject headings (MeSH), a controlled vocabulary. MEDLINE can be searched through both free and paid interfaces.

PubMed is a free search interface for MEDLINE created by the NLM (U.S. NLM, 2015b). Users of PubMed are granted extensive customization options using a service called "My NCBI" (National Center for Biotechnology Information). Using My NCBI within PubMed allows users to save search limiters, to run searches for chronological time intervals, and store user-created bibliographies. The NLM provides several options for those who wish to conduct basic MEDLINE searches from their smartphones. PubMed for Handhelds is available as a mobile application (app) for both the iOS and Android platforms, and also as a mobile website (U.S. NLM, 2015c).

MEDLINE is also available through paid subscriptions from vendors such as Ovid and EBSCO. EBSCOhost, EBSCO's database platform, has an app for iPhone and Android that allows MEDLINE searches on mobile devices.

## CINAHL

CINAHL is an online research database published by EBSCO. With around 3 million citations, including nursing journals, books, multimedia, dissertations, and conference proceedings, CINAHL provides a robust index for midwives (EBSCO Industries, 2015a). CINAHL is accessed through the EBSCOhost interface, which provides the My EBSCOhost tool. Using this tool, searchers are able to save and share citations, create RSS (really simple syndication) feeds of searches, and save search preferences. Articles are indexed in CINAHL using the CINAHL headings controlled vocabulary. The EBSCOhost app makes it possible to search CINAHL from a mobile device.

## The Cochrane Collaboration

Other databases specifically index and house clinical evidence. The Cochrane Collaboration is the leader in this area. It produces the Cochrane Library, which includes the Cochrane Database of Systematic Reviews (CDSR), the Cochrane Central Register of Controlled Trials (CENTRAL), the Database of Abstracts of Reviews of Effects (DARE), the Cochrane Methodology Register (CMR), the Health Technology Assessment (HTA) Database, and the National Health Service Economic Evaluation Database (NHS EED).

Updated monthly, the CDSR, containing Cochrane Reviews, is the leading resource for systematic reviews in health care. Cochrane Reviews are prepared by one of the 53 Cochrane Review groups. Each of these groups focuses on a specific topic area and is responsible for editorial support and peer review; for example, pregnancy and childbirth (Cochrane Library, 2015a, 2015b). Abstracts of Cochrane Reviews are freely available. Many countries, as well as the state of Wyoming, have a provision or subscription to the full library (Cochrane Library, 2015c). In the United States, paid subscriptions are available for both institutions and individuals from Wiley (Cochrane Library, 2015d); EBSCO also offers institutional subscriptions (EBSCO Industries, Inc., 2015b).

## The Joanna Briggs Institute

JBI, housed at the University of Adelaide, Australia, is similar to the Cochrane Collaboration but is more focused on nursing, which may have relevance for midwifery. JBI partners with Wolters Kluwer Health/Ovid and Lippincott Williams and Wilkins to provide access to their resources (JBI, 2014b). JBI databases include the JBI Library of systematic reviews, best practice information sheets, evidence summaries, and evidence-based recommended practices. A limited amount of information is free, with other information available to members of the Institute via JBI ConNect+ Clinical Online Network of Evidence for Care and Therapeutics (JBI, 2014). These resources are also available as a subscription on the Ovid platform (Ovid Technologies, Inc., 2015).

## Meta-Search Engines

Meta-search engines have been created to search multiple evidence sources simultaneously. SUMsearch (sumsearch.org) searches the National Guideline Clearinghouse (NGC), MEDLINE, and DARE simultaneously for systematic reviews, original studies, and practice guidelines (Crom, 2007). The Trip database (www.tripdatabase.com) is a clinical search engine that searches a variety of research evidence to help clinicians answer questions quickly (Trip, n.d.).

## Point-of-Care Tools

Evidence-based information is often needed very quickly. A new generation of databases and other information resources has been created to fill this need. These resources summarize and organize the vast body of clinical literature into electronic, easily readable formats. They are designed to be used at the bedside and are often referred to as point-of-care tools (Ketterman & Besaw, 2010).

The advent of mobile computing devices has greatly accelerated the use of these tools and has given clinicians immediate access to information. The increasing use of smartphones exemplifies this trend. Drug reference software, such as Epocrates, Lexicomp, and Micromedex, were some of the first resources to use handheld platforms, and clinical reference software soon followed.

Widely used, UpToDate was one of the first point-of-care tools available to clinicians. Currently owned by Wolters Kluwer Health, UpToDate provides an overview of clinical topics. The product includes more than 10,500 topics in 22 health care specialties written by expert clinicians and updated continually (UpToDate, 2015a, 2015b). UpToDate has a mobile web page for smartphone users as well as apps for iOS, Android, and Windows (UpToDate, 2015c).

Essential Evidence Plus, originally called InfoRetriever, is produced by Wiley. In addition to Essential Evidence Topics (background, diagnosis, treatment), users can simultaneously search other databases such as EBM Guidelines, CDSR, NGC Guidelines, and Decision Support Tools. Essential Evidence Plus contains Patient-Oriented Evidence that Matters (POEMs) research summaries that synopsize new evidence. An alerting service e-mails this evidence to the user daily. Every recommendation in the database is given a strength-of-evidence rating (Essential Evidence Plus, 2015a, 2015b). There is a mobile-friendly version of the Essential Evidence Plus website.

*DynaMed* is published by EBSCO and provides clinically organized summaries for thousands of topics. It is updated daily (EBSCO Industries, Inc., 2015c). Entries are produced following a seven-step, evidence-based methodology for including and updating content (EBSCO Industries, Inc., 2015d). References are assigned levels in the hierarchy of evidence. This hierarchy includes the quality and source of the evidence. Level 1 is considered reliable evidence, level 2 is mid-level evidence, and level 3 is lacking direct evidence (EBSCO Industries, Inc., 2015e). These levels allow quick assessment of the best available evidence within a topic.

Recommendations not assigned with an evidence level based on the underlying source are labeled strong or weak based on the Grading of Recommendations

Assessment, Development and Evaluation (GRADE) system (EBSCO Industries, Inc., 2015f; The GRADE working group, 2014). A mobile app for *DynaMed* is available. Ketterman and Besaw (2010) compared UpToDate and *DynaMed* and found that the currency of updates was the major difference between the two tools. *DynaMed* has more current updates, but UpToDate has more references per topic. The authors suggest using multiple databases for answering clinical questions (Ketterman & Besaw, 2010).

Released in early 2015, *DynaMed Plus* presents expert synthesis and objective analysis of evidence in addition to the references provided in *DynaMed* (EBSCO Industries, 2015g). The expert opinion offered by many point-of-care tools has become a popular resource for practitioners who prefer synthesized information. In fact, Guyatt, Drummond, Meade, and Cook, credited with coining the term "EBM" and principal editors for *Users' Guides to the Medical Literature: A Manual for Evidence Based Clinical Practice* (2015), stated in an interview in the *Journal of the American Medical Association* that practitioners should "look first for preprocessed evidence in advanced medical texts, summaries, practice guidelines, and online clinical reference tools . . ." (Voelker, 2015, para. 13).

There are many other point-of-care tools available, and the market is growing. Most have a general focus, but some are more specific. *Natural Medicines* (formerly *Natural Standard and Natural Medicines Comprehensive Database*) is an evidence-based resource for complementary and alternative therapies. The professional monographs in *Natural Medicines* provide an evidence table summarizing relevant studies for the use of the selected foods, herbs, or supplements (Therapeutic Research Center, 2015).

With so many point-of-care tools on the market, clinicians may find it difficult to select one to use in their practice. Shurtz and Foster (2011) evaluated eight tools and found that most were similar in terms of content and search options. They found discrepancies, however, in the selection processes and grading systems used for the evidence presented. Evaluation of authorship and possible biases must be a main concern when choosing a system to rely on for clinical information. Users should have a sufficient baseline clinical knowledge to have confidence in the evidence grading system used. Other considerations are cost, mobile availability, and integration with electronic health records (EHRs).

## SEARCHING FOR THE EVIDENCE

Despite the trend toward preprocessed evidence, for best evidence, searching electronic resources, such as bibliographic databases, is a necessary skill for a complete search. This type of searching was once the realm of librarians, who would deliver the results to clinicians. With the advent of the Internet, end-user searching has become more prevalent (Perry & Kronenfeld, 2005). Today, it is common for clinicians to do their own searching, and it is an important time- and labor-saving skill. It is essential for evidence-based midwifery care that clinicians possess skills to find and analyze information. Systematic reviews, RCTs, and

some critically appraised topics are generally published in professional journals. The traditional bibliographic databases index these articles to facilitate
discovery. Database vendors create a record for each article, which contains all
the pertinent information (author, date, title, journal, volume, issue, pages, and
doi). The records are then stored electronically and are machine read, so they can
be searched by elements in the record.

## Search Strategy

Searching for the evidence begins with formulating a comprehensive search strategy. The first step in a search strategy should be forming a clinical question. Rather
than searching broad topics, an evidence-based search strategy attempts to answer
a focused, answerable question. For example, rather than search for information
on morning sickness, a midwife might ask, "Does ginger decrease the severity of
symptoms for women experiencing nausea and vomiting in pregnancy?"

To help build a question, practitioners can use a framework referred to as
PICO:

P = patient, problem, or population
I = intervention
C = comparison
O = outcome

Using the PICO framework as a search strategy has been shown to increase
the percentage of relevant results (Schardt, Adams, Owens, Keitz, & Fontelo,
2007). Applied to the preceding example, the framework results in:

P = pregnant women
I = consumption of ginger
C = no intervention
O = decrease in symptoms, severity, adverse effects

Words from the PICO framework and their synonyms become keywords or
important words used in the search (Reitz, 2014). Keywords are combined with
Boolean operators (Figure 3.2). *Boolean* refers to a system of logic developed by
mathematician George Boole and is commonly used in algebra. There are three
commands or operators used in this logic. The operators tell the database how to
combine terms. The operators are:

AND—includes both terms
OR—includes either term
NOT—excludes terms

The search for keywords can be limited to certain fields. A *field* is an individual piece of information contained within a record (Walker & James, 1993).
Examples of common fields are title, author, source, and subject. Searching can

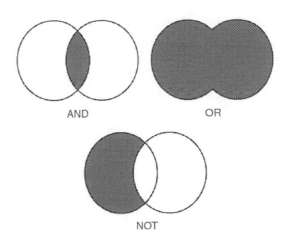

**Figure 3.2**   Boolean operators.

be limited to looking for terms only within the title of a work or only within an abstract. This feature is especially helpful when the citation is already known.

## Subject Headings

Perhaps the most important tool for the searcher is subject headings. Most databases use subject headings, or a thesaurus, for indexing and specialized searching. Subject headings compose a list of preferred terms that a cataloger or indexer must assign to the record of a work. In this way, the terms reflect a controlled vocabulary. They indicate the content of the work in a catalog or database (Reitz, 2014). This process standardizes the terminology. For example, if the subject heading for teenagers is *adolescents*, then an article titled "Dealing With Your Teenager" will have the subject heading of *adolescents*, even though that term is not used in the article. Subject headings can also be used as a search access point.

Subject headings are specific to each database and based on the terminology of the discipline. The standard subject headings for health care disciplines are the MeSH terms. MeSH is the controlled vocabulary thesaurus created and maintained by the NLM. MeSH terms are arranged in a hierarchical structure from general, broad headings to more specific, narrow headings. As of 2015, there were 27,455 descriptors in MeSH. These terms are continually revised and updated, and searchers may suggest new terms (U.S. NLM, 2015d).

Searching with these terms involves choosing the best terms from the list of subject headings. When searching for a term within a database's thesaurus, searchers will be presented with the term in such a way that its hierarchical relationship with other terms is shown. Therefore, the searcher can instantly see which terms are more general (broader) and which are more specific (narrower). If the term selected is not a subject heading, the preferred term will be suggested. In addition, a subject term will also list all other comparable or related terms.

Subject headings usually include a scope note; that is, the term's intended use in the database (Reitz, 2014). The scope note assures the searcher of the term's meaning or alerts the searcher that the database infers a different meaning. For example, the scope note for the MeSH term *young adult* is "a person between 19 and 24 years of age" (U.S. NLM, n.d.). If the searcher wishes to include persons at age 25, the searcher will need to use the MeSH term *adult* instead. Subject headings are particularly useful for alternate spellings. For example, using the preferred term *labor* will also retrieve articles that use *labour.* Subject headings also eliminate the need to search for multiple variations of the same term. *Postpartum depression* may also be referred to as *postnatal depression*, but using the preferred term will retrieve articles that use either term. When the correct subject headings have been identified and selected, those terms can be added to the search. Most databases will run the search automatically, retrieving records with the chosen terms.

## Limiters

Limiters are also very useful tools when searching for evidence-based articles. Limiters allow searchers to set certain parameters on their search results. A very common limiter is the date of publication. For instance, the searcher can elect to retrieve only articles published within the past year or over the past 5 years. Health care databases often include limiters associated with EBP; for example, the publication type can be limited so that only RCTs are retrieved. Limiters are essential for the best search strategy. However, the more limiters placed on a search, the smaller the number of results. It may be preferable to start with a broader search and then apply limiters as needed.

## Indexing

The key to the search-and-retrieval process is proper indexing and maintaining of databases. An indexer reads an article to determine subject and content and then assigns appropriate headings (Reitz, 2014). The standards for indexing of databases require indexers who are well prepared. For example, indexers for the NLM minimally hold a bachelor's degree in biomedical science (U.S. NLM, 2015e). The computerized systems used by the indexers are programed to guard against misspellings and other errors (U.S. NLM, 2015f). Databases include criteria regarding which journals are indexed. A list of the publications indexed is usually available within each database.

## CONCLUSION

Searching for evidence-based information is a best practice skill in providing midwifery care. Developing a search strategy and accessing resources, often at the point of care, can ultimately lead to better patient outcomes.

---

**USING THE EVIDENCE FOR BEST PRACTICE**

**Case Study 3.1    Oral Health in Late Pregnancy: Finding the Evidence**

Justin practices full-scope midwifery in a rural, underserved low-income community where the preterm birth rate is very high, and women frequently do not access prenatal care until well into the second trimester. He has noted a high prevalence of multiple dental caries among many of these women.

Justin has observed the high incidence of preterm labor among this population. He decides to explore the link between oral health and preterm birth. First, he formulated a focused, answerable question. Then he searched for the evidence and evaluated it according to the hierarchy of evidence. Using MeSH, he identified subject headings (dental caries, pregnancy, preterm birth, second trimester) and used limiters (publications in the past 5 years) in major databases, including MEDLINE and the Cochrane Library.

His smartphone with apps enhanced his influence with his colleagues by allowing him to search for and disseminate information at the point of care.

**Exemplar of Best Practice**

Evaluating best practices according to the hierarchy of evidence, Justin offers his patients and colleagues the best information on the management of oral health during late pregnancy. He is respected by his colleagues for his ability to obtain and apply accurate and timely information.

# REFERENCES

Center for Outcomes Research and Education (CORE). (2015). What is the difference between a "systematic review" and a "meta-analysis"? Retrieved from http://researchcore.org/faq/answers.php?recID=5

Crom, V. (2007). SUMsearch. *Journal of the Medical Library Association, 95*(4), 471–473. doi:10.3163/1536-5050.95.4.471

Cochrane Library. (2015a). About the Cochrane Library. Retrieved from http://www.cochrane library.com/about/about-the-cochrane-library.html

Cochrane Library. (2015b). Cochrane review groups. Retrieved from http://www.cochrane library.com/about/cochrane-review-groups.html

Cochrane Library. (2015c). Access options for the Cochrane Library. Retrieved from http://www.cochranelibrary.com/help/access-options-for-cochrane-library.html

Cochrane Library. (2015d). How to order the Cochrane Library. Retrieved from http://www.cochranelibrary.com/help/how-to-order-the-cochrane-library.html

EBSCO Industries. (2015a). CINAHL database. Retrieved from https://health.ebsco.com/products/the-cinahl-database

EBSCO Industries. (2015b). Cochrane Collection Plus. Retrieved from https://health.ebsco.com/products/cochrane-collection-plus

EBSCO Industries. (2015c). DynaMed. Retrieved from http://www.dynamed.com/home/about/dynamed

EBSCO Industries. (2015d). Evidence based methodology. Retrieved from http://www .dynamed.com/home/editorial/evidencebased-content/7-step-editorial-process

EBSCO Industries. (2015e). Levels of evidence. Retrieved from http://www.dynamed.com/ home/editorial/levels-of-evidence

EBSCO Industries. (2015f). Recommendations. Retrieved from http://www.dynamed.com/ home/editorial/evidencebased-content/recommendations

EBSCO Industries. (2015g). DynaMed Plus about. Retrieved from http://www.dynamed.com/ home/about

Essential Evidence Plus. (2015a). Essential Evidence Plus user guide (institutional). Retrieved from http://www.essentialevidenceplus.com/resources/EEP_guidebook_inst.pdf

Essential Evidence Plus. (2015b). Features: Resources & tools. Retrieved from http://www .essentialevidenceplus.com/product/features_ir.cfm

Fahy, K. (2008). Evidence based midwifery and power/knowledge. *Women and Birth, 21*(1), 1–2. doi:10.1016/j.wombi.2007.12.004

GRADE Working Group. (2014). Welcome. Retrieved from http://www.gradeworking group.org

Greenhalgh, T. (2010). *How to read a paper: The basics of evidence based medicine* (4th ed.). Chichester, West Sussex, UK: Wiley.

Guyatt, G., Drummond, R., Meade, M. O., & Cook, D. J. (Eds.). (2015). *Users' guides to the medical literature: A manual for evidence based clinical practice.* New York, NY: McGraw Hill.

Ho, P. M., Peterson, P. N., & Masoudi, F. A. (2008). Evaluating the evidence: Is there a rigid hierarchy? *Circulation, 118*(16), 1675–1684. doi:10.1161/CIRCULATIONAHA.107.721357

Joanna Briggs Institute (JBI). (2014a). The JBI approach. Retrieved from http://joannabriggs .org/jbi-approach.html#tabbed-nav=JBI-approach

Joanna Briggs Institute (JBI). (2014b). Subscribe now. Retrieved from http://joannabriggs .org/subscribe.html

Joanna Briggs Institute (JBI). (2014). Welcome to JBI COnNECT+. Retrieved from http://connect .jbiconnectplus.org

Ketterman, E., & Besaw, M. E. (2010). An evaluation of citation counts, search results, and frequency of updates in DynaMed and UpToDate. *Journal of Electronic Resources in Medical Libraries, 7*(4), 273–280. doi:10.1080/15424065.2010.527238

Kronenfeld, M., Stephenson, P. L., Nail-Chiwetalu, B., Tweed, E. M., Sauers, E. L., McLeod, T. C., . . . Ratner, N. B. (2007). Review for librarians of evidence based practice in nursing and the allied health professions in the United States. *Journal of the Medical Library Association, 95*(4), 394–407. doi:10.3163/1536-5050.95.4.394

Law, K., & Howick, J. (2014). Glossary. Retrieved from http://www.cebm.net/glossary

Ovid Technologies. (2015). Joanna Briggs Institute EBP Database. Retrieved from http://www .ovid.com/site/catalog/databases/11299.jsp

Perry, G. J., & Kronenfeld, M. R. (2005). Evidence based practice: A new paradigm brings new opportunities for health sciences librarians. *Medical Reference Services Quarterly, 24*(4), 1–16. doi:10.1300/J115v24n04_01

Reitz, J. M. (2014). ODLIS—Online Dictionary for Library and Information Science. Retrieved from http://www.abc-clio.com/ODLIS/odlis_a.aspx

Sackett, D. L., Rosenberg, W. M., Gray, J. A., Haynes, R. B., & Richardson, W. S. (1996). Evidence based medicine: What it is and what it isn't. *British Medical Journal*, 312(7023), 71–72. doi:10.1136/bmj.312.7023.71

Sackett, D. L., Straus, S. E., Richardson, W. S., Rosenberg, W., & Haynes, R. B. (2000). *Evidence based medicine: How to practice and teach EBM* (2nd ed.). Edinburgh, Scotland: Churchill Livingstone.

Schardt, C., Adams, M. B., Owens, T., Keitz, S., & Fontelo, P. (2007). Utilization of the PICO framework to improve searching PubMed for clinical questions. *BMC Medical Informatics and Decision Making*, 7(1), 16. doi:10.1186/1472-6947-7-16

Scott, K., & McSherry, R. (2008). Evidence based nursing: Clarifying the concepts for nurses in practice. *Journal of Clinical Nursing*, 18(8), 1085–1095. doi:10.1111/j.1365-2702.2008.02588.x

Shurtz, S., & Foster, M. J. (2011). Developing and using a rubric for evaluating evidence based medicine point-of-care tools. *Journal of the Medical Library Association*, 99, 247–254. doi:10.3163/1536-5050.99.3.012

SUNY Downstate Medical Center. (2002a). SUNY Downstate EBM tutorial: Cohort studies. Retrieved from http://library.downstate.edu/EBM2/2400.htm

SUNY Downstate Medical Center. (2002b). SUNY Downstate EBM tutorial. Case control studies. Retrieved from http://library.downstate.edu/EBM2/2500.htm

Therapeutic Research Center. (2015). Natural medicines. Retrieved from: https://naturalmedicines.therapeuticresearch.com

Trip. (n.d.). What is trip? Retrieved from http://www.tripdatabase.com/about

Trustees of Dartmouth College and Yale University. (2006). Supporting clinical care: An institute in evidence based practice for medical librarians. Retrieved from http://www.dartmouth.edu/~biomed/institute2010/pyramid.html

U.S. National Library of Medicine (U.S. NLM). (n.d.). Young adult (MeSH result). Retrieved from http://www.ncbi.nlm.nih.gov/mesh/68055815

U.S. National Library of Medicine (U.S. NLM). (2015a). Fact sheet: MEDLINE. Retrieved from http://www.nlm.nih.gov/pubs/factsheets/mesh.html

U.S. National Library of Medicine (U.S. NLM). (2015b). PubMed home. Retrieved from http://www.ncbi.nlm.nih.gov/pubmed

U.S. National Library of Medicine (U.S. NLM). (2015c). PubMed for handhelds. Retrieved from http://pubmedhh.nlm.nih.gov/

U.S. National Library of Medicine (U.S. NLM). (2015d). Fact sheet: Medical subject headings (MeSH). Retrieved from http://www.nlm.nih.gov/pubs/factsheets/mesh.html

U.S. National Library of Medicine (U.S. NLM). (2015e). Frequently asked questions about indexing for MEDLINE. Retrieved from http://www.nlm.nih.gov/bsd/indexfaq.html

U.S. National Library of Medicine (U.S. NLM). (2015f). Fact sheet: Online indexing system. Retrieved from http://www.nlm.nih.gov/pubs/factsheets/online_indexing_system.html

UpToDate. (2015a). About us. Retrieved from http://www.uptodate.com/home/about-us

UpToDate. (2015b). What is UpToDate? Retrieved from http://www.uptodate.com/home/help-faq-what-is-utd#updated

UpToDate. (2015c). UpToDate mobile access. Retrieved from http://www.uptodate.com/home/uptodate-mobile-access

Voelker, R. (2015). Everything you ever wanted to know about evidence based medicine. *Journal of the American Medical Association, 313*(18), 1783–1785. doi:10.1001/jama.2015.2845

Walker, G., & James, J. (1993). *Online retrieval: A dialogue of theory and practice* (2nd ed.). Englewood, CO: Libraries Unlimited.

# MIDWIFERY CARE: THE EVIDENCE FOR OPTIMAL OUTCOMES

Rebeca Barroso

*Midwifery care has been identified as a potent solution to changing the staggering inequities and health disparities facing women, children, and families in the United States and globally. Section II, "Midwifery Care: The Evidence for Optimal Outcomes," surveys clinical and social issues that midwives face in implementing change and providing evidence-based care. Chapter 4 focuses on the crucial role of the midwife in providing prenatal and postpartum care to support the "good birth." Chapters 5 to 7 examine the role of nutrition from various perspectives, with special emphasis on the obesity epidemic affecting the world, including the United States. These chapters offer pragmatic, evidence-based best practices. Chapter 8 delves into the public health domain, looking at the vaccination controversy and how to address maternal concerns while providing the most up-to-date evidence. Chapters 9 to 11 address midwifery care within the context of the vulnerable populations of women and infants who midwives serve so well. Chapter 12 explores postpartum mood disorders and the tragedy of mental illness, witnessed daily by the midwife clinician, and Chapter 13 describes mind–body practices as potent tools in midwifery care. Chapters 14 to 16 discuss out-of-hospital birth, both in birth centers and at-home birth, including current evidence from around the world on safety and promotion of physiologic birth sustained by these unique environments as peaceful places for birth.*

# CHAPTER FOUR

# FACILITATING ACCESS TO MIDWIFERY-LED PRENATAL AND POSTPARTUM CARE

Julia C. Phillippi and Melody J. Castillo

## ACCESS TO HEALTH SERVICES

Perinatal care provides women with health screening and education that may improve the woman's health, lessen the possibility of complications for mother and child, and increase the likelihood of infant survival. Prenatal care can assist women in managing chronic conditions, changing health behaviors, and increasing use of community resources. In addition, prenatal care offers women the opportunity for fetal screening and testing, as well as early detection and management of new-onset or pregnancy-related complications.

Current genomic research supports the belief that the health of the mother in pregnancy affects the long-term health of her offspring. For instance, there is growing evidence that the risks for adult obesity and metabolic syndrome are influenced by maternal obesity, underscoring the value of preconception and prenatal care (Lau, Rogers, Desai, & Ross, 2011). However, if prenatal care is only accessible to affluent, mainstream, and socially organized women, then it can increase health disparities (Jackson, Crider, Cragan, Rasmussen, & Olney, 2014; Kucik et al., 2014). Midwives have an ethical obligation to ensure that all women have access to beneficial services during pregnancy (American College of Nurse-Midwives [ACNM], 2004).

Access to health services is defined by the Institute of Medicine (IOM) as the "timely use of personal health services to achieve the best health outcomes" (Millman, 1993, p. 4). Access has three steps: gaining entry to the health care system, gaining access to the site of services, and developing a relationship based on communication and trust with a provider who can meet health care needs (U.S. Department of Health and Human Services [USDHHS], Agency for Healthcare Research and Quality [AHRQ], 2014). Access to prenatal care specifically is defined as "the potential ability of a woman to enter prenatal care services and maintain care for herself and the fetus during the perinatal period" (Phillippi, 2009, p. 220).

Historically, midwives have increased access to health care for women and newborns. In response to increasing demand for primary care services, midwives certified by the American Midwifery Certification Board (AMCB) continue this work (Phillippi & Barger, 2015). Provision of care to vulnerable populations is an ACNM hallmark of midwifery (ACNM, 2012a). The ACNM philosophy states that all people deserve equitable, ethical, accessible quality health care to enable informed health decisions (ACNM, 2004).

Many factors affect access to health care, and particularly midwifery services. Influences include societal, structural, maternal, and medical components (Phillippi & Roman, 2013). Although midwives generally focus on the direct provision of evidence-based care, midwives also work as clinical and research leaders to sculpt clinical, hospital, and public policies (ACNM, 2012a; International Confederation of Midwives [ICM], 2013). In addition, "support of legislation and policy initiatives that promote quality care" is a professional responsibility of certified nurse-midwives (CNMs) and certified midwives (CMs; ACNM, 2012a, p. 2). Such advocacy is an advanced skill in the ICM *Essential Competencies* (ICM, 2013).

## MEASURES OF ACCESS

There are several methods of assessing access to health care, including qualitative and quantitative measures. Clinicians and researchers can examine the experience or perceptions of people needing care using interviews, focus groups, or surveys. This assessment can be done as a quality project designed to improve care or as part of research. Although collecting information from women about their experiences provides exceedingly valuable information, it is less commonly used in studies of access, as qualitative data collection is time-consuming and pregnant women may be reluctant or unable to participate in research. As a result of these constraints, many studies of access use publicly available quantitative data.

One of the most common measures of health care access is the utilization of services. Information about the initiation and number of prenatal care visits is collected on the standard U.S. birth certificate and is available in aggregate from state and national databases. Similar reporting is also used in many international studies (World Health Organization [WHO] & United Nations Children's Fund [UNICEF], 2003). Another common public source of information is the Pregnancy Risk Assessment Monitoring System (PRAMS), a project of the Centers for Disease Control and Prevention (CDC; 2009). Data for PRAMS are obtained from a stratified sample of women in 40 states who have given birth within the past 4 months. Women in the sample complete an in-depth questionnaire and a telephone interview, providing both quantitative and qualitative data (CDC, 2009). Utilization of postpartum services is not well studied, in part related to difficulties in obtaining data, but the PRAMS database includes information on women's self-report of postpartum care utilization.

Access to health care can also be assessed by quantifying the number and location of health care facilities or providers in relation to the geographic distribution of people needing health care. This is one approach utilized by the National Health Service Corps when determining health care provider shortage areas in relation to eligibility for student loan repayment (Office of the Federal Register, 2009). Data on population density can be obtained from the census or other public sources and compared with locations of health care providers (Madkour, Harville, & Xie, 2014). Complex models can overlay these factors with other data, such as rates of timely prenatal care initiation, to further study women's access to maternity services (Shoff, Yang, & Matthews, 2012).

Although these approaches are useful in quantifying women's access to care, they do not demonstrate the effects of midwifery care. The attending provider is listed on the U.S. birth certificate, but there are no mechanisms for identifying women who received midwifery care antepartum, intrapartum, or postpartum but gave birth with another provider type. The ACNM working groups are attempting to rectify this problem so that electronic health systems can be used to track the utilization of midwifery services across the perinatal period (M. Freytsis, personal communication, August 11, 2015).

## Poor Utilization—A Personal or Systemic Problem?

Although access to care is commonly discussed in terms of utilization, these concepts are not interchangeable. Availability of health care services must be considered alongside women's perceptions of access to services, which are not always congruent. It is fairly easy to see poor utilization of prenatal care as a maternal problem. In the United States, services are available within nearly all geographic regions, and a safety-net system of free care can be found in many locations. However, women do not consistently access services available to them.

Placing the blame on women disregards the larger social forces affecting the women's ability to receive prenatal care. Inadequate utilization of prenatal care is nearly always a reflection of a poor fit between the available resources and women's needs (Phillippi & Roman, 2013). This discrepancy between services and needs contributes to the health disparities between mainstream and marginalized groups in the United States and around the world (Bromley, Nunes, & Phipps, 2012; Cox, Zhang, Zotti, & Graham, 2011; Walford, Trinh, Wiencrot, & Lu, 2011). When a population of women has low rates of timely initiation of prenatal care or inadequate use of prenatal or postpartum services, midwives should work to decrease barriers and facilitate care.

## Groups at Risk for Poor Utilization of Prenatal Care

Across all types of health care, including midwifery services, people who are marginalized in society struggle to access services. Women may be marginalized because of their gender; race; ethnicity; sexuality; marital, socioeconomic, or health status; or any trait considered undesirable in their community. Marginalized societal status can make it difficult for women to obtain services for a variety of reasons, including lack of money or time, poor access to the physical location of care, or fear of judgment from health care personnel.

In the United States, women who have a low socioeconomic status often struggle to obtain needed services. Although women who are U.S. citizens often qualify for free or reduced cost prenatal care, women who do not have prepregnancy insurance initiate care later and struggle to obtain needed prenatal care services throughout their pregnancies (Rosenberg, Handler, Rankin, Zimbeck, & Adams, 2007). The Affordable Care Act has made it easier for many nonpregnant women to qualify for reduced cost health insurance. Overall, this change has improved access to primary care services, including preventative gynecologic care (USDHHS, AHRQ, 2015). However, states vary in their approach to funding prenatal care, and it may be difficult for working women to obtain prenatal care at a price they can afford. In addition, women with low socioeconomic status may live in areas with few providers, have irregular transportation, or work in jobs that do not allow time off for medical visits (Phillippi, 2009).

Women with competing personal demands often struggle to obtain early prenatal care and meet the recommended visit schedule. For instance, women with three or more children are less likely to receive early care and have regular visits (Partridge, Balayla, Holcroft, & Abenhaim, 2012). Qualitative studies identify a variety of factors, including feeling that care is not warranted and competes with the needs of existing children (Heaman et al., 2014). Women with preschool-age children report the most difficulty accessing care (Phillippi, 2009).

Also at risk are women who believe that they have to hide certain aspects of their lives. Because pregnancy is linked with sexuality, taboos around sex may impair young women's ability or motivation to obtain care. In order to access care, young women have to know they are pregnant, and often they have to disclose this to their parents to get advice, transportation, or financial help (Teagle & Brindis, 1998). Likewise, women with psychiatric disorders may delay or avoid access to care because of anxiety and fear of stigma (Krans, Davis, & Palladino, 2013; Krans, Davis, & Schwarz, 2013).

Women experiencing unplanned pregnancy may have difficulty accessing prenatal care. Approximately half of all pregnancies in the United States are unplanned and affect women of all childbearing ages (Kost, 2015). Not knowing about a pregnancy, the stresses of an unplanned pregnancy, wanting to hide the pregnancy, and consideration of abortion may contribute to poor access to prenatal care (Heaman et al., 2014).

Some women may be worried about legal ramifications of seeking prenatal care. Women who are actively using illicit drugs or who are physically abused may not obtain needed services in pregnancy as they worry that disclosure may trigger legal action against them or their partners (Krans et al., 2013). Women who are not legal residents may fear legal consequences or deportation if they seek care (White, Yeager, Menachemi, & Scarinci, 2014). These women without legal status may also face challenges related to language and cultural barriers, or exclusion from social programs and resources (Korinek & Smith, 2011).

Women who struggle to access services have higher rates of perinatal morbidity and mortality (Partridge et al., 2012). However, if women from vulnerable groups obtain midwifery services during pregnancy and postpartum, perinatal outcomes can be improved (Raisler & Kennedy, 2005; Sandall, Soltani, Gates, Shennan, & Devane, 2013).

## BARRIERS AND FACILITATORS TO ACCESS

There is an extensive amount of literature on barriers to prenatal care access. Women's comments on barriers are most often found in the qualitative literature. These barriers can be classified into societal, maternal, structural, and medical categories (Phillippi, 2009). Common societal barriers include transportation, payment structures/finances, and the needs/expectations of partners and family members.

Maternal barriers relate to the woman's personal situation. Transportation is a frequent barrier for both rural and urban women. Rural women struggle to have reliable transportation and money for gas, and urban women have difficulty paying for public transportation or clinic parking. Women with children find transportation to be even more of a barrier than women without children who are at home during the day (Phillippi, 2009).

Motivation for prenatal care is another frequently cited barrier. Women may not be aware of pregnancy for many weeks (Haddrill, Jones, Mitchell, & Anumba, 2014). Women with unplanned pregnancies may delay prenatal care entry if considering abortion or until they are emotionally prepared to accept the pregnancy (Heaman et al., 2014; Phillippi, 2009). For some women, especially teens who need advice or help in getting care, disclosure to friends or family can be a strong barrier (Phillippi, Holley, Payne, & Schorn, 2016; Teagle & Brindis, 1998).

Mental health problems may contribute to a lack of motivation. In studies, women state that depression thwarts their entry into prenatal care, even if they know they would benefit from services (Heaman et al., 2014). Some women have anxiety about medical procedures, whereas other women feel that the prenatal care is unnecessary because of cultural reasons or previous uncomplicated pregnancies (Heaman et al., 2014; Phillippi, 2009). Although there are a variety of common barriers, midwives should work to eliminate these barriers whenever possible (Phillippi & Roman, 2013). This work may involve changes at the point of care or advocating for state or national policy change.

The literature on facilitators of access to prenatal care is less robust than information on barriers. Although it can be assumed that elimination of barriers will increase access to care, this needs further testing (Phillippi & Roman, 2013). The literature supports that women are willing to overcome barriers if, upon arrival to care, they are treated with respect and kindness and seen by a clinician who treats them as individuals and answers their questions (Phillippi, Myers, & Schorn, 2014).

## EVIDENCE-BASED STRATEGIES FOR IMPROVING ACCESS

Across sociocultural and age groups, desire for a healthy baby is consistently reported as women's greatest motivator for prenatal care (Heaman et al., 2014; Johnson et al., 2011; Phillippi, 2009). Midwives can capitalize on women's desire for a healthy baby and facilitate their access to needed services during pregnancy and the postpartum period. Best practices incorporate information from research, quality, and customer service.

## Clinic Characteristics

Providing an appointment soon after the woman's initial call is one of the first ways to facilitate care. When women are ready to begin care, they should be seen as soon as possible. Although difficult, especially in busy clinics, midwives can work with the administration to ensure minimal delay in initiation of care. Care can also be facilitated by offering a variety of appointment times, including evenings and times when significant others or support persons can attend visits (Novick, 2009; Phillippi et al., 2014). Additionally, care may be facilitated by providing a variety of payment options and minimizing out-of-pocket costs to women (Phillippi, 2009; Phillippi & Roman, 2013).

Strategic placement of clinic location can facilitate access to prenatal care. Considerations for a location may include proximity to public transportation and minimization of travel time (Novick, 2009; Phillippi, 2009; Phillippi et al., 2014). Transportation assistance can also facilitate access to care. Acceptable transportation assistance includes vouchers to pay for transportation or parking, or free parking (Johnson et al., 2011).

Decreasing wait times at the clinic once women arrive is important as women often have constraints on their transportation or time. Women are more satisfied with care when waits are less than 30 minutes. If unavoidable, women value information about delays. However, an unrushed feel in the clinic environment is also important (Sword et al., 2012).

The clinic environment should be reflective of women's needs: respectful, welcoming, and physically and emotionally safe. Motivation for accessing care is dynamic and every interaction with the clinic or clinic staff is an opportunity to inspire future access to care (Phillippi & Roman, 2013). Women value environments that are clean, comfortable, private, and welcoming to children (Novick, 2009; Sword et al., 2012). Assistance with childcare facilitates prenatal care for women whose children must accompany them to the clinic. Women report that clinics that welcome their children and have child-safe play areas are easier to access, but women are also accepting of other kinds of assistance with child care (Phillippi et al., 2014). Clinic décor, permanent and seasonal, should be sensitive to the social and cultural backgrounds of the women. Home-like décor may facilitate a relaxed and welcoming environment (Proctor, 1998). The qualitative literature specifies that clinic staff who are friendly, welcoming, easy to understand, and receptive to the woman's needs facilitate access (Heaman et al., 2014; Phillippi et al., 2014, 2016).

Creating a safe, welcoming environment is essential in helping women feel safe in disclosing personal information. For example, lesbian women are more likely to share their sexual orientation with health care providers whom they perceive as sensitive and accepting (McManus, Hunter, & Renn, 2006). Disclosing sexual orientation to health care providers increases satisfaction with care, and women with positive perceptions of their providers are more likely to adhere to recommendations and present for follow-up care (Hutchinson, Thompson, & Cederbaum, 2006). Facilitating such an environment starts with careful attention to language on clinic forms, handouts, and in conversations with women (McManus et al., 2006). Midwives may further facilitate access to care by familiarizing themselves with the health care needs of populations they serve, and acting as advocates for women from this population (Hutchinson et al., 2006). A welcoming environment incorporates partner involvement to the full extent desired by the woman, independent of age, sex, gender, or marital status.

The Supreme Court ruling on June 26, 2015, recognized same-sex marriage as a constitutional right (*Obergefell et al. v. Hodges*, 2015). Although not all same-sex couples desire marriage, this ruling may be a catalyst for legal change. Although states explore the ramifications of this ruling, lesbian, gay, bisexual, and transgender parents may still experience challenges (Biblarz & Savci, 2010). Midwives should be sensitive to women's needs and assist as needed with legal resources.

## Provider Characteristics

Populations experience the greatest positive change in health outcomes when they are cared for by providers with similar demographic characteristics (Jackson & Gracia, 2014). In order to improve access to services, the midwifery workforce needs to be more diverse. Although the ACNM Diversity and Inclusion Task Force has been working on issues related to recruiting, retaining, and supporting midwives from diverse backgrounds, this responsibility belongs to all in the profession. Midwives should encourage people with a variety of attributes and skills to enter midwifery, recognizing that our diversity may help us better serve multiple populations.

Qualitative research indicates that women prefer accessing care with a single provider but are open to a variety of providers if their care is personalized, and if they are consistently treated with kindness and respect (Novick, 2009; Phillippi et al., 2015). Practices often balance continuity of care with appointment availability by employing several midwives. Midwifery-led continuity models of care provided by both a single midwife and a group of midwives have demonstrated benefits to women (Sandall et al., 2013). If a woman is not able to establish a relationship with one provider, clinics can increase a woman's sense of connection by disseminating important social and personal aspects of the woman's life among the practicing midwives.

Although women appreciate providers who can speak their language, they are accepting of interpreter services if the provider is genuinely interested in them and provides culturally appropriate care (Heaman et al., 2014; Phillippi et al., 2016; Sword et al., 2012). The literature on prenatal care access overlaps the literature on quality of prenatal care. Women report that high-quality care and competent providers increase their motivation and ability to access services (Phillippi et al., 2016; Sword et al., 2012). Additionally, women value providers who communicate effectively and answer questions (Phillippi et al., 2014).

## Prenatal Care

Prenatal care optimizes perinatal outcomes and is recommended by national and international health organizations, including the CDC (2015) and the WHO (2009). Although utilization is often a measure of prenatal care access, evidence suggests that the quality of care may be more important than the quantity of care. However, there is not a consensus on what constitutes quality prenatal care (Sword et al., 2012), and available measures of prenatal care access do not account for content or quality (Misra & Guyer, 1998). Efforts are being made to address this issue. Renfrew, McFadden et al. (2014) propose a framework for quality maternal and newborn care, outlining effective, evidence-based practices.

The ACNM philosophy provides a broad framework for quality prenatal care, stating that the best model of health care for women "promotes a continuous and compassionate partnership, acknowledges a person's life experiences and knowledge, includes individualized methods of care and healing guided by the best evidence available, [and] involves therapeutic use of human presence and skillful communication" (ACNM, 2004, p. 1). In the United States, prenatal care guidelines are available from several sources, including the American Academy of Pediatrics (AAP) and the American College of Obstetricians and Gynecologists (ACOG; AAP Committee on Fetus and Newborn & ACOG Committee on Obstetric Practice, 2012), and the Institute for Clinical Systems Improvement (Akkerman et al., 2012).

International guidelines are available from several sources, including the U.K.'s National Institute for Health and Care Excellence (NICE) and the WHO (2009). The literature supports that the provision of quality care goes beyond adherence to evidence-based guidelines. The qualitative literature demonstrates that both women and providers include additional components in their assessment of quality, including structural components, such as the physical setting and convenience of the clinic, and interpersonal components such as a provider's approachability, respectfulness, and emotional support (Sword et al., 2012). This highlights the importance of a woman-centered approach to care, a core value of ACNM (ACNM, 2012b).

As the attributes of quality prenatal care continue to be clarified, evidence supports that midwifery care increases access to quality perinatal care (Renfrew, Homer et al., 2014). A recent Cochrane Review found that midwifery-led continuity models of care had no adverse outcomes and demonstrated benefits compared to other models of care (Sandall et al., 2013). The authors conclude that the majority of women need to be offered midwife-led continuity models of care (Sandall et al., 2013). *The Lancet's* Series on Midwifery (2014) explored the role of midwifery in meeting the needs of childbearing women and their families and concluded that trained midwives are essential to improving perinatal care in low-, middle-, and high-resource countries, elaborating that universal access to midwifery services will require a significant increase in the midwifery workforce (Renfrew, Homer et al., 2014).

Women's needs for flexibility in prenatal visit structure, timing, and content were called to the attention of policy makers and health care providers with the publication of "Caring for Our Future: The Content of Prenatal Care" (U.S. Public

Health Service, 1989). Although ideally all prenatal care is based on evidence, historically this has not been true, because of the difficulties of research with pregnant women (IOM, 2010). Newer, emerging models of care, based on research, should be incorporated if they meet population and individual needs.

The standard visit schedule for prenatal care begins in the first trimester and includes at least 12 visits with increasing frequency as pregnancy advances. Designed to prevent maternal deaths from preeclampsia, this schedule has not been changed since the inception of prenatal care in the 1940s (Alexander & Kotelchuck, 2001). However, this schedule does not reflect the need for testing and health promotion in early pregnancy and may not resonate with the perceived needs of women (Krans et al., 2013). Alternate forms of prenatal care, based on current evidence, include reduced frequency of visits as well as group prenatal care models, such as CenteringPregnancy®.

Prenatal care schedules with reduced frequency of visits strategically schedule care to coincide with prenatal screening and health-promotion teaching. The safety of models using approximately eight visits during pregnancy has been established for low-risk women in developed countries (Dowswell et al., 2010). Reduced visits decrease cost, but are also associated with reduced maternal satisfaction (Dowswell et al., 2010). Midwives can customize visit intervals based on maternal needs to ensure a woman's needs are met, within third-party payer limitations.

The CenteringPregnancy model has been shown to have lower rates of preterm birth when compared with individual prenatal care (Ickovics et al., 2007; Picklesimer, Billings, Hale, Blackhurst, & Covington-Kolb, 2012). In addition, participants have greater knowledge of perinatal topics (Baldwin, 2006; Ickovics et al., 2007). Many women are very satisfied with this model of care, feeling it provides a sense of community (Kennedy et al., 2009; Novick et al., 2011). However, this form of care may not be accessible to all women (McDonald et al., 2016), especially those who struggle with anxiety in groups, those with small children, and those who cannot accommodate a fixed group time (Phillippi & Myers, 2013). Midwives should encourage group prenatal care but provide alternatives for women who are unable to attend group visits.

## Postpartum Care

Provision of evidence-based postpartum care is woefully inadequate in the United States. For example, only 8% of women who self-identified as having gestational diabetes reported clinical postpartum testing (Oza-Frank, 2014). Although historically women have returned to the clinic 4 to 6 weeks postpartum, this time frame is not based on evidence. In fact, at this point, it may be too late to promote breastfeeding, encourage use of long-acting contraceptives, or assess for postpartum depression (Fahey & Shenassa, 2013). Although in-person assessment and assistance are preferable, telephone or online contact may be an alternative for women who otherwise would not receive postpartum services (Lavender, Richens, Milan, Smyth, & Dowswell, 2013).

Research suggests that provision of contraception can safely take place much earlier than 4 weeks postpartum (de Bocanegra, Chang, Howell, & Darney, 2014).

Women who desire permanent sterilization can receive a postpartum tubal ligation the day after birth. If a woman has Medicaid and wants a tubal ligation, it is important to assist her in signing an official consent form between 17 and 36 weeks of pregnancy so she can qualify for a Medicaid-funded tubal ligation. Long-acting contraceptives, such as intrauterine devices, can be placed prior to hospital discharge (de Bocanegra et al., 2014). Immediate provision of contraception may improve future perinatal outcomes as it delays subsequent pregnancy and prevents short interpregnancy intervals associated with risks of preterm birth and low birth weight (de Bocanegra et al., 2014). If a woman does not desire a long-acting contraceptive, the midwife can provide a prescription for her chosen method soon after birth to facilitate contraception prior to resumption of intercourse.

Midwifery support for breastfeeding and lactation services is also crucial in the postpartum period. In addition to providing direct breastfeeding support, midwives can facilitate hospital and clinical environments that implement best practices in encouraging breastfeeding. Women may be reluctant to ask for help or see new providers, but a trusted midwife's recommendation can encourage her access to lactation assistance, as needed. Beyond professional care, women, especially those from low-income or marginalized groups, may benefit from support from a peer counselor from her cultural or socioeconomic group (Renfrew, McCormick, Wade, Quinn, & Doswell, 2012; Rozga, Kerver, & Olson, 2015).

The postpartum period involves social and role changes for the woman and her family. Pre-existing stressors are often magnified postpartum as women and their partners have little sleep, many demands, and finances may be tight as women are on leave from paid employment. Midwives should encourage women to mobilize social support from family, friends, or a faith community as these support systems may improve physical and emotional health (Fahey & Shenassa, 2013). Midwives should assess maternal coping and screen for postpartum depression either in person or by phone. Women who struggle to access prenatal care services also struggle to obtain and afford mental health services (Bobo et al., 2014). Referrals as needed should be made to locations that are compatible with the woman's culture, language, and ability to pay.

For many women, free or subsidized health care ends a few weeks following birth. As several conditions in pregnancy are harbingers of increased risk later in life (Brown et al., 2013), midwives can help new mothers to receive as much evidence-based care as possible while they have health insurance. Positive care with a trusted provider increases women's motivation for future care (Phillippi et al., 2016). The final postpartum visit should be a time to reflect on the woman's growth and assist her in planning for her future primary and reproductive health care.

Midwives should provide the woman with clear guidance on where they can obtain affordable future health care. Women may not know that American Midwifery Certification Board (AMCB)-certified midwives can provide primary care services to women beyond pregnancy and postpartum (Phillippi & Barger, 2015). Women should also be directed to appropriate community resources such as mothers' groups, housing support, food pantries, and low-cost or free clinics (Fahey & Shenassa, 2013)

# CONCLUSION

Evidence-based midwifery care can benefit all women, especially those women at risk for poor perinatal outcomes (Renfrew, McFadden et al. 2014). Beyond providing excellent clinical care, midwives work to facilitate access to health services. Facilitation can occur at the individual, clinic, population, or policy level. Although midwives are most known for their care of women during the prenatal, intrapartum, and postpartum periods, AMCB-certified midwives can increase access through providing gynecologic and primary care.

Midwives have a long history of providing high-quality care to vulnerable and marginalized populations around the globe (Ettinger, 2006; Raisler & Kennedy, 2005; United Nations Population Fund, International Confederation of Midwives, & World Health Organization, 2014). Although direct patient care can be rewarding, work with vulnerable groups, especially in resource-poor settings, can contribute to burnout (Mollart, Skinner, Newing, & Foureur, 2013; Yoshida & Sandall, 2013). Strong collegial support is associated with improved midwifery job satisfaction (Jarosova et al., 2016; Warmelink et al., 2015).

## USING THE EVIDENCE FOR BEST PRACTICE

### Case Study 4.1   Facilitating Access to Prenatal Care: The Impact of Midwifery

A small clinic located about 1.5 hours outside of a metropolitan area had an influx of women who were recent U.S. immigrants. Z., one of the clinic midwives, enjoyed caring for this population as the women valued physiologic birth and appreciated midwifery care. However, most women requested the last possible Friday appointment and often arrived late, upsetting the office staff.

Z. asked a woman why she preferred Friday appointments. The woman stated the men in the community work for a city construction company and are paid at 3 p.m. on Fridays. Her husband had to cash his check while the bank was open and get gas before he could bring her to the clinic. Otherwise, they could not get groceries for the weekend. All other days of the week, her husband worked until 4 p.m., making it impossible for her arrive before the clinic closed at 5 p.m.

Once Z. understood the disconnect between the women's needs and the clinic hours, she worked with the administration to develop a solution. Z. offered to come to the clinic at noon on Fridays and stay until 9 p.m. Clinic staff was not available at these times so Z. enlisted C. to work at the front desk during this time frame. C. was a woman from the community who had given birth twice with the midwives, breastfed her children, had an excellent command of English, and was well-respected within her community as a former teacher. C. was honored to be involved with the clinic's work and had many ideas of how to improve her community's health.

The Friday-evening clinic was a resounding success. Under C.'s guidance, the clinic waiting room became a festive community gathering each Friday. Women began bringing food to share and staying for the whole evening to visit with others. C. was able to use this moment to connect women with community resources and explain the value of health care. C. worked with Z. to develop health presentations on topics such

*(continued)*

**USING THE EVIDENCE FOR BEST PRACTICE (continued)**

as breastfeeding, contraception for pregnancy spacing, and well-child visits. Women reported they looked forward to prenatal care as a moment to connect with others and focus on their health. Postpartum women said they enjoyed coming back to share their birth stories with pregnant mothers.

The Friday-evening clinic greatly increased the women's ability to access midwifery care. The rate of women receiving prenatal care increased dramatically, and the number of no-show appointments decreased sharply. The number of women returning postpartum for contraception also increased, resulting in better birth spacing.

**Exemplar of Best Practice**

Z.'s compassionate approach and involvement of stakeholders led to a dramatic increase in access to health services for this population. She found innovative ways to overcome barriers and implemented known facilitators of care to assist women in obtaining needed care. Z. provided personalized, culturally appropriate midwifery services and worked with the administration and community members to facilitate access for a local population.

# REFERENCES

Akkerman, D., Cleland, L., Croft, G., Eskuchen, K., Heim, C., Levine, A., . . . Westby, E. (2012). *Routine prenatal care*. Bloomington, MN: Institute for Clinical Systems Improvement.

Alexander, G. R., & Kotelchuck, M. (2001). Assessing the role and effectiveness of prenatal care: History, challenges, and directions for future research. *Public Health Reports, 116*(4), 306–316. doi:10.1016/S0033-3549(04)50052-3

American Academy of Pediatrics (AAP) & American College of Obstetricians and Gynecologists (ACOG). (2012). *Guidelines for perinatal care* (7th ed.). Elk Village, IL: American Academy of Pediatrics Books.

American College of Nurse-Midwives (ACNM). (2004). Philosophy of the American College of Nurse-Midwives. Retrieved from http://www.midwife.org/index.asp?bid=59&cat=2&button=Search&rec=49

American College of Nurse-Midwives (ACNM). (2012a). Core competencies for basic midwifery practice. Retrieved from http://www.midwife.org/ACNM/files/ACNMLibraryData/UPLOADFILENAME/000000000050/Core%20Comptencies%20Dec%202012.pdf

American College of Nurse-Midwives (ACNM). (2012b). ACNM vision, mission, and core values. Retrieved from http://www.midwife.org/ACNM/files/ACNMLibraryData/UPLOADFILENAME/000000000269/ACNM%20Vision%20Mission%20Core%20Values%20April%202012.pdf

Baldwin, K. A. (2006). Comparison of selected outcomes of CenteringPregnancy versus traditional prenatal care. *Journal of Midwifery and Women's Health, 51*(4), 266–272. doi:10.1016/j.jmwh.2005.11.011

Biblarz, T. J., & Savci, E. (2010). Lesbian, gay, bisexual, and transgender families. *Journal of Marriage and Family, 72*(3), 480–497. doi:10.1111/j.1741-3737.2010.00714.x

Bobo, W. V., Wollan, P., Lewis, G., Bertram, S., Kurland, M. J., Vore, K., & Yawn, B. P. (2014). Depressive symptoms and access to mental health care in women screened for postpartum depression who lose health insurance coverage after delivery: Findings from the translating research into practice for postpartum depression (TRIPPD) effectiveness study. *Mayo Clinic Proceedings, 89*(9), 1220–1228. doi:10.1016/j.mayocp.2014 .05.011

Bromley, E., Nunes, A., & Phipps, M. G. (2012). Disparities in pregnancy healthcare utilization between Hispanic and non-Hispanic White women in Rhode Island. *Maternal and Child Health Journal, 16*(8), 1576–1582. doi:10.1007/s10995-011-0850-5

Brown, M. C., Best, K. E., Pearce, M. S., Waugh, J., Robson, S. C., & Bell, R. (2013). Cardiovascular disease risk in women with pre-eclampsia: Systematic review and meta-analysis. *European Journal of Epidemiology, 28*(1), 1–19. doi:10.1007/s10654-013-9762-6

Centers for Disease Control and Prevention (CDC). (2009). PRAMS model surveillance protocol. Retrieved from http://www.cdc.gov/prams/methodology.htm

Centers for Disease Control and Prevention (CDC). (2015). Safe motherhood: Advancing the health of mothers in the 21st century. Retrieved from http://www.cdc.gov/chronicdisease/ resources/publications/aag/pdf/2015/safe-motherhood-aag-2015.pdf

Cox, R. G., Zhang, L., Zotti, M. E., & Graham, J. (2011). Prenatal care utilization in Mississippi: Racial disparities and implications for unfavorable birth outcomes. *Maternal and Child Health Journal, 15*(7), 931–942. doi:10.1007/s10995-009-0542-6

de Bocanegra, H. T., Chang, R., Howell, M., & Darney, P. (2014). Interpregnancy intervals: Impact of postpartum contraceptive effectiveness and coverage. *American Journal of Obstetrics and Gynecology, 210*(4), 311.e1–311.e8. doi:10.1016/j.ajog.2013.12.020

Dowswell, T., Carroli, G., Duley, L., Gates, S., Gülmezoglu, A. M., Khan-Neelofur, D., & Piaggio, G. G. (2010). Alternative versus standard packages of antenatal care for low-risk pregnancy. *Cochrane Database of Systematic Reviews, 7*. doi:10.1002/14651858.CD000934 .pub3

Ettinger, L. E. (2006). *Nurse-midwifery: The birth of a new American profession.* Columbus, OH: Ohio State University Press.

Fahey, J. O., & Shenassa, E. (2013). Understanding and meeting the needs of women in the postpartum period: The Perinatal Maternal Health Promotion Model. *Journal of Midwifery & Women's Health, 58*(6), 613–621. doi:10.1111/jmwh.12139

Haddrill, R., Jones, G. L., Mitchell, C. A., & Anumba, D. O. (2014). Understanding delayed access to antenatal care: A qualitative interview study. *BMC Pregnancy and Childbirth, 14*(1), 207. doi:10.1186/1471-2393-14-207

Heaman, M. I., Moffatt, M., Elliott, L., Sword, W., Helewa, M. E., Morris, H., . . . Cook, C. (2014). Barriers, motivators and facilitators related to prenatal care utilization among inner-city women in Winnipeg, Canada: A case-control study. *BMC Pregnancy and Childbirth, 14*(1), 227. doi:10.1186/1471-2393-14-227

Hutchinson, M. K., Thompson, A. C., & Cederbaum, J. A. (2006). Multisystem factors contributing to disparities in preventive health care among lesbian women. *Journal of Obstetric, Gynecologic, & Neonatal Nursing, 35*(3), 393–402. doi:10.1111/j.1552-6909.2006.00054.x

Ickovics, J. R., Kershaw, T. S., Westdahl, C., Magriples, U., Massey, Z., Reynolds, H., & Rising, S. S. (2007). Group prenatal care and perinatal outcomes: A randomized controlled trial. *Obstetrics & Gynecology, 110*(2, Pt. 1), 330–339. doi:10.1097/01.AOG.0000275284.24298.23

Institute of Medicine (IOM). (2010). *Women's health research: Progress, pitfalls, and promise.* (Committee on Women's Health Research). Washington, DC: National Academies Press.

International Confederation of Midwives (ICM). (2013). Essential competencies for basic midwifery practice. Retrieved from http://www.internationalmidwives.org/assets/uploads/documents/CoreDocuments/ICM%20Essential%20Competencies%20for%20Basic%20Midwifery%20Practice%202010,%20revised%202013.pdf

Jackson, C. S., & Gracia, J. N. (2014). Addressing health and health-care disparities: The role of a diverse workforce and the social determinants of health. *Public Health Reports, 129*(Suppl. 2), 57–61.

Jackson, J. M., Crider, K. S., Cragan, J. D., Rasmussen, S. A., & Olney, R. S. (2014). Frequency of prenatal cytogenetic diagnosis and pregnancy outcomes by maternal race–ethnicity, and the effect on the prevalence of trisomy 21, Metropolitan Atlanta, 1996–2005. *American Journal of Medical Genetics Part A, 164A*(1), 70–76. doi:10.1002/ajmg.a.36247

Jarosova, D., Gurkova, E., Palese, A., Godeas, G., Ziakova, K., Song, M. S., . . . Babiarczyk, B. (2016). Job satisfaction and leaving intentions of midwives: Analysis of a multinational cross-sectional survey. *Journal of Nursing Management, 24*(1), 70–79. doi:10.1111/jonm.12273

Johnson, A. A., Wesley, B. D., El-Khorazaty, M. N., Utter, J. M., Bhaskar, B., Hatcher, B. J., . . . Rodan, M. F. (2011). African American and Latino patient versus provider perceptions of determinants of prenatal care initiation. *Maternal and Child Health Journal, 15*(1), 27–34. doi:10.1007/s10995-011-0864-z

Kennedy, H. P., Farrell, T., Paden, R., Hill, S., Jolivet, R., Willetts, J., & Rising, S. S. (2009). "I wasn't alone"—A study of group prenatal care in the military. *Journal of Midwifery & Women's Health, 54*(3), 176–183. doi:10.1016/j.jmwh.2008.11.004

Korinek, K., & Smith, K. R. (2011). Prenatal care among immigrant and racial-ethnic minority women in a new immigrant destination: Exploring the impact of immigrant legal status. *Social Science & Medicine, 72*(10), 1695–1703. doi:10.1016/j.socscimed.2011.02.046

Kost, K. (2015). Unintended pregnancy rates at the state level: Estimates for 2010 and trends since 2002. Retrieved from https://www.guttmacher.org/pubs/StateUP10.pdf

Krans, E. E., Davis, M. M., & Palladino, C. L. (2013). Disparate patterns of prenatal care utilization stratified by medical and psychosocial risk. *Maternal and Child Health Journal, 17*(4), 639–645. doi:10.1007/s10995-012-1040-9

Krans, E. E., Davis, M. M., & Schwarz, E. B. (2013). Psychosocial risk, prenatal counseling and maternal behavior: Findings from PRAMS, 2004–2008. *American Journal of Obstetrics and Gynecology, 208*(2), 141.e1–141.e7. doi:10.1016/j.ajog.2012.11.017

Kucik, J. E., Cassell, C. H., Alverson, C. J., Donohue, P., Tanner, J. P., Minkovitz, C. S., . . . Kirby, R. S. (2014). Role of health insurance on the survival of infants with congenital heart defects. *American Journal of Public Health, 104*(9), e62–e70. doi:10.2105/AJPH.2014.301969

Lau, C., Rogers, J. M., Desai, M., & Ross, M. G. (2011). Fetal programming of adult disease: Implications for prenatal care. *Obstetrics & Gynecology, 117*(4), 978–985. doi:10.1097/AOG.0b013e318212140e

Lavender, T., Richens, Y., Milan, S. J., Smyth, R., & Dowswell, T. (2013). Telephone support for women during pregnancy and the first six weeks postpartum. *Cochrane Library, 7.* doi:10.1002/14651858.CD009338.pub2

Madkour, A. S., Harville, E. W., & Xie, Y. (2014). Neighborhood disadvantage, racial concentration and the birthweight of infants born to adolescent mothers. *Maternal and Child Health Journal, 18*(3), 663–671. doi:10.1007/s10995-013-1291-0

McDonald, S. D., Sword, W., Eryuzlu, L. N., Neupane, B., Beyene, J., & Biringer, A. B. (2016). Why are half of women interested in participating in group prenatal care? *Maternal and Child Health Journal, 20*(1), 97–105.

McManus, A. J., Hunter, L. P., & Renn, H. (2006). Lesbian experiences and needs during childbirth: Guidance for health care providers. *Journal of Obstetric, Gynecologic, & Neonatal Nursing, 35*(1), 13–23. doi:10.1111/j.1552-6909.2006.00008.x

Millman, M. (Ed.). (1993). Access to healthcare in America (Committee on Monitoring Access to Personal Health Care Services). Retrieved from http://www.ncbi.nlm.nih.gov/books/NBK235882/pdf/Bookshelf_NBK235882.pdf

Misra, D. P., & Guyer, B. (1998). Benefits and limitations of prenatal care: From counting visits to measuring content. *Journal of the American Medical Association, 279*(20), 1661–1662. doi:10.1001/jama.279.20.1661

Mollart, L., Skinner, V. M., Newing, C., & Foureur, M. (2013). Factors that may influence midwives work-related stress and burnout. *Women and Birth, 26*(1), 26–32. doi:10.1016/j.wombi.2011.08.002

National Institute for Health and Clinical Excellence. (2008). Antenatal care: Routine care for the healthy pregnant woman *NICE Clinical Guideline 62*, 1–56. Retrieved from http://www.rcpch.ac.uk/system/files/protected/page/CG062NICEguideline.pdf

Novick, G. (2009). Women's experience of prenatal care: An integrative review. *Journal of Midwifery & Women's Health, 54*(3), 226–237. doi:10.1016/j.jmwh.2009.02.003

Novick, G., Sadler, L. S., Kennedy, H. P., Cohen, S. S., Groce, N. E., & Knafl, K. A. (2011). Women's experience of group prenatal care. *Qualitative Health Research, 21*(1), 97–116. doi:10.1177/1049732310378655

Obergefell et al. v. Hodges. (2015). Retrieved from http://www.supremecourt.gov/opinions/14pdf/14-556_3204.pdf

Office of the Federal Register. (2009). *Code of Federal Regulations, Title 42, Public Health, Pt. 1-399* (Revised October 1, 2009). Washington, DC: U.S. Government Printing Office.

Oza-Frank, R. (2014). Postpartum diabetes testing among women with recent gestational diabetes mellitus: PRAMS 2009–2010. *Maternal and Child Health Journal, 18*(3), 729–736. doi:10.1007/s10995-013-1299-5

Partridge, S., Balayla, J., Holcroft, C. A., & Abenhaim, H. A. (2012). Inadequate prenatal care utilization and risks of infant mortality and poor birth outcome: A retrospective analysis of 28,729,765 US deliveries over 8 years. *American Journal of Perinatology, 29*(10), 787–793. doi:10.1055/s-0032-1316439

Phillippi, J. C. (2009). Women's perceptions of access to prenatal care in the United States: A literature review. *Journal of Midwifery & Women's Health, 54*(3), 219–225. doi:S1526-9523(09)00004-X

Phillippi, J. C., & Barger, M. (2015). Midwives as primary care providers for women. *Journal of Midwifery & Women's Health, 60*(3), 250–257. doi:10.1111/jmwh.12295

Phillippi, J. C., Holley, S., Payne, K., & Schorn, M. (2016). Facilitators of prenatal care in an exemplar urban clinic. *Women & Birth, 29*(2), 160–167. doi:10.1016/j.wombi.2015.09.007

Phillippi, J. C., & Myers, C. R. (2013). Reasons women in Appalachia decline Centering-Pregnancy care. *Journal of Midwifery & Women's Health, 58*(5), 516–522. doi:10.1111/jmwh.12033

Phillippi, J. C., Myers, C., & Schorn, M. (2014). Facilitators of prenatal care access in rural Appalachia. *Women and Birth, 27*(4), e28–e35. doi:10.1016/j.wombi.2014.08.001

Phillippi, J. C., & Roman, M. W. (2013). The motivation–facilitation theory of prenatal care access. *Journal of Midwifery & Women's Health, 58*(5), 509–515. doi:10.1111/jmwh.12041

Picklesimer, A. H., Billings, D., Hale, N., Blackhurst, D., & Covington-Kolb, S. (2012). The effect of CenteringPregnancy group prenatal care on preterm birth in a low-income population. *American Journal of Obstetrics and Gynecology, 206*(5), 415.e1–415.e7. doi:10.1016/j.ajog.2012.01.040

Proctor, S. (1998). What determines quality in maternity care? Comparing the perceptions of childbearing women and midwives. *Birth, 25*(2), 85–93. doi:10.1046/j.1523-536x.1998.00085.x

Raisler, J., & Kennedy, H. (2005). Midwifery care of poor and vulnerable women, 1925–2003. *Journal of Midwifery & Women's Health, 50*(2), 113–121. doi:10.1016/j.jmwh.2004.12.010

Renfrew, M. J., Homer, C., Downe, S., McFadden, A., Muir, N., & Prentice, T. (2014). Midwifery: An executive summary for *The Lancet*'s series. *Lancet, 20,* 1–8.

Renfrew, M. J., McCormick, F. M., Wade, A., Quinn, B., & Dowswell, T. (2012). Support for healthy breastfeeding mothers with healthy term babies. *Cochrane Database of Systematic Reviews, 5.* doi:10.1002/14651858.CD001141.pub4

Renfrew, M. J., McFadden, A., Bastos, M. H., Campbell, J., Channon, A. A., Cheung, N. F., . . . Declercq, E. (2014). Midwifery and quality care: Findings from a new evidence-informed framework for maternal and newborn care. *Lancet, 384*(9948), 1129–1145. doi:10.1016/S0140-6736(14)60789-3

Rosenberg, D., Handler, A., Rankin, K. M., Zimbeck, M., & Adams, E. K. (2007). Prenatal care initiation among very low-income women in the aftermath of welfare reform: Does pre-pregnancy Medicaid coverage make a difference? *Maternal & Child Health Journal, 11*(1), 11–17. doi:10.1007/s10995-006-0077-z

Rozga, M. R., Kerver, J. M., & Olson, B. H. (2015). Impact of peer counselling breast-feeding support programme protocols on any and exclusive breast-feeding discontinuation in low-income women. *Public Health Nutrition, 18*(03), 453–463. doi:10.1017/S1368980014000603

Sandall, J., Soltani, H., Gates, S., Shennan, A., & Devane, D. (2013). Midwife-led continuity models versus other models of care for childbearing women. *Cochrane Database of Systematic Reviews, 8.* doi:10.1002/14651858.CD004667.pub3

Shoff, C., Yang, T. C., & Matthews, S. A. (2012). What has geography got to do with it? Using GWR to explore place-specific associations with prenatal care utilization. *GeoJournal, 77*(3), 331–341. doi:10.1007/s10708-010-9405-3

Sword, W., Heaman, M. I., Brooks, S., Tough, S., Janssen, P. A., Young, D., . . . Hutton, E. (2012). Women's and care providers' perspectives of quality prenatal care: A qualitative descriptive study. *BMC Pregnancy and Childbirth, 12*(1), 29. doi:10.1186/1471-2393-12-29

Teagle, S. E., & Brindis, C. D. (1998). Perceptions of motivators and barriers to public prenatal care among first-time and follow-up adolescent patients and their providers. *Maternal & Child Health Journal, 2*(1), 15–24.

United Nations Population Fund, International Confederation of Midwives, and World Health Organization. (2014). The state of the world's midwifery 2014: A universal pathway. A woman's right to health. Retrieved from http://www.unfpa.org/sites/default/files/pubpdf /EN_SoWMy2014_complete.pdf

U.S. Department of Health and Human Services (USDHHS), Agency for Healthcare Research and Quality (AHRQ). (2014). *2013 National Healthcare Quality Report* (AHRQ Publication No. 14-0005). Retrieved from http://www.ahrq.gov/sites/default/files/publications/files/ 2013nhqr.pdf

U.S. Department of Health and Human Services (USDHHS), Agency for Healthcare Research and Quality (AHRQ). (2015). *2014 National Healthcare Quality & Disparities Report* (AHRQ Publication No. 15-0007). Retrieved from http://www.ahrq.gov/sites/default/files/wysi wyg/research/findings/nhqrdr/nhqdr14/2014nhqdr.pdf

U.S. Public Health Service. (1989). *Caring for our future: The content of prenatal care.* Washington, DC: U.S. Department of Health and Human Services. Retrieved from http://files.eric.ed .gov/fulltext/ED334018

Walford, H. H., Trinh, S., Wiencrot, A., & Lu, M. C. (2011). What is the role of prenatal care in reducing racial and ethnic disparities in pregnancy outcomes? In A. Handler & J. Kennelly (Eds.), *Reducing racial/ethnic disparities in reproductive and perinatal outcomes* (pp. 151–179). New York, NY: Springer Publishing Company.

Warmelink, J. C., Hoijtink, K., Noppers, M., Wiegers, T. A., de Cock, T. P., Klomp, T., & Hutton, E. K. (2015). An explorative study of factors contributing to the job satisfaction of primary care midwives. *Midwifery, 31*(4), 482–488. doi:10.1016/j.midw.2014.12.003

White, K., Yeager, V. A., Menachemi, N., & Scarinci, I. C. (2014). Impact of Alabama's immigration law on access to health care among Latina immigrants and children: Implications for national reform. *American Journal of Public Health, 104*(3), 397–405. doi:10.2105/ AJPH.2013.301560

World Health Organization (WHO). (2009). *WHO recommended interventions for improving maternal and newborn health* (2nd ed., WHO/MPS/07.05). Geneva, Switzerland: Author. Retrieved from http://apps.who.int/iris/bitstream/10665/69509/1/WHO_MPS_07.05_eng .pdf

World Health Organization (WHO) & United Nations Children's Fund (UNICEF). (2003). Antenatal care in developing countries: Promises, achievement, and missed opportunities. An analysis of trends, levels and differentials, 1990–2001. Retrieved from http://www .childinfo.org/files/antenatal_care.pdf

Yoshida, Y., & Sandall, J. (2013). Occupational burnout and work factors in community and hospital midwives: A survey analysis. *Midwifery, 29*(8), 921–926. doi:10.1016/j.midw .2012.11.002

# CHAPTER FIVE

# NUTRITION AND EPIGENETICS IN PREGNANCY

Mary K. Barger

## EPIGENETICS AND PREGNANCY

When we mapped the human genome, we thought we would have a major understanding of the role of genes in health and disease. However, we learned that the reasons why certain genes are expressed and others are not are more complex. Hence, the field of epigenetics (a term that was first used in the 1990s) began to explore the role environment plays on gene phenotype. With our increased understanding of the complex interplay between genes and the environment, we now understand that the in utero environment of the fetus can play an important role on the long-term health of the person. Hence, there has been a renewed focus on nutrition during pregnancy and its role in determining a newborn's genetic phenotype.

Barker was one of the first to link low birth weight, a proxy for insufficient nutrition in utero, to development of adult diseases such as hypertension, heart disease, and diabetes (Barker, 1990). Since then, extensive work has been done examining pregnancy to childhood birth cohorts and using animal models in understanding programing of fetal metabolism and other physiological processes. Control of gene expression is mediated through methylation of bases on the DNA molecule or through histone modification. Evidence shows that too little methyl-donating folic acid or choline just before and during early pregnancy causes certain genes coding for development of particular body areas to be under-methylated for life. Therefore, a person's genetic phenotype is not only influenced by the in utero environment but also the lactation environment, the postnatal environment, and ongoing environmental influences. The epigenetic alterations are also transgenerational in that the reproductive cells, especially of the female fetus, can be altered, influencing her fertility and her offspring (Hanley et al., 2010). Other exposures besides maternal nutrition can alter the fetal epigenome and these include stress, toxins, and even antibiotics.

This DNA methylation process is influenced by undernutrition, micronutrient deficiency or excess, obesity, and diabetes during pregnancy (Lau, Rogers, Desai, & Ross, 2011). In addition, the timing of a deficiency or excess plays an important role on what changes to the epigenome will occur (Ojha, Fainberg, Sebert, Budge, & Symonds, 2015). For example, a growth-restricted baby with low birth weight will develop a *thrifty phenotype*, altered insulin–glucose metabolism, in utero, which, when exposed to the postnatal environment of adequate or excess calories, triggers abnormal responses. These responses result in adult chronic diseases. These infants can also experience poor development of neurons that control satiety, another mechanism for obesity later in life (Lau et al., 2011). Maternal obesity, with high circulating lipids, also leads to fetal programing of obesity and metabolic abnormalities (Lau et al., 2011).

Maternal diet influences a child's food preferences. Evidence shows that fetuses experience odor and taste from the amniotic fluid flavored by what the mother eats. This influences flavor preferences for four of the five basic tastes: sweet, bitter, sour, and umami (savory), and also volatile odors, such as carrots and garlic (Beauchamp & Mennella, 2011; Mennella, Jagnow, & Beauchamp, 2001).

In summary, the uterine environment plays a crucial role in determining the phenotype of a fetus' genome. The amount and timing of exposure to crucial elements needed for proper methylation of DNA determines the outcome. Maternal diet plays a role, along with the quality of placental implantation and development and the presence or absence of maternal diseases. Fetal exposure to a varied diet, especially strong-flavored vegetables, can influence food preferences in childhood.

## NUTRITION IN PREGNANCY: THE EVIDENCE

There are very few high-level studies (meta-analyses or randomized controlled trials [RCT]) regarding nutrition interventions in pregnancy. Most of the knowledge of nutrition in pregnancy is derived from observational studies. In many instances, it would be unethical to randomly assign women to lower quality diets compared to higher quality ones. Women enter pregnancy with a history of dietary eating patterns as well as a variety of health habits. The problem with observational studies is factors, other than diet, that can confound results. For example, women with poor diet are more likely to engage in risk habits, such as smoking and the use of drugs. In addition, dietary patterns vary not only by culture or ethnicity but also by social class and other factors associated with common adverse perinatal outcomes such as preterm birth.

Many observational studies of diet and pregnancy come from long-standing cohorts, such as the Nurses' Health Study, or from specific cohorts that have followed pregnant women and their children over time, such as Project Viva in Boston or the Avon Longitudinal Study of Parents and Children in England. Typically, these studies compare outcomes in women in the lowest quartile on an identified health-eating index to those in the highest quartile. These healthy eating indices generally are based on some form of the Mediterranean diet.

A Mediterranean diet is one rich in whole fruits and vegetables (generally at least five servings a day), whole grains, legumes, low-fat proteins, such as chicken and fish, with less intake of red meat and processed food, and use of monounsaturated fats such as olives or olive oil. Some indices, such as those based on the Dietary Approaches to Stop Hypertension diet, also give points for decreased sodium intake ($< 2,300$ mg/d).

The evidence for nutrition in pregnancy is derived from studies on populations from developed countries where undernutrition is rarely a problem but overnutrition is an issue. Nutrition issues for women from low- and middle-income countries not only include undernutrition but also high prevalence of chronic disease secondary to parasite and infectious disease, including malaria and HIV.

## The Body's Physiologic Response to Food

The food we eat is made up of macronutrients: protein, carbohydrates, fats, water, and micronutrients. Unfortunately, many intervention studies on the effects of diet in pregnancy have manipulated a single nutrient. However, it is the food combinations at any one meal that affect our production of hormones, such as insulin, cortisol, and eicosanoids (locally produced hormones). Eicosanoids are important because they exert a powerful effect on the production of cyclic adenosine monophosphate (AMP). Cyclic AMP is needed for peptide hormones to exert their effect within a cell. Peptide hormones, such as luteinizing hormone, follicle-stimulating hormone, human chorionic gonadotropin, oxytocin, insulin, and leptin, are key to pregnancy and fetal growth and development. Cyclic AMP, essential in pregnancy, is required to mobilize glucose from the liver. The glycemic index, a measure of blood sugar response 2 hours after eating carbohydrate, has been shown to affect not only glucose and insulin levels but also the production of pro-inflammatory or anti-inflammatory hormones (Ludwig, 2002).

Studies indicate that the typical American diet, high in refined sugar and omega-6 fatty acids, causes high levels of pro-inflammatory hormones to be produced, possibly explaining the increase in chronic health conditions such as arthritis, heart disease, and cancer. Individual nutrients are discussed later in the chapter, but the reader should keep in mind that it is the complex interaction of dietary nutrients that affects pregnancy outcomes. Therefore, information from RCT and meta-analyses of a single nutrient supplementation in pregnancy are less likely to demonstrate an effect than observational studies or animal studies manipulating the whole diet.

## Macronutrients

### Protein

Protein is essential for pregnancy and, more important, for the fetus to make the astonishing amount of DNA needed to produce a healthy newborn. American women do not appear to be at risk for inadequate protein intake. Pregnant women should eat 1.1 g/kg/d of protein, most of which is needed in the last 6 months of pregnancy (Food and Nutrition Board, 2011[2004]). Ideally, protein sources should be mostly from poultry, fish, legumes, grains, and less processed meats. A protein source that should be limited in pregnancy is liver, which has high levels of vitamin A as retinol, a teratogen at levels greater than 10,000 IU (international units; Rothman et al., 1995).

### Carbohydrates

High levels of glucose appear to be teratogenic for a growing embryo. Evidence is clear that among women with type 1 diabetes, glucose control at the very beginning of pregnancy is key to avoiding two risks: spontaneous abortion and congenital heart malformations. Women whose hemoglobin A1C (HbA1C) levels are higher than 1% above normal have a risk of neural tube defects or congenital heart defects and spontaneous abortion rates at three to four times that of healthy women (Greene, Hare, Cloherty, Benacerraf, & Soeldner, 1989; Macintosh et al., 2006). The rates significantly increase for women with HbAICs greater than 11%. Other evidence that a diet higher in carbohydrates increases early pregnancy loss comes from a study of healthy, normal-weight women seeking fertility treatments. Women whose diets were higher in protein (>25% kcal) and lower in carbohydrates (<40% kcal) had over twice the pregnancy rate and five times the live birth rate compared to women eating lower protein and higher carbohydrate diets (Russell et al., 2012).

The evidence on the effects of high-glycemic diets on pregnancy outcomes is limited. Using data from the Nurses' Health Study II cohort, Tobias and colleagues found adherence to any healthy-eating diets, such as Mediterranean or Dietary Approaches to Stop Hypertension, lowered gestational diabetes mellitus (GDM) by 24% to 46% (Tobias et al., 2012). A review of the use of low glycemic index diets by women with GDM identified four RCTs (Louie, Brand-Miller, & Moses, 2013). There was a modest decrease in birth weight in one study (Grant, Wolever, O'Connor, Nisenbaum, & Josse, 2011), and less need for the use of insulin in another (Moses, Barker, Winter, Petocz, & Brand-Miller, 2009), but no differences in weight gain. The interventions in these studies were only able to achieve a lower glycemic index level of eight to nine units between groups and most of the studies had small sample sizes, ranging from 12 to 99 women (Louie et al., 2013).

### Fats

Essential unsaturated fatty acids that cannot be made by the body must come from diet. These are linoleic acid (an omega-6) and α-linolenic acid (ALA; an omega-3). Two other important omega-3 fatty acids, eicosapentaenoic acid (EPA) and docosahexaenoic acid (DHA), can be converted from ALA, but this pathway has low conversion efficiency. They are, however, found in adequate amounts in food. These essential fatty acids are essential for normal placental functioning and play key roles in regulating eicosanoid metabolism. In addition, DHA accumulates in the fetal/neonatal brain, retina, and nervous system and is essential, especially during the last trimester and the first 6 weeks of the infant's life, for normal cognitive and visual development.

Because of the importance of fatty acid, and particularly DHA, studies have examined the association between omega-3 intake and both pregnancy and neonatal outcomes. A 2013 meta-analysis pooled results from 15 RCTs (a total of over 114,000 women) with 12 trials from upper income countries (Imhoff-Kunsch, Briggs, Goldenberg, & Ramakrishnan, 2012). Most trials provided supplements as fish oil (DHA + EPA) or DHA alone with daily amounts of DHA ranging from 80 mg to 2.2 g, in either drink or food. The results for effects of supplementation on pregnancy outcomes that included 2,000 to 3,300 women showed no differences in maternal blood pressure, preeclampsia, or fetal growth restriction. They did show a small increase in birth weight (42 g), 26% lower risk of preterm birth at less than 34 weeks (RR [relative risk] = 0.74; 95% CI [0.58, 0.94]), and a suggestive decrease in overall preterm birth (RR = 0.91; 95% CI [0.82, 1.01]; Imhoff-Kunsch et al., 2012). These results are similar to an RCT, not included in this analysis, which randomized 350 women to placebo or 600 mg DHA, finding that supplemented women had 4.2% less incidence of preterm births at less than 34 weeks (0.6% vs. 4.8%; Carlson et al., 2013).

Gould, Smithers, and Makrides (2013) examined the effects of omega-3 pregnancy supplementation on early childhood cognitive and visual development. Eleven trials with more than 5,000 subjects were included but many of the studies were of low quality. Results of the effect of visual acuity in children could only be evaluated in six trials, with four of the six finding no difference and two studies excluded for high attrition rates. Many studies used measures of visual function that could not be compared. Results for effects on cognitive outcomes only showed an increase of 3.92 points on the Developmental Standard Score among the DHA-supplemented group at 2 to 5 years but no differences at less than 12 months, 12 to 24 months, or 5 to 12 years (Gould et al., 2013).

In summary, intake of omega-3 fatty acid, found in fatty fish, is important during pregnancy. The Institute of Medicine (IOM) recommends a minimum of 200 mg/d in pregnancy although their recommendation for healthy nonpregnant adults is 250 mg/d (Food and Nutrition Board, 2011). The European Food Safety Authority recommends 100 to 200 mg/d for pregnant women in addition to the 250 mg/d of EPA plus DHA recommended for healthy adults (European Food Safety Authority [EFSA], 2012). Two to three servings of fish per week (12 oz) would meet this latter recommendation. Concern regarding heavy metals found in large fish and warning from the U.S. Environmental Protection Agency for pregnant women to avoid tilefish, shark, swordfish, and king mackerel have resulted in a dramatic decrease in intake of all fish in pregnant women (Oken et al., 2003). However, a study from the Seychelles Islands in the Indian Ocean is highly reassuring. Pregnant women at this location consumed the equivalent of 12 fish meals a week and there was no effect on child cognitive function despite the presence of mercury exposure (Strain et al., 2015). Women unwilling to consume fish or DHA-enriched eggs can meet requirements with a daily supplement of 500 mg of EPA and 300 mg of DHA.

### Water and Fluids

The primary fluid women should consume in pregnancy is water. Increased water needs in pregnancy depend on increased calorie requirements. Therefore, women need an increase of 300 to 400 mL in pregnancy or eight to 10 glasses a day (Montgomery, 2002). Water is not only essential for blood volume expansion but it also helps prevent constipation.

The intake of other beverages should be limited or avoided. It is well known that women should avoid alcohol intake during pregnancy. Caffeine, as tea or coffee, probably accounts for the highest fluid intake after water. There is controversy regarding the effect of caffeine intake on pregnancy outcomes, especially miscarriage. Caffeine intake may be associated with other behaviors or factors that also affect outcomes but are not well controlled in observational studies. The assessment of exposure is crude and not at the biologic level as liver enzymes that metabolize caffeine into active metabolites vary widely based on genetics (Greenwood et al., 2014). A systematic review of two intervention studies limiting caffeine intake in pregnancy was of low quality and showed nonsignificant effects (Greenwood et al., 2014). The conclusion is that an intake of 200 mg of caffeine a day (about two cups of coffee) does not result in any adverse pregnancy effects (American College of Obstetricians and Gynecologists, 2010).

## Micronutrients

Micronutrients, with higher requirements in pregnancy, are essential for normal fetal development and healthy pregnancy. Eating a varied diet rich in whole grains, fruits, and vegetables will provide these needed requirements. Table 5.1, a review of the latest National Health and Nutrition Exam Survey (NHANES) survey data, identifies the recommended levels of some important micronutrients for pregnant women compared to the actual status of American women (see Table 5.1).

Vitamins A and E, fat-soluble vitamins, are generally consumed in sufficient amounts in the American diet with less than 1% of the population below recommended amounts (Centers for Disease Control and Prevention [CDC], 2012). This section discusses selected micronutrients with a focus on those more commonly deficient among reproductive-age women.

### Vitamins

*Vitamin A*
Although vitamin A deficiency is rare in the United States, it is much more common in developing countries. Vitamin A is essential for both maternal health and immune functioning as well as for normal embryonic and fetal development, particularly the heart, eyes, ears, and limbs. Consuming preformed vitamin A in amounts greater than 3,000 mcg (10,000 IU) daily can result is birth defects. The defects also occur with use of pharmaceutical retinoids, such as isotretinoin (Accutane). Preformed vitamin A is found in organ meats, but there is no problem with large intakes of vitamin A as beta-carotene.

**TABLE 5.1  Recommended Pregnancy Intakes and Actual Current Status of Selected Micronutrients in U.S. Women Ages 20 to 39 by Race/Ethnicity, National Nutrition and Health Examination Survey Years 2003 to 2006**

| Micronutrient | Adequate Levels in Pregnant Women | Actual Status for Women Ages 20–39 Geometric Mean Values | | | |
| --- | --- | --- | --- | --- | --- |
| | | All Women Ages 20–39 | Non-Hispanic White | Non-Hispanic Black | Mexican American |
| Vit A mcg/dL | > 20 | 50.0 | 52.5 | 49.9 | 45.0 |
| Vit E mcg/dL | > 500 | 1,010 | 1,040 | 917 | 1,000 |
| Vit $B_6$: PLP nmol/L | > 20 | 42.4 | 44.6 | 35.4 | 37.3 |
| Vit $B_{12}$ pg/mL | > 400 | 439 | 414 | 469 | 501 |
| Folate: RBC folate ng/mL | 220 | 253 | 263 | 213 | 256 |
| Vit D as 25(OH)D ng/mL | 20–32 | 55.3 | 66.7 | 32.7 | 43.9 |
| Iron: Ferritin ng/mL | > 15 | 38.1 | 41.0 | 30.1 | 33.7 |
| Iodine—urinary excretion ng/mL | 150–249 | 118 Pregnancy 125 (95% CI 86–198) | 112 | 118 | 171 |

CI, confidence interval; 25 (OH)D, 25-hydroxyvitamin D; PLP, pyridoxal 5′-phosphate; RBC, red blood cell; Vit, vitamin.

*Source*: CDC (2012).

*B Vitamins*

Folate was identified in the mid-20th century as critical to embryonic and fetal growth and metabolism. It is necessary for amino acid, DNA, and ribonucleic acid (RNA) synthesis. The incidence of neural tube defects has decreased dramatically following both the public health campaign to assure women have adequate preconception folic acid supplementation and the folic acid fortification of wheat and cereals. NHANES surveys show folate deficiency has dropped from 12%, pre-fortification, to now less than 1% in the population, including reproductive-age women of all races (CDC, 2012). There are populations of women who need to consume higher doses than the pregnancy requirement of 600 mcg either because of drug interactions with medication, such as anticonvulsants, or malabsorption disorders, such as inflammatory bowel disease or bariatric surgery.

Vitamin $B_6$ has many roles, it is necessary for nucleic acid synthesis and the functioning of red blood cells, steroid hormones, and the nervous system. In pregnancy, it is essential in fetal development through its effects on the folate pathway for DNA methylation. It is also used to alleviate nausea and vomiting during pregnancy. Three RCTs examining vitamin $B_6$ supplementation showed an increase in birth weight of around 220 g (Dror & Allen, 2012). Although mean intakes of vitamin $B_6$ appear adequate (see Table 5.2), 10% of women are deficient, that is, below 20 nmol/L of pyridoxal 5'-phosphate (PLP; CDC, 2012).

Vitamin $B_{12}$ is also needed for DNA methylation to modulate gene expression and organ formation, especially of the brain and spinal cord during embryonic and fetal development. This is the explanation for the identified association with neural tube defects (Molloy et al., 2009). However, there have been no supplementation studies of vitamin $B_{12}$ during preconception or pregnancy. Although $B_{12}$ deficiency is typically associated with the older age group, recent data have shown that there are not large differences among age groups (Tucker et al., 2000). The latest U.S. surveys show that American women, except for non-Hispanic Whites, have mean serum levels of $B_{12}$ above an adequate level. Non-Hispanic White women have minimum levels with nearly half at below pregnancy-required levels (CDC, 2012). In addition, as $B_{12}$ is only found in foods from animals, there is a concern that lacto-ova vegetarians and vegans will not achieve pregnancy-required intakes of 2.6 mcg/d (Piccoli et al., 2015). Vegans can obtain $B_{12}$ from fortified soy or rice beverages, other fortified foods, or nutritional yeast supplements. Eating a fortified food three times a day or taking a 10 mcg supplement daily or 2,000 mcg weekly can meet the requirement. Women with gastric surgery, such as bypass surgery, are also at risk for deficiency and may need injectable $B_{12}$.

### Vitamin D

Vitamin D is a fat-soluble vitamin that is not only essential for fetal skeletal growth but also for placental implantation and functioning. It addition, vitamin D is important in glucose metabolism. Because of the rich number of vitamin D receptor sites important to pregnancy, there has been a new focus on its role in pregnancy. Two recent systematic reviews of RCTs examined vitamin D in varying amounts of 2,000 or 4,000 mg in addition to the 600 mg found in prenatal vitamins. The results showed increased serum vitamin D levels among the pregnant women and increased birth weights (Harvey et al., 2014; Perez-Lopez et al., 2015). The evidence is mixed as to whether vitamin D has any effect on lowering preeclampsia rates with only one RCT from India showing a difference. Only three studies found an effect on gestational diabetes; none of the studies were RCTs and none accounted for important confounders (Harvey et al., 2014).

None of these reviews included a paper on preterm birth from the South Carolina RCT of safety of vitamin supplements in pregnancy and lactation (Wagner et al., 2015). This analysis showed that women with 25(OH)D concentrations greater than 40 ng/mL had 59% less preterm birth compared with those less than 20 ng/mL (RR = 0.41; 95% CI [0.20, 0.86]; Wagner et al., 2015).

There are several large, ongoing multicenter trials in the United States examining vitamin D supplementation, which may answer important questions. The importance of this information is shown in Table 5.1, which demonstrates that large groups of American women have an inadequate serum level of vitamin D. There is some controversy about how to define *deficiency*. The IOM defines deficiency as 25(OH)D levels less than 20 ng/mL and the Endocrine Society and the CDC argue for less than 30 ng/mL with levels between 30 and 50 ng/mL being insufficient (CDC, 2012). Using less than 30 ng/mL, 30% of non-Hispanic Blacks and 12% of Mexican Americans are vitamin D deficient (CDC, 2012).

Because of the lack of strong RCTs demonstrating improved pregnancy outcomes with vitamin D supplementation, most systematic reviews agreed there is not enough evidence for routine measuring of 25(OH) D levels in pregnant women. However, some practices serving high-risk women, for example, women with minimum skin exposure resulting from dark skin and living in northern climates or cultural customs of heavy draping, do measure vitamin D levels. The current IOM recommendation for vitamin D intake in pregnancy is 600 mg but the Endocrine Society recommends 2,000 mg daily, especially in light of the high levels of deficiency (Holick et al., 2011). The best method of obtaining vitamin D is through exposure to sunlight, but climate, dark skin, and customs of cultural dress may preclude obtaining adequate levels. Foods fortified with vitamin D, such as cereals, milk, orange juice, and eggs, are important dietary elements for adequate intake.

## Minerals

### Calcium

Calcium intake in pregnancy is important for both maternal and fetal skeletal needs. Among populations with low calcium intake, the risk of pregnancy-induced hypertensive disorders increases. Systematic meta-analyses show calcium intake reduces risk of preeclampsia by 55% to 78% for low-risk and high-risk women, respectively (Hofmeyr, Lawrie, Atallah, Duley, & Torloni, 2014). In general, it is felt that U.S. women are not calcium deficient, although there are groups with low calcium intake, such as adolescent girls. The latest NHANES data show daily intakes for reproductive-age women 19 to 30 years to range from 600 mg for those not taking supplements to 1,000 mg for those who take supplements (Mangano, Walsh, Insogna, Kenny, & Kerstetter, 2011). The recommended intake in pregnancy is 1,000 mg except for 1,300 mg in women younger than 19 years (Food and Nutrition Board, 2011).

### Iodine

Iodine is essential for maternal and fetal thyroid function and it plays a crucial role in fetal/neonatal brain development. The World Health Organization (WHO) has identified iodine deficiency as the most preventable cause of mental retardation (WHO, 2007). Geographical areas with moderate to severe iodine deficiency are associated with decreased cognitive function in children and may account for as much as 12 to 13.5 IQ points (Zimmermann, 2012). In addition, studies have shown even mild deficiency is associated with some cognitive impairment. The requirements for iodine increase 50% in pregnancy. The recommended intake in pregnancy is 220 to 250 mcg/d with the higher range recommended by WHO and three major professional groups: the American Dietetic Association, the American Thyroid Association, and the American Association of Pediatrics (Craig & Mangels, 2009; Public Health Committee of the American Thyroid

Association et al., 2006; Rogan et al., 2014). The NHANES data demonstrate that many U.S. women have insufficient iodine intakes. One third of women ages 20 to 39 have levels below 100 ng/mL, indicative of mild deficiency and 57% fall below the recommended pregnancy level. From 1970 to the early 1990s, American intake of iodine declined 50% (CDC, 2012). Reasons for the decline include public health messaging to decrease salt intake, the use of noniodized salts, such as Kosher and gourmet sea salts, and, among pregnant women, decrease in fish intake resulting from heavy metal concerns. Although a 2009 survey showed that 50% of prenatal vitamins did not contain iodine (Leung, Pearce, & Braverman, 2009), the focus on iodine deficiency in pregnancy has been noted by pharmaceutical makers and a recent Internet search of common prenatal vitamins showed all contained the recommended 150 mcg of potassium iodide. Supplements that use kelp for iodine are not reliable sources for adequate levels of iodine (Public Health Committee of the American Thyroid Association et al., 2006).

*Iron*

Iron in pregnancy is needed for fetal growth and development, to meet the need to increase blood volume, and to decrease the risk for postpartum hemorrhage. There is increased dietary iron absorption in the second and third trimesters of pregnancy to meet this growing need providing there is dietary iron intake. However, if iron intake is low or a woman enters pregnancy in an iron-depleted state, iron supplementation is needed. Table 5.1 shows U.S. women have adequate iron intake. However, 14% of all women are iron deficient with serum ferritin less than 15 ng/mL. Among Non-Hispanic Whites, 11% have low levels whereas among Mexican Americans and non-Hispanic Black, 21% have low levels (CDC, 2012). Vegan vegetarians are also at higher risk for iron deficiency (Piccoli et al., 2015). Most prenatal vitamins contain 30 mg of elemental iron, the recommended amount of supplementation.

### Other Micronutrient

*Choline*

It was not until 1998 that choline was identified as a needed micronutrient. It is essential for normal functioning of all cells, especially for brain development and function. Low choline intake has been identified with a four times increase in neural tube defects (Shaw, Carmichael, Yang, Selvin, & Schaffer, 2004). There is also evidence that maternal choline intake may exert an epigenetic effect on the fetal hypothalamus by modulating cortisol activity (Jiang et al., 2012). One observational study examined the effects of maternal choline intake during pregnancy on children at 7 years of age (Boeke et al., 2013). This study found a modest increase in visual memory among children whose mothers were in the highest quartile of choline intake. In this study, the mean daily choline intake during pregnancy was 328 mg, well below the recommended intake (Boeke et al., 2013). The current recommended intake of choline in pregnancy is 450 mg/d (Food and Nutrition Board, 2011[2004]). The mean daily intake of choline among women of reproductive age in the United States is 260 mg, well below the recommendation. This level is similar for Whites, Blacks, and Hispanics (Chester, Goldman, Ahuja, & Moshfegh, 2011). The foods richest in choline are eggs, particularly the yolk, liver, milk, and peanuts.

## BEST PRACTICES: NUTRITION GUIDELINES IN PREGNANCY

### Energy Requirements in Pregnancy

Contrary to the popular adage, pregnant women are *not* eating for two. In the first trimester, there are no increased calorie needs and in subsequent trimesters, the increased calorie needs are 350 to 400 cal/d (National Research Council [NRC], 2009). The latest synthesis of studies argues that the needed increase in calories in the second half of pregnancy is only 166 cal/d (Butte & King, 2005). A 350 to 400 calorie increase is equivalent to one apple and 2 oz of cheese, one cup of black beans, and one corn tortilla, or 8 oz of skim milk, a banana, and one and a half tablespoons of peanut butter, not an additional meal.

### Gestational Weight Gain

Not all countries have gestational weight gain recommendations. Scott-Pillai and colleagues reviewed recommendations of 66 countries, finding that 40% had no or only informal recommendations and only 80% advocated weighing women at each prenatal visit (Scott-Pillai, Spence, Cardwell, Hunter, & Holmes, 2013). In the United States, there have been recommendations for recommended weight gain in pregnancy by body mass index (BMI) since 1990. The original concern was that inadequate weight gain was associated with small-for-gestational-age infants. In 2009, the IOM revised recommendations based on the rising obesity epidemic in the general population and concern that weight gain in pregnancy was contributing to obesity (NRC, 2009; see Table 5.2). The IOM has stated that there is not enough evidence to provide specific recommendations for weight gain in pregnancy by BMI; yet 36% of American women are obese (Ogden, Carroll, Fryar, & Flegal, 2015). This is a key public health problem.

Obesity is associated with several adverse perinatal outcomes such as stillbirth, birth defects, gestational diabetes, pregnancy-induced hypertension, assisted or surgical delivery, and shoulder dystocia (Heslehurst et al., 2008; Kominiarek & Chauhan, 2015; Scott-Pillai et al., 2013). Faucher and Barger's (2015) systematic review (*n* = 740,000 pregnant obese women) from four countries makes the case for considering weight gain recommendations by obesity class. The current guidelines of 5 to 9 kg (11–20 lbs) may be most appropriate for women with class I obesity but lesser weight gains may optimize outcomes for women with class II and III obesity (Faucher & Barger, 2015).

The evidence is strong that excessive gestational weight gain contributes to macrosomia and retained postpartum weight, and, among obese women, an increased risk for cesarean section (Heslehurst et al., 2008; Kominiarek & Chauhan, 2015; Scott-Pillai et al., 2013). A recent meta-analysis also showed

TABLE 5.2 Recommended Weight Gain in Pregnancy by Body Mass Index

| Body Mass Index (BMI) | Category | Singleton Pregnancy Weight Gain in Pounds | Multiple-Pregnancy Weight Gain in Pounds |
|---|---|---|---|
| < 18.5 | Underweight | 28–40 (12.5–18.0 kg) | No recommendation |
| 18.5–24.9 | Normal | 25–35 (11.5–16.0 kg) | 37–54 (17–25 kg) |
| 25.0–29.9 | Overweight | 15–25 (7.0–11.5 kg) | 31–50 (14–23 kg) |
| ≥ 30 | Obese | 11–20 (5.0–9.0 kg) | 25–42 (11–19 kg) |

Source: NRC (2009).

women with excessive weight gain had a 40% risk of gestational diabetes (OR [odds ratio] 1.40; 95% CI [1.21, 1.61]; Brunner et al., 2015). Using 2012 to 2013 U.S. birth certificate data, Deputy, Sharma, and Kim (2015) found only 32% of women gained the recommended amount of weight during pregnancy with 20% having inadequate gain and 48% having excessive gain. Excessive weight gain was much higher among overweight and obese women (62% and 56%) compared to 38% for those with normal BMI (Deputy et al., 2015).

In two short studies, 30% of obstetric providers (obstetricians, family practice, and nurse-midwives) did not provide women with any weight gain targets during pregnancy (Cogswell, Scanlon, Fein, & Schieve, 1999; Stotland et al., 2005). In addition, when women did receive advice, 25% of overweight women were advised to gain more than the recommended amount and 50% of women with low BMI were not advised to gain adequate weight (Stotland et al., 2005). Controlling for other factors, inadequate information on weight gain was associated with not gaining the recommended amount (Chang, Llanes, Gold, & Fetters, 2013). Many providers stated they only discussed weight gain after a woman had gained an excessive amount of weight and only 41% of providers routinely discussed weight gain at the beginning of the pregnancy (Chang et al., 2013; Herring et al., 2010). Two qualitative studies with multidisciplinary groups of obstetric providers showed that discussion of gestational weight gain is not a priority, providers are uncertain about guidelines, lacked resources for their clients, and were uncomfortable with discussing the sensitive topic of excessive weight gain (Chang et al., 2013; Stotland et al., 2010). For obese women, providers may avoid both the topic of weight gain and other recommended aspects of prenatal care counseling. A study of low-income women in Illinois found obese women were less likely to receive eight recommendations for prenatal care content, including depression screening, referral to family services, and Women, Infants, and Children (WIC) programs (Kominiarek, Rankin, & Handler, 2014).

Two qualitative analyses among low-income women, one of which examined African American women, revealed that weight gain in pregnancy is synonymous with a healthy pregnancy and low weight gain is concerning (Groth, Morrison-Beedy, & Meng, 2012; Kominiarek, Vonderheid, & Endres, 2010). Most

---

**Gestational Weight Gain Graphic**
   Available in English and Spanish from http://www.midwife.org/
   Share-With-Women
   This site also has a food safety handout for patients in English and Spanish

**Diet Assessment Resources**
*Brown University Nutrition Academic Award Center:* http://med.brown.edu/nutrition

   - Rate My Plate: Used to educate or hand out to patients
   - Rapid Eating Assessment for Patients (REAP) tool
   - WAVE Assessment: Tool used to assess weight, activity, and variety of foods
     eaten on one page

*The Nutrition Source, Harvard University School of Public Health:*
www.hsph.harvard.edu/nutritionsource

**Healthy Eating Plate Graphic**: ChooseMyPlate.gov: U.S. government
website with eating in pregnancy tools and resources

**Figure 5.1**  Resources for nutritional counseling of pregnant women.
*Source:* Barger (2010).

women were unaware of the risks of excessive weight gain. Most women perceived a 20-plus-pounds weight gain as fine. The term *obesity* was not part of their language and larger body type was culturally valued; yet they demonstrated interest in learning nutritional and culturally normative ways to prepare food. After taking a survey, 75% of the participants wanted more information related to obesity, pregnancy outcomes, and weight loss between pregnancies (Kominiarek et al., 2010).

The midwife needs to be clear about recommended weight gain, including starting a graphic chart at the first prenatal visit so both the woman and the midwife can sequentially plot and monitor gain providers. The midwife needs to deliver clear, positive messages about gestational weight gain without admonishing or stigmatizing patients (see Figure 5.1). Group prenatal care has been shown to decrease excess gestational weight gain by 54% compared to traditional care (Tanner-Smith, Steinka-Fry, & Gesell, 2014).

## Frequent Eating

The IOM recommends three meals and at least two snacks per day during pregnancy, and there appears to be substantial research in support of this recommendation (Committee on Nutritional Status during Pregnancy, Food and Nutrition Board, & Institute of Medicine, 1992). Fasting or prolonged periods without eating has been associated with preterm birth especially from premature rupture of membranes (Herrmann, Siega-Riz, Hobel, Aurora, & Dunkel-Schetter, 2001). An increase in spontaneous births has been noted after the Jewish Yom Kippur fast (Kaplan, Eidelman, & Aboulafia, 1983). Additionally, among Muslim women choosing to maintain the Ramadan fast, there is an increased rate of gestational diabetes, lower biophysical profile scores compared to the women who are eating, and twice the rate of medically necessary labor induction (Mirghani & Hamud, 2006; Mirghani, Weerasinghe, Ezimokhai, & Smith, 2003). All major religions that have a tradition of periodic fasting exempt pregnant women. Rationale for this exemption should be communicated to women during these proscribed periods.

## Food Safety in Pregnancy

Because pregnant women are at increased risk for intracellular infection, avoidance of foodborne illnesses that can adversely affect the mother and/or the fetus is essential. The primary infections of concern are toxoplasmosis, *Listeria monocytogenes*, *Salmonella enterica*, and *Campylobacter*. The first three infections are the leading causes of foodborne illness deaths in the United States (Painter et al., 2013). In 2011, salmonella caused 1 million reported infections in the United States and was the leading cause of foodborne hospitalizations and deaths (Painter et al., 2013). It has been well documented that toxoplasmosis, listeria, and brucellosis have transplacental transfer. The mechanism by which salmonella results in fetal infection, preterm labor, and abortion is less well studied. Case studies have shown both transplacental fetal infections and vaginally acquired neonatal infection among mothers with *Campylobacter*. Animal studies show the infection causes significant placental dysfunction (Noto Llana et al., 2014).

Consuming contaminated and raw or undercooked foods is the source of the infection. Public health measures for prevention include meticulous handwashing when preparing food, thoroughly cleaning cutting boards, and cleaning all raw fruits and vegetables. Raw sprouts should be avoided as it is nearly impossible to clean them adequately. Pregnant women should avoid all raw meat, eggs, and unpasteurized dairy products, including meat spreads, pâtés, and smoked seafood. Meat should be cooked thoroughly and monitored by using a cooking thermometer. Processed delicatessen meat and hot dogs should be heated to the steaming point. Raw seafood and shellfish, although potentially causing gastrointestinal illness, have not been implicated in fetal or pregnancy complications.

## Nutrition Counseling

### Low-Glycemic Diet

A cholesterol-lowering diet during pregnancy may have an influence on the outcome. An RCT in Norway studied nonsmoking women with BMIs between 19 and 32 and pregnant with singletons (*n* = 290; Khoury, Henriksen, Christophersen, & Tonstad, 2005). They were randomized at 17 to 20 weeks gestation into an intervention group and a control group. The intervention group met with a dietician four times during pregnancy. They were counseled to limit cholesterol to 150 mg/d, limit saturated fats to 8%, and replace them with fatty fish and monounsaturated fats such as olive oil, avocado, and nuts. In addition, they were advised to eat six servings of fruits and vegetables daily, choose low-fat dairy, and limit red meat to twice a week. This diet is essentially the Mediterranean diet with low glycemic index. The intervention group made significant changes in their diet (Khoury et al., 2005).

At the end of the study, the intervention group had a lower calorie intake; ate 2% less fat but had higher mono- and polyunsaturated fats; had slightly higher carbohydrate intake but 2% less sugar; consumed 215 mg of cholesterol a day, significantly lower than preintervention; and had higher intake of vitamins A, C, and calcium and magnesium. Although there were no differences in the primary outcome, lipid levels in neonatal cord blood, there was a remarkable 90% decrease in preterm birth in the intervention group (0.7% vs. 7.4%; Khoury et al., 2005). Although midwives may not have the resources to send women for such close follow-up, information about the Mediterranean diet is readily available.

Several meta-analyses show that dietary interventions can effect gestational weight gain but not neonatal outcomes (Muktabhant, Lawrie, Lumbiganon, & Laopaiboon, 2015; Streuling, Beyerlein, & von Kries, 2010; Thangaratinam et al., 2012). Dietary intervention from 44 RCTs with a total of 7,300 women resulted in an 8.5-pound (4 kg) difference in gestational weight gain. If providers discussed diet at all, there was a 3-pound (1.5 kg) difference (Thangaratinam et al., 2012). There is also a suggestion that these interventions can decrease pregnancy-related hypertension (Muktabhant et al., 2015). Therefore, contrary to what providers might think, dietary advice does have an effect on gestational weight gain and evidence shows women want to know how much they should gain.

Pregnancy is a teachable opportunity when women are often open to making lifestyle changes for the health of their infants. An RCT in Ireland randomized women with their second pregnancy to standard care or to an intervention group learning about low glycemic diet. One 2-hour teaching session resulted is 1.7 kg less gestational weight gain and lower glucose levels at 28 weeks. In addition, the women in the intervention group were more likely to continue this dietary pattern into the postpartum period (Walsh & McAuliffe, 2015). This exemplifies how even limited counseling can influence decision making about dietary choices in pregnancy.

### Preconception Nutrition Counseling and Assessment

Prior to pregnancy, the midwife should assure that women are meeting daily requirements for folic acid and choline either through a varied diet or multivitamin supplement. Women at high risk for nutritional absorption problems or metabolic disturbances should obtain serum levels or relevant markers. This would include HbA1C for diabetic women. Women with inflammatory bowel disease, bariatric surgery, or other malabsorption disorders should have an assessment of the status of vitamins A and D, iron, folic acid, and $B_{12}$ status prior to pregnancy. Some women with these disorders may need up to 4 mg of folic acid to maintain adequate serum folate levels (Kaska et al., 2013).

### Prenatal Counseling

At the first prenatal visit, along with the recommended gestational weight gain based on the woman's BMI, the midwife should explain that pregnancy is a time for women to help their infants lay a good foundation for lifelong health. This includes influencing later food preferences based on exposure to a variety of foods in utero. Explaining the increased calorie requirement as equivalent to an extra snack, not a meal, may alter preconceived notions about "eating for two." A brief handout outlining summary recommendations for healthy eating in pregnancy and food safety is helpful (Figure 5.2). This handout can be coupled with a listing of online information resources (see Figure 5.1).

Midwives should choose resources that are culturally appropriate. If group prenatal care is available, women who are at high risk for excessive gestational weight, that is, overweight or obese, should be particularly encouraged to enroll. Another method to help women self-monitor their weight gain is to encourage them to weigh themselves weekly at home. For women who are gaining too much weight, one method to assess their diet is to ask them to take pictures of everything they eat for 1 to 3 days (Martin et al., 2014). Midwives can spot non-nutrient, calorie-dense foods and make recommendations for small dietary changes.

There are specific subpopulations of women with increased dietary requirements in pregnancy. Women who have had bariatric surgery and other malabsorption disorders need may need higher requirement of vitamins and micronutrients. After bariatric surgery, long-term use of a multivitamin is encouraged but only 59% of women do so (Kaska et al., 2013). Pregnant women who have undergone bariatric surgery need increased intake of the following: calcium (2,000 mg/d), iron (ferrous form 40–65 mg/d), vitamin A (retinol < 5,000 IU/d), folic acid (4 mg), and vitamin $B_{12}$ (sublingual cobalamin 19 mcg/d; Kaska et al., 2013). These may also apply to women with other malabsorption disorders.

A woman pregnant with twins or higher order gestation has increased nutritional needs. Their pattern of gestational weight gain is important. Adequate early gestational weight gain is essential as 80% of the fetus' weight is acquired by 28 weeks (Luke, Minogue, Witter, Keith, & Johnson, 1993). For women with multiple pregnancies and normal BMI, an intake of 3,000 to 3,500 kcal divided into 175 g protein, 330 g carbohydrate, and 156 g fat is recommended. The following nutrient requirements are increased: folic acid 1 mg, zinc 30 mg, magnesium 800 mg, and vitamin D 1,000 IU (compared to the IOM of 600 IU for singletons; Goodnight & Newman, 2009). The recommendation is to take two prenatal vitamins daily, as long as the vitamin A intake does not exceed 5,000 IU of retinol or the tablets are formulated with beta-carotene (Goodnight & Newman, 2009).

## CONCLUSION

The evidence is strong for the role of adequate preconception folic acid in preventing neural tube defects and for calcium supplementation, among women with low calcium intakes, in preventing preeclampsia. Exposure to certain foods in utero appears to influence food preferences in children, strengthening the case for encouraging the woman to eat a varied diet, especially high in vegetables. The evidence also shows that diet counseling, even at a modest level, can decrease gestational weight gain by about 3 pounds. Pregnancy is an ideal time to influence

**Gain the recommended weight for your body mass index by eating the following:**
- Three meals and two snacks a day to avoid long periods of fasting
- Five servings of fruits and vegetables, at minimum, per day
- Whole-grain carbohydrates; limit high-sugar foods such as desserts, fruit juices, and sodas
- Healthy fats, such as olive oil, olives, avocado, or canola oil; and limit butter intake
- Adequate amount of protein with at least two meals from plant-based sources
- Two servings of omega-3-rich fish a week or use an omega-3 supplement
    - Avoid the following fish: tilefish, shark, swordfish, and king mackerel
    - Limit tuna to twice a week

**Drink eight to 10 glasses of water a day:**
- Limit caffeine to 200 mg a day (two cups of coffee or four cups of black tea)
- Avoid alcoholic drinks
- Limit sweetened drinks

**Ensure adequate intake of these micronutrients and minerals:**
- Vitamin A as beta-carotene and limit food sources with preformed vitamin A such as liver (< 4 oz/wk) or cod liver oil
- Vitamin D from sunshine exposure; if not feasible, supplement with vitamin $D_3$ (1,000–4,000 IU depending on intake of vitamin D fortified dairy products and vitamin serum levels)
- Folic acid through a multivitamin supplement
- Women adhering to a strict vegan diet will need vitamin $B_{12}$ supplements or consciously consume vitamin $B_{12}$-fortified products
- Iodine through diet (fish or iodized salt) or in a multivitamin with 150 mcg of iodine
- Iron through diet, multivitamin, or additional low-dose supplement, if anemic
- Calcium through diet with higher levels suggested for women at risk for preeclampsia
- Choline-rich food sources such as meat, poultry, and eggs (this is not typically in prenatal vitamins)

**Avoid foodborne illnesses that can cause maternal or fetal disease:**
- Eat well-cooked meat, poultry (including eggs), and fish
- Eat only pasteurized dairy and fruit juices
- Avoid soft cheeses, processed meats such as bologna or hot dogs unless heated until steaming, and raw sprouts
- Thoroughly wash hands, cutting boards, and fruits and vegetables

**Figure 5.2** Dietary recommendations for pregnant women.
*Source:* Barger (2010). Reprinted with permission from *Journal of Midwifery and Women's Health.*

long-term dietary patterns as women are interacting with the health care system on a regular basis and are usually invested in protecting the health of the fetus.

# REFERENCES

American College of Obstetricians and Gynecologists. (2010). Moderate caffeine consumption during pregnancy. Committee opinion No. 462. *Obstetrics & Gynecology, 116,* 467–468.

Barger, M. K. (2010). Maternal nutrition and perinatal outcomes. *Journal of Midwifery and Women's Health, 55*(6), 502–511.

Barker, D. J. (1990). The fetal and infant origins of adult disease. *British Medical Journal, 301*(6761), 1111.

Beauchamp, G. K., & Mennella, J. A. (2011). Flavor perception in human infants: Development and functional significance. *Digestion, 83*(Suppl. 1), 1–6. doi:10.1159/000323397

Boeke, C. E., Gillman, M. W., Hughes, M. D., Rifas-Shiman, S. L., Villamor, E., & Oken, E. (2013). Choline intake during pregnancy and child cognition at age 7 years. *American Journal of Epidemiology, 177*(12), 1338–1347. doi:10.1093/aje/kws395

Brunner, S., Stecher, L., Ziebarth, S., Nehring, I., Rifas-Shiman, S. L., Sommer, C., . . . von Kries, R. (2015). Excessive gestational weight gain prior to glucose screening and the risk of gestational diabetes: A meta-analysis. *Diabetologia, 58*(10), 2229–2237. doi:10.1007/s00125-015-3686-5

Butte, N. F., & King, J. C. (2005). Energy requirements during pregnancy and lactation. *Public Health Nutrition, 8*(7A), 1010–1027.

Carlson, S. E., Colombo, J., Gajewski, B. J., Gustafson, K. M., Mundy, D., Yeast, J., . . . Shaddy, D. J. (2013). DHA supplementation and pregnancy outcomes. *American Journal of Clinical Nutrition, 97*(4), 808–815. doi:10.3945/ajcn.112.050021

Centers for Disease Control and Prevention (CDC). (2012). Second national report on biochemical indicatiors of diet and nutrition in the U.S. population. Retrieved from http://www.cdc.gov/nutritionreport/pdf/Nutrition_Book_complete508_final.pdf

Chang, T., Llanes, M., Gold, K. J., & Fetters, M. D. (2013). Perspectives about and approaches to weight gain in pregnancy: A qualitative study of physicians and nurse midwives. *BMC Pregnancy and Childbirth, 13*, 47. doi:10.1186/1471-2393-13-47

Chester, D. N., Goldman, J. D., Ahuja, J. K., & Moshfegh, A. J. (October, 2011). Dietary intakes of choline: What we eat in America, NHANES 2007–2008. Retrieved from http://ars.usda.gov/Services/docs.htm?docid=19476

Cogswell, M. E., Scanlon, K. S., Fein, S. B., & Schieve, L. A. (1999). Medically advised, mother's personal target, and actual weight gain during pregnancy. *Obstetrics & Gynecology, 94*(4), 616–622.

Committee on Nutritional Status during Pregnancy, Food and Nutrition Board, & Institute of Medicine. (1992). *Nutrition during pregnancy and lactation: An implementation guide.* Washington, DC: National Academies Press.

Craig, W. J., & Mangels, A. R. (2009). Position of the American Dietetic Association: Vegetarian diets. *Journal of the American Dietetic Association, 109*(7), 1266–1282.

Deputy, N., Sharma, A., & Kim, S. (2015). Gestational weight gain—United States 2012 and 2013. *Morbidity and Mortality Weekly Report, 64*(43), 1215–1220.

Dror, D. K., & Allen, L. H. (2012). Interventions with vitamins B6, B12 and C in pregnancy. *Paediatric and Perinatal Epidemiology, 26*(Suppl. 1), 55–74. doi:10.1111/j.1365-3016.2012.01277.x

European Food Safety Authority (EFSA). (2012). Panel on dietetic products, nutrition and allergies—Scientific opinion related to the tolerable upper intake level of eicosapentaenoic acid (EPA), docosahexaenoic acid (DHA) and docosapentaenoic acid (DPA). *EFSA Journal, 10*(7), 2815. doi:10.2903/j.efsa.2012.2815

Faucher, M. A., & Barger, M. K. (2015). Gestational weight gain in obese women by class of obesity and select maternal/newborn outcomes: A systematic review. *Women and Birth, 28*(3), e70–e79. doi:10.1016/j.wombi.2015.03.006

Food and Nutrition Board. (2011). *Dietary reference intakes (DRIs): Recommended intakes for individuals.* Washington, DC: National Academies Press.

Goodnight, W., & Newman, R. (2009). Optimal nutrition for improved twin pregnancy outcome. *Obstetrics and Gynecology, 114*(5), 1121–1134. doi:10.1097/AOG.0b013e3181bb14c8

Gould, J. F., Smithers, L. G., & Makrides, M. (2013). The effect of maternal omega-3 (n-3) LCPUFA supplementation during pregnancy on early childhood cognitive and visual development: A systematic review and meta-analysis of randomized controlled trials. *American Journal of Clinical Nutrition, 97*(3), 531–544. doi:10.3945/ajcn.112.045781

Grant, S. M., Wolever, T. M., O'Connor, D. L., Nisenbaum, R., & Josse, R. G. (2011). Effect of a low glycaemic index diet on blood glucose in women with gestational hyperglycaemia. *Diabetes Research and Clinical Practice, 91*(1), 15–22. doi:10.1016/j.diabres.2010.09.002

Greene, M. F., Hare, J. W., Cloherty, J. P., Benacerraf, B. R., & Soeldner, J. S. (1989). First-trimester hemoglobin A1 and risk for major malformation and spontaneous abortion in diabetic pregnancy. *Teratology, 39*(3), 225–231. doi:10.1002/tera.1420390303

Greenwood, D. C., Thatcher, N. J., Ye, J., Garrard, L., Keogh, G., King, L. G., & Cade, J. E. (2014). Caffeine intake during pregnancy and adverse birth outcomes: A systematic review and dose-response meta-analysis. *European Journal of Epidemiology, 29*(10), 725–734. doi:10.1007/s10654-014-9944-x

Groth, S. W., Morrison-Beedy, D., & Meng, Y. (2012). How pregnant African American women view pregnancy weight gain. *Journal of Obstetrical, Gynecological, and Neonatal Nursing, 41*(6), 798–808. doi:10.1111/j.1552-6909.2012.01391.x

Hanley, B., Dijane, J., Fewtrell, M., Grynberg, A., Hummel, S., Junien, C., . . . van Der Beek, E. M. (2010). Metabolic imprinting, programming and epigenetics—A review of present priorities and future opportunities. *British Journal of Nutrition, 104*(Suppl. 1), S1–25. doi:10.1017/s0007114510003338

Harvey, N. C., Holroyd, C., Ntani, G., Javaid, K., Cooper, P., Moon, R., . . . Cooper, C. (2014). Vitamin D supplementation in pregnancy: A systematic review. *Health Technology Assessment, 18*(45), 1–190. doi:10.3310/hta18450

Herring, S. J., Platek, D. N., Elliott, P., Riley, L. E., Stuebe, A. M., & Oken, E. (2010). Addressing obesity in pregnancy: What do obstetric providers recommend? *Journal of Women's Health, 19*(1), 65–70. doi:10.1089/jwh.2008.1343

Herrmann, T. S., Siega-Riz, A. M., Hobel, C. J., Aurora, C., & Dunkel-Schetter, C. (2001). Prolonged periods without food intake during pregnancy increase risk for elevated maternal corticotropin-releasing hormone concentrations. *American Journal of Obstetrics and Gynecology, 185*, 403–412.

Heslehurst, N., Simpson, H., Ells, L. J., Rankin, J., Wilkinson, J., Lang, R., . . . Summerbell, C. D. (2008). The impact of maternal BMI status on pregnancy outcomes with immediate short-term obstetric resource implications: A meta-analysis. *Obesity Review, 9*(6), 635–683. doi:10.1111/j.1467-789X.2008.00511.x

Hofmeyr, G. J., Lawrie, T. A., Atallah, A. N., Duley, L., & Torloni, M. R. (2014). Calcium supplementation during pregnancy for preventing hypertensive disorders and related problems. *Cochrane Database of Systematic Reviews, 6*. doi:10.1002/14651858.CD001059.pub4

Holick, M. F., Binkley, N. C., Bischoff-Ferrari, H. A., Gordon, C. M., Hanley, D. A., Heaney, R. P., . . . Weaver, C. M. (2011). Evaluation, treatment, and prevention of vitamin D deficiency: An Endocrine Society clinical practice guideline. *Journal of Clinical Endocrinology and Metabolism, 97*(7), 1911–1930.

Imhoff-Kunsch, B., Briggs, V., Goldenberg, T., & Ramakrishnan, U. (2012). Effect of n-3 long-chain polyunsaturated fatty acid intake during pregnancy on maternal, infant, and child health outcomes: A systematic review. *Paediatric and Perinatal Epidemiology, 26*(Suppl. 1), 91–107. doi:10.1111/j.1365-3016.2012.01292.x

Jiang, X., Yan, J., West, A. A., Perry, C. A., Malysheva, O. V., Devapatla, S., . . . Caudill, M. A. (2012). Maternal choline intake alters the epigenetic state of fetal cortisol-regulating genes in humans. *Federation of American Societies for Experimental Biology Journal, 26*(8), 3563–3574. doi:10.1096/fj.12-207894

Kaplan, M., Eidelman, A. I., & Aboulafia, Y. (1983). Fasting and the precipitation of labor. *Journal of the American Medical Association, 250,* 1317–1318.

Kaska, L., Kobiela, J., Abacjew-Chmylko, A., Chmylko, L., Wojanowska-Pindel, M., Kobiela, P., . . . Stefaniak, T. (2013, January 30). Nutrition and pregnancy after bariatric surgery. *International Scholarly Research Notices Obesity, 2013.* doi:10.1155/2013/492060

Khoury, J., Henriksen, T., Christophersen, B., & Tonstad, S. (2005). Effect of a cholesterol-lowering diet on maternal, cord, and neonatal lipids, and pregnancy outcome: A randomized clinical trial. *American Journal of Obstetrics and Gynecology, 193,* 1292–1301.

Kominiarek, M. A., & Chauhan, S. P. (2015). Obesity before, during, and after pregnancy: A review and comparison of five national guidelines. *American Journal of Perinatology, 33*(5), 433–441. doi:10.1055/s-0035-1567856

Kominiarek, M. A., Rankin, K., & Handler, A. (2014). Provider adherence to recommended prenatal care content: Does it differ for obese women? *Maternal and Child Health Journal, 18*(5), 1114–1122. doi:10.1007/s10995-013-1341-7

Kominiarek, M. A., Vonderheid, S., & Endres, L. K. (2010). Maternal obesity: Do patients understand the risks? *Journal of Perinatology, 30*(7), 452–458. doi:10.1038/jp.2010.52

Lau, C., Rogers, J. M., Desai, M., & Ross, M. G. (2011). Fetal programming of adult disease: Implications for prenatal care. *Obstetrics and Gynecology, 117*(4), 978–985. doi:10.1097/AOG.0b013e318212140e

Leung, A. M., Pearce, E. N., & Braverman, L. E. (2009). Iodine content of prenatal multivitamins in the United States. *New England Journal of Medicine, 360*(9, 939–940. doi:10.1056/NEJMc0807851

Louie, J. C., Brand-Miller, J. C., & Moses, R. G. (2013). Carbohydrates, glycemic index, and pregnancy outcomes in gestational diabetes. *Current Diabetes Reports, 13*(1), 6–11. doi:10.1007/s11892-012-0332-1

Ludwig, D. S. (2002). The glycemic index: Physiological mechanisms relating to obesity, diabetes, and cardiovascular disease. *Journal of the American Medical Association, 287*(18), 2414–2423.

Luke, B., Minogue, J., Witter, F. R., Keith, L. G., & Johnson, T. R. (1993). The ideal twin pregnancy: Patterns of weight gain, discordancy, and length of gestation. *American Journal of Obstetrics and Gynecology, 169*(3), 588–597.

Macintosh, M. C., Fleming, K. M., Bailey, J. A., Doyle, P., Modder, J., Acolet, D., . . . Miller, A. (2006). Perinatal mortality and congenital anomalies in babies of women with type 1 or type 2 diabetes in England, Wales, and Northern Ireland: Population based study. *British Medical Journal, 333*(7560), 177. doi:10.1136/bmj.38856.692986.AE

Mangano, K. M., Walsh, S. J., Insogna, K. L., Kenny, A. M., & Kerstetter, J. E. (2011). Calcium intake in the United States from dietary and supplemental sources across adult age groups: New estimates from the National Health and Nutrition Examination Survey 2003–2006. *Journal of the American Dietetic Association, 111*(5), 687–695. doi:10.1016/j .jada.2011.02.014

Martin, C. K., Nicklas, T., Gunturk, B., Correa, J. B., Allen, H. R., & Champagne, C. (2014). Measuring food intake with digital photography. *Journal of Human Nutrition and Dietetics, 27*(Suppl. 1), 72–81. doi:10.1111/jhn.12014

Mennella, J. A., Jagnow, C. P., & Beauchamp, G. K. (2001). Prenatal and postnatal flavor learning by human infants. *Pediatrics, 107*(6), E88.

Mirghani, H. M., Weerasinghe, D. S., Ezimokhai, M., & Smith, J. R. (2003). The effect of maternal fasting on the fetal biophysical profile. *International Journal of Gynaecology & Obstetrics, 81*(1), 17–21.

Mirghani, H. M., & Hamud, O. (2006). The effect of maternal diet restriction on pregnancy outcome. *American Journal of Perinatology, 23*(1), 21–24.

Molloy, A. M., Kirke, P. N., Troendle, J. F., Burke, H., Sutton, M., Brody, L. C., . . . Mills, J. L. (2009). Maternal vitamin B12 status and risk of neural tube defects in a population with high neural tube defect prevalence and no folic acid fortification. *Pediatrics, 123*(3), 917–923. doi:10.1542/peds.2008-1173

Montgomery, K. S. (2002). Nutrition column: An update on water needs during pregnancy and beyond. *Journal of Perinatal Education, 11*(3), 40–42. doi:10.1624/105812402x88830

Moses, R. G., Barker, M., Winter, M., Petocz, P., & Brand-Miller, J. C. (2009). Can a low-glycemic index diet reduce the need for insulin in gestational diabetes mellitus? A randomized trial. *Diabetes Care, 32*(6), 996–1000. doi:10.2337/dc09-0007

Muktabhant, B., Lawrie, T. A., Lumbiganon, P., & Laopaiboon, M. (2015). Diet or exercise, or both, for preventing excessive weight gain in pregnancy. *Cochrane Database of Systematic Reviews, 6*. doi:10.1002/14651858.CD007145.pub3

National Research Council (NRC). (2009). *Weight gain during pregnancy: Reexamining the guidelines*. Washington, DC: National Academies Press.

Noto Llana, M., Sarnacki, S. H., Aya Castaneda Mdel, R., Pustovrh, M. C., Gartner, A. S., Buzzola, F. R., . . . Giacomodonato, M. N. (2014). *Salmonella enterica* serovar *enteritidis* enterocolitis during late stages of gestation induces an adverse pregnancy outcome in the murine model. *PLoS One, 9*(11), e111282. doi:10.1371/journal.pone.0111282

Ogden, C. L., Carroll, M. D., Fryar, C. D., & Flegal, K. M. (2015). Prevalence of obesity among adults and youth: United States, 2011–2014. *National Center for Health Statistics Data Briefs #219*, 1–8.

Ojha, S., Fainberg, H. P., Sebert, S., Budge, H., & Symonds, M. E. (2015). Maternal health and eating habits: Metabolic consequences and impact on child health. *Trends in Molecular Medicine, 21*(2), 126–133. doi:10.1016/j.molmed.2014.12.005

Oken, E., Kleinman, K. P., Berland, W. E., Simon, S. R., Rich-Edwards, J. W., & Gillman, M. W. (2003). Decline in fish consumption among pregnant women after a national mercury advisory. *Obstetrics and Gynecology, 102*(2), 346–351.

Painter, J. A., Hoekstra, R. M., Ayers, T., Tauxe, R. V., Braden, C. R., Angulo, F. J., & Griffin, P. M. (2013). Attribution of foodborne illnesses, hospitalizations, and deaths to food commodities by using outbreak data, United States, 1998–2008. *Emerging Infectious Diseases, 19*(3), 407–415. doi:10.3201/eid1903.111866

Perez-Lopez, F. R., Pasupuleti, V., Mezones-Holguin, E., Benites-Zapata, V. A., Thota, P., Deshpande, A., & Hernandez, A. V. (2015). Effect of vitamin D supplementation during pregnancy on maternal and neonatal outcomes: A systematic review and meta-analysis of randomized controlled trials. *Fertililty and Sterility*, *103*(5), 1278–1288. doi:10.1016/j .fertnstert.2015.02.019

Piccoli, G. B., Clari, R., Vigotti, F. N., Leone, F., Attini, R., Cabiddu, G., . . . Avagnina, P. (2015). Vegan-vegetarian diets in pregnancy: Danger or panacea? A systematic narrative review. *British Journal of Obstetrics and Gynaecology*, *122*(5), 623–633. doi:10.1111/1471-0528.13280

Public Health Committee of the American Thyroid Association, Becker, D. V., Braverman, L. E., Delange, F., Dunn, J. T., Franklyn, J. A., . . . Rovet, J. F. (2006). Iodine supplementation for pregnancy and lactation—United States and Canada: Recommendations of the American Thyroid Association. *Thyroid*, *16*(10), 949–951.

Rogan, W. J., Paulson, J. A., Baum, C., Brock-Utne, A. C., Brumberg, H. L., Campbell, C. C., . . . Trasande, L. (2014). Iodine deficiency, pollutant chemicals, and the thyroid: New information on an old problem. *Pediatrics*, *133*(6), 1163–1166. doi:10.1542/peds.2014-0900

Rothman, K. J., Moore, L. L., Singer, M. R., Nguyen, U. S., Mannino, S., & Milunsky, A. (1995). Teratogenicity of high vitamin A intake. *New England Journal of Medicine*, *333*(21), 1369–1373.

Russell, J. B., Abboud, C., Williams, A., Gibbs, M., Pritchad, S., & Chalfant, D. (2012). Does dietary protein and carbohydrate intake influence blastocyst development and pregnancy rates? *Fertility and Sterility*, *98*(3), S233–234.

Scott-Pillai, R., Spence, D., Cardwell, C. R., Hunter, A., & Holmes, V. A. (2013). The impact of body mass index on maternal and neonatal outcomes: A retrospective study in a UK obstetric population, 2004–2011. *British Journal of Obstetrics and Gynecology*, *120*(8), 932–939. doi:10.1111/1471-0528.12193

Shaw, G. M., Carmichael, S. L., Yang, W., Selvin, S., & Schaffer, D. M. (2004). Periconceptional dietary intake of choline and betaine and neural tube defects in offspring. *American Journal of Epidemiology*, *160*(2), 102–109. doi:10.1093/aje/kwh187

Stotland, N. E., Gilbert, P., Bogetz, A., Harper, C. C., Abrams, B., & Gerbert, B. (2010). Preventing excessive weight gain in pregnancy: How do prenatal care providers approach counseling? *Journal of Women's Health*, *19*(4), 807–814. doi:10.1089/jwh.2009.1462

Stotland, N. E., Haas, J. S., Brawarsky, P., Jackson, R., Fuentes-Afflick, E., & Escobar, G. (2005). Body mass index, provider advice, and target gestational weight gain. *Obstetrics & Gynecology*, *105*(3), 633–638.

Strain, J. J., Yeates, A. J., van Wijngaarden, E., Thurston, S. W., Mulhern, M. S., McSorley, E. M., . . . Davidson, P. W. (2015). Prenatal exposure to methyl mercury from fish consumption and polyunsaturated fatty acids: Associations with child development at 20 months of age in an observational study in the Republic of Seychelles. *American Journal of Clinical Nutrition*, *101*(3), 530–537. doi:10.3945/ajcn.114.100503

Streuling, I., Beyerlein, A., & von Kries, R. (2010). Can gestational weight gain be modified by increasing physical activity and diet counseling? A meta-analysis of interventional trials. *American Journal of Clinical Nutrition*, *92*(4), 678–687. doi:10.3945/ajcn.2010.29363

Tanner-Smith, E. E., Steinka-Fry, K. T., & Gesell, S. B. (2014). Comparative effectiveness of group and individual prenatal care on gestational weight gain. *Maternal and Child Health Journal*, *18*(7), 1711–1720. doi:10.1007/s10995-013-1413-8

Thangaratinam, S., Rogozinska, E., Jolly, K., Glinkowski, S., Roseboom, T., Tomlinson, J. W., . . . Khan, K. S. (2012). Effects of interventions in pregnancy on maternal weight and obstetric outcomes: Meta-analysis of randomised evidence. *British Medical Journal, 344*, e2088. doi:10.1136/bmj.e2088

Tobias, D., Hu, F., Chavarro, J., Rosner, B., Mozaffarian, D., & Zhang, C. (2012). Healthful dietary patterns and type 2 diabetes mellitus risk among women with a history of gestational diabetes mellitus. *Archives of Internal Medicine, 17*(20), 1566–1572.

Tucker, K. L., Rich, S., Rosenberg, I., Jacques, P., Dallal, G., Wilson, P. W., & Selhub, J. (2000). Plasma vitamin B-12 concentrations relate to intake source in the Framingham offspring study. *American Journal of Clinical Nutrition, 71*(2), 514–522.

Wagner, C. L., Baggerly, C., McDonnell, S. L., Baggerly, L., Hamilton, S. A., Winkler, J., . . . Hollis, B. W. (2015). Post-hoc comparison of vitamin D status at three timepoints during pregnancy demonstrates lower risk of preterm birth with higher vitamin D closer to delivery. *Journal of Steroid Biochemistry and Molecular Biology, 148*, 256–260. doi:10.1016/j.jsbmb.2014.11.013

Walsh, J. M., & McAuliffe, F. M. (2015). Impact of maternal nutrition on pregnancy outcome—Does it matter what pregnant women eat? *Best Practices & Research Clinical Obstetrics & Gynaecology, 29*(1), 63–78. doi:10.1016/j.bpobgyn.2014.08.003

World Health Organization (WHO). (2007). Assessment of iodine deficiency disorders and monitoring their elimination: A guide for programme managers. Retrieved from http://www.who.int/nutrition/publications/micronutrients/iodine deficiency/9789241595827/en

Zimmermann, M. B. (2012). The effects of iodine deficiency in pregnancy and infancy. *Paediatric and Perinatal Epidemiology, 26* (Suppl. 1), 108–117. doi:10.1111/j.1365-3016.2012.01275.x

# CHAPTER SIX

# EVIDENCE-BASED MIDWIFERY CARE FOR OBESE CHILDBEARING WOMEN

Laura A. Aughinbaugh and Nicole S. Carlson

## THE RISKS OF OBESITY IN CHILDBEARING

The United States is in the midst of an obesity epidemic that has rapidly evolved over the past 25 years (Centers for Disease Control and Prevention [CDC], 2015). Currently, more than 60% of adults in the United States are overweight or obese (Flegal, Carroll, Kit, & Ogden, 2012). One third of childbearing-age women are obese with higher rates among racial and ethnic minority groups:

- 31.9% obesity among childbearing women in general
- 34.4% among Hispanic women
- 58.5% among non-Hispanic Black women (Flegal et al., 2012)

The trend in maternal obesity in the United States is consistent with other developed nations (Vahratian, Zhang, Troendle, Savitz, & Siega-Riz, 2004; World Health Organization [WHO], 2015; Yeh & Shelton, 2005). Overweight and obesity are linked to numerous health conditions, including cardiovascular disease, diabetes, musculoskeletal disorders, and some cancers (WHO, 2015).

The WHO identifies Class I obesity as body mass index (BMI) greater than 30 kg/m$^2$; Class II obesity as BMI greater than or equal to 35 kg/m$^2$, and Class III obesity as BMI greater than or equal to 40 kg/m$^2$ (WHO, 2015). When a woman meets the criteria of Class I obesity prior to pregnancy, her pregnancy has increased risks for both her child and herself. If the woman's BMI prior to pregnancy is Class III, the likelihood of less than optimal outcomes is even greater as both she and her offspring may experience short-term and long-term adverse health conditions. Significant social factors associated with obesity in women of childbearing age are lower formal educational attainment, low household income, and inadequate health insurance status (Vahratian et al., 2004). See Tables 6.1 and 6.2 for studies of the literature on childbearing outcomes related to obesity.

**TABLE 6.1   Short-Term Health and Situational Risks of Obesity in Childbearing: A Synthesis of the Literature**

| Risk | Studies |
| --- | --- |
| First trimester miscarriage | Lashen, Fear, and Sturdee (2004); Ramsay, Greer, and Sattar (2006) |
| Limitations with ultrasound | Phatak and Ramsay (2010); Troya-Nutt et al. (2003); Yeh and Shelton (2005) |
| Limitations with conventional care | ACOG (2013); Hawkins, Koonin, Palmer, and Gibbs (1997); Hood and Dewan (1993); Ockenden (2008); Saravanakumar, Rao, and Cooper (2006); Swan and Davies (2012) |
| Gestational diabetes | Bhattacharya, Campbell, Liston, and Bhattacharya (2007); Sebire et al. (2001) |
| Gestational hypertensive disorders | Bhattacharya et al. (2007); Sebire et al. (2001) |
| Induction of labor | Sebire et al. (2001) |
| Slower progress of labor | Vahratian et al. (2004) |
| Cesarean delivery | Chu et al. (2007a) |
| Emergency cesarean delivery | Sebire et al. (2001) |
| Wound infection | Myles, Gooch, and Santolaya (2006); Sebire et al. (2001) |
| Prematurity | Bhattacharya et al. (2007) |
| Thromboembolic disorders | Larson, Sorensen, Gislum, and Johnsen (2007) |
| Macrosomnia | Cedergren (2004); Sebire et al. (2001) |
| Shoulder dystocia | Cedergren (2004) |
| Admission to NICU | Sebire et al. (2001) |
| Maternal postpartum hemorrhage | Bhattacharya et al. (2007); Sebire et al. (2001) |
| Maternal depression | Dotlic et al. (2014); Usha-Kiran, Hemmadi, Bethel, and Evans (2005) |
| Breastfeeding difficulties | Amir and Donath (2007); Lepe, Bascardi-Gascon, Castaneda-Gonzalez, Perez-Morales, and Jimenez-Cruz (2011); Mok et al. (2008); Rasmussen and Kjolhede (2004) |
| Congenital anomalies | O'Reilly and Reynolds (2013); Rasmussen et al. (2008); Stothard et al. (2009) |
| Stillbirth | Chu et al. (2007b) |
| Neonatal death | Chu et al. (2007b); Kristensen, Vestergaard, Wisborg, Kesmodel, and Secher (2005) |

*(continued)*

**TABLE 6.1   Short-Term Health and Situational Risks of Obesity in Childbearing: A Synthesis of the Literature (*continued*)**

| Risk | Studies |
|------|---------|
| Preterm labor, both medically induced and spontaneous | Cnattingius et al. (2013); Suidan, Apuzzio, and Williams (2012) |
| Prolonged pregnancy, cervical ripening failure | Arrowsmith, Wray, and Quenby (2012); Bhattacharya et al. (2007); Bogaerts, Witters, Van den Bergh, Jans, and Devlieger (2013) |
| Increased risk of postpartum hemorrhage | Bloomberg (2011); Wetta et al. (2013) |
| Delayed lactogenesis (> 60–72 hours) | Lepe et al. (2011) |
| Postpartum depression and anxiety | Molyneaux, Poston, Ashurst-Williams, and Howard (2014) |
| Newborn depressed innate and adaptive immune response | Wilson and Messaoudi (2015) |

NICU, neonatal intensive care unit.
Compiled by Auginbaugh and Carlson (2016).

**TABLE 6.2   Long-Term Risks of Obesity in Childbearing: A Synthesis of the Literature**

| Risk | Studies |
|------|---------|
| Infertility | Ramsay et al. (2006); Kelly et al. (2001); Zain and Norman (2008) |
| Long-term obesity—mother and chronic illness | WHO (2015); Rasmussen and Yaktine (2009) |
| Long-term obesity and diabetes of the child | O'Reilly and Reynolds (2013) |
| Cardiovascular disease of the child | O'Reilly and Reynolds (2013) |
| Higher incidence diabetes and asthma to children born to obese women | Wilson and Messaoudi (2015) |
| Stress incontinence for the mother | Dwyer, Lee, and Hoy (1988) |
| Parenting a child born prematurely or born with birth defects | Lindbald, Rasmussen, and Sandman (2005); Ray (2002); Kirk (1999) |

Compiled by Auginbaugh and Carlson (2016).

The increasing rates of overweight and obesity in women of childbearing age, combined with the risks of poor outcomes for the mother–child dyad, make it imperative for midwives to be aware of the evidence. In this chapter, evidence-based best practices for the preconception, antepartum, intrapartum, and postpartum care of the obese woman are described. In addition, in providing care to the normal-weight pregnant woman with a history of gastric surgery for weight loss, the midwife needs to be cognizant of unique clinical considerations that deviate from routine care.

## OBESITY PRIOR TO PREGNANCY

### Preconception Concerns

The most ideal time to reduce obesity-associated risks is prior to pregnancy (American College of Obstetricians & Gynecologists [ACOG] 2013; Jevitt, 2009; Modder & Fitzsimons, 2010). A pregnancy complicated by obesity is at greater risk for fetal neural tube defects (NTDs; Rasmussen, Chu, Kim, Schmid, & Lau, 2008; Stothard, Tennant, Bell, & Rankin, 2009). However, there is strong evidence that obese women who take high doses of folic acid supplementation prior to pregnancy can minimize the risk of NTDs (Lumley, Watson, Watson, & Bower, 2001; Modder & Fitzsimons, 2010; Mojtabai, 2004; Rassmussen et al., 2008; Scholl & Johnson, 2000).

### Midwifery Best Practices

During preconception/well-woman visits, the midwife needs to obtain accurate height and weight measurements, determine BMI, and tactfully discuss BMI outside the defined limits as a risk in pregnancy. To supplement the discussion, the obese woman should be given written material. The ACOG has a number of excellent patient education fact sheets available online (see www.acog.org/Resources-And-Publications/Patient-Education-FAQs-List).

The woman contemplating pregnancy should begin supplementation with folic acid. ACOG guidelines (ACOG, 2013) and the joint guidelines of the Centre for Maternal and Child Enquiries (CMACE) and the Royal College of Obstetricians and Gynaecologists (RCOG; Modder & Fitzsimons, 2010) agree on an increased preconception folic acid dose for obese women. To prevent NTDs, women with a BMI greater than or equal to 30 kg/m$^2$ should supplement with 5 mg of folic acid daily, as compared to 4 mg daily among normal-weight women.

## ANTEPARTUM OBESITY

### Antepartum Concerns

#### Gestational Diabetes

Women with a pregnant BMI greater than or equal to 30 kg/m$^2$ are at greater risk for developing gestational diabetes mellitus (GDM; Bhattacharya et al., 2007; Sebire et al., 2001).

### Congenital Anomalies

Obese women are at greater risk of giving birth to an infant with a congenital anomaly. Ultrasonography is a cost-effective and widely available tool for evaluating fetal well-being, screening and detection of fetal anomalies, and assessing potential aneuploidy. However, the accuracy of ultrasonography is not equivalent across all BMI categories as the distance from the image and the presence of adipose tissue disrupt the clarity of the image. In 1990, Wolf, Sokol, Martier, and Sador conducted a prospective study ($n = 1,622$ singleton pregnancies) at a mean gestational age of 28.5 weeks. All the fetuses were anatomically normal. High BMI was the best predictor of poor ultrasound visualization. With increasing gestation or increasing examination length of time, visualization of organs did not improve. Despite significant advances, ultrasound technology is still unable to adequately navigate through adipose tissue.

In 2015, Tsai, Loichinger, and Zalud published a meta-analysis identifying the challenges in the use of ultrasound among obese pregnant women. The authors confirmed that, in detecting certain congenital anomalies and aneuploidy, maternal obesity makes ultrasound less useful as a screening tool. Especially in the second trimester, there may be suboptimal visualization as a result of the increased thickness of the abdominal wall (Tsai et al., 2015).

The limitations of ultrasound to detect fetal anomalies and aneuploidy markers, in combination with the significant increase in rates of fetal anomalies, make it logical to offer the *triple screen* or *quad screen*. These serum analyte tests screen the mother's blood for biochemical markers for certain fetal anomalies and aneuploidy. The analytes measured are pregnancy-associated plasma protein (PAPP-A), alpha-fetoprotein (AFP), unconjugated estriol (uE3), beta-human chorionic gonadotrophin (beta-hCG), and inhibin A (inhA). The concentrations of these markers in the maternal serum are expressed in a gestation-specific multiple of the median (MoM). The levels of these markers are constantly changing during pregnancy, making the testing time specific. The testing results are dependent upon maternal age, race, single versus multiple gestation, maternal diabetes mellitus, in vitro fertilization, smoking, and previous testing. The most significant variable, however, is maternal weight. The increased blood volume in the women with higher BMIs decreases the concentration of analyte levels (Tsai et al., 2015).

### Place and Type of Birth

Although the safety and cost-efficiency of out-of-hospital birth, as well as vaginal birth after cesarean (VBAC) for low-risk pregnancy, has been established, obesity increases the level of risk for women contemplating either an out-of-hospital birth or a VBAC. With the increase in the level of BMI and in the number of VBAC attempts, the safety index decreases for the obese pregnant woman (Jevitt, 2009; Modder & Fitzsimons, 2010).

Currently available data indicate that, even if VBAC is successful, the neonatal risks are increased (Belogolovkin et al., 2012). In addition, medical costs and the rate of puerperal infections are increased (Edwards, Harnsberger, Johnson,

Treloar, & Cruz, 2003). However, the authors of a recent study concluded that VBAC success is increased among overweight and obese women who lose weight between the first and second pregnancy (Callegari, Sterling, Zelek, Hawes, & Reed, 2014).

### Consideration of Intrapartum Anesthesia

The greatest risks for both regional and general anesthesia complications occur in the obese pregnant woman with BMI greater than or equal to 40 kg/m² (ACOG, 2013; Jevitt, 2009; Modder & Fitzsimons, 2010). With regional anesthesia, the woman with a BMI greater than or equal to 40 kg/m² may have problems with positioning, distorted anatomical landmarks, and significant layers of adipose tissue that can interfere with anesthesia placement (ACOG, 2013). With general anesthesia, the woman can have difficult or failed endotracheal intubation from edema and excessive tissue in the airway (ACOG, 2013).

### Pregnancy After Bariatric Surgery

As the obesity epidemic increases among women of childbearing age, so has bariatric surgery. According to the American Society for Metabolic and Gastric Surgery, there were 179,000 gastric weight-loss surgeries performed in 2013, 50% of the surgeries among women of childbearing age (18–45 years old; Maggard et al., 2008). Women with exclusively Class III obesity (BMI 40 or above) or Class I and II obesity (BMI 30–39) in conjunction with one or more co-morbid conditions are eligible for gastric weight-loss surgery. Co-morbid conditions include insulin-resistant type 2 diabetes mellitus, chronic hypertension, hyperlipidemia, obstructive sleep apnea, osteoarthritis, or cardiovascular disease (Landsberger & Gurewitsch, 2007).

Gastric procedures to enhance weight loss are either constrictive or malabsorptive. The constrictive procedures (the lap-band or gastric sleeve) changes the capacity and emptying time of the gastrointestinal tract. The malabsorptive procedure (Roux-en-Y gastric bypass) changes the absorption of macro- and micronutrients. Both the constrictive and malabsorption procedures alter sensations of hunger and satiety (Landsberger & Gurewitsch, 2007).

Women who conceive and give birth after gastric weight-loss surgery have specific risks depending upon which gastric procedure was performed (Maggard et al., 2008). Essentially, the procedures that cause malabsorption tend to cause greater weight loss while also causing significantly more nutrient deficiency (Landsberger & Gurewitsch, 2007). The literature is evolving on this topic.

The literature on pregnancy after weight-loss surgery (PWLS) addresses whether risk increases, decreases, or just differs with pregnancy. At this juncture, the studies on PWLS are observational and must be appraised with caution. In a meta-analysis, Galazis, Docheva, Simillis, and Nicolaides (2014) found that, compared to matched controls, in PWLS women there was a reduction in large-for-gestational-age (LGA) neonates, a decrease in incidences of preeclampsia, and a decrease in gestational diabetes. However, the authors also found that there were increases in maternal anemia, small-for-gestational-age (SGA) neonates, preterm birth, and admission to the neonatal intensive care unit

(NICU) in the PWLS women and their newborns (Galazis et al., 2014). The authors concluded that there was no significant difference between PWLS women and matched controls for perinatal mortality or incidence of cesarean section delivery (Galazis et al., 2014).

With both constrictive and malabsorption procedures, outcomes for both the PWLS mother and her child are slightly less risky compared to the woman whose pregnancy is complicated by obesity, providing the PWLS mother has adequate nutrition and vitamin supplementation to offset malabsorption (Maggard et al., 2008). However, it must be noted that many women who have undergone gastric surgery still have BMIs greater than or equal to 30 kg/m$^2$ despite significant weight reduction. The likelihood of complications related to gastric surgery is small but can include internal hernia and obstruction of the small intestine, pouch rupture, necrosis of gastric remnants, and slippage of the band or sleeve. Because both restrictive and malabsorptive procedures change hunger and satiety sensations, both protein and micronutrient deficiencies are likely to occur, especially in the first 18 months postprocedure and possibly long term (Landsberger & Gurewitsch, 2007).

## Best Practices in Midwifery During the Antepartum Period

### Nutrition and Glucose Management

At the first prenatal visit, accurate height, weight, and BMI should be obtained and recorded. Based on the woman's BMI, the midwife should explain appropriate weight gain and the risks associated with obesity in pregnancy (ACOG, 2013; Jevitt, 2009; Moddler & Fitzsimons, 2010). The 1-hour 50-g glucose tolerance test should be administered in the first trimester or at the first pregnancy encounter to all women with prepregnancy obesity. If the result is negative, the test should be repeated at 26 to 28 weeks gestation (ACOG, 2013; Jevitt, 2009). British guidelines recommend that women with prepregnancy obesity complete a 75-g 2-hour glucose tolerance test at 24 to 28 weeks gestation (Modder & Fitzsimons, 2010). The WHO recommends that all women have a glucose screen at 24 to 28 weeks gestation (1999).

### Monitoring for Congenital Anomalies and Fetal Well-Being

The midwife needs to counsel the obese pregnant woman about options available for screening for congenital anomalies, including information about the limitations of ultrasound among pregnant obese women (ACOG, 2013; Jevitt, 2009; Modder & Fitzsimons, 2010). These limitations include less accuracy in detection of aneuploidy markers. With the obese woman, the ultrasonagrapher needs to use higher frequency and lower frequency probes, image brightness alternation, and scanning where there is less subcutaneous fat (the umbilical window or suprapubic/under the pannus; Tsai et al., 2015). Despite the limitations of maternal serum analyte testing, the midwife should offer this testing to all obese pregnant women as the rates of congenital anomalies in this population are increased (ACOG, 2013; Jevitt, 2009; Modder & Fitzsimons, 2010).

### Planning for Place and Type of Birth

Women with a prepregnancy BMI greater than or equal to 35 should plan to give birth in a hospital for maternal and fetal safety. As for women with BMI between 30 and 34, individual risk assessment can determine the safety of out-of-hospital birth (Modder & Fitzsimons, 2010). The increased risks of both shoulder dystocia and postpartum hemorrhage should be considered when offering hydrotherapy or water birth. In water-birth conditions, the midwife may be limited with maneuvers and must be ready for the possibility of having to lift the woman out of the tub without her full cooperation. For obese women requesting VBAC, the midwife must inform the women and family of both maternal and neonatal risks, especially with very high BMI (Jevitt, 2009).

### Discussion About Intrapartum Anesthesia

If needed, the ACOG (2013) recommends regional rather than general anesthesia for the obese pregnant woman. The midwife should counsel the woman on anesthesia options and limitations as well as request, if at all possible, an anesthesia consultation prior to the onset of labor.

### Midwifery Care of the Post-Bariatric Pregnant Woman

Women should wait at least 12 to 18 months after bariatric surgery before attempting pregnancy (ACOG, 2013). Once pregnancy occurs, the midwife should request a nutrition consultation (Jevitt, 2009). The PWLS woman should be screened for anemia by measuring serum iron, ferritin, folate, and vitamin $B_{12}$ levels. In addition, serum levels of calcium, phosphate, and 25-OH vitamin D should be assessed and, if abnormal, parathyroid hormone levels should be tested. If serum albumin levels are low, the woman may have insufficient protein intake and will need dietary counseling (Landsberger & Gurewitsch, 2009).

As with the pregnant obese woman, the midwife should recommend that the PWLS woman with a prepregnant BMI of 30 or higher be screened for gestational diabetes in the first trimester or at the first prenatal encounter (Jevitt, 2009). Most PWLS women cannot tolerate the 50-g glucose tolerance test because this technique is likely to cause dumping syndrome. Instead, a viable option is to test fasting blood glucose level and 2-hour postprandial glucose level using cut-offs of 95 and 120, respectively (Landsberger & Gurewitsch, 2007).

## LABOR, BIRTH, AND OBESITY

Compared to normal-weight women, initiation and progression of labor in obese women are more difficult and more likely to result in unplanned cesarean section (Chu et al., 2007a; Poobalan, Aucott, Gurung, Smith, & Bhattacharya, 2009). Although comprehensive guidelines for the intrapartum care of obese women do not yet exist, reported clinical studies demonstrate that careful labor management strategies can decrease the potential for unnecessary interventions, including unplanned cesarean section (Abenhaim & Benjamin, 2011; Leeman & Leeman, 2003).

## Cervical Ripening

Obesity may cause delay in cervical ripening at the end of pregnancy (Wendremaire et al., 2012). In general, obese women have lower Bishop scores in late pregnancy compared to nonobese women (Zelig, Nichols, Dolinsky, Hecht, & Napolitano, 2013). These women are more likely to have prolonged pregnancies (> 41 weeks; Arrowsmith, Wray, & Quenby, 2011; Usha-Kiran et al., 2005) and comorbidities such as hypertension and preeclampsia (Mission, Marshall, & Caughey, 2013). Obese women are more than twice as likely to have induced labor compared to nonobese women (Sebire et al., 2001). In addition, induction is twice as likely to fail because they may start the induction with low Bishop scores (< 3; Gauthier et al., 2011; Zelig et al., 2013).

## Labor Progression

Time of labor lengthens as maternal BMI increases, with labors (4–10 cm dilation) among morbidly obese nulliparous women lasting up to 7 hours longer than those of nonobese women (Carlhäll, Källén, & Blomberg, 2013; Hirshberg, Levine, & Srinivas, 2014; Kominiarek et al., 2011; Walsh, Foley, & O'Herlihy, 2011). Slow labor in obese women was initially thought to be caused by excess adipose tissue causing obstruction of the pelvis in late labor and at birth (Crane, Wojtowycz, Dye, Aubry, & Artal, 1997). More recent findings are that labor in obese women is actually slowest during latent and early first-stage labor, from 4 to 7 cm of cervical dilation (Fyfe et al., 2011; Kominiarek et al., 2011; Vahratian et al., 2004).

Obese women are more likely than normal-weight women to have slightly larger babies. Yet in studies that control for maternal diabetes, heavier fetal weight is not associated with labor arrest or slowing of the labor curve (Verdiales, Pacheco, & Cohen, 2009; Zhang, Bricker, Wray, & Quenby, 2007). Slow labor progress in the obese woman is theorized to be the result of abnormalities in the powers of labor, or myometrial dysfunction. Multiple physiologic alterations appear to cause inefficient myometrial contraction in obese women (Bogaerts et al., 2013; Parkington et al., 2014; Zhang et al., 2007). Cervical exams in obese women, especially morbidly obese women, can be difficult for both woman and provider. Excess vaginal and perineal adipose tissue can obscure pelvic landmarks, leading to the impression that fetal station is artificially high (Schmied, Duff, Dahlen, Mills, & Kolt, 2011).

## Second-Stage Labor and Birth

Once obese women reach the second stage of labor, their vaginal birth rate is the same as normal-weight women's (Buhimschi, Buhimschi, Malinov, & Weiner, 2004; Robinson et al., 2011). Second-stage labor is not lengthened in obese women (Kominiarek et al., 2011). In fact, multiparous obese women have significantly shorter second-stage labors compared to multiparous, nonobese women (Suidan, Rondon, Apuzzio, & Williams, 2015). Maternal obesity is not an independent risk factor for shoulder dystocia (Tsur, Sergienko, Wiznitzer, Zlotnik, & Sheiner, 2012). However, obesity combined with gestational diabetes is associated with a 70% increased risk of shoulder dystocia (Catalano et al., 2012).

## Best Practices in the Intrapartum Period

### Cervical Ripening

When caring for the obese woman during labor induction, the midwife should provide anticipatory guidance that the process may take several days (Gauthier et al., 2011). As with all women undergoing induction of labor, cervical ripening methods should be continued until the obese woman achieves active labor or the Bishop score is greater than or equal to 6 (Suidan, Rondon, Apuzzio, & Williams, 2015). When choosing a cervical ripening agent for the obese woman, the midwife should avoid dinoprostone (Cervidil or Prepidil), as this agent has a 50% failure rate among obese women. With these cervical ripening agents, there are no differences in nonreassuring fetal heart rate tracing, NICU admission, or postpartum hemorrhage (Suidan, Rondon, Apuzzio, & Williams, 2015). Vaginal examination should be minimized during cervical ripening among obese women, as the longer length of labor may increase their risks of developing chorioamnionitis (Briese, Voigt, Wisser, Borchardt, & Straube, 2010).

### Labor Progression

Some obese women feel stigmatized and humiliated during labor by their clinicians (Furber & McGowan, 2011). It is crucial that the midwife sensitively supports obese women through labor. Because their labors may proceed more slowly than normal-weight women, obese women frequently have a more lengthy admission in early labor, augmentation with synthetic oxytocin (Pitocin), artificial rupture of membranes, and unplanned cesarean birth (Abenhaim & Benjamin, 2011; Carlson & Lowe, 2014a). Oxytocin augmentation, the leading treatment for slow labor, is less likely to end with vaginal birth in obese women compared to normal-weight women (Usha-Kiran et al., 2005). Adjusting synthetic oxytocin dosage for maternal BMI is not practiced, although several studies of induction protocols show that obese women require longer administration times, larger total doses, and greater per minute titrations to achieve cervical change or vaginal delivery in comparison with normal-weight women (Hill, Reed, & Cohen, 2014; Pevzner, Powers, Rayburn, Rumney, & Wing, 2009; Walsh et al., 2011). The midwife should be prepared for the increased likelihood of postpartum hemorrhage when synthetic oxytocin is used.

The higher a woman's BMI at the time of labor, the slower her labor is likely to proceed. In the presence of reassuring maternal and fetal status, midwives can encourage the obese woman to rest, ambulate, and use hydrotherapy or massage in early labor. In most obese women, it is best to delay hospital admission until the active phase of labor, usually after 6 cm (Kominiarek et al., 2011). Because obese women have longer labors, the midwife should avoid frequent vaginal exams: using these evaluations only when labor progress is abnormally slow in view of the woman's BMI or if other problems are suspected. Artificial rupture of membranes should be avoided and, if used, should be performed only with the active phase of labor. If synthetic oxytocin augmentation is used, it is important that the midwife allows more time for cervical change than with nonobese women.

Monitoring fetal heart rate and contraction characteristics is often challenging in obese women, especially when BMI is greater than or equal to 35 kg/m². Obese women are eligible for intermittent fetal heart rate monitoring as per the Association of Women's Health, Obstetric and Neonatal Nurses (AWHONN) high-risk guidelines (AWHONN, 2015). If continuous fetal heart rate monitoring is needed, abdominal fetal electrocardiogram, if available, is more reliable than ultrasound Doppler systems (Cohen & Hayes-Gill, 2014). Internal fetal heart rate monitoring is very reliable, yet should be avoided because it may increase obese women's already higher risk of chorioamnionitis (Briese et al., 2010).

Obese women's labor contractions can be monitored externally using palpation, tocodynamometer, or electrohysterogram (EHG; Cohen & Hayes-Gill, 2014). Intrauterine pressure catheters (IUPCs) provide the most accurate contraction monitoring but require membranes to be ruptured for insertion, which, like internal fetal heart rate monitoring, increases the obese women's already higher risk of the potential for chorioamnionitis (Euliano et al., 2013). When continuous contraction monitoring is necessary, EHG provides a reliable, noninvasive contraction-monitoring alternative to IUPC and is not affected by obesity. The midwife should be cautious when using IUPC to judge the adequacy of contractile force in obese women. Although the IUPC readings in late first-stage labor are equivalent to nonobese women, obese women still require more time than nonobese women to make cervical changes (Chin, Henry, Holmgren, Varner, & Branch, 2012). Watchful waiting is the key to successful labor assistance when working with obese women (Carlson & Lowe, 2014b).

### Second-Stage Labor and Birth

Genital tract trauma following vaginal birth is not increased among obese compared to nonobese women, even among nulliparas (Gallagher et al., 2014). Because gestational diabetes risk rises with each increase in BMI and the current GDM screening fails to identify some women who are diabetic, midwives should be especially vigilant for possible shoulder dystocia. With increased risk of both shoulder dystocia and postpartum hemorrhage among the obese women with gestational diabetes, water birth is a concern because the maneuvers used by the midwife are limited in water and tubs (Jevitt, 2009). Because birth is more frequently complicated in obese women with BMI greater than or equal to 35 kg/m², neonatal intensive care services should be available (Modder & Fitzsimons, 2010). When caring for the morbidly obese woman, it is important that the midwife alerts consulting physicians and hospital teams so that arrangements can be made to acquire special hospital beds or special tables, blood products, and extra personnel in the birth or operating room, if necessary.

## OBESITY IN THE POSTPARTUM

### Postpartum Hemorrhage

The obese pregnant woman is at greater risk for atonic and nonatonic postpartum hemorrhage (Bloomberg, 2011; Wetta et al., 2013). Establishing intravenous (IV) access may be more complicated in women with obesity and access should be established before it becomes imperative (Modder & Fitzsimons, 2010).

### Postnatal Thromboprophylaxis

The obese woman is at greater risk for thromboembolism during the postpartum period. The risk of thromboembolism increases even further in the event of an operative delivery, prolonged hospitalization, or immobility (Larson et al., 2007).

### Breastfeeding and Lactation

Obese women are at greater risk for poor breastfeeding outcomes with poor initiation and duration rates, difficult positioning, and impaired lactogenesis (Amir & Donath, 2007; Lepeet al., 2011; Mok et al., 2008; Rasmussen & Kjolhede, 2004).

### Depression and Anxiety

Pregnancy is a time of emotional vulnerability and increased need for social support. Higher BMI both before and at the end of the childbearing cycle is positively associated with depression. Social support may be lower, reaching lowest levels among morbidly obese women (Dotlic et al., 2014).

### Postpartum Follow-Up Care

The prime time to decrease the risks of obesity and pregnancy is prior to the pregnancy itself. A modest 10-pound weight loss prior to a subsequent pregnancy has shown to decrease the likelihood of gestational diabetes in the subsequent pregnancy (ACOG, 2013). Obese women with a history of gestational diabetes have a significant risk of developing type 2 diabetes after pregnancy even though the diabetic state often does not develop for several years (Bellamy, Casas, Hingorani, & Williams, 2009; Kim, Newton, & Knopp, 2002; Lauenborg et al., 2004).

### Best Practices in the Postpartum

#### Postpartum Hemorrhage

Women with BMI greater than or equal to 40 $kg/m^2$ should have IV access established prior to the third stage of labor. The midwife should consider active management of the third stage of labor (AMTSL), including prophylactic misoprostol for women with BMI greater than or equal to 30 (Modder & Fitzsimons, 2010). Use of synthetic oxytocin in obese women may require higher titrations to produce desired results, but postpartum hemorrhage risk is increased and preparations should be in place.

### Postpartum Thromboprophylaxis

All women with prepregnancy BMI greater than or equal to 30 should be encouraged to ambulate as soon as possible after the birth. Thromboprophylaxis, depending on mode of delivery and other risk factors, is recommended (ACOG, 2013; Jevitt, 2009; Modder & Fitzsimons, 2010). For women with a BMI of 40, full postnatal thromboprophylaxis should be prescribed regardless of the mode of delivery. Fractionated and low molecular weight heparin for postnatal thromboprophylaxis is recommended (ACOG, 2013; Modder & Fitzsimons, 2010).

### Breastfeeding and Lactation

Lactation can facilitate weight loss. Decreasing caloric intake by 500 cal/d during breastfeeding does not affect the quality or quantity of the mother's milk. The midwife should request a lactation specialist referral immediately in the postpartum period to promote maternal confidence and address potential lactation difficulties (Jevitt, Hernandez, & Groer, 2007; Modder & Fitzsimmons, 2010).

### Depression and Anxiety

The midwife should administer the Edinburgh Postnatal Depression Scale (or use a similar validated tool) in the postpartum period to identify obese women at risk for depression (Jevitt, Zapata, Harrington, & Berry, 2006).

### Postpartum Follow-Up

Women with BMI greater than or equal to 30 kg/m$^2$ and the diagnosis of gestational diabetes should have a diabetic surveillance at 6 weeks postpartum and be screened for insulin-resistance risk factors at least annually. Attention to diet and exercise is essential to decrease BMI prior to a subsequent pregnancy (ACOG, 2013; Jevitt, 2009; Modder & Fitzsimons, 2010).

---

**USING THE EVIDENCE FOR BEST PRACTICE**

**Case Study 6.1    Best Practices With the Obese Pregnant Woman**

M.K. is a 31-year-old, single, Caucasian primigravida. She seeks care at a midwifery-run clinic in rural Appalachia staffed by three midwives who attend births at the local community hospital. Two obstetricians at the hospital provide consultation, collaboration, and referral.

At her first visit, M.K. is 10 weeks gestation by last normal menstrual period and the midwife calculates her current BMI to be 39 kg/m$^2$. M.K. states that she probably

*(continued)*

## USING THE EVIDENCE FOR BEST PRACTICE (*continued*)

has lost 5 to 10 pounds over the past month as a result of nausea and occasional episodes of heartburn. Adhering to best-practice guidelines for the care of obese women during pregnancy, the midwife counsels M.K. about the risks associated with obesity in pregnancy for her and her child, including the limitations of ultrasound. The midwife informs M.K. about ways to decrease some risks by minimizing weight gain and ensuring daily intake of a prenatal vitamin daily, 5 mg of folic acid, and 10 mcg of vitamin D. The midwife discusses adequate physical activity during pregnancy and refers M.K. to a dietician for guidance on food choices to maximize nutrition and minimize weight gain. In addition to obtaining HgbA1C as part of the initial labs, the midwife also advises having a 50-g glucose tolerance test done now and again at 26 weeks gestation. A maternal serum marker screening is scheduled and the midwife explains the test in light of maternal obesity. The midwife also provides anticipatory guidance on planned place of birth.

M.K.'s pregnancy proceeds uneventfully and, at 39 weeks gestation, she arrives at the hospital with spontaneous rupture of membranes and clear amniotic fluid. Her total pregnancy weight gain has been 11 pounds, her blood pressure has remained normotensive, and all blood sugar screenings have been normal. Keenly aware that M.K.'s prepregnancy BMI was 39 kg/m$^2$, the midwife consults with the obstetrician on call. M.K.'s initial assessment reveals normal vital signs, category 2 fetal heart tracing, cervix at 4 cm, 100% effacement, and fetal head at zero station with estimated fetal size 8.5 to 9.0 pounds. The midwife and obstetrician agree to watchful waiting because it is likely that M.K.'s labor progression will be slower than normal as a result of her obesity. The midwife notifies the anesthesiologist on-call and the nurse places an IV access lock. M.K.'s labor progresses slower than expected but her vital signs remain stable and her baby tolerates labor well. At 15 hours after admission, M.K.'s cervix is completely dilated and she feels the urge to bear down. After 25 minutes of spontaneous pushing, M.K. gives birth to a vigorous infant weighing 9 pounds, 1 ounce and sustains a first-degree perineal laceration. The midwife institutes AMTSL while M.K. and her infant have skin-to-skin contact. The infant nurses well and the midwife orders lactation consultation as needed to help M.K. with breastfeeding. The midwife encourages M.K. to ambulate as soon as possible.

### Exemplar of Best Practice

At her 6-week postpartum visit, M.K. is exclusively breastfeeding, has lost 15 pounds since the time of birth, and feels well. The Edinburgh Postnatal Depression Scale is within defined limits, as is her 75-g glucose tolerance test. The midwife praises M.K. and counsels her about weight management during the postpartum period and prior to subsequent pregnancies. The midwife also encourages M.K. to follow up with her primary care physician for periodic evaluation of blood sugars.

With careful midwifery management, M.K. has had a healthy pregnancy and infant.

## REFERENCES

Abenhaim, H., & Benjamin, A. (2011). Higher caesarean section rates in women with high body mass index: Are we managing differently? *Journal of Obstetrics and Gynaecology*, *33*(5), 443–448.

American College of Obstetricians & Gynecologists (ACOG). (2013). ACOG Committee opinion no. 549: Obesity in pregnancy. *Obstetrics & Gynecology, 121*(1), 213–217. doi:http://10.1097/01.AOG.0000425667.10377.60

Amir, L. H., & Donath, S. (2007). A systematic review of maternal obesity and breastfeeding intention, initiation, and duration. *MC Pregnancy and Childbirth, 7*(1), 9. doi:10.1186/1471-2393-7-9

Arrowsmith, S., Wray, S., & Quenby, S. (2011). Maternal obesity and labour complications following induction of labour in prolonged pregnancy. *BJOG: An International Journal of Obstetrics & Gynaecology, 118*(5), 578–588. doi:10.1111/j.1471-0528.2010.02889.x

Arrowsmith, S., Wray, S, & Quenby, S. (2012). Maternal obesity and labor complications after induction of labor in prolonged pregnancy. *Obstetric Anesthesia Digest, 32*(1), 39. doi:10.1097/01.aoa.0000410800.85641.94

Association of Women's Health, Obstetric and Neonatal Nurses (AWHONN). (2015). Fetal heart monitoring: AWHONN position statement. *Journal of Obstetric, Gynecologic, & Neonatal Nursing, 44*(5), 683–686. doi:10.1111/1552-6909.12743

Bellamy, L., Casas, J. P., Hingorani, A. D., & Williams, D. (2009). Type 2 diabetes mellitus after gestational diabetes: A systematic review and meta-analysis. *Lancet, 373*(9677), 1773–1779. doi:10.1016/S0140-6736(09)60731-5

Belogolovkin, V., Crisan, L., Lynch, O., Weldeselasse, H., August, E. M., Alio, A. P., & Salihu, H. M. (2012). Neonatal outcomes of the successful VBAC among obese and super-obese mothers. *Journal of Maternal–Fetal Medicine and Neonatal Medicine, 25*(6), 711–718. doi:10.3109/14767058.2011.596594

Bhattacharya, S., Campbell, D. M., Liston, W. A., & Bhattacharya, S. (2007). Effect of body mass index on pregnancy outcomes in nulliparous women delivering singleton babies. *BMC Public Health, 7*(1), 168. doi:10.1186/1471-2458-7-168

Bloomberg, M. (2011). Maternal obesity and risk of postpartum hemorrhage. *Obstetrics and Gynecology, 118*(3), 561–568. doi:10.1097/AOG.0b013e31822a6c59

Bogaerts, A., Witters, I., Van den Bergh, B., Jans, G., & Devlieger, R. (2013). Obesity in pregnancy: Altered onset and progression of labour. *Midwifery, 29*(12), 1303–1313. doi:10.1016/j.midw.2012.12.013

Briese, V., Voigt, M., Wisser, J., Borchardt, U., & Straube, S. (2010). Risks of pregnancy and birth in obese primiparous women: An analysis of German perinatal statistics. *Archives of Gynecology and Obstetrics, 283*(2), 249–253. doi:10.1007/s00404-009-1349-9

Buhimschi, C. S., Buhimschi, I., Malinow, A., & Weiner, C. (2004). Intrauterine pressure during the second stage of labor in obese women. [Erratum: *Obstetrics & Gynecology* (2004, May), *103*(5, Pt. 1), 1019]. *Obstetrics & Gynecology, 103*(2), 225–230. doi:10.1097/01.AOG.0000102706.84063.C7

Callegari, L. S., Sterling, L. A., Zelek, S. T., Hawes, S. E., & Reed, S. D. (2014). Interpregnancy body mass index change and success of term vaginal birth after cesarean section. *American Journal of Obstetrics and Gynecology, 210*(4), 330.e1–330.e7. doi:10.1016/j.ajog.2013.11.013

Carlhäll, S., Källén, K., & Blomberg, M. (2013). Maternal body mass index and duration of labor. *European Journal of Obstetrics, Gynecology, and Reproductive Biology, 171*(1), 49–53. doi:10.1016/j.ejogrb.2013.08.021

Carlson, N. S., & Lowe, N. K. (2014a). Intrapartum management associated with obesity in nulliparous women. *Journal of Midwifery and Women's Health, 59*(1), 43–53. doi:10.1111/jmwh.12073

Carlson, N. S., & Lowe, N. K. (2014b). A concept analysis of watchful waiting among providers caring for women in labour. *Journal of Advanced Nursing, 70*(3), 511–522. doi:10.1111/jan.12209

Catalano, P. M., McIntyre, H. D., Cruickshank, J. K., McCance, D. R., Dyer, A. R., Metzger, B. E., . . . Hapo Study Cooperative Research Group. (2012). The hyperglycemia and adverse pregnancy outcome study: Associations of GDM and obesity with pregnancy outcomes. *Diabetes Care, 35*(4), 780–786. doi:10.2337/dc11-1790

Cedergren, M. I. (2004). Maternal morbid obesity and the risk of adverse pregnancy outcome. *Obstetrics and Gynecology, 103*(2), 219–224. doi:10.1097/01.AOG.0000107291.46159.00

Centers for Disease Control and Prevention (CDC). (2015, September 21). Adult obesity facts. Retrieved from http://www.cdc.gov/obesity/data/adult.html

Chin, J., Henry, E., Holmgren, C., Varner, M., & Branch, D. (2012). Maternal obesity and contraction strength in the first stage of labor. *American Journal of Obstetrics and Gynecology, 207*(2), 129.e1–129.e6. doi:10.1016/j.ajog.2012.06.044

Chu, S. Y., Kim, S. Y., Schmid, C. H., Dietz, P. M., Callaghan, W. M., Lau, J., & Curtis, K. M. (2007a). Maternal obesity and risk of cesarean delivery: A meta-analysis. *Obesity Reviews, 8*(5), 385–394. doi:10.1111/j.1467-789X.2007.00397.x

Chu, S. Y., Kim, S. Y., Schmid, C. H., Dietz, P. M., Callaghan, W. M., Lau, J., & Curtis, K. M. (2007b). Maternal obesity and risk of stillbirth: A meta-analysis. *American Journal of Obstetrics and Gynecology, 197*(3), 223–228. doi:http://dx.doi.org/10.1016/j.ajog.2007.03.027

Cnattingius, S., Villamor, E., Johansson, S., Edstedt Bonamy, A. K., Persson, M., Wikstrom, A. K., & Granath, F. (2013). Maternal obesity and risk of preterm delivery. *Journal of the American Medical Association, 309*(22), 2362–2370. doi:10.1001/jama.2013.6295

Cohen, W. R., & Hayes-Gill, B. (2014). Influence of maternal body mass index on accuracy and reliability of external fetal monitoring techniques. *Acta Obstetricia & Gynecologica Scandinavica, 93*(6), 590–595. doi:10.1111/aogs.12387

Crane, S. S., Wojtowycz, M. A., Dye, T. D., Aubry, R. H., & Artal, R. (1997). Association between pre-pregnancy obesity and the risk of cesarean delivery. *Obstetrics and Gynecology, 89*(2), 213–216. doi:10.1016/S0029-7844(96)00449-8

Dotlic, J., Terzic, M., Babic, D., Vasiljevic, N., Janosevic, S., Janosevic, L., & Pekmezovic, T. (2014). The influence of body mass index on the perceived quality of life during pregnancy. *Applied Research in the Quality of Life, 9*(2), 387–399. doi:10:1007/s11482-013-9224-z

Dwyer, P. L., Lee, E. T., & Hoy, D. M. (1998). Obesity and urinary incontinence in women. *British Journal of Obstetrics and Gynaecology, 95*(1), 91–96. doi:10.1111/j.1471-0528.1988.tb06486.x

Edwards, R. K., Harnsberger, D. S., Johnson, I. M., Treloar, R. W., & Cruz, A. C. (2003). Deciding route of delivery for obese women with a prior cesarean delivery. *American Journal of Obstetrics and Gynecology, 189*(2), 385–390. doi:10.1067/S0002-9378(03)00710-5

Euliano, T. Y., Nguyen, M. T., Darmanjian, S., McGorray, S. P., Euliano, N., Onkala, A., & Gregg, A. R. (2013). Monitoring uterine activity during labor: A comparison of 3 methods. *American Journal of Obstetrics and Gynecology, 208*(1), 66.e1–66.e6. doi:10.1016/j .ajog.2012.10.873

Flegal, K. M., Carroll, M. D., Kit, B. K., & Ogden, C. L. (2012). Prevalence of obesity and trends in the distribution of body mass index among US adults, 1999–2010. *Journal of the American Medical Association, 307*(5), 491–497. doi:10.1001/jama.2012.39

Furber, C. M., & McGowan, L. (2011). A qualitative study of the experiences of women who are obese and pregnant in the UK. *Midwifery, 27*(4), 437–444. doi:10.1016/j.midw.2010 .04.001

Fyfe, E. M., Anderson, N. H., North, R. A., Chan, E. H., Taylor, R. S., Dekker, G. A., & McCowan, L. M. (2011). Risk of first-stage and second-stage cesarean delivery by maternal body mass index among nulliparous women in labor at term. *Obstetrics & Gynecology, 117*(6), 1315–1322. doi:10.1097/AOG.0b013e318217922a

Galazis, N., Docheva, N, Simillis, C., & Nicolaides, K. H. (2014). Maternal and neonatal outcomes in women undergoing bariatric surgery: A systematic review and meta-analysis. *European Journal of Gynecology and Reproductive Biology, 181*, 45–53. doi:10.1016/j.ejogrb .2014.07.015

Gallagher, K., Migliaccio, L., Rogers, R. G., Leeman, L., Hervey, E., & Qualls, C. (2014). Impact of nulliparous women's body mass index or excessive weight gain in pregnancy on genital tract trauma at birth. *Journal of Midwifery & Women's Health, 59*(1), 54–59. doi:10.1111/jmwh.12114

Gauthier, T. Mazeau, S., Dalmay, F., Eyraud, J., Catalan, C., Marin, B., & Aubard, Y. (2011). Obesity and cervical ripening failure risk. *Journal of Maternal–Fetal and Neonatal Medicine, 25*(3), 304–307. doi:10.3109/14767058.2011.575485

Hawkins, J. L., Koonin, L. M., Palmer, S. K., & Gibbs, S. P. (1997). Anesthesia-related deaths during obstetric delivery in the United States, 1979–1990. *Anesthesiology, 86*(2), 277–284. doi:10.1097/00000542-199710000-00046

Hill, M., Reed, K. L., & Cohen, W. R. (2014). Oxytocin utilization for labor induction in obese and lean women. *Journal of Perinatal Medicine, 43*(6), 703–706. doi:10.1515/jpm -2014-0134

Hirshberg, A., Levine, L. D., & Srinivas, S. (2014). Labor length among overweight and obese women undergoing induction of labor. *Journal of Maternal–Fetal & Neonatal Medicine, 27*(17), 1771–1775. doi:10.3109/14767058.2013.879705

Hood, D. D., & Dewan, D. M. (1993). Anesthetic and obstetric outcome in morbidly obese parturients. *Anesthesiology, 79*(6), 1210–1218. doi:10.1097/00000542-199312000-00011

Jevitt, C. (2009). Pregnancy complicated by obesity: Midwifery management. *Journal of Midwifery and Women's Health, 54*(6), 445–451. doi:10.1016/j.jmwh.2009.02.002

Jevitt, C., Hernandez, I., & Groer, M. (2007). Lactation complicated by overweight and obesity: Supporting the mother and newborn. *Journal of Midwifery and Women's Health, 52*(6), 606–613. doi:10.1016/j.jmwh.2007.04.006

Jevitt, C., Zapata, L., Harrington, M., & Berry, E. (2006). Screening for perinatal depression with limited psychiatric resources. *American Psychiatric Nurses Association, 11*(6), 359–363. doi:10.1177/1078390305284530

Kelly, C. C., Lyall, H., Petrie, J. R., Gould, G. W., Connell, J. M., & Sattar, N. (2001). Low grade chronic inflammation in women with polycystic ovarian syndrome. *Journal of Clinical Endocrinology and Metabolism, 86*(6), 2453–2455. doi:10.1210/jcem.86.6.7580

Kim, C., Newton, K. M., & Knopp, R. H. (2002). Gestational diabetes and the incidence of type 2 diabetes: A systematic review. *Diabetes Care, 25*(10), 1862–1868. doi:10.2337/diacare.25.10.1862

Kirk, S. (1999). Caring for children with specialized healthcare needs in a community: The challenges for primary care. *Health & Social Care in the Community, 7*(5), 350–357. doi:10.1046/j.1365-2524.1999.00197.x

Kominiarek, M., Zhang, J., VanVeldhuisen, P., Troendle, J., Beaver, J., & Hibbard, J. (2011). Contemporary labor patterns: The impact of maternal body mass index. *American Journal of Obstetrics and Gynecology, 205*(3), 244.e1–248.e8. doi:10.1016/j.ajog.2011.06.014

Kristensen, J., Vestergaard, M., Wisborg, K., Kesmodel, U., & Secher, N. J. (2005). Pre-pregnancy weight and the risk of stillbirth and neonatal death. *BJOG: An International Journal of Obstetrics and Gynaecology, 112*(4), 403–408. doi:10.1111/j.1471-0528.2005.00437.x

Landsberger, E. J., & Gurewitsch, E. D. (2007). Reproductive implications of bariatric surgery: Pre-and postoperative considerations for extremely obese women of childbearing age. *Current Diabetes Reports, 7*(4), 281–288. doi:10.1007/s11892-007-0045-z

Larson, T., Sorensen, H., Gislum, M., & Johnsen, S. (2007). Maternal smoking, obesity, and risk of venous thromboembolism during pregnancy and the puerperium: A population-based nested case-control study. *Thrombosis Research, 120*(4), 505–509. doi:10.1016/j.thromres.2006.12.003

Lashen, H., Fear, K., & Sturdee, D. W. (2004). Obesity is associated with increased risk of first trimester and recurrent miscarriage: A matched case-control study. *Human Reproduction, 19*(7), 1644–1646. doi:10.1093/humrep/deh277

Lauenborg, J., Hansen, T., Jensen, D. M., Vestergaard, H., Molsted-Pedersen, L., Hornnes, P., . . . Damm, P. (2004). Increasing incidence of diabetes after gestational diabetes: A long-term follow-up in a Danish population. *Diabetes Care, 27*(5), 1194–1199. doi:10.2337/diacare.27.5.1194

Leeman, L., & Leeman, R. (2003). A Native American community with a 7% cesarean delivery rate: Does case mix, ethnicity, or labor management explain the low rate? *Annals of Family Medicine, 1*(1), 36–43. doi:10.1370/afm.8

Lepe, M., Bascardi-Gascon, L. M., Castaneda-Gonzalez, M., Perez-Morales, E. P., & Jimenez-Cruz, A. J. (2011). Effect of maternal obesity on lactation: Systematic review. *Nutricion Hospitalaria, 26*(6), 1266–1269. doi:10.1590/S0212-16112011000600012

Lindbald, B. M., Rasmussen, B., & Sandman, P. O. (2005). Being invigorated in parenthood: Parents lived experiences of professional support when having a disabled child. *Journal of Pediatric Nursing, 20*(4), 288–297. doi:10.1016/j.pedn.2005.04.015

Lumley, J., Watson, L., Watson, M., & Bower, C. (2001). Periconceptional supplementation with folate and/or multivitamins for preventing neural tube defects. *Cochrane Database of Systematic Reviews, 3.* doi:10.1002/14651858.CD001056.pub2

Maggard, M., Li, Z., Yermilov, I., Maglione, M. Suttorp, M., Carter, J., . . . Shekelle, B. (2008). *Bariatric surgery in women of reproductive age: Special concerns for pregnancy* (Evidence Reports/Technology Assessments No. 169. Prepared by the Southern California

Evidence-Based Practice Center). Rockville, MD: Agency for Healthcare Research and Quality.

Mission, J. F., Marshall, N. E., & Caughey, A. B. (2013). Obesity in pregnancy: A big problem and getting bigger. *Obstetrical & Gynecological Survey, 68*(5), 389–399. doi:10.1097/OGX.0b013e31828738ce

Modder, J., & Fitzsimons, K. J. (2010). *Joint guideline: Management of women with obesity in pregnancy* (Centre for Maternal and Child Enquiries and Royal College of Obstetricians and Gynaecologists). Retrieved from https://www.rcog.org.uk/globalassets/documents/guidelines/cmacercogjointguidelinemanagementwomenobesitypregnancya.pdf

Mojtabai, R. (2004). Body mass index and serum folate in childbearing women. *European Journal of Epidemiology, 19*(11), 1029–1036. doi:10.1007/s10654-004-2253-z

Mok, E., Multon, C., Piguel, L., Barroso, E., Goua, V., Christin, P., . . . Hankard, R. (2008). Decreased full breastfeeding, altered practices, perceptions, and infant weight change of prepregnant obese women: A need for extra support. *Pediatrics, 121*(5), e1319–e1324. doi:10.1542/peds.2007-2747

Molyneaux, E., Poston, L., Ashurst-Williams, S., & Howard, L. M. (2014). Obesity and mental disorders during pregnancy and postpartum: A systematic review and meta-analysis. *Obstetrics and Gynecology, 123*(4), 857–867. doi:10.1097/AOG.0000000000000170

Myles, T. D., Gooch, J., & Santolaya, J. (2002). Obesity as an independent risk factor for infectious morbidity in patients who undergo Cesarean delivery. *Obstetrics and Gynecology, 100*(5, Pt. 1), 959–964. doi:10.1016/S0029-7844(02)02323-2

Ockenden, J. (2008). Midwifery basics: Diet matters (5). Obesity and complications of pregnancy and birth. *Practising Midwife, 11*(3), 36–39.

O'Reilly, J. R., & Reynolds, R. M. (2013). The risk of maternal obesity to the long-term health of the offspring. *Clinical Endocrinology, 78*(1), 9–16. doi:10.1111/cen.12055

Parkington, H. C., Stevenson, J., Tonta, M. A., Paul, J., Butler, T., Maiti, K., . . . Smith, R. (2014). Diminished hERG K+ channel activity facilitates strong human labour contractions but is dysregulated in obese women. *Nature Communication, 5*, 4108. doi:10.1038/ncomms5108

Phatak, M., & Ramsay, J. (2010). Impact of maternal obesity on procedure of mid-trimester anomaly scan. *Journal of Obstetrics and Gynaecology, 30*(5), 447–450. doi:10.3109/01443611003797679

Pevzner, L., Powers, B. L., Rayburn, W. F., Rumney, P., & Wing, D. A. (2009). Effects of maternal obesity on duration and outcomes of prostaglandin cervical ripening and labor induction. *Obstetrics & Gynecology, 114*(6), 1315–1321. doi:10.1097/AOG.0b013e3181bfb39f

Poobalan, A. S., Aucott, L. S., Gurung, T., Smith, W. C., & Bhattacharya, S. (2009). Obesity as an independent risk factor for elective and emergency caesarean delivery in nulliparous women: Systematic review and meta-analysis of cohort studies. *Obesity Reviews, 10*(1), 28–35. doi:10.1111/j.1467-789X.2008.00537.x

Ramsay, J. E., Greer, I., & Sattar, N. (2006). ABC of obesity. Obesity and reproduction. *British Journal of Medicine, 333*(7579), 1159–1162. doi: 10.1136/bmj.39049.439444.DE1

Rasmussen, K. M., & Kjolhede, C. L. (2004). Prepregnant overweight and obesity diminish the prolactin response to suckling in the first week postpartum. *Pediatrics, 113*(5), e465–e471. doi:10.1542/peds.113.5.e465

Rasmussen, K. M., & Yaktine, A. L. (Eds.) (2009). *Weight gain during pregnancy: Reexamining the guidelines* (Committee to Reexamine IOM Pregnancy Weight Guidelines). Washington, DC: National Academies Press. Retrieved from http://www.nap.edu/catalog/12584/weight-gain-during-pregnancy-reexamining-the-guidelines

Rasmussen, S. A., Chu, S. Y., Kim, S. Y., Schmid, C. H., & Lau, J. (2008). Maternal obesity and the risk of neural tube defects: A meta-analysis. *American Journal of Obstetrics and Gynecology, 198*(6), 611–619. doi:10.1016/j.ajog.2008.04.021

Ray, L. (2002). Parenting and childhood chronicity: Making visible the invisible work. *Journal of Pediatric Nursing, 17*(6), 424–438. doi:10.1053/jpdn.2002.127172

Robinson, B. K., Mapp, D. C., Bloom, S. L., Rouse, D. J., Spong, C. Y., Varner, M. W., . . . Eunice Kennedy Shriver National Institute of Child Health and Human Development of the Maternal–Fetal Medicine Units Networks. (2011). Increasing maternal body mass index and characteristics of the second stage of labor. *Obstetrics & Gynecology, 118*(6), 1309–1313. doi:10.1097/AOG.0b013e318236fbd1

Saravanakumar, K., Rao, S. G., & Cooper, G. M. (2006). The challenges of obesity and obstetric anesthesia. *Current Opinion in Obstetrics and Gynecology, 18*(6), 631–635. doi:10.1097/GCO.0b013e3280101019

Schmied, V. A., Duff, M., Dahlen, H. G., Mills, A. E., & Kolt, G. S. (2011). "Not waving but drowning": A study of the experiences and concerns of midwives and other health professionals caring for obese childbearing women. *Midwifery, 27*(4), 424–430. doi:10.1016/j.midw.2010.02.010

Scholl, T. O., & Johnson, W. G. (2000). Folic acid: Influence on the outcome of pregnancy. *American Journal of Clinical Nutrition, 71*(5), 1295S–1303S.

Sebire, N. J., Jolly, M., Harris, J. P., Wadsworth, J., Joffe, M., Beard, R. W., . . . Robinson, S. (2001). Maternal obesity and pregnancy outcome: A study of 287,213 pregnancies in London. *International Journal of Obesity and Related Metabolic Disorders, 25*(8), 1175–1182. doi:10.1038/sj.ijo.0801670

Stothard, K. J., Tennant, P. W., Bell, R., & Rankin, J. (2009). Maternal overweight and obesity and risk of congenital anomalies: A systematic review and meta-analysis. *Journal of the American Medical Association, 301*(6), 636–650. doi:10.1001/jama.2009.113

Suidan, R. S., Apuzzio, J. J., & Williams, S. F. (2012). Obesity, comorbidities, and the Cesarean delivery rate. *American Journal of Perinatology, 29*(8), 623–628. doi:10.1055/s-0032-1319808

Suidan, R. S., Rondon, K. C., Apuzzio, J. J., & Williams, S. F. (2015). Labor outcomes of obese patients undergoing induction of labor with misoprostol compared to dinoprostone. *American Journal of Perinatology, 30*(2), 187–192. doi:10.1055/s-0034-1381721

Swan, L., & Davies, S. (2012). The role of midwives in improving normal birth rates in obese women. *British Journal of Midwifery, 20*(1), 7–12. doi:10.12968/bjom.2012.20.1.7

Troya-Nutt, M., Hendler, I., Blackwell, S., Treadwell, M., Bujold, E., Sokol, R., & Sorokin, Y. (2003). The accuracy of prenatal diagnosis of fetal heart anomalies in the obese gravida. *American Journal of Obstetrics and Gynecology, 189*(6), S239. doi:10.1016/j.ajog.2003.10.670

Tsai, S. P., Loichinger, M., & Zalud, I. (2015). Obesity and the challenges of ultrasound fetal abnormality diagnosis. *Best Practice & Research in Clinical Obstetrics & Gynecology, 29*(3), 320–327. doi:10.1016/j.bpobgyn.2014.08.011

Tsur, A., Sergienko, R., Wiznitzer, A., Zlotnik, A., & Sheiner, E. (2012). Critical analysis of risk factors for shoulder dystocia. *Archives of Gynecology & Obstetrics, 285*(5), 1225–1229. doi:10.1007/s00404-011-2139-8

Usha-Kiran, T. S., Hemmadi, S., Bethel, J., & Evans, J. (2005). Outcome of pregnancy in a woman with an increased body mass index. *BJOG: An International Journal of Obstetrics and Gynaecology, 112*(6), 768–772. doi:10.1111/j.1471-0528.2004.00546.x

Vahratian, A., Zhang, J., Troendle, J. F., Savitz, D. A., & Siega-Riz, A. M. (2004). Maternal prepregnancy overweight and obesity and the pattern of labor progression in term nulliparous women. *Obstetrics & Gynecology, 104*(5, Pt. 1), 943–951. doi:10.1097/01.AOG.0000142713.53197.91

Verdiales, M., Pacheco, C., & Cohen, W. R. (2009). The effect of maternal obesity on the course of labor. *Journal of Perinatal Medicine, 37*(6), 651–655. doi:10.1515/JPM.2009.110

Walsh, J., Foley, M., & O'Herlihy, C. (2011). Dystocia correlates with body mass index in both spontaneous and induced nulliparous labors. *Journal of Maternal–Fetal & Neonatal Medicine, 24*(6), 817–821. doi:10.3109/14767058.2010.531313

Wendremaire, M., Goirand, F., Barrichon, M., Lirussi, F., Peyronel, C., Dumas, M., . . . Bardou, M. (2012). Leptin prevents MMP activation in an in vitro model of myometrial inflammation. *Fundamental and Clinical Pharmacology, 26*, 82–83.

Wetta, L. A., Szychowski, J. M., Seals, S., Mancuso, M. S., Biggio, J. R., & Tita, A. T. (2013). Risk factors for unterine atony/postpartum hemorrhage requiring treatment after vaginal delivery. *American Journal of Obstetrics and Gynecology, 209*(1), 51.e1–51.e6. doi:10.1016/j.ajog.2013.03.011

Wilson, R., & Messaoudi, I. (2015). The impact of maternal obesity during pregnancy on offspring immunity. *Molecular and Cellular Endocrinology, 418*(Pt. 2), 134–142. doi:10.1016/j.mce.2015.07.028

Wolf, H. M., Sokol, R. J., Martier, S. M., & Sador, I. E. (1990) Maternal obesity: A potential source of error in sonographic prenatal diagnosis. Obstetrics and Gynecology, 76(3), 339–342.

World Health Organization (WHO). (1999). *Definition, diagnosis and classification of diabetes mellitus and its complications.* Retrieved from http://apps.who.int/iris/bitstream/10665/66040/1/WHO_NCD_NCS_99.2.pdf

World Health Organization (WHO). (2015). *Obesity and overweight. Fact Sheet No. 311* (Updated January 2015). Retrieved from http://www.who.int/mediacentre/factsheets/fs311/en

Yeh, J., & Shelton, M. A. (2005). Increasing prepregnancy body mass index: Analysis of trends and contributing variables. *American Journal of Obstetrics and Gynecology, 193*(6), 1994–1998. doi:10.1016/j.ajog.2005.05.001

Zain, M. M., & Norman, R. J. (2008). Impact of obesity on female fertility and fertility treatment. *Women's Health, 4*(2), 183–194. doi:10.2217/17455057.4.2.183

Zelig, C. M., Nichols, S. F., Dolinsky, B. M., Hecht, M. W., & Napolitano, P. G. (2013). Interaction between maternal obesity and Bishop score in predicting successful induction of labor in term, nulliparous patients. *American Journal of Perinatology, 30*(1), 75–80. doi:10.1055/s-0032-1322510

Zhang, J., Bricker, L., Wray, S., & Quenby, S. (2007). Poor uterine contractility in obese women. *British Journal of Obstetrics and Gynaecology, 114*(3), 343–348. doi:10.1111/j.1471-0528.2006.01233.x

# CHAPTER SEVEN

# WEIGHT MANAGEMENT COUNSELING WITH OVERWEIGHT AND OBESE PREGNANT WOMEN

Cecilia M. Jevitt

## OVERWEIGHT AND OBESITY IN PREGNANCY

The health challenges and obesity-related morbidity associated with overweight and obesity (body mass index [BMI] > 30) during pregnancy affects not only the mother, but also the fetus. Emerging research indicates that genetic switches that can mold fetal metabolism are turned on and off in utero in response to maternal blood glucose levels and general nutrition (Lau, Rogers, Desai, & Ross, 2011; Williams, Mackenzie, & Gahagan, 2014). Optimizing maternal nutrition and weight gain during pregnancy can improve the health of mother and infant for a lifetime, yet more than 50% of women in the United States gain excessive weight during pregnancy and women who are overweight or obese before pregnancy have the highest risk for excess gestational weight gain. Excessive gestational weight gain imposes the same risks on pregnancy outcomes as pregravid obesity (Deputy, Sharma, & Kim, 2015).

To be effective, weight management strategies must be tailored to the individual woman and used by her daily for months. The midwife offers advice but has no control over implementation. This lack of a quick fix can be professionally frustrating. The midwife may avoid frank discussions about weight management, fearing offense, psychological stress, or driving the woman to seek a different health care provider. With 30% of women in the United States overweight and 30% obese (Centers for Disease Control and Prevention [CDC], 2015), midwives need to be comfortable in talking about weight management with women. The American College of Obstetricians and Gynecologists (ACOG) issued a *Committee Opinion on Obesity in Pregnancy* (ACOG, 2013). It recommends giving women specific information about the risks to mother and fetus posed by obesity in pregnancy (ACOG, 2013). A BMI greater than or equal to 30 increases risks for spontaneous abortion, urinary tract infection, gestational diabetes and hypertension, preeclampsia, prolonged pregnancy, prolonged labor, and cesarean birth. Additionally, risks are increased for placental abruption, fetal death in utero, stillbirth, and postpartum hemorrhage. Furthermore, the fetus is at risk for neural tube defects and macrosomia and its accompanying birth complications (ACOG, 2013; National Research Council [NRC], 2009). Women with BMIs greater than or equal to 30 have delays in lactogenesis II, placing them at risk for breastfeeding difficulties and early weaning (Anstey & Jevitt, 2011).

There is a linear relationship between increasing BMI and perinatal health complications. However, if the midwife discusses only the risks and potential problems, only half the job is done. The woman needs evidence-based weight gain goals, strategies for weight optimization, and support for her efforts. The conversation about weight gain in pregnancy must change. This chapter reviews methods to assist women in reaching optimal prenatal weight gain through use of research-proven weight management behaviors, unbiased language in weight counseling, culturally aware food counseling, an advantage list, and motivational interviewing (MI) techniques. This chapter limits the discussion to the high frequency of obesity and excessive weight gain in pregnancy and does not address optimizing weight gain for underweight women or those with inadequate weight gain.

## BEHAVIORS ASSOCIATED WITH WEIGHT MAINTENANCE

Decades of weight loss and weight maintenance research have established frustrating facts that apply to weight maintenance during pregnancy. Wing and Phelan (2005) describe them as follows:

- Eating is learned during infancy and is one of the most difficult behaviors to change.
- Eating, as a problematic behavior, cannot be extinguished like smoking during pregnancy; it must be modified. This is especially true in pregnancy when the mother needs to maintain nutritious intake rather than dieting.
- Weight maintenance is more than calories in and calories out. A person's weight demonstrates a relationship with the bio-psycho-cultural-political environment. The built environment and federal food subsidies impact individual weight as much as the individual's food choices.
- Changed eating and activity behaviors are difficult to sustain with about 80% of individuals relapsing after 6 to 12 months of restrained behavior (Wing & Phelan, 2005).

Weight management research, dating back some three decades, documents strategies that are used for successful weight loss and long-term weight maintenance (Table 7.1). These strategies can be safely used by pregnant women to optimize prenatal weight gain. Most women tried one or more of these strategies outside of pregnancy and are in an ideal position to work with a midwife in designing a self-managed eating and activity program for pregnancy. The subtle but central fact is that all these strategies are patient centered. The midwife can provide an evidence-based target weight gain recommendation, help the woman to select possible strategies, and support her through the pregnancy in sustaining or

**TABLE 7.1   Evidence-Based Strategies for Weight Maintenance: Literature Review**

| Strategy | Reference |
| --- | --- |
| Prepares own meals | Jacobs (2006); Milsom, Middleton, and Perri (2011); Wansink and van Kleef (2014); Zoumas-Morse, Rock, Sobo, and Neuhouser (2001) |
| Eats with family at least four times a week | Hammons and Fiese (2011); Taveras et al. (2012); Wansink and van Kleef (2014) |
| Eats intentionally with TV turned off | Brunstrom and Mitchell (2006); Fitzpatrick, Edmunds, and Dennison (2007) |
| Loses or maintains weight by reducing intake | Andreyeva, Long, Henderson, and Grode (2010); Juanola-Falgarona et al. (2014); Weiss et al. (2015) |
| Loses or maintains weight by using low glycemic index foods | Boden, Sargrad, Homko, Mozzoli, and Stein (2005); Horan, McGowen, Gibney, Donnelly, and McAuliffe (2014); Juanola-Falgarona et al. (2014) |
| Loses or maintains weight by eating high-fiber foods | Horan et al. (2014) |
| Loses or maintains weight by following ADA or My Plate diet | Boden et al. (2005); Horan et al. (2014) |
| Loses or maintains weight by eating low-fat foods | Tobias et al. (2015); Juanola-Falgarona et al. (2014) |
| Eats canned or frozen low-calorie, portion-controlled meals | Foster et al. (2013); Gudzune et al. (2015) |
| Drinks water instead of sugared beverages | Malik, Schulze, and Hu (2006); Schulze et al. (2004) |
| Uses a smartphone or computer program to support a weight management program | Archarya, Elci, Sereika, Styn, and Burke (2011) |
| Eats five fruit or vegetable servings daily | Byrd-Bredbenner, Abbot, and Cussler (2011); de Jong, Visscher, HiraSing, Seidell, and Renders (2014) |
| Counts calories to plan intake | Andreyeva et al. (2010); Weiss et al. (2015) |
| Weighs self regularly | Milsom et al. (2011) |
| Remained within NRC 2009 guidelines for weight gain during a prior pregnancy | Waring, Moore Simas, and Liao (2013) |

*(continued)*

**TABLE 7.1 Evidence-Based Strategies for Weight Maintenance: Literature Review (*continued*)**

| Strategy | Reference |
|---|---|
| Returned to prepregnancy weight following the birth of a baby | Nehring et al. (2011); Jain et al. (2013) |
| Breastfed a baby (exclusively) for at least 3 months | Ruiz et al. (2013) |
| Sleeps at least 7 hours each night | Chaput, Klingenberg, and Sjodin (2010); Patel, Malhotra, White, Gottlieb, and Hu (2006) |
| Does planned physical activity at least 30 minutes a day 5 days a week | CDC (2015) |

ADA, American Diabetes Association; CDC, Centers for Disease Control; NRC, National Research Council.

adapting weight management behaviors. In well-woman care, midwives can prescribe weight loss medications and arrange bariatric surgery but, in order to be successful, these weight management strategies need to be followed with the behaviors described in Table 7.1. Once the woman is pregnant, obesity medications and bariatric surgery are contraindicated and she must rely on other strategies.

# CHANGING THE CONVERSATION

## Unbiased Language and Attitude in Weight Management

Changing the conversation in weight management starts with changing the language. It is best to use scientific terms whenever possible, such as BMI greater than or equal to 30, instead of obesity, and class III obesity instead of morbid obesity. Euphemisms, such as "big girls" or "extra padding," signal that the topic is to be avoided. Developing novel terms, such as "a woman of size," that try to sound unbiased further obfuscate the medical risks associated with obesity. Person-centered language recognizes the individual before the disease process. Instead of saying, "the obese woman," it is better to say, "the woman with a body mass index ≥ 30." This is consistent with the change in language from "a diabetic" to "a woman with diabetes." Therapeutic conversation in weight management is not about size or image; it is about reducing health risks and behaviors that support current and future health for mother and baby.

This chapter uses the term "weight management" instead of "weight control" because the body is primed for growth particularly in pregnancy and weight control eludes most people. "Eating plan" has been used more often than "diet." Pregnant women with pregravid BMIs greater than or equal to 30 may not gain weight in pregnancy if they are following healthy eating patterns or following a diabetic diet, but restricting calories to lose weight during pregnancy is not recommended (ACOG, 2013). The term "physical activity" will be used in sample conversations rather than "exercise." Many women associate exercise with the discomfort, sweating, and pain of past efforts to use exercise to burn calories for weight loss. Physical activity is stressed more for aerobic fitness during pregnancy than weight management.

Advice from primary care providers can have a significant effect on patient's weight management activities (Rose, Poynter, Anderson, Noar, & Conigliaro, 2013). Midwives need to move beyond the concept of weight being the personal responsibility of the woman and excess weight being the consequence of poor intake and activity choices. Personal responsibility situates the conversation in blame, weakness, and individual moral failing instead of recognizing the social and environmental conditions that thwart an individual's physical and psychological regulatory systems (Brownell et al., 2010). These include nutrition-poor school lunch programs, food deserts, that is, areas in regions or urban settings where nutritious food is not available, and environments inhospitable to walking. Salt, sugar, and flavorings in processed food are ways to sell the product and are designed to overcome appetite regulatory systems. The midwife needs to acknowledge these issues that erode the patient's ability and responsibility to manage her own weight, while offering ideas and support to overcome those conditions. When patients perceive antiobesity bias or judgmental attitudes in midwives, weight management success is reduced (Gudzune, Bennett, Cooper, & Bleich, 2014).

## Culturally Aware Food Counseling

The midwife who counsels a woman about nutrition without knowing her favorite and available foods is not providing the most useful information. If a midwife, for example, is developing a meal plan using bread when the woman regularly uses rice as her carbohydrate, the woman is not likely to use the plan. This chapter uses the term *culturally aware* for food counseling as only persons within their own culture or professional chefs are likely to be culturally competent in the food uses of a particular ethnic group.

A midwife working in a culturally diverse location can improve communication by identifying the distinct cultural groups served by the practice and knowing, as specifically as possible, the immigrants' origins, and food customs. Once a woman's ethnic origin is known, the midwife can research generally available and preferred foods. Knowing the dominant carbohydrate, protein, and fat used by a group will assist the midwife in making culturally appropriate recommendations. For example, women with south Italian heritage who cook in the traditional manner use bread or pasta as their carbohydrate, chicken or fish as the protein source, and olive oil as the fat (Edelstein, 2011).

Culturally aware food counseling also encompasses knowing ethnic food intolerances, such as lactose intolerance (Edelstein, 2011), and the cultural significance of foods. All cultures use foods ceremonially or for celebrations. A midwife who knows holiday feasting customs may give anticipatory guidance to women in order to optimize their eating during feasting. Times of fasting are equally important to know and incorporate in eating plans.

## The Advantage List

Lawrence Weed developed the Problem-Oriented Medical Record in the 1960s as a method of organizing medical information, systematically assessing patient data to make a diagnosis, and making a management plan. Medical data were organized into a *problem list*. The problem list documented actual problems, such as hypertension, but evolved to include potential problems or risk status, especially after computerization facilitated the analysis of large data sets yielding associations and risks. The Problem-Oriented Medical Record became the communication route for health care providers, shifting attention from the patient to the problems. A woman can be defined by her problem list. When a woman has a BMI exceeding 29, the prenatal problem list may include potential problems related to maternal obesity. Unless the midwife is diplomatic, reviewing a problem list can be a negative experience for a woman. Weight management counseling traditionally consists of expert opinion that correctly applies evidence-based risks, but tells women what is wrong and what not to do. Women may feel victims of negative stereotyping and scolding.

Conversely, an *advantage list* is a list of self-management behaviors that have been demonstrated through research to successfully help in coping with a health challenge or chronic problem. The advantage list is not a new intervention but an instrument based on compiled research findings used in counseling. In weight maintenance during pregnancy, the list contains strategies that maintain weight during pregnancy or facilitate weight loss in the postpartum period (see Table 7.1) by providing a way for the midwife to support a woman's self-care. These strategies include activities such as intentional eating with the television off. The midwife can discover which advantages a woman brings to care through interview or by having the woman complete an advantage list self-assessment before the first visit (Table 7.2).

The sample advantage list in Table 7.2 not only records information for the midwife to use during the weight management conversation, but shows the woman evidence-based weight management strategies. This alleviates the need for the midwife to recite a laundry list of weight management behaviors, imposing a plan on the patient. The patient can concentrate on what has worked for her in the past and consider other strategies. The advantage list exemplifies values embedded in the American College of Nurse-Midwives (ACNM) philosophy, which urges midwives to utilize a woman's life experience and knowledge as well as individualizing her care (ACNM, 2015).

The midwife can avoid being discouraged by remembering that most people regain and lose weight throughout their lives. The focus during prenatal care is not the mother's current or final weight but a weight gain that is healthiest for the baby, within the NRC prenatal weight gain guidelines (NRC, 2009). A mother who is successful in prenatal weight management is primed to attempt postpartum weight loss.

Acknowledging advantageous behaviors has its roots in the principles of person-centered care in MI (Miller & Rollnick, 2013). These principles include:

- Change is fundamentally self-change
- People are experts on themselves
- People have their own strengths, motivations, and resources that are vital to activate in order for change to occur
- Motivation for change is not installed but is evoked (Miller & Rollnick, 2013)

Every woman has some weight maintenance advantage or has used an advantage behavior in the past. Although the prenatal care midwife must discuss the risks associated with obesity and pregnancy for the woman to be fully informed, knowledge of a woman's advantage list shifts the focus from problem labels to self-help. Table 7.3 compares one woman's problem list with her advantage list.

| TABLE 7.2   An Advantage List for Weight Management |
|---|
| **Advantage List Survey** |
| The answers to these questions will help us work with you to plan your health care. Please place a check mark to the left of statements that describe your eating and activity now or in the past. |

| Check √ if yes | About Your Eating and Activity |
|---|---|
| | 1. I prepare most of my own meals. |
| | 2. My family eats together at least four times a week. |
| | 3. The TV is turned off when I eat. |
| | 4. I have lost weight before by decreasing what I eat. |
| | 5. I have followed a low-glycemic diet before. |
| | 6. I have eaten a high-fiber diet before. |
| | 7. I have used the American Diabetes Association My Plate diet before. |
| | 8. I have eaten a low-fat diet before. |
| | 9. I have followed a diabetic diet before. |
| | 10. I use frozen or prepared low-calorie meals often. |
| | 11. I usually eat at least five servings of fruits or vegetables a day. |
| | 12. I have counted calories or portions before to decide how much to eat. |
| | 13. I have used a phone or computer app to decide what to eat. |
| | 14. I weigh myself on a scale at home or on a public scale. |
| | 15. I weigh myself on a public scale. |
| | 16. After my last baby was born, I got back to the weight I was before the pregnancy started. |
| | 17. I breastfed a baby for at least 3 months. |
| | 18. I usually get 7 hours of sleep a night. |
| | 19. I do some kind of physical activity, like walking or bicycling, for 30 minutes at least 5 days a week. |

Passive sentences 3%.

Flesch reading ease 81.1%.

Flesch–Kincaid reading grade level 4.5.

Average words per sentence 10.4.

*Source:* Jevitt (2015).

Documenting an advantage list in the medical record along with the problem list is recommended so that advantages are continually acknowledged during prenatal care. An advantage list template can be formatted within an electronic medical record. The problem list and the advantage list both aim to improve maternal and newborn prenatal health outcomes, but they focus on different aspects: risk or advantage (Figure 7.1). Each is an essential component of health assessment and communication. The person-centered, holistic focus of midwifery supports the use of an advantage list. Use of an advantage list is not limited to weight management. The advantage list can also be used in counseling for gestational diabetes or other health challenges requiring self-management.

A written advantage list also communicates the woman's strengths to other providers. A woman can complete an advantage list survey before the first prenatal visit. The survey provides a starting point for the conversation about weight management during pregnancy. The advantage list survey can be scanned into an electronic medical record. The conversation in Case Study 7.1 shows the use of the advantage list survey with the woman described in Table 7.3, a 35-year-old G3P1011.

**TABLE 7.3　Comparison of a Problem List and an Advantage List**

| 35-year old, G3P1011, singleton pregnancy, BMI 38 | |
| --- | --- |
| **Problems** | **Advantages** |
| Advanced maternal age | Exercises in gym 5 days a week |
| Trisomy risk increased | Cooks own meals |
| Obese | Daily family dinners |
| At risk for gestational diabetes | Has six fruit or vegetable servings a day |
| At risk for preeclampsia | Drinks water instead of soda |
|  | Has counted calories before |

BMI, body mass index.

*Source:* Jevitt (2015).

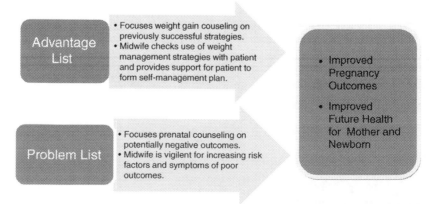

**Figure 7.1**　The advantage list compared with the problem list.
*Source:* Jevitt (2015).

## CASE STUDY 7.1  USING THE ADVANTAGE LIST SURVEY

| Midwife (During First Prenatal Visit) | Woman (BMI 40 at 8 Weeks Gestation) |
|---|---|
| Thank you for filling out the survey on eating and activity. You have practice in several ways to eat healthful, like cooking family dinners and drinking water instead of soda. | Yeah, I try but it isn't easy. I just put on weight—already have, 5 pounds. |
| Weight management isn't easy. | You got that right. |
| Let's talk some about what the baby needs during pregnancy and some ways for you to get that without gaining too much. | I already started my prenatal vitamin. |
| That's great. That will help with vitamins and minerals but you also need them from foods. I see from the advantage list that you have six fruit or vegetable servings a day. What are your favorites? | Oh, apples, grapes, oranges, strawberries. |
| And vegetables? | Peas, green beans, corn, tomatoes, salsa, peppers. |
| It sounds as if you have a variety of fruits and vegetables that you like. Is your stomach settled enough to continue to have at least five servings of them a day? | Yeah, I'm a little nauseous but I can eat. |
| Good, because fruits and vegetables are great baby-building foods. Another way is fill half your plate at each meal with fruits or vegetables. | That's a lot. |
| It is a lot but it's a reliable way of keeping your weight gain healthy for the baby. Based on your weight today, a healthy weight gain would be 11 to 15 pounds over the pregnancy. | That doesn't seem like enough for the baby. |
| We'll show you how the baby is growing. Gaining too much weight can push you toward diabetes and high blood pressure during pregnancy as well as other complications. I see that you've also weighed yourself and counted calories before. Can we make a plan from things you've done before to watch your weight during this pregnancy? | Well, yeah, I guess. |
| You've done these things before: cook family meals, eat fruits and vegetables, weigh yourself, drink water instead of soda, and count calories. Which of those do you think would be most helpful in planning eating for this month coming up? | |

BMI, body mass index.

*Source:* Jevitt (2015).

The advantage list is not only used during the first prenatal visit but becomes a tool that is reviewed at each prenatal visit (Figure 7.2). An advantage list can be used along with MI conversational techniques to assist women in taking charge of their own weight maintenance and supporting their ongoing weight maintenance work during pregnancy and the postpartum period.

## Motivational Interviewing

Once the midwife and woman have assembled an advantage list, the midwife can use principles from MI to continue the conversation. MI is a collaborative, person-centered, goal-oriented style of communication that uses the language of change (Miller & Rollnick, 2013). MI has a long history in change counseling. Originally developed for substance abuse counseling, it has been studied in tobacco cessation, dental decay prevention, weight loss, and many other medical conditions (Lundahl et al., 2013). Two meta-analyses demonstrated the usefulness of MI interventions in obesity management (Burke, Arkowitz, & Menchola, 2003; Rubak, Sandbaek, Lauritzen, & Christensen, 2005). MI used for weight management has been shown

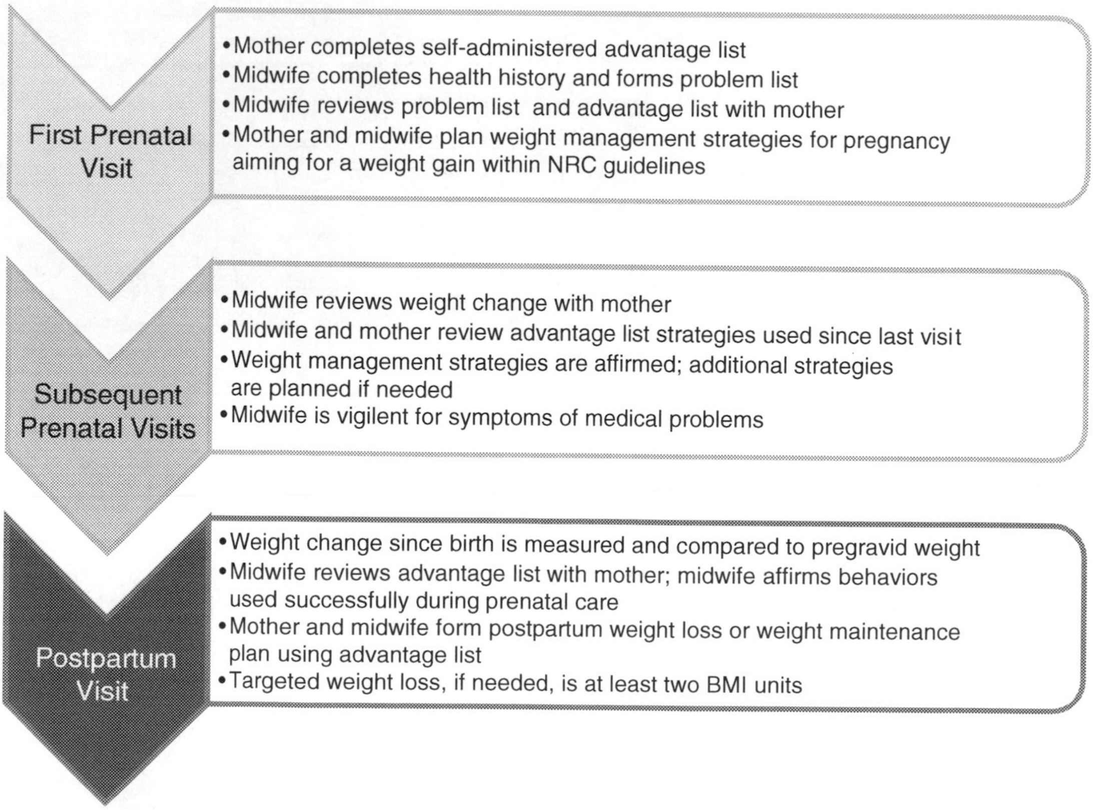

**First Prenatal Visit**
- Mother completes self-administered advantage list
- Midwife completes health history and forms problem list
- Midwife reviews problem list and advantage list with mother
- Mother and midwife plan weight management strategies for pregnancy aiming for a weight gain within NRC guidelines

**Subsequent Prenatal Visits**
- Midwife reviews weight change with mother
- Midwife and mother review advantage list strategies used since last visit
- Weight management strategies are affirmed; additional strategies are planned if needed
- Midwife is vigilent for symptoms of medical problems

**Postpartum Visit**
- Weight change since birth is measured and compared to pregravid weight
- Midwife reviews advantage list with mother; midwife affirms behaviors used successfully during prenatal care
- Mother and midwife form postpartum weight loss or weight maintenance plan using advantage list
- Targeted weight loss, if needed, is at least two BMI units

**Figure 7.2** The advantage list used in prenatal and postpartum care.
BMI, body mass index; NRC, National Research Council.
*Source:* Jevitt (2015).

to be most effective when treatment lasts longer than 6 months (Armstrong et al., 2011). This is particularly relevant for the extended midwife–patient relationship, which exists throughout a pregnancy and the postpartum period.

A midwife using MI seeks to explore a person's own reasons for change while demonstrating acceptance and compassion. The collaborative, person-centered approach of MI is consistent with the ACNM philosophy of care, which focuses on continuity, compassion, and communication (ACNM, 2015).

## MI Key Processes

MI has four key processes: engaging, focusing, evoking, and planning.

### Engaging
Engaging refers to establishing connection and relationship (Miller & Rollnick, 2013). This is the heart of the first prenatal visit: establishing a helping relationship with a woman. A rapport that facilitates the changes needed for a healthy pregnancy and the start of parenting is the aim of the midwife/patient relationship.

### Focusing
Focusing refers to a specific direction taken to bring about change (Miller & Rollnick, 2013). Midwives typically want to give women every shred of their knowledge. Learning to focus a conversation gives women useable chunks of information directly related to their immediate needs. This abbreviated but targeted conversation helps to keep the midwife on schedule.

### Evoking
Evoking refers to eliciting the motivation for change (Miller & Rollnick, 2013). Instead of the midwife offering one-way expert advice to the woman, MI tilts the conversation, placing the woman's perceptions of her own need for health care change at the center of the relationship. If the woman is barraged with questions such as, "Are you exercising?" and "How many fruits and vegetables do you eat each day?" she is likely to mentally withdraw from the conversation. Evoking subtly explores what a woman thinks about an area where change could occur.

### Planning
Planning includes commitment to change and making a plan of action (Miller & Rollnick, 2013). Midwives generally excel at developing and implementing a safe and efficient plan of action as part of the midwifery management process (King et al., 2015). In MI, the process of change is centered on the patient. The midwife cannot assume that evidence-based information will necessarily affect the decision-making process with the patient.

## MI Key Communication Skills

MI technique uses five key communication skills: asking open questions, affirming, reflecting, providing information and advice with permission, and summarizing

(Miller & Rollnick, 2013). These communication skills will be described and demonstrated using MI techniques.

### Open Questions

Most midwives are skilled in the use of open questions but this skill can be minimized during a busy clinic day. Open questions related to eating and weight management can be particularly challenging. Here are some examples:

- Can you tell me about your usual eating, your meals, and what you like to eat?
- Pregnancy changes appetite and tastes. Tell me about ways you've managed changes in eating before.
- Imagine that you needed to make a plan for eating during pregnancy. Can you think of two or three changes you might be able to make?
- Describe to me parts of your usual meals that you would like to keep.

Learning what the patient knows about a topic before asking further questions or delivering standardized information shows respect for the patient. This can be done through an open question such as, "Can you tell me what you know about weight gain in pregnancy?"

### Affirming

Affirming is more than responding "good job" to every action taken by the patient. Affirming is sincere recognition of effort, an attitude of looking for the positive instead of focusing on missteps or inaction by the patient. Affirming supports and encourages while building the midwife/patient relationship. Affirming statements include:

- You stayed right on target for your planned weight gain this month. Good for you. Tell me what you did to achieve that (*affirmations followed by an open, information seeking question*).
- I can hear from your description of grocery shopping and cooking this week that you tried really hard to change your eating. That's a lot of work.
- You did gain more weight than expected but you tried new foods and made your portions smaller this month (*fact-based assessment delivered with neutral tone*). Your intentions were good even though the results weren't exactly what you wanted (*affirmation*).

### Reflecting

Reflecting is a good listening skill. It acknowledges the patient's own thought without imposing a value judgment or requiring the midwife to have an authoritative answer to everything the patient says. Sometimes what the patient says is unclear or may have multiple meanings. Reflecting helps the midwife to determine what the patient means and can evoke additional information. Reflective responses often begin with "you." Reflective responses do not have to be exact mirrors of what the patient says. In fact, a conversation that is dominated by mirrored reflections can annoy the patient. Here are some examples of reflection:

> Patient: I hate vegetables. Don't even talk to me about vegetables.
> Midwife: You hate vegetables.

> Patient: I can't believe I gained so much weight this month.
> Midwife: You're surprised by today's weight.

> Patient: I don't think I'm eating too much for this baby. This baby needs to grow.
> Midwife: You think the baby needs a lot of food to grow.

### Providing Information and Advice With Permission

Knowledge acquisition assumes that if patients have correct information, they will be motivated to put that knowledge to use in maintaining or improving their own health. These theories do not account for the multiple variables involved in change, including resources to effect change, social support for change, difficulty of the change required, and various motivations for change. Knowledge acquisition prompts midwives to provide bags of pamphlets and booklets with pregnancy and labor information at the first prenatal visit. This approach pressures midwives to try to deliver every prenatal fact to every patient. Asking permission to give information or advice helps the midwife and patient to work together on knowledge acquisition. Some ways to ask permission include:

- May I talk to you about foods that we know provide nutrients for the baby?
- I don't know if these will apply to you, but may I talk about some simple ways to increase your activity while you work?
- I noticed you didn't talk much about physical activity. Could I fill in some pieces of information from new research that might help you?

### Summarizing

Summaries can serve several functions. They can pull similar topics together while indicating the important points of the conversation. Summaries can also focus a conversation or begin wrapping up a conversation. Summaries often reflect and affirm statements made by the patient. Examples of conversation summaries include:

- We've talked about your weight gain with your first pregnancy, how difficult it was for you to lose that weight postpartum and your favorite foods. We're straying into what you're thinking about for coping during labor. May we return to prenatal weight gain? We'll come back to labor coping. Can you describe to me what you were thinking about in terms of eating and activity during this pregnancy?
- We've talked about a lot of prenatal information today: lab testing, ultrasounds, baby-building foods, and rest. Here's what I remember you planning

to do. I'm going to write this in your medical record so we can review it at our next visit in a month. You're going to have blood drawn in 2 weeks at the time of your ultrasound. You're going to change from white-wheat tortillas to whole-wheat tortillas and have one less tortilla per day. And last, you're going to get to bed an hour earlier at least 4 days a week. Did I get everything?

## BEST PRACTICES FOR MIDWIVES IN WEIGHT MANAGEMENT COUNSELING

### Mutually Established Weight Management Goals

Recommended prenatal weight gain is based on prepregnancy BMI. The NRC-recommended weight gain in pregnancy advises weight gain according to BMI, adjusted for singleton and multiple-birth pregnancy (see Table 5.2, Chapter 5). Weight gain for women with a BMI greater than or equal to 30 should not exceed 11 to 20 pounds (5–9 kg) with the lower end of the range being most advantageous for maternal–fetal health. Weight gain beyond the NRC recommendations, even when a woman starts pregnancy with a normal BMI, poses the same health risks as prepregnancy obesity.

A midwife who begins the conversation with the statement, "Based on your BMI, you should gain only 11 to 20 pounds during this pregnancy," has made an authoritative statement and closes down the conversation. The goal is to strengthen the woman's efficacy, build upon her prior experiences with weight management, and to help her to understand her responsibility to individualize her weight gain plan. Statements such as, "An 11- to 20-pound weight gain during this pregnancy is healthy for you and the baby. What are your thoughts about weight gain in this pregnancy?" opens dialogue and enlists the woman in her own care. A prenatal weight gain plan set without the woman's input is a plan that is likely to fail. An MI concept is that the patient is the expert in her own care. The midwife needs to be able to step back and relinquish the expert's role, but to offer information and support efforts to change. Vesco et al. (2014) used calorie goals, planned physical activity, and weekly group meetings for women with BMIs greater than or equal to 30, demonstrating that calorie restriction and support-facilitated weight gain resulted in outcomes closer to NRC recommendations than routine prenatal care (Vesco et al., 2014). In the extended prenatal relationship, support from one prenatal midwife is ideal. Often prenatal care is provided by a group of professionals, that is, midwives, advanced practice nurses, and physicians. When 1:1 midwife continuity of care is not possible, the following steps help foster continuity of management:

- Midwives and prenatal care providers within the group meet regularly, discuss prenatal weight gain attitudes, beliefs, and management, and develop a group consensus on messaging
- Providers select and consistently offer handouts for patients that reinforce the information

● Providers document the patient's goals, weight management plan, successes, obstacles, and revised plans for clear communication in subsequent visits

# Using MI

### *Practicing MI Skills*

The latest work by psychologists Miller and Rollnick is *Motivational Interviewing: Helping People Change* (2013). It provides background in change, motivation theory, and the precepts of MI conversations (2013). In addition to this source, the midwife might practice conversations with a colleague who has MI experience.

Another helpful technique for learning MI is to do a classic process recording such as those used in psychiatric/mental health or social work clinical learning. In a process recording, the midwife would attempt an MI conversation with a patient. Following the visit, the midwife would write out the conversation phrase by phrase, to the best of her memory. Writing down a conversation stimulates the memory to think about practice reflectively. The midwife can then review the conversation against the principles of MI. If some elements of conversation could be improved, the midwife can practice new phrases out loud or in front of a mirror like an actor learning lines, and then apply them the next time they are needed clinically.

### *One-to-One Counseling*

The dialogue in Case Study 7.2 outlines a conversation that steers the prenatal visit into discussion of weight gain. This dialogue, "Using Motivational Interviewing to Start Prenatal Weight Gain Discussion," could be used with any woman but is a gentle entry into the topic of weight for clinicians who feel awkward discussing this topic with obese or overweight women.

In the next dialogue (Case Study 7.3, "Using Motivational Interviewing When a Patient's Plan Does Not Seem to Work") the patient has gained more weight than planned since the previous prenatal visit. The midwife must acknowledge the excess weight gain while still affirming whatever strategies the patient did try. The midwife learns more about the patient as a person while gathering data and giving information that will assist the patient to take responsibility for revising her plan.

Not all patients will effortlessly take charge of their own self-care. The midwife will encounter women who are resistant to change. The midwife needs to avoid what Miller and Rollnick call *the righting reflex*. The righting reflex is the tendency of health care providers to offer a quick fix, to make the situation *right* by prescribing what should be done. Patients who seem resistant to change or to accept aspects of their own care instead should bring out the MI skills of the midwife. Case Study 7.4, "Using Motivational Interviewing to Assist a Patient When the Patient Seems Resistant," portrays a young woman with excessive weight gain between prenatal visits. Her self-efficacy is challenged by the influence of her mother.

**CASE STUDY 7.2  USING MOTIVATIONAL INTERVIEWING TO START PRENATAL WEIGHT GAIN DISCUSSION**

| Midwife | Woman | MI Concept | Comments |
|---|---|---|---|
| We've discussed the testing that we usually do during pregnancy. May we talk about prenatal weight gain? | Yeah, I have so much trouble with my weight. | Summarizing. Asking permission to discuss a potentially sensitive concept. | |
| You have trouble with your weight. Can you describe that more for me? | Well, I just look at food and my hips pop out. I've tried everything. | Reflecting what patient says. Asking for clarification and engaging patient in the conversation. | |
| It sounds as if you have experience managing your own weight. What sorts of things have you tried? | Oh, herbal teas, exercise, diets—all kinds: vegetable soups, low carb, low fat, Weight Watchers, fasting, fruit smoothies . . . | Affirming patient's experience and self-management. Asking for further clarification. | |
| You have a lot of experience with weight management. Of the weight management strategies that you've tried before, which do you think were successful? | My low-carb days and Weight Watchers were the best for me but I can't get to Weight Watchers because of work. | Affirming patient's experience. Asking for what the patient thinks is most successful instead of imposing one's own preferences or expert advice. | Use weight management instead of dieting. Weight management includes more options than dieting. |
| What did you need to do make those food plans work for you? | Well, hmmm. I guess I was careful about counting portions or what kinds of food I ate. | Asking for clarification and the patient's perception of what worked. This midwife could have said, "The Weight Watcher's plan is the proven way to manage weight." That would have closed the conversation and moved efficacy from the patient to the eating plan. | Give the patient time to consider answers to the question. Pauses in conversation give both parties time to think and increases engagement. |

*(continued)*

**CASE STUDY 7.2   USING MOTIVATIONAL INTERVIEWING TO START PRENATAL WEIGHT GAIN DISCUSSION (*continued*)**

| Midwife | Woman | MI Concept | Comments |
|---|---|---|---|
| That's good. You have experience thinking about food that will help you choose foods that are good for you and the baby during this pregnancy. What do you know about prenatal weight gain? | That you're eating for two. | Affirming, complementing the patient on something done well and tying it to current needs. Asking about patient's own knowledge. | |
| In a way you're eating for two. Mother's need vitamins and nutrients for themselves and the baby, but not calories for two. May I show you our recommendations for prenatal weight gain tailored to you? | | Affirming patient's information and filling in gaps in knowledge. Asking permission to give more information. This requests the patient's participation and encourages engagement. The patient will shape her plan instead of passively listening to information. | Avoid totally contradicting the patient. This midwife could have said, "Eating for two is too much," or "Eating for two is an old wives' tale," which would have closed the conversation. |

*Source:* Jevitt (2015).

### MI in Group Prenatal Care

An advantage list is an ideal tool for use during group prenatal care. Women can complete the advantage list in group time, and then compare strategies they have used in the past. Because so many women struggle with weight management, this generally starts a lively debate about what works and how much weight should be gained during pregnancy. Women then choose their own strategies and make a written plan. Women become their own weight management support group as they check-in on weights at each visit (Brumley & Jevitt, 2012).

It is tempting to design a special prenatal care group for women with BMIs greater than or equal to 30. However, this can have the effect of making overweight and obese women feel stigmatized. With 30% of reproductive-age women

**CASE STUDY 7.3 USING MOTIVATIONAL INTERVIEWING WHEN A PATIENT'S PLAN DOES NOT SEEM TO WORK**

| Midwife | Woman (Prepregnancy BMI of 36) | MI Concept | Comments |
|---------|-------------------------------|------------|----------|
| (Looking at the medical record) You've had a larger weight gain this month than the last 2 months. It's above the target weight gain that's in your plan. What do you think was different this month? | It was slow at work so my shifts at the restaurant got divided. I worked 3 hours in the morning and then 4 or 5 hours at night. I got called off sometimes just before the shift started. It was hellish at home trying to get the kids to school and make dinner, well it happened whenever. | The midwife in a matter-of-fact way indicates that the weight gain is outside of the plan and gives ownership of the plan to the patient. The midwife asks the patient what was different instead of saying what must change now. | The open-ended question from the midwife prompted a long, detailed response. |
| You had a lot of change to deal with. How did you manage to fit your own meals into all that? | Who knows? I just ate whenever. (Pause) And whatever. That was the last thing on my mind. | Affirms the patient's challenges. Asks for further information. | |
| So, if you used a scale of 1 to 10 this month, with 10 being the most important, where would your eating be this month in importance? | One to 10? I wasn't even on a scale. I was just getting by one day at a time. Crazy, crazy. | This is called the "Importance Ruler" in MI. Its usefulness comes not from the numerical value but how it is used to stimulate further thought and action. | |
| Ah, on autopilot. (Nodding in agreement) Mother survival mode. | Yeah. | Affirming patient's reality and obstacles. | |
| What might be done this month to move the importance of nourishing yourself and the baby from 1 to say, maybe 5? | (Heavy sigh) Well, it's a better day when I'm not so tired at work. Then I don't eat so much at the restaurant, like the fries. | Gives the patient a numerical indicator of the importance of changing this month, while asking the patient what she might be able to do. | |

(continued)

**CASE STUDY 7.3   USING MOTIVATIONAL INTERVIEWING WHEN A PATIENT'S PLAN DOES NOT SEEM TO WORK (*continued*)**

| Midwife | Woman (Prepregnancy BMI of 36) | MI Concept | Comments |
|---|---|---|---|
| Sleep is important to weight management. The ideal is 7 hours of sleep a night. What's sleep been like for you with those scattered work hours? | Hmmmm, I guess I usually go to bed about 12 and get up at 6 to get the kids to school. | Offers information. Then asks for additional information from patient while again acknowledging the difficulty in the patient's schedule related to self-care. | |
| Hmmm. That might be leaving you a little short. | I just can't get things done before midnight. I wish I could sleep more. | Mirrors patient's style while tentatively assessing sleep. | |
| You wish you could sleep more. What changes might you make that would give you more sleep, at least on the nights before you work? | Well, I could teach the kids to make their own lunches. I've been meaning to do that. I could watch less TV with Mark but that's my time with him. I guess I could drop my Bible studies until work settles down. | Reflecting the patient's desire. Asks patient for ideas. This will generate ideas that might actually work for the patient instead of ideas imposed from the outside that might fail because of the major changes required to fit the measure into the patient's routine. | "Wish" indicates a low-level motivation to change, along with words such as "hope," "want" or "would like." Words indicating a stronger motivation to change are, "need to," "must," "got to," "have to." |
| You have some ideas of what you could try. Of those, which do you think would be the easiest one for you to try this month? | Missing Bible study a week or two wouldn't hurt. I'm going to get those kids making their own lunches. That will help when the new baby comes too. | Affirms the patient's ideas without putting a good or bad value on them. Acknowledges that these are the patient's ideas. Uses patient's own self-help measures and helps patient choose a priority. Sets a time frame for the change: this month. | |

(*continued*)

**CASE STUDY 7.3   USING MOTIVATIONAL INTERVIEWING WHEN A PATIENT'S PLAN DOES NOT SEEM TO WORK (*continued*)**

| Midwife | Woman (Prepregnancy BMI of 36) | MI Concept | Comments |
|---|---|---|---|
| Those sounds like ideas that will work. So before the next visit, you'll skip Bible studies if your work schedule is jumbled and you're going to teach the kids to make their own lunches. I'll be eager to hear how those work for you. | | Affirming patient's own ideas. Summarizing the plan. Engaging the patient by stating interest in the patient's outcomes. | |

*Source:* Jevitt (2015).

having a BMI greater than or equal to 30 and another 30% being overweight (BMI of 25–29.9) and at risk for obesity following the pregnancy, women who need special eating and activity support during pregnancy will be present in any prenatal care group. During prenatal meeting times, the group facilitator uses the principles of MI to elicit women's experiences and feelings. Modeling MI language gives the entire group the opportunity to learn open-ended questions and supportive dialogue (Brumley & Jevitt, 2012).

## Counseling for Weight Management in the Postpartum Period

For most women, weight management in the postpartum will involve weight loss. The advantage list (see Table 7.2) can be revisited during the postpartum period using techniques from MI to assist the woman in making a plan for weight management during and after the postpartum period (see Figure 7.2).

Breastfeeding can be an important weight-loss tool in the postpartum period. Women can reduce intake by 500 calories per day without affecting infant growth or the quality or quantity of breast milk, enabling a gradual, 1-pound weight loss per week (Anstey & Jevitt, 2011). Women who return to their pregravid weight between pregnancies are at low risk for future obesity and are most likely to have future prenatal weight gains within the NRC recommendations (Jain et al., 2013; Nehring, Schmoll, Beyerlein, Hauner, & von Kries, 2011).

**CASE STUDY 7.4   USING MOTIVATIONAL INTERVIEWING TO ASSIST A PATIENT WHEN THE PATIENT SEEMS RESISTANT**

| Midwife | Woman (Prepregnancy BMI of 36) | MI Concept | Comments |
|---|---|---|---|
| It looks like sticking to the prenatal eating plan was tough this month. | Well, no. I mean, it's OK. The baby needs food. | Affirms the tough work of weight management. | |
| The baby needs more food. | Yeah. (*Pause and eye contact broken as patient looks at floor.*) | Reflecting the patient's statement. | |
| Can we talk about what the baby needs? | My mother talks about it all the time. | Asking permission to talk about a topic. | |
| Pregnant women get so much advice. Tell me what she tells you. | She is such a pain sometimes. She is always after me about this and that, like she has nothing else to do. She doesn't go after my sister like that. | Affirming that the patient receives a lot of opinions. Asking for additional information with an open request. | Once a rapport is established through interest in what a patient thinks, it's easy for conversations to stray. A social worker or counselor might continue to delve into the mother–daughter relationship but the prenatal care conversation has to be more focused. |
| It sounds like your mother can be difficult but what we need to talk about now is what she's told you. | She says she can't see me getting bigger so the baby must not be growing. The only way I can look pregnant is to gain more weight. | Affirming the patient's difficulties with her mother but refocusing the conversation. | |
| She says the baby isn't growing. That could worry you. | I am worried. If I don't eat enough how will the baby grow? | Reflecting patient's statement and affirming potential stress. | |

*(continued)*

**CASE STUDY 7.4   USING MOTIVATIONAL INTERVIEWING TO ASSIST A PATIENT WHEN THE PATIENT SEEMS RESISTANT (continued)**

| Midwife | Woman (Prepregnancy BMI of 36) | MI Concept | Comments |
|---|---|---|---|
| Let me review what tells me the baby is growing well. You have gained weight so you and the baby are getting enough calories. The size of your uterus when I palpate it and measure it tell me the baby is growing and 2 weeks ago you had an ultrasound that showed the baby was growing just the size he should be. | But no one else can see that I'm pregnant. | Reviewing for patient and summarizing information. | |
| Looking pregnant is important to you and pregnant women get special attention. | Yeah. My cousin is pregnant and they're always loving on her belly and fussing over her. | Reflecting patient's statement and opening the dialogue for additional information. | |
| Can you think of things that might show your mother that the baby is growing; things that make you look more pregnant? | Well, I'm going to buy one of those tops that says "Baby" with the arrow pointing to the belly and I'm going to keep wearing smaller tops so you can see the baby. | Evoking ideas with open question. | Often, assisting patients with weight management has less to do with eating dictums than facilitating lifestyle changes. |
| Let's keep thinking about ways to show her that the baby is healthy while you follow the eating plan. | That'll be hard. I'm only supposed to gain 11–15 pounds and she says the baby needs 30 pounds. | Open request. | |

(continued)

| CASE STUDY 7.4   USING MOTIVATIONAL INTERVIEWING TO ASSIST A PATIENT WHEN THE PATIENT SEEMS RESISTANT (*continued*) | | | |
| --- | --- | --- | --- |
| **Midwife** | **Woman (Prepregnancy BMI of 36)** | **MI Concept** | **Comments** |
| You have an ultrasound today. Let's ask the ultrasonographer to give you a copy with a label on it that says something like, "Baby Jackie, perfect size!" | | Reviewing care and planning. | |

*Source:* Jevitt (2015).

## Billing for Weight Management Work

The amount of conversation involved in using the language and techniques in this chapter might seem impossible to fit into a prenatal or postpartum visit. With practice, these techniques become automatic to the midwife and the conversation can continue while the midwife does an abdominal exam. However, women with BMIs greater than or equal to 30 may require extra prenatal visits for closer weight management follow-up. Most insurers, including Medicaid programs, list a BMI greater than or equal to 30 as a risk factor that permits additional prenatal visits.

Additional International Classification of Diseases, 10th revision, Clinical Modification (ICD-10-CM) codes that apply to weight management work during pregnancy and the postpartum period are included in Table 7.4. Use of these codes, in addition to prenatal care codes, should reimburse the midwife for time spent in counseling. A summary of the counseling and time spent in counseling must be documented in the medical record.

## CONCLUSION

This chapter has reviewed several evidence-based methods for assisting women in weight management during prenatal care: culturally aware food counseling, use of an advantage list, MI, goal setting, and breastfeeding during the postpartum period. No single technique alone can fully achieve weight management during pregnancy or the postpartum period, but using a combination of these methods can provide satisfying results for both the patient and the midwife.

**TABLE 7.4  ICD-10-CM Codes for Reimbursement of Weight Management Work**

| Code | Description |
|---|---|
| O99.210 | Obesity complicating pregnancy, unspecified trimester |
| O99.211 | Obesity complicating pregnancy, first trimester |
| O99.212 | Obesity complicating pregnancy, second trimester |
| O99.213 | Obesity complicating pregnancy, third trimester |
| O26.00 | Excessive weight gain in pregnancy, unspecified trimester |
| O26.01 | Excessive weight gain in pregnancy, first trimester |
| O26.02 | Excessive weight gain in pregnancy, second trimester |
| O26.03 | Excessive weight gain in pregnancy, third trimester |
| Z71.89 | Other specified counseling. This includes:<br>● Health advice, education, or counseling done<br>● Nutrition and exercise counseling<br>● Breastfeeding counseling<br>● Weight-loss counseling |

ICD-10-CM, International Classification of Diseases, 10th revision, Clinical Modification.
*Source:* Centers for Medicare & Medicaid Services (2015).

# REFERENCES

Acharya, S, D., Elci, O. U., Sereika, S. M., Styn, M. A. & Burke, L. E. (2011). Using a personal digital assistant for self-monitoring influences diet quality in comparison to a standard paper record among overweight/obese adults. *Journal of the American Dietetic Association, 111*(4), 583–588.

American College of Nurse-Midwives (ACNM). (2015). Our philosophy of care. Retrieved from http://www.midwife.org/Our-Philosophy-of-Care

American College of Obstetricians and Gynecologists (ACOG). (2013). *Obesity in pregnancy. ACOG Committee Opinion #549.* Washington, DC: Author.

Andreyeva, T., Long, M., Henderson, K., & Grode, G. (2010). Trying to lose weight: Diet strategies among Americans with overweight or obesity in 1996 and 2003. *Journal of the American Dietetic Association, 110,* 535–542.

Anstey, E., & Jevitt, C. (2011). Maternal obesity and breastfeeding: A review of the evidence and implications for practice. *Clinical Lactation, 2–3,* 11–16.

Armstrong, M., Mottershead, T., Ronksley, P., Sigal, R., Campbell, T., & Hemmelgarn, B. (2011). Motivational interviewing to improve weight loss in overweight and/or obese patients: A systematic review and meta-analysis of randomized controlled trials. *Obesity Reviews, 12*(9), 709–723.

Boden, G., Sargrad, K., Homko, C., Mozzoli, M., & Stein, T. P. (2005). Effect of a low-carbohydrate diet on appetite, blood glucose levels, and insulin resistance in obese patients with type 2 diabetes. *Annals of Internal Medicine, 142*(6), 403–411.

Brownell, K. D., Kersh, R., Ludwig, D. S., Post, R. C., Puhl, R. M., Schwartz, M. B., & Willett, W. C. (2010). Personal responsibility and obesity: A constructive approach to a controversial issue. *Health Affairs, 29*(3), 379–387. doi:10.1377/hlthaff.2009.0739

Brumley, J., & Jevitt, C. (2012). Optimizing prenatal weight gain through group prenatal care. *Journal of Obstetric Gynecologic and Neonatal Nursing, 41*(S1), S21. doi:10.1111/j.1552-6909 .2012.01359_24.x

Brunstrom, J. M., & Mitchell, G. L. (2006). Effects of distraction on the development of satiety. *British Journal of Nutrition, 96*(4), 761–769.

Burke, B., Arkowitz, J., & Menchola, M. (2003). The efficacy of motivational interviewing: A meta-analysis of controlled clinical trials. *Journal of Consulting and Clinical Psychology, 71*(5), 843–861.

Byrd-Bredbenner, C., Abbot, J. M., & Cussler, E. (2011). Relationship of social cognitive theory concepts to mothers' dietary intake and BMI. *Maternal and Child Nutrition, 7*(3), 241–252.

Centers for Disease Control and Prevention (CDC). (2015). Physical activity for healthy pregnant or postpartum women. Retrieved from http://www.cdc.gov/physicalactivity/ basics/pregnancy/index.htm

Centers for Medicare & Medicaid Services. (2015). ICD-10 codes for reimbursement of weight management work. Retrieved from https://www.cms.gov/medicare-coverage-database/static pages/icd-10-code-lookup.aspx

Chaput, J. P., Klingenberg, I., & Sjodin, A. M. (2010). Do all sedentary activities lead to weight gain: Sleep does not. *Current Opinion in Clinical and Metabolic Care, 13*(6), 601–607. doi:10.1097/MCO.0b013e32833ef30e

de Jong, E., Visscher, T. L., HiraSing, R. A., Seidell, J. C., & Renders, C. M. (2015). Home environmental determinants of children's fruit and vegetable consumption across different SES backgrounds. *Pediatric Obesity, 10*(2), 134–140.

Deputy, N., Sharma, A., & Kim, S. (2015). Gestational weight gain—United States 2012 and 2013. *Morbidity and Mortality Weekly Report, 64*(43), 1215–1220.

Edelstein, S. (2011). *Food, cuisine, and cultural competency for culinary, hospitality, and nutrition professionals.* Sudbury, MA: Jones & Bartlett Learning.

Fitzpatrick, E., Edmunds, L. S., & Dennison, B. A. (2007). Positive effects of family dinner are undone by television viewing. *Journal of the American Dietetic Association, 107*(4), 666–671.

Foster, G. D., Wadden, T. A., LaGrotte, C. A., Vander Veur, S. S., Hesson, L. A., Homko, C. J., . . . Vetter, M. L. (2013). A randomized comparison of a commercially available portion-controlled weight loss intervention with a diabetes self-management education program. *Nutrition & Diabetes, 3*, e63.

Gudzune, K. A., Bennett, W. L., Cooper, L. A., & Bleich, S. N. (2014). Perceived judgement about weight can negatively influence weight loss: A cross-sectional study of overweight and obese patients. *Preventative Medicine, 62*, 103–107.

Gudzune, K. A., Doshi, R. S., Mehta, A. K., Chaudhry, Z. W., Jacobs, D. K., Vakil, R. M., . . . Clark, J. M. (2015). Efficacy of commercial weight-loss programs: An updated systematic review. *Annals of Internal Medicine, 162*(7), 501–512.

Hammons, A. J., & Fiese, B. H. (2011). Is frequency of shared family meals related to the nutritional health of children and adolescents? *Pediatrics, 127*(6), e1565–574.

Horan, M. K., McGowan, C. A., Gibney, E. R., Donnelly, J. M., & McAuliffe, F. M. (2014). Maternal diet and weight at 3 months postpartum following a pregnancy intervention with a low glycemic index diet: Results from the ROLO randomized controlled trial. *Nutrients*, 6(7), 2946–2955.

Jacobs, D. R. (2006). Fast food and sedentary lifestyle: A combination that leads to obesity. *American Journal of Clinical Nutrition*, 83, 189–190.

Jain, A. P., Gavard, J. A., Rice, J. J., Catanzaro, R. B., Artal, R., & Hopkins, S. A. (2013). The impact of interpregnancy weight change on birthweight in obese women. *American Journal of Obstetrics and Gynecology*, 208(3), 1–7. doi:10.1016/j.ajog.2012.12.018

Juanola-Falgarona, M., Salas-Salvado, J., Ibarrola-Jurado, N., Rabassa-Soler, A., Diaz-Lopez, A., Guasch-Ferr, M., . . . Bullo, M. (2014). Effect of the glycemic index of the diet on weight loss, modulation of satiety, inflammation, and other metabolic risk factors: A randomized controlled trial. *American Journal of Clinical Nutrition*, 100(1), 27–35. doi:10.3945/ajcn.113.081216

King, T., Brucker, M., Kriebs, J., Fahey, J., Gegor, C., & Varney, J. (2015). *Varney's midwifery* (5th ed.). Sudbury, MA: Jones & Bartlett Learning.

Lau, C., Rogers, J. M., Desai, M., & Ross, M. G. (2011). Fetal programming of adult disease: Implications for prenatal care. *Obstetrics and Gynecology*, 117(4), 978–985. doi:10.1097/AOG.0b013e318212140e

Lundahl, B., Moleni, T., Burke, B., Tollefson, D., Butler, C., & Rollnick, S. (2013). Motivational interviewing in medical care settings: A systematic review and meta-analysis of randomized controlled trials. *Patient Education and Counseling*, 93(2), 157–168.

Malik, V. S., Schulze, M. B., & Hu, F. B. (2006). Intake of sugar-sweetened beverages and weight gain: A systematic review. *American Journal of Clinical Nutrition*, 84(2), 274–288.

Miller, W. R., & Rollnick, S. (2013). *Motivational interviewing: Helping people change* (3rd ed.). New York, NY: Guildford Press.

Milsom, V. A., Middleton, K. M., & Perri, M. G. (2011) Successful long-term weight loss maintenance in a rural population. *Clinical Interventions in Aging*, 6, 303–309.

National Research Council (NRC). (2009). *Weight gain during pregnancy: Reexamining the guidelines*. Washington, DC: National Academies Press.

Nehring, I., Schmoll, S., Beyerlein, A., Hauner, H., & von Kries, R. (2011). Gestational weight gain and long-term postpartum weight retention: A meta-analysis. *American Journal of Clinical Nutrition*, 94(5), 1225–1231.

Patel, S. R., Malhotra, A., White, D. P., Gottlieb, D., & Hu, F. (2006). Association between reduced sleep and weight gain in women. *American Journal of Epidemiology*, 164(10), 947–954.

Rose, S. A., Poynter, P. S., Anderson, J. W., Noar, S. M., & Conigliaro, J. (2013). Physician weight loss advice and patient weight loss behavior change: A literature review and meta-analysis of survey data. *International Journal of Obesity*, 37, 118–128.

Rubak, S., Sandbaek, A., Lauritzen, T., & Christensen, B. (2005). Motivational interviewing: A systematic review and meta-analysis. *British Journal of General Practice*, 55(513), 305–312.

Ruiz, J. R., Perales, M., Pelaez, M., Lopez, C., Lucia, A., & Barakat, R. (2013). Supervised exercise-based intervention to prevent excessive gestational weight gain: A randomized controlled trial. *Mayo Clinic Proceedings*, 88(12), 1388–1397.

Schulze, M. B., Manson, J. E., Ludwig, D. S., Colditz, G. A., Stampfer, M. J., Willett, W. D., & Hu, F. B. (2004). Sugar-sweetened beverages, weight gain, and incidence of type 2 diabetes in young and middle-aged women. *Journal of the American Medical Association, 292*(8), 927–934. doi:10.1001/jama.292.8.927

Taveras, E. M., McDonald, J., O'Brien, A., Haines, J., Sherry, B., Bottino, C. J., . . . Koziol, R. (2012). Healthy habits, happy homes: Methods and baseline data of a randomized controlled trial to improve household routines for obesity prevention. *Preventative Medicine, 55*(5), 418–426.

Tobias, D. K., Chen, M., Manson, J. E., Ludwig, D. S., Willett, W., & Hu, F. B. (2015). Effect of low-fat diet interventions versus other diet interventions on long-term weight change in adults: A systematic review and meta-analysis. *Lancet Diabetes Endocrinology, 3*(12), 968–979.

Vesco, K., Karanja, N., King, J., Gillman, M., Leo, M., Perrin, N., . . . Stevens, V. (2014). Efficacy of a group-based dietary intervention for limiting gestational weight gain among women: A randomized trial. *Obesity, 22*(9), 1989–1996.

Wansink, B., & van Kleef, E. (2014). Dinner rituals that correlate with child and adult BMI. *Obesity, 22*, E91–95.

Waring, M. E., Moore Simas, T. A., & Liao, X. (2013). Gestational weight gain within recommended ranges in consecutive pregnancies: A retrospective cohort study. *Midwifery, 29*(5), 550–556.

Weiss, E. P., Albert, S. G., Reeds, D. N., Kress, K. S., Ezekiel, U. R., McDaniel, J. L., . . . Villareal, D. T. (2015). Calorie restriction and matched weight loss from exercise: Independent and additive effects on glucoregulation and the incretin system in overweight women and men. *Diabetes Care, 38*(7), 1253–1262.

Williams, C. B., Mackenzie, K. C., & Gahagan, S. (2014). The effect of maternal obesity on the offspring. *Clinical Obstetrics and Gynecology, 57*(3), 508–515.

Wing, R. R., & Phelan, S. (2005). Long-term weight loss maintenance. *American Journal of Clinical Nutrition, 82*(Suppl. 1), 222S–225S.

Zoumas-Morse, C., Rock, C. L., Sobo, E. J., & Neuhouser, M. L. (2001). Children's patterns of macronutrient intake and associations with restaurant eating and home eating. *Journal of the American Dietetic Association, 101*(8), 923–925.

# CHAPTER EIGHT

# MATERNAL CONCERNS AND KNOWLEDGE ABOUT VACCINATION DURING PREGNANCY: COUNSELING CHILDBEARING WOMEN

Deborah M. Brickner

## THE VACCINATION CONTROVERSY

### Parental Concerns

Although immunization is considered to be one of the greatest benefits of modern health care, parents have concerns regarding the safety of the current childhood immunization schedule (Glanz et al., 2013). These concerns lead parents to seek information on childhood vaccines from multiple sources, including potentially unreliable sources such as friends, websites, and celebrities (Freed, Clark, Butchard, Singer, & Davis, 2011).

Antivaccination groups use fear tactics such as claiming that vaccines contain poison, cause diseases of unknown origin, and erode immunity (Kata, 2009). Parents who have heard these claims may become overly suspicious of any health care provider claiming that vaccines are safe (Kata, 2009). Current evidence has demonstrated that parents who are hesitant to accept vaccines are more likely to form their resistance during pregnancy and reassess that resistance frequently (Glanz et al., 2013). This pattern would suggest a need for childhood immunization education to begin during pregnancy and continue during pediatric visits throughout the first few years of the child's life.

The American College of Nurse-Midwives (ACNM) has partnered with the Centers for Disease Control and Prevention (CDC) to improve vaccine uptake in women, and the National Vaccine Advisory Committee (NVAC) has worked to reduce patient and provider barriers to maternal immunization (ACNM, 2014; NVAC, 2014). It is recommended that women be up to date on all adult vaccinations prior to pregnancy, and that they receive the influenza injection and the Tdap (tetanus, diphtheria, pertussis) vaccine in each pregnancy (March of Dimes, 2015). Yet, immunization coverage rates among pregnant women remain low (ACNM, 2014; NVAC, 2014).

## Herd Immunity

Vaccines develop immunity by imitating infection without causing illness, leading the immune system to produce lymphocytes and antibodies that remember how to fight exposure in the future (CDC, 2012). The immune response may cause minor reactions such as injection site tenderness, low-grade fever, and irritability. However, the prevention benefits far outweigh side effects for almost all children; although a link between vaccines and autism has been suggested, scientific studies continue to show no relationship.

According to the CDC (2012), concerns regarding immune system overload are also unfounded as the amount of antigens contained in vaccines is only a fraction of the antigens normally encountered each day in an infant's usual environment. Although some individuals hold the opinion that natural immunity formed by actually having the disease offers a stronger and better immune response, natural immunity has the risk of significant complications, lasting damage, or even death (CDC, 2012).

There are several types of vaccines. *Live attenuated vaccines*, including the measles, mumps, and rubella (MMR), varicella, and nasal flu vaccine contain live viruses. Theses vaccines are weakened so that they cannot cause disease in those with healthy immune systems. These live vaccines teach the immune system how to repel the disease but should not be given to anyone with a weakened immune system or during pregnancy (CDC. 2012). *Inactivated vaccines*, such as polio, contain the dead virus and often need multiple doses to build up immunity (CDC, 2012). *Toxoid vaccines*, such as diphtheria and tetanus, contain weakened toxins or toxoids and teach the body how to repel these toxins (CDC, 2012). *Subunit vaccines* contain only the essential antigen part of a virus or bacteria, such as that used for pertussis or whooping cough, and are less likely to cause side effects (CDC, 2012). *Conjugated vaccines* are designed to combat specific bacteria, such as *Haemophilus influenzae* (Hib), that have antigens with a polysaccharide coating to disguise them from recognition by a young child's immature immune system. These vaccines connect or conjugate the coating to the antigen allowing the immature immune system to react and develop an immune response (CDC, 2012).

*Herd immunity* is defined as a sufficiently high percentage of a population with immunity to an infectious disease so that infectious disease will not be able to spread (CDC, 2014). Herd immunity allows those who cannot be vaccinated because of age or weakened immune systems to have the benefit of protection against vaccine-preventable diseases (VPDs). Vaccinations are not ever completely effective and herd immunity helps to protect those who cannot mount an immune response to a vaccine (CDC, 2014). As vaccine refusal increases among certain populations, herd immunity levels may decrease below that which is needed to protect the most vulnerable populations (CDC, 2014).

## THE HISTORY AND UPTAKE OF VACCINATIONS

### Political Issues

The safety of vaccines has remained a volatile political issue since the beginning of their use. In Britain, by the 1850s, fearing that the vaccine was more dangerous than the disease, an antivaccination league was formed to oppose compulsory smallpox vaccination, fearing that the vaccine was more dangerous than the disease (Poland & Jacobson, 2012). According to Poland and Jacobson (2012), antivaccination arguments have remained similar through time. Those concerns include that vaccines cause antigen overload and autoimmune disorders, and that immunizations are more dangerous than the infectious diseases they prevent.

The public health success of vaccines has caused incidence rates of VPDs to become so low that fear of potentially deadly infectious diseases has been replaced with fear of vaccine side effects (Olpinski, 2012). Although it seems the unconfirmed information distributed through the antivaccination movement is accepted at face value, vaccine-hesitant parents have expressed a low level of trust in vaccine information from clinicians (Glanz et al., 2013). Besides providing misinformation on vaccine safety and effectiveness, some present antivaccine arguments are based on civil liberty rights, conspiracy theories, and perceived levels of morality (Kata, 2009).

In the 1960s, federal laws providing funding for vaccines and mandatory state immunization laws appeared (Harris, Hughbanks-Wheaton, Johnston, & Kubin, 2007). However, all state laws currently allow medical exemptions; religious exemptions exist in 46 states, and philosophical exemptions are accepted in 19 states (CDC, 2011). As vaccine refusal increases, a growing public health concern is that herd immunity levels may decrease to the level of failure of immunization coverage (Brunson, 2013; Kata, 2009; Sadaf, Richards, Glanz, Salmon, & Omer, 2013).

Following a measles outbreak traced back to Disneyland, the state of California went from being one of the most accommodating states regarding vaccine exemptions to one of the strictest when California Senate Bill No. 277 (2015) was signed into law by Governor Jerry Brown on June 30, 2015. This law removed all vaccine exemptions other than medical thus requiring all immune-competent children to receive all recommended childhood vaccines in order to attend public school.

### Cost–Benefit

Analyses of the cost of immunization and attendant education to decrease vaccine hesitancy are minor compared with the cost of treating VPDs (World Health Organization [WHO], 2004; Zhou et al., 2014). Zhou et al. (2014) calculated that vaccinating all the children born in the United States according to the current childhood immunization schedule in 1 year (2009) alone would result in 42,000 lives saved and 20 million cases of infectious diseases prevented. This level of intervention would save $13.5 billion in direct cost and $68.8 billion in total societal costs (Zhou et al., 2014).

Currently, in the United States, all children may receive vaccines at no cost either through their health insurance company or through the vaccines for children (VFC) program. The VFC program, administered by the CDC and managed at the state level, distributes childhood immunizations at no cost to eligible providers (CDC, 2014).

## Cultural Factors Affecting Uptake

The NVAC recently published recommendations on reducing patient and provider barriers to maternal immunizations. There were several recommendations for increasing knowledge and self-efficacy among prenatal care providers (NVAC, 2014). ACNM has now partnered with the CDC and the Association of State and Territorial Health Officials (ASTHO) in implementing a national program to improve vaccination rates in both pregnant woman and women who identify themselves as racial–ethnic minorities (ACNM, 2014).

However, recent evidence indicates that only 43% of certified nurse-midwives (CNMs) currently accept the influenza vaccine for themselves, refusing the flu vaccine because of doubts about necessity, safety, and effectiveness (Ishola, Permalloo, Cordery, & Anderson, 2013). In one study, 48% of midwives identified that integrating pertussis vaccine education and administration into their practice would be moderately easy, with 22% responding that it would be moderately difficult (Cooper-Robbins, Lesak, Hayles, & Sinn, 2011). In a study by Bean and Catania (2013), 47% of Oregon health care providers interviewed (physicians, nurses, chiropractors, and midwives) voiced concerns about one or more of the vaccines currently included in the childhood immunization schedule. The provided reasons for concern encompassed that natural immunity has a greater benefit, vaccines may cause immune system overload, and that evidence for vaccination is skewed by a profit motive (Bean & Catania, 2013).

A survey conducted by ACNM in July 2014 indicated that 21% of midwives had changed their practice since the CDC/ACNM/ASTHO partnership program was implemented. As of the time of the survey, 44% of midwives stated that they were now asking every woman about her immunization status, and 76% were recommending the appropriate vaccines. Among the midwives who have not changed their practice, 12% report that they do not think vaccines are safe. ACNM is continuing to expand its program to promote vaccines and has received funding from the CDC for another year (ACNM, 2014).

In an unpublished doctoral capstone project, Brickner (2014) conducted an online survey of 87 midwife members of the Tennessee State Affiliate of ACNM. Brickner queried members on their current practices and attitudes toward vaccines. With a response rate of 25.3% (n = 22), Brickner reported that 95.5% of the respondents frequently recommended the influenza vaccine to their pregnant patients, 82% frequently recommended the Tdap vaccine in the third trimester, and 81% frequently recommended Tdap in the postpartum period (Brickner, 2014).

Bricker's results indicated that only 23% of these midwives frequently discussed childhood vaccines with their pregnant patients, with 54% sometimes discussing, and 23% never discussing childhood vaccinations (Brickner, 2014). When the midwives were asked to provide all reasons as to why they do not offer childhood vaccine information to their pregnant patients, these responses were provided:

- 45.5% stated they lacked time
- 31.8% indicated this health education content was a pediatric role
- 31.8% never thought about it
- 27.3% expressed lack of confidence in answering questions on childhood vaccines
- 13.6% expressed fear of upsetting vaccine-hesitant patients
- 4.5% cited concerns over vaccine safety (Brickner, 2014)

Among the midwife respondents, 82% indicated interest in a continuing-education module on the safety and benefits of the current infant and toddler immunization schedule, and 91% stated they were interested in a module on how to discuss childhood vaccines with vaccine-hesitant parents (Brickner, 2014). When the midwives were asked whether they were willing to encourage their patients to accept vaccines for their children, only 9% of the midwives responded that they were unwilling to encourage vaccine acceptance (Brickner, 2014).

## BEST PRACTICES IN PROMOTING VACCINATION UPTAKE

### Role of the ACNM in Promoting Vaccination Uptake

The ACNM is committed to improving vaccination rates among pregnant women (ACNM, 2014). Public health efforts to increase vaccination rates among pregnant women became critical during the 2009 H1N1 outbreak when pregnant women were disproportionately affected with severe complications (NAVC, 2014).

In partnership with the CDC and ASTHO, ACNM has a national-level initiative that strives to improve vaccination rates in women. The initiative includes access to professional resources and patient education materials on vaccination for midwives to use. The ACNM initiative, Our Moment of Truth, provides clear, readable information and works in tandem with the ACNM focus on vaccination (ACNM, 2014; see www.ourmomentoftruth.com). Midwives are encouraged to use these resources, readily available on the ACNM website.

### Maternal Immunization and Cocooning

Maternal immunization, as a means of protecting infants from VPDs, has been used globally since the 1970s. Young infants have very naïve immune systems that rely on maternal antibodies transferred in utero or during breastfeeding. Maternal antibodies transfer through the placenta beginning at week 17 and peak at week 30 (NVAC, 2014).

Cocooning is the process of protecting infants too young to be vaccinated by vaccinating all those in contact with the infant. Although this strategy is recommended, studies have shown that it is difficult to implement logistically. Cocooning should be used as an adjunct to maternal immunization (NVAC, 2014).

Since 1999, the United Nations Children's Fund (UNICEF) has reported a 90% decrease in neonatal tetanus mortality as a result of encouraging nations to establish a policy vaccinating pregnant women with two or more doses of tetanus toxoid (NVAC, 2014). Authors of multiple studies have concluded that maternal influenza immunization can decrease the incidence of the disease in infants younger than 6 months of age by up to 63%. Maternal vaccination results in decreased hospitalization rates among infants who do contact influenza and it is a contributing factor in decreasing preterm and small-for-gestational-age babies (NVAC, 2014). Maternal antibodies to pertussis cross the placenta readily. Neonates and infants up to 2 months of age have significantly higher serum antibody concentrations if mothers are vaccinated during pregnancy compared to the postpartum period (NVAC, 2014). At present, the recommendation is to vaccinate every pregnant woman against pertussis during the second half of every pregnancy (NVAC, 2014).

## Vaccination Counseling

Midwives and other providers of prenatal care have the opportunity to provide counseling on vaccinations during preconception, pregnancy, and the postpartum period. Vaccine hesitancy forms prior to parenthood, therefore counseling should include information on childhood vaccines as well as adult vaccine recommendations (Glanz et al., 2013). Klein et al. (2009) found that vaccine-hesitant mothers who were surveyed after giving birth would have preferred to have received childhood immunization information during pregnancy. A randomized controlled trial by Saitoh et al. (2013) concluded that perinatal immunization education increased women's knowledge of vaccines and their intention to vaccinate, and resulted in increased vaccine uptake with their children.

There is a growing need for trusted clinicians, like midwives, to engage in the discussion of vaccine safety with their clients (Fairbrother, Fuentes-Afflick, Ross, & Thomas, 2013). Vaccine-hesitant parents may be suspicious of the health care environment (Glanz et al., 2013) and their need to seek out midwifery care, especially for out-of-hospital birth, may speak to this distrust of the mainstream medical culture.

Midwives are committed to a philosophy of individualized and self-guided care, generally supporting nonintervention in physiologic processes (ACNM, 2010). Midwives spend considerable time with their prenatal patients, which often offers opportunities for midwives to discuss issues and for patients to consider choices; for example, intermittent fetal monitoring, what to eat while in labor, water birth, out-of-hospital birth, and extended breastfeeding. Although midwives may be hesitant to forge into an area of patient doubt, the trust women place in midwives and the midwives' respect for autonomy provide an avenue for the midwife to help women objectively examine the evidence on vaccine safety. Because trust in the source of the information is critical in vaccination decision making, the midwife's expressed confidence in the benefits of immunization may ease the women's concerns (Glanz et al., 2013).

## Current Vaccination Recommendations

The CDC (2015b) recommends that all adults be current on the following vaccines:

- Influenza
- Tetanus, diphtheria, pertussis (Td or Tdap)
- Varicella
- Human papilloma virus (HPV)
- MMR
- Both pneumococcal pneumonia vaccines and vaccines for meningococcal meningitis, hepatitis A, hepatitis B, and Hib are dependent upon medical, occupational, or lifestyle risk factors

Preconception counseling should include assessment of vaccination or immunity status for the MMR, varicella, Tdap, HPV, and influenza vaccines. Currently, the Tdap vaccine is recommended in every pregnancy after the first trimester. Influenza is more likely to cause serious illness in pregnant women. It is now recommended that all pregnant women routinely be given the flu shot (not the nasal mist) at any stage of pregnancy (CDC, 2015a; March of Dimes, 2015). Vaccination for hepatitis A and B may be administered if the woman is at high risk (CDC, 2015b). All adult immunizations are considered to be safe while breastfeeding (March of Dimes, 2015). The current childhood immunization schedule is revised by the CDC regularly and available on the CDC website as well as state health department and immunization websites.

## Vaccination Resources

Several reliable websites offer vaccine information for clinicians as well as teaching materials for patients. As recommendations are continually being revised, midwives may also subscribe to e-mail updates. Some key websites include:

- CDC: www.cdc.gov/vaccines
- ACNM: www.ourmomentoftruth.com
- March of Dimes: www.marchofdimes.org/pregnancy/vaccinations
- The Children's Hospital of Philadelphia: www.chop.edu/centers-programs/vaccine

## USING THE EVIDENCE FOR BEST PRACTICE

### Case Study 8.1   The Vaccine-Hesitant Primipara

Jenna is a 28-year-old gravida 1 para 0 who entered prenatal care at 7 weeks and has been compliant with all her visits and testing to this point. On her visit at 24 weeks, she received teaching material on influenza and Tdap vaccines. When the midwife enters the room, Jenna expresses concern over the safety of vaccines in pregnancy. She states she has heard that there is mercury and other poisons in vaccines, which could harm the baby or cause him to be autistic. Jenna also states she has never gotten the flu vaccine before and has always been fine. She states she does not feel safe risking her baby's health by agreeing to be vaccinated in pregnancy. While listening to her concerns, the midwife is also aware that two other women are already waiting in exam rooms after Jenna's appointment.

### Exemplar of Best Practice

A difficult juggling act for the midwife, she must give accurate information on the benefits and safety of vaccines, but not alienate Jenna, and keep on schedule with her other patients. The midwife first attempts to dispel some myths. She assures Jenna that links between autism and vaccines have been thoroughly disproven. She explains that mercury (thimerosal) is not used in vaccines given to pregnant women.

She provides a simple explanation of the potential risks of serious complications of flu in pregnancy and points to some recent outbreaks of VPDs. The midwife provides a brief explanation on how placental transfer of antibodies will protect her newborn from potentially fatal pertussis. This information may help Jenna to make an informed choice.

Finally, in a nonjudgmental fashion, the midwife encourages Jenna to read the teaching material again. Jenna agrees to take the material home and reread it. The midwife makes a note on the record to address Jenna's concerns and offer the vaccines again at her next visit.

# REFERENCES

American College of Nurse-Midwives (ACNM). (2010). Philosophy of care. Retrieved from http://www.midwife.org/index.asp?bid=18

American College of Nurse-Midwives (ACNM). (2014). Immunization recommendations. Retrieved from http://www.midwife.org/ImmunizeWomen

Bean, S., & Catania, J. (2013). Vaccine perceptions among Oregon health care providers. *Qualitative Health Research*, 23(9), 1251–1266. doi:10.1177/1049732313501891

Brickner, D. (2014). *Certified nurse-midwives practices and attitudes toward prenatal education on childhood vaccines* (Unpublished doctor of nursing practice capstone project). Frontier Nursing University, Hyden, Kentucky.

Brunson, E. (2013). How parents make decisions about their children's vaccinations. *Vaccine*, 31(46), 5466–5470. doi:10.1016/j.vaccine.2013.08.104

California Senate Bill 277 Legislative Counsel's Digest. (2015). Retrieved from http://leginfo.legislature.ca.gov/faces/billTextClient.xhtml?bill_

Centers for Disease Control and Prevention (CDC). (2011). School and childcare vaccination surveys: School vaccination requirements, exemptions and web links. Retrieved from http://www2a.cdc.gov/nip/schoolsurv/schImmRqmtReport.asp?s=grantee&d=4&w=WHERE%20a.gradeID=1%20AND%20a.vaccineID=1

Centers for Disease Control and Prevention (CDC). (2012). Infant immunization FAQs. Retrieved from http://www.cdc.gov/vaccines/parents/parent-questions.html

Centers for Disease Control and Prevention (CDC). (2014). Vaccines for children program (VFC). Retrieved from http://www.cdc.gov/vaccines/programs/vfc/index.html

Centers for Disease Control and Prevention (CDC). (2015a). Flu vaccine safety and pregnancy: Questions and answers. Retrieved from http://www.cdc.gov/flu/protect/vaccine/qa_vacpregnant.htm

Centers for Disease Control and Prevention (CDC). (2015b). Vaccine information for adults: These are vaccines you need as an adult. Retrieved from http://www.cdc.gov/vaccines/adults/index.html

Cooper-Robbins, S. C., Lesak, J., Hayles, E. H., & Sinn, J. K. (2011). Midwife attitudes: An important determinant of maternal postpartum pertussis booster vaccine. *Vaccine, 29*(34), 5591–5594. doi:10.1016/j.vaccine.2011.05.049

Fairbrother, G., Fuentes-Afflick, E., Ross, L. F., & Thomas, P. A. (2013). Communicating with parents about immunization safety: Messages for pediatricians in the IOM report "The childhood immunization schedule and safety: Stakeholder concerns, scientific evidence, and future studies." *Academic Pediatrics, 13*(5), 387–398. doi:10.1016/j.acap.2013.06.002

Freed, G. L., Clark, S. J., Butchart, A. T., Singer, D. C., & Davis, M. M. (2011). Sources and perceived credibility of vaccine-safety information for parents. *Pediatrics, 127*(Suppl. 1), s107–s112. doi:10.1542/peds.2010-1722P

Glanz, J. M., Wagner, N. M., Narwaney, K. J., Shoup, J. A., McClure, D. L., McCormick, E. V., & Daley, M. F. (2013). A mixed methods study of parental vaccine decision making and parent-provider trust. *Academic Pediatrics, 13*(5), 481–488. doi:10.1016/j.acap.2013.05.030

Harris, K. M., Hughbanks-Wheaton, D. K., Johnston, R., & Kubin, L. (2007). Parental refusal or delay of childhood immunization: Implications for nursing and health education. *Teaching and Learning in Nursing, 2*(4), 126–132. doi:10.1016/j.teln.2007.07.005

Ishola, D. A., Jr., Permalloo, N., Cordery, R. J., & Anderson, S. R. (2013). Midwives influenza vaccine uptake and their views on vaccination of pregnant women. *Journal of Public Health, 35*(4), 570–577. doi:10.1093/pubmed/fds109

Kata, A. (2009). A postmodern Pandora's box: Anti-vaccination misinformation on the internet. *Vaccine, 28*(7), 1709–1716. doi:10.1016/j.vaccine.2009.12.022

Klein, N. P., Kissner, J., Aguirre, A., Sparks, R., Campbell, S., Edwards, K. M., . . . Gust, D. A. (2009). Differential maternal responses to a newly developed vaccine information packet. *Vaccine, 28*(2), 323–328. doi:10.1016/j.vaccine.2009.10.046

March of Dimes. (2015). Vaccinations and pregnancy. Retrieved from http://www.marchofdimes.org/pregnancy/vaccinations-during-pregnancy.aspx#

National Vaccine Advisory Committee (NVAC). (2014). Reducing patient and provider barriers to maternal immunizations [Reports and Recommendations]. *Public Health Reports, 130*, 10–42. Retrieved from http://www.hhs.gov/nvpo/nvac/reports/nvac_reducing_patient_barriers_maternal_immunizations.pdf

Olpinski, A. (2012). Anti-vaccination movement and parental refusals of immunization of children in USA. *Pediatria Polska, 87*(4), 381–385. doi:10.1016/j.pepo.2012.05.003

Poland, G. A., & Jacobson, R. M. (2012). The clinician's guide to the anti-vaccinationists' galaxy. *Human Immunology, 73*(8), 859–866. doi:10.1016/j.humimm.2012.03.014

Sadaf, A., Richards, J. L., Glanz, J., Salmon, D. A., & Omer, S. B. (2013). A systematic review of interventions for reducing parental vaccine refusal and vaccine hesitancy. *Vaccine, 31*(40), 4293–4304. doi:10.1016/j.vaccine.2013.07.013

Saitoh, A., Nagata, S., Saitoh, A., Tsukahara, Y., Vaida, F., Sonobe, T., . . . Murashima, S. (2013). Perinatal immunization education improves immunization rates and knowledge: A randomized controlled trial. *Preventive Medicine, 56*(6), 398–405. doi:10.1016/j.ypmed .2013.03.003

World Health Organization (WHO). (2004). Economics of immunization: A guide to the literature and other resources. Retrieved from http://apps.who.int/iris/bitstream/10665/68526/1/ WHO_V-B_04.02_eng.pdf?ua=1

Zhou, F., Shefer, A., Wenger, J., Messioner, M., Wang, L. Y., Lopez, A., . . . Rodewald, L. (2014) Economic evaluation of the routine childhood immunization program in the United States, 2009. *Pediatrics, 133*(4), 577–585. doi:10.1542/peds.2013-0698

# CHAPTER NINE

# WOMEN IN MIGRATION: BEST PRACTICES IN MIDWIFERY

Jane M. Dyer

## WOMEN IN MIGRATION

The United States is home to women in migration from many countries who have come through a variety of mechanisms and for a variety of reasons. These women frequently are underinsured or uninsured, may prefer a female provider, and often access care in systems serving underserved populations. As more than 70% of women who receive care from midwives are considered vulnerable by virtue of their socioeconomic status, age, education, ethnicity, or residence, midwives are often the providers of midwifery care to women in migration (American College of Nurse-Midwives [ACNM], n.d.). These women bring beliefs about health, illness, healing, and pregnancy. It is imperative that midwives develop an approach to assure that these women receive culturally appropriate and quality care.

## Terminology

An alien is any person who is not a citizen of the United States (U.S. Citizenship and Immigration Services [USCIS], 2015), but migration terminology is confusing. Persons may come to the United States as foreign born, immigrants, or aliens. Immigrants are people who choose to resettle or migrate to another country. They may become naturalized citizens or lawful permanent residents, or they may have entered as undocumented persons (USCIS, 2015).

Others come with refugee status. The United States has resettled more refugees than any other country in the world (Zong & Batalova, 2015a), until perhaps the recent events resulting from the Syrian migration and settlement in Jordan. Refugees and those seeking asylum may be lumped under one term, but they are actually different. The *1951 Convention Relating to the Status of Refugees* (United Nations General Assembly, 1951) specifies that a refugee is someone who:

[O]wing to a well-founded fear of being persecuted for reasons of race, religion, nationality, membership of a particular social group or political opinion, is outside the country of his nationality, and is unable to, or owing to such fear, is unwilling to avail himself of the protection of that country. (p. 14)

A person with asylum status meets the definition of refugee but is already on U.S. soil at the time of application or alternately, seeks admission as an asylee at a port of entry. An asylee is one who has suffered persecution or fears persecution because of race, religion, nationality, or membership in a particular social group or political opinion (USCIS, 2015). There are many types of visas and once here, a new resident may hold any one of these visas, potentially be eligible for permanent residency, or engage in the process of becoming a naturalized citizen. The services and types of assistance available differ by legal status, state of residence, and length of time in the United States.

## The Scope of Immigration

The American Community Survey (2012) estimates that 40 million or 13% of the total U.S. population are immigrants, with almost 12 million entering after the year 2000, although the actual numbers are difficult to capture. Although statistics are kept for the numbers of those entering under refugee or asylum status, there are only estimates for the numbers of those entering without documentation. Also, secondary migration, people moving from initial site of relocation to another location within the United States, accentuates the problem of accurate statistics. Actual numbers of secondary migration are unknown.

In 2013, more than 25,000 people were granted asylum status and almost 70,000 were admitted under refugee status (Zong & Batalova, 2015b). Since 1980, consistently just over half of the immigrants have been women (Zong & Batalova, 2015b). Although the largest proportion (42.2%) of people who migrated to the United States come from an increasingly diverse group of countries, 60% of people who migrated to the United States in 2013 came from only 10 countries, including Mexico, India, Philippines, China, El Salvador, Vietnam, Cuba, Korea, Dominican Republic, and Guatemala (Zong & Batalova, 2015b). In 2014, the largest numbers of people of refugee origin were from Afghanistan, Iraq, Somalia, Democratic Republic of Congo, Myanmar, Colombia, Sudan, Vietnam, Eritrea, and China. The largest number of people holding asylee status are in Pakistan, Iran, Syria, Germany, Jordan, Kenya, Chad, China, the United States, and the United Kingdom (Centers for Disease Control and Prevention [CDC], 2012, para. 1). Within each country of origin, there are a variety of cultures, health practices, and belief systems. In this chapter, the term "immigrant" has been used for women born outside the United States regardless of status, be it legal or undocumented, refugee or under asylum.

## Strengths of Women in Migration

Immigrant women have challenges, but many are resilient survivors (Ahmad, Rai, Petrovic, Erickson, & Stewart, 2013; Campbell, 2008; Gagnon & Stewart, 2014). Most find ways to cope with their new world, seeking balance and harmony (Catolico, 2013). Many refugee communities form their own self-help organizations or community organizations. Women form new support systems or use existing support systems to help them integrate into their new communities (Ahmad et al., 2013; Sossou, Craig, Ogren, & Schnak, 2008). Local assistance agencies also contribute to strengthening immigrant women's survival, often hiring both immigrant men and women as interpreters, as well as providing microloans to support immigrant businesses and larger purchases such as vehicles. The resilience of immigrant women is often tied to their spiritual and religious beliefs, no matter what their religion (Byrskog, Olsson, Essen, & Allvin, 2014; Ross-Sheriff, 2006; Sossou et al., 2008). Although immigrant women face many barriers and challenges, they also have strengths to help them address those barriers and challenges.

## Challenges in Accessing Health Care

Health issues faced by immigrant women differ by group and geographic area of origin. Although immigrant women under refugee and asylum status undergo thorough medical examination, testing, and treatment for acute conditions both overseas and in the United States, they still have health challenges. Acute infections common to immigrant women may include tuberculosis, HIV status, hepatitis B, and intestinal parasites (Pottie, Janakiram, Topp, & McCarthy, 2007). Chronic conditions are often recognized once the acute conditions are treated and the immigrant women resettle in the United States. These conditions include diabetes, hypertension, nutritional deficiencies, and cardiovascular disease (Terasaki, Ahrenholz, & Haider, 2015).

Immigrant women face isolation, depression, anxiety, grief, separation from family and social supports, breakdown of family, loss of respect for elderly, and the effects of violence, witnessing atrocities, and posttraumatic stress disorder (PTSD). These mental health issues may be exacerbated by experiences in migration and may contribute to increased vulnerability to family violence (Costa, 2007). Screening for mental health issues is challenging and screening tools are not diagnostic. Although some screening tools have been translated and validated across languages and cultures, they are not available for all cultures and languages. Simply translating a tool does not assure validity and reliability. The Refugee Health Screener-15 (RHS-15) is a brief screening instrument that detects anxiety, depression, and PTSD across populations. It has been validated in Arabic (Iraqi), Burmese, and Nepali and additionally translated into Farsi, Karen, Russian, Somali, French, Amharic, Tigrinya, and Swahili (Johnson-Agbakwu, Allen, Nizigiyimana, Ramirez, & Hollifield, 2014; Lutheran Community Services Northwest, 2013). The widely used Edinburgh Postnatal Depression Scale has been translated into many languages; however, it has been validated in English and Mexican Spanish (Gibson, McKenzie-McHarg, Shakespeare, Price, & Gray, 2009).

Immigrant women's reproductive issues may be unique to their country of origin, such as the circumcision/cutting/genital mutilation known as female genital mutilation (FGM) practiced in many African countries, as well as some countries in Asia and the Middle East. Midwives in the United States have demonstrated some factual knowledge of FGM, depending on their experience level. However, they lack knowledge about legal and cultural aspects of FGM (Hess, Weinland, & Saalinger, 2010). Other reproductive challenges include histories of poor perinatal outcomes, birth traumas such as fistulas, frequent pregnancies, and lack of cancer screening. Immigrant women may also have a variety of health conditions resulting from previous living and working conditions, such as living in poverty, dangerous agricultural work, or living in under-resourced locations.

There are challenges when providing care for immigrant women. The most obvious challenge is communication and its impact on health care access, utilization, and understanding (Gurnah, Khoshnood, Bradley, & Yuan, 2011; Kenny et al., 2010; Paternotte, van Dulmen, van der Lee, Scherpbier, & Scheele, 2015; Tobin & Murphy-Lawless, 2014). The most common languages spoken by immigrant women in the United States are Spanish, Chinese (both Mandarin and Cantonese), Tagalog (Philippines), Vietnamese, Korean, German, French, Arabic, and Russian (Zong & Batalova, 2015b). These communication challenges make navigating the complex U.S. health care system difficult for immigrant women. These challenges include calling for appointments, completing registration information, understanding diagnosis and treatment, filling and taking prescriptions, and using over-the-counter medications (Morris, Popper, Rodwell, Brodine, & Brouwer, 2009).

Health care providers and systems are legally responsible to provide language access for all immigrant women (Chen, Youdelman, & Brooks, 2007) and interpreters are commonly used to address these language issues. Interpretive services include trained persons within a health care system, interpreters provided by local agencies, or through language-line telephone services. Interpreters may not be gender appropriate or, while speaking the congruent language, may not speak the correct dialect (Tobin & Murphy-Lawless, 2014). Although family members should not be used as interpreters, some women prefer them, especially if given the option of a male interpreter who is a stranger.

In addition to language barriers, cultural differences present the second most common set of challenges for immigrant women. Causes of illness, how symptoms are described, the meaning of a diagnosis, beliefs about medications, consequences of treatment, the woman's role in the family and in health care decision making are culturally defined (Esegbona-Adeigbe, 2011). These cultural beliefs may differ dramatically from the midwife's culture, adding to the challenges of care.

Other challenges include a lack of familiarity with how care is provided in the United States, such as making an appointment and arriving on time. Women may assume that multiple types of providers (front-office staff, clinical staff, physician assistants, physicians, nurse practitioners, and midwives) are "doctors" and that all sites of care are "hospitals." Provision of routine preventive health care and screening may not have been available in their country of origin, even if the women understood this care (Barnes & Harrison, 2004; Morris et al., 2009). Women may have experienced disrespect and abuse when receiving maternity care in their country of origin (Bohren et al., 2015) and discrimination once in the United States (Derose, Escarce, & Lurie, 2007; Thorburn, Kue, Keon, & Lo, 2012), further complicating their motivation to receive care. Although some immigrant women may drive and have access to a vehicle, others do not. Public transportation may not be available, convenient, timely, affordable, or accessible without an escort. Additional access barriers may include lack of insurance coverage, gaps in insurance coverage, and financial difficulties in affording copays or over-the-counter medications (Morris et al., 2009).

These challenges can result in immigrant women being labeled by health providers as noncompliant or the opposite, overly agreeable (LaMancuso, Goldman, & Nothnagle, 2016). Western health care practices around pregnancy, labor, and birth may be especially problematic for immigrant women, who believe that pregnancy is normal and approach labor and birth with a preference for little medical intervention (Tobin & Murphy-Lawless, 2014). Traditionally, immigrant women are expected to adapt to the U.S. health care system rather than the system adapting to meet the needs of immigrant women. All of these challenges contribute to immigrant women's difficulties in accessing health care.

## BEST PRACTICES

### Cultural Understanding

The first best practice is for the midwife to learn about various cultures, developing a broad understanding of diversity (Tobin & Murphy-Lawless, 2014), and exploring reproductive health as an issue of social justice (Gilliam, Neustadt, & Gordon, 2009). Midwives should develop a general awareness of the cultures of immigrant women specifically residing in the local area. Although it is not possible to know all cultures in depth, the goal is to recognize that cultures deserve to be respected and validated.

At the same time, midwives must avoid adopting stereotypes of any culture (Burgess, 2004). There are many resources available to develop these understandings. First, the best way midwives can learn is to listen to the immigrant women themselves explain about their various cultures. Once a trusting relationship is established, immigrant women are usually interested in sharing their cultural beliefs. Depending on a midwife's location, immigrant communities may be hidden; however, cultural celebrations, school-based events, and religious celebrations provide opportunities to learn about the local immigrant communities. Often there are well-known formal and informal community leaders who can provide insight, information, knowledge, and access to these communities. These leaders and other community representatives can act as cultural ambassadors to add to a midwife's cultural knowledge. Local education systems of all levels and many types of media offer additional opportunities to learn. Accessing these resources may be time-consuming for the busy midwife, but will improve care to immigrant women.

## Listening to Immigrant Women

Immigrant women want what most women want in their health care: establishing a trusting relationship with their provider, positive and respectful interpersonal interactions, ability to navigate the health care system, adequate and appropriate information, participation in care decisions, and sensitivity to needs (Houle, Harwood, Watkins, & Baum, 2007; McKinnon, Prosser, & Miller, 2014). In a systematic review of 34 multinational research studies of women's maternity care experiences, Small et al. (2014) found few differences between immigrant and nonimmigrant women. They proposed a mnemonic from their research:

- Q—quality care that promotes well-being for mothers and babies with a focus on individual needs
- U—unrushed caregivers with enough time to give information, explanations, and support; begin by acquiring cultural knowledge to do a cultural assessment
- I—involvement in decision making about care and procedures, explore clients' views and the restrictions that these views place on care
- C—continuity of care with caregivers who understand women's individual needs and communicate effectively
- K—kindness and respect (Small et al., 2014)

## Culturally Appropriate Care

Midwives should access specific current health resources to assure appropriate midwifery care, based upon the evidence. There are a variety of health guidelines and provider education resources easily available to midwives that provide background information about immigrants, health issues of immigrants, health care guidelines, and health education resources. These include:

- Office of Refugee Resettlement, U.S. Department of Health and Human Services (2015)
- Centers for Disease Control and Prevention, Immigrant and Refugee Health (CDC, 2012)
- Refugee Health Technical Assistance Center (2015)
- EthnoMed (University of Washington Health Sciences Libraries & Harborview Medical Center's Interpreter Services Department/Community House Calls Program, 2015)

The community- and health-focused resources assist the midwife in determining the immigrant woman's expectations about care during childbearing and help the midwife provide care that is congruent with the woman's culture (Esegbona-Adeigbe, 2011).

Reproductive health care is often the main focus of an immigrant woman's visit to a midwife and can be the most challenging to provide. Immigrant women are at risk for sexually transmitted diseases, intimate partner or family violence, and poor perinatal outcomes. Maintaining vigilance regarding these issues is important; a careful health history is the first step (Costa, 2007). Perinatal care should also include appropriate, gender-aligned interpreters, assurance of modesty, culturally appropriate education materials, modification of standardized visit content, and information about what to expect during childbirth (Herrel et al., 2004). As immigrant women with FGM are likely to seek midwifery care because of a preference for a female provider, this necessitates that midwives must be knowledgeable about unique aspects of their care. Midwives should engage in open discussions with these women, document preferences in the medical record, and assure them that there are appropriate female interpreters who will be present during childbirth. Midwives should also learn anterior episiotomy or de-infibulation skills (releasing the infibulation during childbirth) and repair techniques to improve outcomes (Jacoby & Smith, 2013).

Mental health issues of immigrant women may be particularly challenging for midwives (Kirmayer et al., 2011). Screening for mental health issues can be difficult because of communication issues and, yet, these women are at increased risk for these issues, including postpartum depression (O'Mahony & Donnelly, 2010). Screening tools should be used as appropriate and, if possible, validated in the woman's language and culture. Given the concerns about validated screening tools, a midwife's cultural knowledge, observations, and impressions are important diagnostic tools for mental health issues.

Finally, midwives should advocate for change within communities and in the health care systems to meet the needs of all women, including immigrant women. Providers need time, resources, accurate data-collection systems, and training to provide appropriate care for an increasingly diverse population. Midwives should advocate for tailored programs for immigrant women and other diverse communities with an active program of outreach services (Carolan & Cassar, 2010; Esegbona-Adeigbe, 2011). Midwives need to collaborate with immigrant community associations and woman's social networks in their communities. Health care and social service systems need to invest in adequate personnel, translated material, and mediators (Sandín-Vázquez, Larraz-Antón, & Río-Sánchez, 2014). Recognizing the importance of communication, midwives need to help improve the quality and appropriateness of interpreters, as well as the availability of other methods of communication such as videos, drawings, or written materials (Tobin & Murphy-Lawless, 2014).

Two congruent sets of standards clearly describe the role of the midwife in the care of immigrant women: the ACNM's *Core Competencies for Basic Midwifery Practice* (ACNM, 2012), and the *Position Statement on Heritage and Culture in Childbearing*, offered by the International Confederation of Midwives (ICM; 2005). Among the ACNM Hallmarks of Midwifery, the first of the core competencies, cultural humility is listed—a key quality in working with immigrant women (ACNM, 2012). The ICM document speaks to the need for knowledge about cultural traditions and knowing when traditional practices can cause harm, urging the midwife to work with the community to eliminate these practices (ICM, 2005).

## CONCLUSION

Midwives frequently care for the growing number of immigrant women residing in the United States. In any midwifery health care encounter, there are two main participants—the woman and the midwife, both with their own unique cultural perspective that may be accentuated when experiences, beliefs, and culture are diverse. Immigrant women want information about how care is provided in their new country and they need respectful, nondiscriminatory, safe, high-quality, attentive, and individualized care (Small et al., 2014). In general, they prefer care and interpretive services from female providers. Preserving standards of modesty dictated by social and/or religious norms exists among women of many cultures, including American women (Gurnah et al., 2011).

Midwives need to know about cultural diversity, specifically, the diet, leisure, alternative therapies, health practices, illness perceptions, and illness-prevention practices of the immigrant populations they serve. Lack of this knowledge generates fear and insecurity for health care providers and leads to perceptions of noncompliance when women do not follow recommendations (Gurnah et al., 2011; Plaza, Grau, Cegri, Domínguez, & Casanovas, 2014; Sandín-Vázquez et al., 2014). Immigrant women come with pre-existing illnesses, both acute and chronic, mental health issues, unique reproductive health concerns, and, equally important, a set of cultural beliefs that inform health care practices. Communication and issues with access to care can be major barriers in caring for immigrant women. These women demonstrate admirable resilience. Given the diversity of cultures, countries of origin, and health issues immigrants present with, it is difficult for a midwife to master knowledge of them all. However, there are many resources available to help the midwife caring for a diverse population, the most important of which is listening to the beliefs and experiences of these women.

---

**USING THE EVIDENCE FOR BEST PRACTICE**

**Case Study 9.1   Caring for an Immigrant Woman From Somalia**

S.A., a 19-year-old woman from Somalia, will be coming for her first prenatal visit. Although the midwife has provided care to women from many countries, she has never cared for an immigrant woman from Somalia. Although there are many languages spoken in Somalia, the most common one is Somali. The nurse printed some literature in the Somali language for the new patient and identified several websites that could be helpful for the midwife to review before the visit.

*(continued)*

**USING THE EVIDENCE FOR BEST PRACTICE (continued)**

First, the midwife meets briefly with the office staff to plan for S.A.'s care and arranges to meet S.A. in an administrative office with a table and several chairs, instead of the usual examination room. When S.A. arrives, she is accompanied by her father and mother. A petite young woman in a head scarf, she smiles readily and giggles often. The local refugee resettlement agency has provided a linguistically congruent, female interpreter. As no one in S.A.'s family extends a hand for a handshake, neither does the midwife. Through the interpreter, the midwife learns that S.A. has lived in a Kenyan refugee camp for the past 7 years, was married about 4 months ago, and has been in the United States for 2 months. She does not speak or read English, but she speaks three African languages, including Somali. Her husband remains in the Kenyan camps and she now lives with her parents, another sister, and the sister's two children in a four-bedroom apartment. S.A. and her family express happiness about the pregnancy. S.A. has public insurance coverage for her health care and pregnancy.

The midwife invites the family to sit at the table in the administrative office. Through the interpreter, she introduces herself and shares a little about herself and her career. S.A. and her family are invited to tell the midwife about life and pregnancy care in Somalia and the Kenyan camps. The midwife briefly explains Western prenatal care, focusing on early pregnancy care. At this time, S.A.'s father elects to wait in the car.

S.A.'s medical history does not identify any risk factors, including FGM. S.A. thinks her last menstrual period was about a month before she left Kenya. She has not felt fetal movement. S.A. and her mother decide to postpone the examination, focusing on gestational age assessment and laboratory tests at this visit. S.A.'s uterus is well below the umbilicus and fetal heart tones are easily heard. Everyone is excited and claps.

The midwife provides written information but not the websites as the family has no access to the electronics needed view them. A 1-hour follow-up visit is scheduled in 2 weeks with the same midwife for the remaining testing and physical examination, including an ultrasound for gestational age. The same interpreter arranges to attend that future appointment.

The midwife expresses happiness that S.A. has come to see her. S.A. and her mother tell her, through the interpreter, that they are very happy with the visit and are excited to return in 2 weeks.

# REFERENCES

Ahmad, F., Rai, N., Petrovic, B., Erickson, P. E., & Stewart, D. E. (2013). Resilience and resources among South Asian immigrant women as survivors of partner violence. *Journal of Immigrant and Minority Health*, *15*(6), 1057–1064. doi:10.1007/s10903-013-9836-2

American College of Nurse-Midwives (ACNM). (n.d.). About the midwifery profession. Retrieved from http://midwife.org/About-the-Midwifery-Profession

American College of Nurse-Midwives (ACNM). (2012). Core competencies for basic midwifery practice. Retrieved from http://www.midwife.org/ACNM/files/ACNMLibraryData/UPLOADFILENAME/000000000050/Core%20Comptencies%20Dec%202012.pdf

American Community Survey. (2012). The foreign-born populations in the United States: 2010. Retrieved from https://www.census.gov/prod/2012pubs/acs-19.pdf?cssp=SERP

Barnes, D. M., & Harrison, C. L. (2004). Refugee women's reproductive health in early resettlement. *Journal of Obstetric, Gynecologic, and Neonatal Nursing, 33*(6), 723–728. doi:10 .1177/0884217504270668

Bohren, M. A., Vogel, J. P., Hunter, E. C., Lutsiv, O., Makh, S. K., Souza, J. P., . . . Gulmezoglu, A. M. (2015). The mistreatment of women during childbirth in health facilities globally: A mixed-methods systematic review. *PLoS Medicine, 12*(6), e1001847. doi:10.1371/journal .pmed.1001847

Burgess, A. (2004). Health challenges for refugees and immigrants. *Refugee Reports, 25*(2), 1–4.

Byrskog, U., Olsson, P., Essen, B., & Allvin, M. K. (2014). Violence and reproductive health preceding flight from war: Accounts from Somali born women in Sweden. *BMC Public Health, 14*(892), 1–11. doi:10.1186/1471-2458-14-892

Campbell, W. (2008). Lessons in resilience: Undocumented Mexican women in South Carolina. *Journal of Women and Social Work, 23*(3), 231–241.

Carolan, M., & Cassar, L. (2010). Antenatal care perceptions of pregnant African women attending maternity services in Melbourne, Australia. *Midwifery, 26*(2), 189–201. doi: 10.1016/j.midw.2008.03.005

Catolico, O. (2013). Seeking life balance: The perceptions of health of Cambodian women in resettlement. *Journal of Transcultural Nursing, 24*(3), 236–245. doi:10.1177/1043659613481624

Centers for Disease Control and Prevention (CDC). (2012). Immigrant and refugee health. Retrieved from http://www.cdc.gov/immigrantrefugeehealth/about-refugees.html

Chen, A. H., Youdelman, M. K., & Brooks, J. (2007). The legal framework for language access in healthcare settings: Title VI and beyond. *Journal of General Internal Medicine, 22*(Suppl. 2), 362–367. doi:10.1007/s11606-007-0366-2

Costa, D. (2007). Health care of refugee women. *Australian Family Physician, 36*(3), 151–154. Retrieved from http://www.ncbi.nlm.nih.gov/pubmed/17339979

Derose, K., Escarce, J., & Lurie, N. (2007). Immigrants and health care: Sources of vulnerability. *Health Affairs, 26*(5), 1258–1268. doi:10.1377/hlthaff.26.5.1258

Esegbona-Adeigbe, S. (2011). Acquiring cultural competency in caring for black African women. *British Journal of Midwifery, 19*(8), 489–496.

Gagnon, A. J., & Stewart, D. E. (2014). Resilience in international migrant women following violence associated with pregnancy. *Archives of Women's Mental Health, 17*(4), 303–310. doi:10.1007/s00737-013-0392-5

Gibson, J., McKenzie-McHarg, K., Shakespeare, J., Price, J., & Gray, R. (2009). A systematic review of studies validating the Edinburgh Postnatal Depression Scale in antepartum and postpartum women. *Acta Psychiatrica Scandinavica, 119*(5), 350–364. doi:10.1111/j.1600 -0447.2009.01363.x

Gilliam, M. L., Neustadt, A., & Gordon, R. (2009). A call to incorporate a reproductive justice agenda into reproductive health clinical practice and policy. *Contraception, 79*(4), 243–246. doi:10.1016/j.contraception.2008.12.004

Gurnah, K., Khoshnood, K., Bradley, E., & Yuan, C. (2011). Lost in translation: Reproductive health care experiences of Somali Bantu women in Hartford, Connecticut. *Journal of Midwifery and Women's Health, 56*(4), 340–346. doi:10.1111/j.1542-2011.2011.00028.x

Herrel, N., Olevitch, L., DuBois, D. K., Terry, P., Thorp, D., Kind, E., & Said, A. (2004). Somali refugee women speak out about their needs for care during pregnancy and delivery. *Journal of Midwifery and Women's Health*, 49(4), 345–349. doi:10.1016/j.jmwh.2004.02.008

Hess, R. F., Weinland, J., & Saalinger, N. M. (2010). Knowledge of female genital cutting and experience with women who are circumcised: A survey of nurse-midwives in the United States. *Journal of Midwifery and Women's Health*, 55(1), 46–54. doi:10.1016/j.jmwh.2009.01.005

Houle, C., Harwood, E., Watkins, A., & Baum, K. D. (2007). What women want from their physicians: A qualitative analysis. *Journal of Women's Health*, 16(4), 543–550. doi:10.1089/jwh.2006.M079

International Confederation of Midwives (ICM). (2005). Position statement: Heritage and culture in childbearing. Retrieved from http://www.internationalmidwives.org/assets/uploads/documents/Position%20Statements%20-%20English/PS2011_009%20ENG%20Heritage%20and%20Culture%20in%20Childbearing.pdf

Jacoby, S. D., & Smith, A. (2013). Increasing certified nurse-midwives' confidence in managing the obstetric care of women with female genital mutilation/cutting. *Journal of Midwifery and Women's Health*, 58(4), 451–456. doi:10.1111/j.1542-2011.2012.00262.x

Johnson-Agbakwu, C. E., Allen, J., Nizigiyimana, J. F., Ramirez, G., & Hollifield, M. (2014). Mental health screening among newly arrived refugees seeking routine obstetric and gynecologic care. *Psychological Services*, 11(4), 470–476. doi:10.1037/a0036400

Kenny, D. A., Veldhuijzen, W., Weijden, T., Leblanc, A., Lockyer, J., Legare, F., & Campbell, C. (2010). Interpersonal perception in the context of doctor-patient relationships: A dyadic analysis of doctor-patient communication. *Social Science and Medicine*, 70(5), 763–768. doi:10.1016/j.socscimed.2009.10.065

Kirmayer, L. J., Narasiah, L., Munoz, M., Rashid, M., Ryder, A. G., Guzder, J., . . . Refugee, H. (2011). Common mental health problems in immigrants and refugees: General approach in primary care. *Canadian Medical Association Journal*, 183(12), E959–967. doi:10.1503/cmaj.090292

LaMancuso, K., Goldman, R. E., & Nothnagle, M. (2016, February 28). "Can I ask that?". Perspectives on perinatal care after resettlement among Karen refugee women, medical providers, and community-based doulas. *Journal of Immigrant and Minority Health*, 18(2), 428–435. doi:10.1007/s10903-015-0172-6

Lutheran Community Services Northwest. (2013). Pathways to wellness: Refugee Health Screener-15 (RHS-15): Development and use. Retrieved from http://www.lcsnw.org/pathways/pdf/RefugeeHealthScreener.pdf

McKinnon, L. C., Prosser, S. J., & Miller, Y. D. (2014). What women want: Qualitative analysis of consumer evaluations of maternity care in Queensland, Australia. *BMC Pregnancy and Childbirth*, 14(366), 1–14. doi:10.1186/s12884-014-0366-2

Morris, M. D., Popper, S. T., Rodwell, T. C., Brodine, S. K., & Brouwer, K. C. (2009). Healthcare barriers of refugees post-resettlement. *Journal of Community Health*, 34(6), 529–538. doi:10.1007/s10900-009-9175-3

O'Mahony, J., & Donnelly, T. (2010). Immigrant and refugee women's post-partum depression help-seeking experiences and access to care: A review and analysis of the literature. *Journal of Psychiatric Mental Health Nursing*, 17(10), 917–928. doi:10.1111/j.1365-2850.2010.01625.x

Paternotte, E., van Dulmen, S., van der Lee, N., Scherpbier, A. J., & Scheele, F. (2015). Factors influencing intercultural doctor–patient communication: A realist review. *Patient Education and Counseling, 98*(4), 420–445. doi:10.1016/j.pec.2014.11.018

Plaza, I., Grau, J., Cegri, F., Domínguez, N., & Casanovas, C. (2014). The difficulties met by primary healthcare professionals providing care to patients from culturally diverse communities. Perceptions of healthcare professionals and basis for improvement strategies. *Procedia—Social and Behavioral Sciences, 132*, 209–215. doi:10.1016/j.sbspro.2014.04.300

Pottie, K., Janakiram, P., Topp, P., & McCarthy, A. (2007). Prevalence of selected preventable and treatable diseases among government-assisted refugees: Implications for primary care providers. *Canadian Family Physician, 53*(11), 1928–1934. Retrieved from http://www.ncbi.nlm.nih.gov/pubmed/18000270

Refugee Health Technical Assistance Center. (2015). Retrieved from http://refugeehealthta.org

Ross-Sheriff, F. (2006). Afghan women in exile and repatriation: Passive victims or social actors? *Journal of Women and Social Work, 21*(2), 206–219.

Sandín-Vázquez, M., Larraz-Antón, R., & Río-Sánchez, I. (2014). Immigrant patient care inequalities: The importance of the intercultural approach. *Procedia—Social and Behavioral Sciences, 132*, 277–284. doi:10.1016/j.sbspro.2014.04.310

Small, R., Roth, C., Raval, M., Shafiei, T., Korfker, D., Heaman, M., . . . Gagnon, A. (2014). Immigrant and non-immigrant women's experiences of maternity care: A systematic and comparative review of studies in five countries. *BMC Pregnancy and Childbirth, 14*, 152. doi:10.1186/1471-2393-14-152

Sossou, M. A., Craig, C. D., Ogren, H., & Schnak, M. (2008). A qualitative study of resilience factors of Bosnian refugee women resettled in the southern United States. *Journal of Ethnic and Cultural Diversity in Social Work, 17*(4), 365–385. doi:10.1080/15313200802467908

Terasaki, G., Ahrenholz, N. C., & Haider, M. Z. (2015). Care of adult refugees with chronic conditions. *Medical Clinics of North America, 99*(5), 1039–1058. doi:10.1016/j.mcna.2015.05.006

Thorburn, S., Kue, J., Keon, K. L., & Lo, P. (2012). Medical mistrust and discrimination in health care: A qualitative study of Hmong women and men. *Journal of Community Health, 37*(4), 822–829. doi:10.1007/s10900-011-9516-x

Tobin, C. L., & Murphy-Lawless, J. (2014). Irish midwives' experiences of providing maternity care to non-Irish women seeking asylum. *International Journal of Women's Health, 6*, 159–169. doi:10.2147/IJWH.S45579

United Nations General Assembly. (1951). 1951 convention relating to the status of refugees. Retrieved from http://www.unhcr.org/3b66c2aa10.html

U.S. Citizenship and Immigration Services (USCIS). (2015, November 2). *Glossary of terms.* Washington, DC: Department of Homeland Security. Retrieved from http://www.uscis.gov/tools/glossary

U.S. Department of Health and Human Services. (2015). Office of Refugee Resettlement. Retrieved from http://www.acf.hhs.gov/programs/orr

University of Washington Health Sciences Libraries & Harborview Medical Center's Interpreter Services Department/Community House Calls Program (2015). EthnoMed. Retrieved from https://ethnomed.org/about

Zong, J., & Batalova, J. (2015a). Refugees and asylees in the United States. Retrieved from http://www.migrationpolicy.org/article/refugees-and-asylees-united-states

Zong, J., & Batalova, J. (2015b). *Frequently requested statistics on immigrants and immigration in the United States.* Retrieved from http://www.migrationpolicy.org/article/frequently -requested-statistics-immigrants-and-immigration-united-states?gclid=CMrzpuevrMkC FRRlfgodIDgJEA

# CHAPTER TEN

# RACIAL AND ETHNIC DISPARITIES IN BIRTH OUTCOMES: THE CHALLENGE TO MIDWIFERY

Patricia O. Loftman

Racism would not exist in an ideal world. In an ideal world, equity would govern institutions, structural systems, and policies that affect all phases of life—political, economic, health, and social. Equity emanates from systems of power that govern the distribution of necessary resources, guaranteeing equal access to all. With equity, everyone would have impartial and unimpeded access to effective political representation, quality education and health care, employment opportunity, merit-based compensation, and decent housing. "Achieving health equity requires valuing all individuals and populations equally, recognizing and rectifying historical injustices, and providing resources according to need. Health disparities in racial and ethnic communities would be eliminated if health equity were achieved" (Jones, 2014, p. S74).

By any indices measuring equity by race and ethnicity, people of color are at the bottom. In October 2015, the U.S. unemployment rate was 5%. The rate varied by race and ethnicity: Whites (4.4%), Hispanics (6.3%), and African Americans (9.2%; U.S. Department of Labor, 2015). In 2014, the median income in the United States was $53,657. Median income also varied by race and ethnicity: Whites ($60,256), Hispanics ($42,491), and African Americans ($35,398; U.S. Department of Commerce, 2015). The overall national poverty rate was 15% (U.S. Census Bureau, 2015). The poverty rate was 26% for African Americans, 24% for Hispanics, and 10% for Whites (U.S. Census Bureau, 2015). Racial and ethnic disparities in economic well-being parallel health disparities.

## WEATHERING AND ALLOSTATIC LOAD

### Racial and Ethnic Disparities In Birth Outcomes Among African American Women

African American women experience health disparities, including maternal and infant mortality, preterm birth, and low birth weight, at a rate two to three times that of White women. These disparities have persisted over decades. Although medical advances and the emergence of evidence-based health practices have improved the quality of medical care rendered to everyone, including the quality of women's health care, the racial gap in maternal and infant outcomes remains unacceptably high for women of color (Colon, Geronimus, Bound, & James, 2006; Dominguez, 2008; Dominguez, Dunkel-Schetter, Glynn, Hobel, & Sandman, 2008; Health Resources and Services Administration, 2013).

Historically, women at risk for a poor pregnancy outcome have been categorized as those with no prenatal care; low income; low literacy; engaging in unhealthy behaviors such as tobacco, alcohol, and/or illegal drug use; exposed to intimate partner violence; and having mental health challenges. Although socioeconomic factors and individual behaviors contribute to negative birth outcomes, evidence now supports that, when controlling for these factors, racism and personal experiences of discriminatory events play an even greater role in poor birth outcomes. The 1992 sentinel study by Schoendorf, Hogue, Kleinman, and Rowley (1992) published in the *New England Journal of Medicine* demonstrated that being a college-educated, middle-class African American woman was not protective against poor birth outcomes (Schoendorf et al., 1992). Among these women, the infant mortality, prematurity, and low birth rates were comparable to rates seen for African American women in the general population. Further, infant mortality was two times higher compared to White college-educated women (Schoendorf et al. 1992).

## The Weathering Hypothesis

The weathering hypothesis, proposed by Geronimus (1996), attempted to explain this racial disparity in birth outcomes among college-educated, middle-class African American women, considered at low risk for a poor outcome. She postulated that among African American women, repeated exposure to discrimination, social or economic adversity, and environmental insults resulted in early physiological changes and health deterioration that compounded with age. She observed that among African American women, African American adolescents aged 15 to 19 experienced the lowest rates of poor birth outcomes; the rate increased among African American women in their early and mid-twenties. She termed this premature health deterioration *weathering*, and also noted that health deterioration was more pronounced among African American women with low and average income compared to African American women with higher incomes (Geronimus, 1996). Geronimus (1996) and Lu and Halfon (2003) further noted that weathering was not observed among White women (Geronimus, 1996; Lu & Halfon, 2003).

After controlling for medical and sociodemographic risk, Dominguez et al. (2008) proposed that exposure to perceived racism, either as a child or indirectly through parental influence, could heighten a child's perception of vulnerability, resulting in a stress-induced chronic state of hyperarousal with health consequences, including poor birth outcomes in their offspring. She further suggested that African American women, regardless of education and socioeconomic level, feel the fear of and the need to protect their children from racism, a factor that could significantly increase stress hormone levels during pregnancy, with resultant risk of poor birth outcomes. African American women fear for the safety of their children outside of the home and understand the need to instruct their children, especially sons, at a very young age on strategies for interacting safely with the police (Dominguez et al., 2008).

Lu and Halfon (2003) posited that racial disparities in birth outcomes represent two synergistic processes that occur simultaneously over the course of one's entire lifetime. The first is the body's adaptation to weathering, the early physiologic and health deterioration resulting from the stress of living in a race-based society. The second is the body's normal physiologic, adaptive response to chronic stress, the cumulative allostatic load (wear and tear on the body) of living in a race-based society. This physiologic response is mediated through the sympathetic nervous system and the hypothalamic–pituitary–adrenal axis with the release of norepinephrine, epinephrine, cortisol, and dehydroepiandrosterone sulfate. The body returns to its usual state of hormonal equilibrium once the stressor abates. However, exposure to chronic stress and an ongoing high-alert situation creates an internal state of hormonal hyperactivity and dysregulation that leads to the creation of an allostatic load on the body's systems (Lu & Halfon, 2003). Early and ongoing negative risk exposures influence future reproductive health, and weathering accelerates the decline in reproductive health (Geronimus, Hicken, Keene & Bound, 2006; Lu et al., 2010; Lu & Halfon, 2003).

Maternal stress increases norepinephrine and cortisol levels, triggering the release of placental corticotropin-releasing hormone. This forms a pattern: the higher the intensity of maternal stress, the higher the levels of norepinephrine, cortisol, and corticotropin-releasing hormone (Geronimus et al., 2006). Stress potentially alters immune function in African American women, predisposing them to intra-amniotic infection or inflammation, degradation of amnion–chorion integrity, preterm premature rupture of membranes, preterm delivery, very-low-birth-weight or low-birth-weight infants. Common, pervasive, daily stressors in the lives of African American women include the burden of raising children as single parents, poverty, poor employment and housing opportunities, discrimination, social isolation, and the stress of partners incarcerated at alarmingly high rates. African American women carry a heavy burden in their families and communities (Geronimus et al., 2006).

During sensitive fetal developmental periods in utero, early life exposures and experiences in sufficient quantity may alter an organ or system function later in adult life also influencing future reproductive potential. Throughout this time, elevated stress hormone levels potentially alter immune maturation and function resulting in increased vulnerability to infectious or inflammatory processes later in life. Maternal stress could potentially prime the developing fetus' hypothalamic–pituitary–adrenal axis and immune system with stress hormones, resulting in higher stress reactivity and immune–inflammatory dysregulation that could increase the woman's female infant's susceptibility to preterm labor and low birth weight later on in life (Hanley et al., 2010; Lu et al., 2010; also see Chapter 5).

Three variables are of note. In comparison with White women, African American women are less likely to use tobacco during pregnancy, a factor associated with poor birth outcome. Yet African American infant mortality is still higher. Second, among African American women, those who initiated prenatal care in the first trimester compared to White women with late or no prenatal care, African American infant mortality is still higher. These variables are not sufficient to explain disparate racial birth outcomes (Lu et al., 2010). Of interest is that preconception stress has been suggested as an important variable in the outcome (Hogan et al., 2013; Kramer, Hogue, Dunlop, & Menon, 2011). The third variable is a generational increase in family income. Among poor White women, increased income decreased the likelihood of a low-birth-weight infant. The same effect was not seen among poor African American women (Colen et al., 2006). Vinikoor, Kaufman, MacLehose, and Laraia (2008) found that high income and residing in a wealthier neighborhood was not protective against preterm birth and low-birth-weight infants for African American women. The potential benefits in perinatal outcome were offset by racism, racial stigma, isolation, and lack of social support. The beneficial effect of higher income on pregnancy outcomes for African American women occurred only if they lived in neighborhoods with a population of African American residents greater than 90% (Vinikoor et al., 2008).

The story of racial and ethnic disparities is a sad chapter in the history of the United States and distrust in the health care system among women of color is a reality. One of the most pressing needs in the care of mothers and infants is to increase the number of midwives of color who may be able to provide a level of cultural comfort that others cannot (Institute of Medicine [IOM], 2004; see discussion of this workforce issue in Chapter 2).

## MISTRUST AND DISTRUST OF THE HEALTH CARE SYSTEM

Midwives need to understand the pervasive effects of historical events that have eroded the trust among women of color in the health care system. Some examples of medical abuses are presented.

### The Tuskegee Study of Untreated Syphilis in the African American Male

The Tuskegee Syphilis Experiment was a federally funded clinical experiment that was conducted for 40 years between 1932 and 1972 by the U.S. Public Health Service. Rural, uneducated, poor African American men in Alabama ($n = 600$) were enrolled in the study. Among them, 399 had latent syphilis and 201 were syphilis free. They were enticed with promises of free medical care, transportation to and from the clinic, hot meals on the study days, free burial insurance, and funeral benefits if they agreed to undergo autopsy after death. Although the men were told they were being treated for "bad blood," a term the men associated with anemia, fatigue, or syphilis, the goal of the experiment was to study the natural history and progression of untreated syphilis. Although the clinical manifestations of untreated syphilis were already known, based on reports of untreated syphilis in White males in Oslo, Norway, it was believed that African Americans would respond differently biologically.

The infected men were never told they had syphilis, that they would never be treated, or that by 1947, penicillin had become the standard cure for the disease. During World War II, the U.S. Public Health Service attempted to prevent treatment among this population of drafted men who screened positive for syphilis. The men were given a placebo as the intent was to follow the men until death. At the end of the experiment in 1972, 74 men were alive, 28 had died of neurosyphilis and syphilitic cardiac complications, 40 wives had been infected, and 19 children had been born with congenital syphilis (Centers for Disease Control and Prevention [CDC], 1997; Thomas & Quinn, 1991; Tuskegee University, 2015). The erosion of trust in the health care system among the African American population was enormous.

## Sterilization of Women of Color—Past and Present

The history of medical interventions designed to control the reproductive rights of women of color is extensive. It dates back to slavery and continues into the 21st century (Roberts, 1997). Between 1930 and 1970, more than a third of the women of childbearing age living in the U.S. territory of Puerto Rico were sterilized without informed consent. These women, primarily working class, poor, and uneducated, were never informed that having the procedure meant they would never be able to have biological children in the future. Funded by the U.S. government at little to no cost, the procedure was so common it was known by the familiar name of "La Operacion" and contributed to Puerto Rico having the highest sterilization rate in the world (Krase, 2014; Nittle, 2014).

In 1964, House Bill No. 180 was passed in regular session of the Mississippi House of Representatives but failed to pass in the Senate. Entitled "An Act to Discourage Immorality of Unmarried Females by Providing for Sterilization of the Unwed Mother Under Conditions of this Act and for Related Purposes," it specifically targeted women of color (Carter G. Woodson Institute, 2004). One might also ask about the meaning of *related purposes*.

In 1976, the U.S. government admitted that through the 1960s and 1970s, the Indian Health Service sterilized more than 3,400 Native American women between the ages of 15 to 45, without informed consent. Young women entered Indian Health Service hospitals for appendectomies and instead received tubal ligations. The government acknowledged that 36 women younger than the age of 21 had been forcibly sterilized during this period, despite a court-ordered moratorium on the sterilization of women younger than the age of 21 (Lawrence, 2000; U.S. National Library of Medicine, 1976).

California state law mandates that all tubal ligations occurring in a situation of incarceration must be approved by the State Medical Board. Between 2006 and 2012, almost 500 incarcerated women in California were sterilized through tubal ligations without informed consent. A review documented that none of these tubal ligations had been submitted to the medical board for review. Another 378 women underwent radical hysterectomies or endometrial ablation without State Medical Board approval. Women were told they had fibroids and the only treatment was a hysterectomy. The review demonstrated that most of the women did not have fibroids (Law, 2014).

## The Unlikely Story of Henrietta Lacks

Henrietta Lacks was a young, working-class African American woman who was diagnosed in 1951 with a virulent, aggressive form of cervical cancer. Without her knowledge and without informing her family, her treating physician took a biopsy of the cancer cells and cultured them. Attempts to grow human cells in a Petri dish and keep them alive had previously been unsuccessful. However, her cells reproduced on a 24-hour cycle continuously. They are the first eternal strain of human cells reproduced in a laboratory setting. They were subsequently identified as HeLa cells, becoming a key part of genome research and understanding of the human telomerase. Her cells have been used in investigating drugs for herpes, leukemia, influenza, hemophilia, and Parkinson's disease, as well as many other studies (Skloot, 2011).

More than 20 years after her death from cervical cancer, researchers began conducting studies on Henrietta's children, drawing and analyzing their blood, even though they were unaware of the nature of the research and did not know that her cells had been harvested. The children believed they were being tested to see whether they had the cancer that killed Henrietta but researchers were actually studying the Lacks family to obtain more information about Henrietta's cells. Her cells have been commercialized and have generated millions of dollars in profit for the researchers who patented her tissue. Unfortunately, neither Henrietta nor her family ever derived any financial benefit from the commercialization of her cells (Skloot, 2011). At this point, the National Institutes of Health has negotiated an agreement with the family on the release of HeLa genomic data while agreeing to abide by the wishes of the relatives (Callaway, 2013).

## MIDWIFERY RESPONSE TO WEATHERING: BEST PRACTICES

Women of color have experienced significant threats to trust by abuses within the health care system. The effect has been weathering, an erosion of well-being over time that has consequences for birth outcomes. The Special Prenatal Clinic model midwifery program is presented as a strategy for addressing the effects of weathering.

## The Special Prenatal Clinic Model

Behavioral responses to chronic and racial stressors vary for women of color. For some, coping mechanisms include drug use. Although perinatal drug use is accepted as a contributor to poor birth outcomes, quantifying its contribution is difficult. In 2013, an estimated 5.4% of all pregnant women, aged 15 to 44, used illegal drugs (U.S. Department of Health and Human Services [USDHHS], 2015).

However, rates of drug use across all racial and ethnic groups have been found to be similar (Chasnoff, Landress, & Barett, 1990; USDHHS, 2015).

A Cochrane Review evaluated the evidence for the effectiveness of interventions for chemically dependent pregnant women on birth and neonatal outcomes, attendance and retention in treatment, and maternal and neonatal drug abstinence (Terplan, Ramanadhan, Locke, Longinaker, & Lui, 2015). Originally conducted in 2007, the review was updated in 2015. The reviews included randomized controlled trials that compared psychological intervention, contingency management, and motivational interviewing. Contingency management utilizes supportive reinforcement with incentives, such as baby strollers, if predetermined endpoints are met. Motivational interviewing involves patient-centered counseling. Terplan et al. (2015) concluded there was no difference in treatment outcomes. Other researchers have reported that limited use of contingency management appears the most successful option (Forray & Foster, 2015; Yonkers et al., 2012).

Designing effective interventions for chemically dependent pregnant women is extremely complex. It demands a cultural lens knowledgeable about the affected population or community. The author was unable to locate any intervention similar to the successful Special Prenatal Clinic. Anecdotal information, although least reliable in the hierarchy of evidence (see Chapter 3), is valuable in providing clinical observations, experiences, and outcomes. With that disclaimer, this material represents the author's 30-year experience working with women of color and in the Special Prenatal Clinic. These experiences have guided best practices in providing safe, culturally relevant, and satisfying health care to women of color and women with special needs, including drug use.

The author was one of two midwives who were care providers in the Harlem Hospital Center, Special Prenatal Clinic, located in New York City, from 1985 to 1999. The Special Prenatal Clinic was created and designed in response to the large numbers of pregnant women without prenatal care presenting to the obstetrical unit in precipitous labor. Drug use among all women, including pregnant women of color, prior to the crack-cocaine epidemic of the 1980s, was rare. The arrival of crack-cocaine heralded a new era in drug history. Prior to the 1960s, tobacco use by women was less common. When cigarette smoking increased among women, the tobacco companies eagerly responded to this new market with flavored, menthol cigarettes and heavy advertising to women. Tobacco was a gateway drug to smoking crack (Carrington et al., 1994).

Although the focus of the clinic at inception was narrow, providing care to pregnant, drug-using women, the scope was subsequently expanded to include women whose pregnancies were complicated by HIV. At that time, a woman's drug use was the main risk factor for acquiring HIV. Today, the risk of acquiring HIV for women of color is sexual contact with a partner who is HIV positive. The challenges to caring for women whose pregnancies are affected by drug use and HIV are multifaceted and complex. Although affected by the same race-based stressors that college-educated middle-class African American women experience, these most vulnerable women have access to fewer resources to protect them from weathering (Carrington et al., 1994).

The clinic was strategically located apart from the regular obstetrical clinic and the term "special" was adopted to reduce the stigma attached to the clinic's purpose and to encourage participation. The model was multidisciplinary in order to address the women's addiction as the principal issue. Their pregnancy and medical complications were secondary. The core care providers included the midwives as the primary care providers, a perinatologist available for consultation as needed, a nutritionist, an addiction counselor, and a social worker. Linkages were established with on-site and off-site drug rehabilitation services, pediatrics, psychiatric services, and infectious disease care. Each woman was assigned a midwife and given the midwife's business card. This signaled the initial bond between the woman and the midwife (Carrington et al., 1994).

Dual commitment was necessary for success. The midwife had already declared her intention and the woman needed to declare her commitment. The women would frequently refer to her midwife as "my doctor" despite the midwives' repeated correction of their professional identity. The women were seen weekly by their assigned midwife, from whom they received prenatal care for the duration of the pregnancy. By the end of the pregnancy, a comprehensive plan for both the woman and infant had been developed. In the event that the infant's urine toxicology was positive at birth, the plan clearly outlined the need for disposition. The pregnant woman and her providers were all aware of the plan. During the pregnancy, the midwives and the women developed mutually satisfying relationships. The relationships were built on the continuity of care provided by the midwives as well as mutual trust, respect, and the midwives' knowledge of the circumstances affecting the women (Carrington et al., 1994).

Characteristics of these pregnant drug-using women of color as well as of HIV-positive pregnant women in the Special Prenatal Clinic were that they:

- Perceived themselves as victims of "the system"
- Were economically and environmentally vulnerable
- Had few resources to move from their geographic location even though remaining in the environment reinforced their vulnerability
- Lacked confidence that they could survive apart from abusive relationships increasing feelings of helplessness, hopelessness, low self-esteem, and fear
- Were unable to engage in mature communication describing feelings and needs
- Were in a state of denial (Carrington et al., 1994)

The women stated a strong belief that both of the midwives, who were race concordant, cared about their general well-being. Continuity of care contributed to high adherence with weekly care appointments in this group of women who traditionally had been outside of the health care system. Adherence was high despite rigid clinic rules, weekly drug testing, and the consequences of "dirty urine." These conditions were outlined at the first visit. Referrals to supportive services were coordinated with frequent communication, including regularly scheduled care conferences. The trust established not only with the midwives but the entire clinic staff was transferred to the referring specialty services.

The women knew they were being referred to safe environments (Carrington et al., 1994).

The target outcomes were negative maternal and neonatal urine toxicologies at birth (Carrington et al., 1994). Prematurity and low birth rates were low. Before leaving the hospital after giving birth, the woman was given a scheduled appointment to see both her midwife and the pediatrician connected to the Special Prenatal Clinic within 2 weeks. The woman continued well-woman care with her midwife for a period of 2 years, at which time she was returned to the traditional gynecology clinic. Most women chose to remain with their designated midwife, who also provided care in the traditional gynecology clinic (Carrington et al., 1994).

The Special Prenatal Clinic's success was based on a model that provided individualized, comprehensive, interdisciplinary care to chemically dependent and HIV-positive pregnant women, offering an opportunity for behavior change. The environment created was informative, sensitive, culturally competent, nonjudgmental, supportive, and caring, all of which contributed to the women's trust in the health care system. The most important ingredient in the clinic's success was the relationships that developed with the administrative and clinical staff as there were many components involved in rendering health care. Direct patient services were only one element (Carrington et al., 1993, 1994; Carrington, Loftman, Jones, Williams, & Mitchell, 1998).

The philosophy of the Special Prenatal Clinic places women at the center with all services offered based upon the women's self-identified needs. The clinic is an exemplar of best practices in midwifery.

## Women-Centered Care

### Centrality and Totality

Rodriguez-Trias (1992) described the concepts of centrality and totality in the context of women-centered care. *Centrality* refers to health problems as women themselves define and experience them within their families of origin, community, and society. *Totality* describes women as totally entangled with their families and communities. It involves women as active participants in their health care. Nonetheless, health issues identified by the provider as pressing are valid and deserve attention. Centrality and totality are inextricably intertwined and linked. Racism is a system of power, oppression, and privilege. Race operates as a social stratifier within group hierarchies and is characterized by marked inequalities in receipt of resources and opportunity (Dominguez, 2008). Racial disparities in perinatal outcome are a symptom of racism. Lu and Halfon (2003) describe racial and ethnic disparities in birth outcomes as the result of inequities present over a lifetime; they cannot be completely resolved in the short period of time available during a pregnancy (Lu & Halfon, 2003).

A large focus of health care for reproductive-age women centers on maximizing infant outcomes. Policies, strategies, and practices are directed toward prevention or elimination of risk for poor outcome, and financial services available during pregnancy usually disappear after the birth. The benefits of preconception

## USING THE EVIDENCE FOR BEST PRACTICE

### Case Study 10.1  The Special Prenatal Clinic

P.L. is one of the two midwives in the Special Prenatal Clinic. Her client, D.A., a 29-year-old para 0414, registers at 18 weeks gestation for prenatal care. She admits that her drug of choice is crack. D.A. is instructed regarding the clinic rules, including the required weekly prenatal attendance and urine toxicology testing, and she is referred to the addiction counselor who matches her with a residential drug treatment program. D.A.'s four children are in her mother's custody and D.A. states she lives with her mother. However, during a case conference, D.A.'s mother shares that she does not want D.A. to be a negative influence on the children and consequently she does not allow D.A. to reside in the home. D.A. reluctantly reports living on the street and engaging in prostitution.

D.A. appears to be adjusting well to the residential drug treatment program's routine and is compliant with the weekly prenatal appointments. After 6 weeks, she decides the program is too regimented and leaves. The Special Prenatal Clinic addiction counselor is notified and we await D.A.'s arrival for her next prenatal visit. D.A. does not keep her scheduled weekly prenatal appointment for 4 weeks.

As the midwife is driving home from the hospital one evening, she stops for a red light near a place where prostitutes and "johns" congregate. Her car window is down. "Ms. L, Ms. L," the midwife hears her name. Suddenly D.A. appears with a huge smile on her face. She is always friendly and pleasant. If she is anticipating a lecture, it does not show. P.L. states, "We miss you in clinic." D.A. replies, "I'll see you next week."

D.A. misses her appointment the next week, appears 2 weeks later, comes for 3 weeks, and disappears again. This pattern continues for the entire pregnancy. D.A. presents in labor and delivers a low-birth-weight infant with urine toxicology positive for cocaine. D.A. knows the infant will be placed in her mother's custody when medically ready for discharge. P.L. provides D.A. with a 2-week postpartum appointment, which D.A. keeps.

### Exemplar of Best Practice

When D.A. initially disappeared, P.L. knew she would probably have limited opportunity to help D.A. before she came to the hospital in labor. Each prenatal visit had to be maximized. Although pregnancy motivates many chemically dependent women to cease their drug use, for others addiction is difficult to interrupt. D.A. communicated she was cognizant that her addiction was a problem, one she was not yet ready to relinquish. The established relationship provided the vehicle for D.A. to know she could return to the clinic at any time, no judgments. The primary goal of the staff was addressing her addiction and getting her back into a therapeutic environment. Success in promoting a healthy lifestyle might not be achieved in this pregnancy, but retaining her in the health care system offered the staff the continued opportunity to engage her in behavior change over time.

and interconception care have recently gained traction as strategies to improve birth outcomes. The preconception and interconception periods, however, do not provide sufficient time to restore allostasis and optimize women's health in anticipation of pregnancy. The goal must be to minimize cumulative allostatic load by focusing on the totality of women's health, throughout her lifetime (Lu et al., 2010).

### The Midwife as Primary Care Provider

The midwife, as primary care provider, plays a critical role in assisting a woman to achieve a state of optimal health. Women access midwifery care at multiple life points—reproductive care, preconception, pregnancy, and well-woman care. At the initial encounter, the midwife has the opportunity to define her ability to address a woman's total health needs. This requires knowledge of the standard of care components for adult well-woman care, including immunization and vaccine schedules and age-specific laboratory analysis. Development of a referral network of trusted colleagues to whom women can be referred, when necessary, complements the midwife's capacity in providing total care. Continuity of care and engaging the woman as an active, empowered participant in her health care is essential.

The relationship the woman has with her midwife is central to quality of care, utilization of services, and health care outcomes. This relationship is built on trust and evolves over time. The Special Prenatal Clinic project demonstrated that the midwives who believed in this relationship of trust:

- Involved women as active rather than passive participants in health care, including decisions regarding treatment plans and options
- Communicated clearly and interactively with exchange of ideas
- Demonstrated respect for the women
- Connected with the women on a personal level, earning confidence and trust (Carrington et al., 1998)

### Race Concordance in Care

Women of color often prefer providers who are racially and ethnically concordant with themselves. Race-concordant providers frequently reside in the same community and possess shared experience of daily life, language, values, customs, and cultural norms. The IOM (2004) and the Sullivan Report (2004) state that upon graduation, professionals of color consistently return to work and serve in their communities (IOM, 2004; Sullivan, 2004). Among clients who could choose their providers, there was a preference for race concordance. This factor facilitated increased adherence with appointments and treatment plans. Patients reported feeling more connected and comfortable, respected and trusted, and had more confidence in these providers. They also had the highest level of satisfaction with these providers. Negative attitudes about providers from other ethnic groups were reported, reflecting internalization of broader issues around societal racism (Boulware, Cooper, Ratner, LaVeist, & Powe, 2003; LaVeist & Carroll, 2002; LaVeist & Nuru-Jeter, 2002; Meghani et al., 2009).

In a nationally representative sample of ($n = 6,722$ adults 18 years or older), researchers from George Washington University and the RAND Corporation reported that 14% of African Americans, 19% of Hispanics, and 20.2% of Asian Americans believed they had been treated with disrespect by their health care providers (Blanchard & Lurie, 2004). In cumulative data sets from 1972 through 2014, the General Society Survey (2015) of the University of Chicago reports that 43% of White respondents stated they believed that African Americans have worse jobs, income, and housing than Whites because they lacked the motivation or willpower to pull themselves out of poverty. Among these respondents, 55% stated these differences were not caused by a lack of education, 62% felt discrimination was not the cause, 28% stated African Americans were lazy, and 69% stated that African Americans are not intelligent (University of Chicago, 2015). To reiterate, there is a pressing need to increase the number of midwives of color who may be able to provide a level of cultural comfort and trust that others cannot (IOM, 2004).

## Implicit Bias and Cultural Humility

Implicit bias is an unconscious or intangible belief or preconception about a racial or ethnic group that an individual may be unwilling or unable to report. Implicit bias represents the internalization of the culture of one's family of origin, extended family, peer group, community, and social institutions to which one has been exposed throughout life. With implicit bias, providers enter the clinical environment laden with assumptions and stereotypes. Such assumptions can compromise the midwife–patient interactions.

Cooper et al. (2012) reported that unconscious racial biases and stereotypes existed among a group of providers working in urban Baltimore. These providers had expressed a desire to provide care in low-income communities and did not regard themselves as having a race-based preference or harboring racial stereotypes (Cooper et al., 2012). The providers participated in the Implicit Association Test (implicit.harvard.edu), a validated test that measures how quickly an individual associates good or bad words or positive or negative images. One of the tests examines the unconscious response to persons from different racial groups. Cooper and colleagues note that although it is difficult to change subconscious attitudes, awareness can help providers to change behavior (Cooper et al., 2012).

The increasing racial and ethnic diversity of the U.S. population will continue to present a challenge to midwives. The dearth of midwives of color suggests that the majority of women of color will continue to receive their health care from White midwives (Schuiling, Sipe, & Fullerton, 2013). White midwives are well educated, skilled, and competent. They are also committed and dedicated to providing excellent women's health care without prejudice or racial bias. However, bias may seep into patient encounters, impacting the satisfaction and utilization of health services by women of color. Central to this dilemma is understanding the barriers that impede trust.

Culture, as the aggregate rules of behavior and values informing norms, defines a social group and is transmitted across generations. The increasing diversity of the U.S. population precludes any midwife from achieving total cultural competence with any one group. The challenge for midwives is to provide high-quality care that is culturally based and acceptable. This requires acquisition of information about the cultural community of women receiving services and developing skills that advance cross-cultural communication in clinical encounters (Eiser & Elis, 2007). It also requires incorporating protective cultural practices, encouraging women to use their support networks, and, as possible, strengthening relationships with community outreach organizations.

James (1993) notes that all U.S. racial and ethnic minorities have experienced varying levels of discrimination but the exposure level for African Americans has a particularly prolonged history, contributing to the racial and ethnic disparities in birth outcomes. Supportive midwifery care of women of color at any socioeconomic strata and the care of women vulnerable to the effects of weathering must include consideration of current life events in the framework of cultural histories (James, 1993).

---

**USING THE EVIDENCE FOR BEST PRACTICE**

**Case Study 10.2   Cultural Sensitivity and Implicit Bias**

In 2015, the author attended a conference of doulas, midwives (certified nurse-midwives [CNMs], certified professional midwives [CPMs], lay midwives), traditional birth attendants, and consumers who were primarily women of color. During a workshop on maternal mortality, a consumer who was approximately 32 weeks pregnant shared a recent pregnancy experience. The consumer stated this was her second pregnancy and she had initiated her prenatal care with a physician. However, as they never established a relationship, she decided to transfer her care to a midwife. Unable to locate her first choice, a midwife of color in her community, she located a midwifery practice staffed by Caucasian midwives.

During the initial visit with the midwife, the consumer expressed her belief that the midwife would be discussing preparations for her impending birth. Instead, the midwife asked her about the birth control method she intended to use after delivery. Expressing ire and consternation, the woman asked the conference participants, "Did she think that because I am Black, I shouldn't have more babies? What was she saying?" The consumer ended by saying, "That's why it's so important to have more Black midwives."

**Exemplar of Best Practice**

The consumer was questioning whether the midwife believed that most African American women are single and have many children they cannot afford. Many health care providers acquire such stereotypes about women of color during their educational training. Medical education teaches students that a risk factor for poor perinatal outcomes for communities of color is being a single female head of household. An understanding that many women of color are single by circumstance, not by choice, is lacking. This event exemplifies institutional and educational propagation of racial stereotypes and the pervasive power of implicit bias.

---

# REFERENCES

Blanchard, J., & Lurie, N. (2004). Patient reports of disrespect in the health care setting and its impact on care. *Journal of Family Practice, 53*(9), 721–730.

Boulware, L. E., Cooper, L. S., Ratner, L. E., LaVeist, T. A., & Powe, N. R. (2003). Race and trust in the health care system. *Public Health Reports, 118*(4), 358–365.

Callaway, E. (2013, August 7). NIH director explains HeLa agreement. *Nature: The International Weekly Journal of Science*. Retrieved from http://www.nature.com/news/nih-director -explains-hela-agreement-1.13521. doi.10.1038/nature.2013.13521

Carrington, B. W., Loftman, P. O., Boucher, E., Irish, G., Piniaz, D. K., & Mitchell, J. L. (1994). Modifying a childbirth education curriculum for two specific populations: Inner-city adolescents and substance-using women. *Journal of Nurse Midwifery*, 39(5), 312–320.

Carrington, B. W., Loftman, P. O., Jones, K., Williams, D., & Mitchell, J. L. (1998). The special prenatal clinic: One approach to women and substance abuse *Journal of Women's' Health*, 7(2), 189–193.

Carrington, B. W., Thompson, R. L., Mitchel, J. L., Namerow, P. B., Gordon, T., Loftman, P. O., & Williams, S. B. (1993). The need for family planning services for women delivering with little or no prenatal care. *Women & Health*, 20(1), 1–9.

Carter, G. Woodson Institute. (2004). The case for genocide in Mississippi: SNCC pamphlet, 1964. Retrieved from http://civilrights.woodson.virginia.edu/exhibits/show/caseforgenocide/genocide

Centers for Disease Control and Prevention (CDC). (1997). U.S. Public Health Service Syphilis Study at Tuskegee: Presidential apology [Press release]. Retrieved from http://www.cdc.gov/tuskegee/clintonp.htm

Chasnoff, I. J., Landress, H., & Barett, M. E. (1990). The prevalence of illicit-drug or alcohol use during pregnancy and discrepancies in mandatory reporting in Pinellas County, Florida. *New England Journal of Medicine*, 332, 1202–1206.

Colen, C., Geronimus, A. T., Bound, J., & James, S. A. (2006). Maternal upward socioeconomic mobility and Black–White disparities in infant birth weight. *American Journal of Public Health*, 96(11), 2032–2039.

Cooper, L. A., Roter, D. L. Carson, D. A., Beach, M. C. Sabin, J. A., Greenwald, A. G., & Inui, D. S. (2012). The associations of clinicians' implicit attitudes about race with medical visit communication and patient ratings of interpersonal care. *American Journal of Public Health*, 102(5), 979–987.

Dominguez, T. P. (2008). Race, racism, and racial disparities in adverse birth outcomes. *Clinical Obstetrics and Gynecology*, 51(2), 360–370.

Dominguez, T. P., Dunkel-Schetter, C., Glynn, L. M., Hobel, C., & Sandman, C. A. (2008). Racial differences in birth outcomes: The role of general, pregnancy, and racism stress. *Health Psychology*, 27(2), 194–203.

Eiser, A. R., & Elis, G. (2007). Cultural competence and the African American experience with health care: The case for specific content in cross-cultural education. *Academic Medicine*, 82(2), 176–183.

Forray, A., & Foster, D. (2015). Substance use in the perinatal period. *Current Psychiatry Reports*, 17(11), 91.

Geronimus, A. T. (1996). Black/White differences in the relationship of maternal age to birthweight: A population-based test of the weathering hypothesis. *Social Science and Medicine*, 42(4), 589–597.

Geronimus, A. T., Hicken, M., Keene, D., & Bound, J. (2006). "Weathering" and age patterns of allostatic load scores among Blacks and Whites in the United States. *American Journal of Public Health, Research and Practice*, 96(5), 826–833.

Hanley, B., Dijane, J., Fewtrell, M., Grynberg, A., Hummel, S., Junien, C., . . . van Der Beek, E. M. (2010). Metabolic imprinting, programming and epigenetics: A review of present priorities and future opportunities. *British Journal of Nutrition*, 104(Suppl. 1), S1–S25. doi:10.1017/s0007114510003338

Health Resources and Services Administration. (2013). Maternal and Child Health Bureau: Perinatal health status indicators. Retrieved from http://mchb.hrsa.gov/chusa13/perinatal -health-status-indicators/.html

Hogan, V. K., Culhane, J. F., Crews, K. J., Mwaria, C. B., Rowley, D. L., Levenstein, L., & Mullings, L. P. (2013). The impact of social disadvantage on preconception health, illness, and well-being: An intersectional analysis. *American Journal of Health Promotion*, 27(3, Suppl.), eS32–eS42. doi:10.4278/ajhp.120117-QUAL-43

Institute of Medicine (IOM). (2004). In the nation's compelling interest: Ensuring diversity in the health care workforce. Retrieved from http://iom.nationalacademies.org/Reports/2004/ In-the-Nations-Compelling-Interest-Ensuring-Diversity-in-the-Health-Care-Workforce.aspx

James, S. A. (1993). Racial and ethnic differences in infant mortality and low birth weight. *Annals of Epidemiology*, 7(3), 130–136.

Jones, C. (2014). Systems of power, axes of inequity: Parallels, intersections, braiding the strands. *Medical Care*, 52(10, Suppl. 3), S71–S75.

Kramer, M. R., Hogue, J. H., Dunlop, A. L., & Menon, R. (2011). Preconceptional stress and racial disparities in preterm birth: An overview. *Acta Obstetricia et Gynecologica Scandinavica*, 90(12), 1307–1316. doi:10.1111/j.1600-0412.2011.01136

Krase, K. (2014). History of forced sterilization and current U.S. abuses. Retrieved from http:// www.ourbodiesourselves.org/health-info/forced-sterilization

LaVeist, T. A., & Carroll, T. (2002). Race of physician and satisfaction with care among African American patients. *Journal of the National Medical Association*, 94, 937–943.

LaVeist, T. A., & Nuru-Jeter, A. (2002). Is doctor–patient race concordance associated with greater satisfaction with care? *Journal of Health and Social Behavior*, 43, 296–306.

Law, V. (2014, January 14). It's 2014. Why do we still need laws banning coerced sterilization? Retrieved from http://www.truth-out.org/news/item/27121-it-s-2014-why-do-we-still-need -laws-banning-coerced-sterilization

Lawrence, J. (2000). The Indian Health Service and the sterilization of Native American women. *American Indian Quarterly*, 24(3), 400–419. Retrieved from http://bixby.ucla.edu/ journal_club/Lawrence_s2.pdf

Lu, M. C., & Halfon, N. (2003). Racial and ethnic disparities in birth outcomes: A life course perspective. *Maternal and Child Health Journal*, 7(1), 13–30.

Lu, M. C., Kotelchuck, M., Hogan, V., Jones, L., Wright, K., & Halfon, N. (2010). Closing the Black–White gap in birth outcomes: A life-course approach. *Ethnicity and Disease*, 20(Suppl. 2), 62–76.

Meghani, S. H., Brooks, J. M., Gipson-Jones, T., Waite, R., Whitefield-Harris, L., & Deatric, J. (2009). Patient–provider race concordance: Does it matter in improving minority patients' health outcomes? *Ethnicity and Health*, 14(1), 107–130.

Nittle, N. K. (2014). The U.S. Government's role in sterilizing women of color. Retrieved from http://racerelations.about.com/od/historyofracerelations/a/The-U-S-Governments-Role-In-Sterilizing-Women-Of-Color.htm

Roberts, D. (1997). *Killing the Black body: Race, reproduction and the meaning of liberty*. New York, NY: Pantheon Books.

Rodriguez-Trias, H. (1992). Women's health, women's lives, women's rights. *American Journal of Public Health*, 82(5), 663–664.

Schoendorf, K. C., Hogue, C. J., Kleinman, J. C., & Rowley, D. (1992). Mortality among infants of Black as compared with White college-educated parents. *New England Journal of Medicine*, *326*, 1522–1526.

Schuiling, K. D., Sipe, T. A., & Fullerton, J. (2013). Findings from the analysis of the American College of Nurse-Midwives' membership surveys: 2009 to 2011. *Journal of Midwifery and Women's Health*, *58*(4), 404–415.

Skloot, R. (2011). *The immortal life of Henrietta Lacks*. New York, NY: Random House.

Sullivan, L. W. (2004). Missing persons: Minorities in the health professions. The Sullivan Report. Retrieved from http://www.aacn.nche.edu/media-relations/SullivanReport.pdf

Terplan, M., Ramanadhan, S., Locke, A., Longinaker, N., & Lui, S. (2015). Psychosocial interventions for pregnant women in outpatient illicit drug treatment programs compared to other interventions (review). The Cochrane Collaboration. *Cochrane Library*, (4). Retrieved from http://www.Thecochranelibrary.com

Thomas, S. B., & Quinn, S. C. (1991). Public health then and now. The Tuskegee Syphilis Study, 1932 to 1972: Implications for HIV education and AIDS risk education programs in the Black community. *American Journal of Public Health*, *81*(11), 1498–1504.

Tuskegee University. (2015). 18th anniversary of U.S. syphilis study apology to be marked at Tuskegee University. Retrieved from http://www.tuskegee.edu/Articles/18th_anniversary_of_us_syphilis_study_apology_to_be_marked_at_tuskegee_university.aspx

University of Chicago. (2015). General Society Survey 2015 data set 1971–2014 cumulative file. Chicago, IL: NORC. Retrieved from https://gssdataexplorer.norc.org/variables/vfilter

U.S. Census Bureau. (2015). Income, poverty, and health insurance coverage in the United States: 2014. Retrieved from https://www.census.gov/hhes/www/hlthins/data/incpovhlth

U.S. Department of Commerce. (2015). Income and poverty in the United States: 2014. Retrieved from http://www.census.gov/content/dam/Census/library/publications/2015/demo/p60-252.pdf.

U.S. Department of Health and Human Services (USDHHS). (2015). Substance Abuse and Mental Health Services Administration: Results from the 2013 National Survey on Drug Use and Health: Summary of national findings. Retrieved from http://www.samhsa.gov/data/sites/default/files/NSDUHresultsPDFWHTML2013/ Web/NSDUHresults2013.htm#2.7

U.S. Department of Labor. (2015). Bureau of Labor Statistics: The employment situation—October 2015. Retrieved from http://www.bls.gov/news.release/pdf/empsit.pdf

U.S. National Library of Medicine. (1976). Native voices: 1976: Government admits forced sterilization of Indian women. Retrieved from https://www.nlm.nih.gov/nativevoices/timeline/543.html

Vinikoor, L. C., Kaufman, J. S., MacLehose, R. F., & Laraia, B. A. (2008). Effects of racial density and income incongruity on pregnancy outcomes in less segregated communities. *Social Science and Medicine*, *66*(2), 255–259.

Yonkers, K. A., Forray, A., Howell, H. B., Gotman, N., Kershaw, T., Rounsaville, B. J., & Carroll, K. M. (2012). Motivational enhancement therapy coupled with cognitive behavioral therapy versus brief advice: A randomized trial for treatment of hazardous substance use in pregnancy and after delivery. *General Hospital Psychiatry*, *34*(5), 439–449.

# CHAPTER ELEVEN

# CIRCLES OF CHANGE: CENTERINGPREGNANCY®, HEALTH DISPARITIES, AND VULNERABLE WOMEN

Margaret S. Hutchison and Melanie R. Thomas

Concern about adverse outcomes among poor and vulnerable populations has long been a part of the national health care conversation. Health disparity affects people who have experienced barriers based on the following: racial or ethnic group; religion; socioeconomic status; gender; age; impaired mental health; cognitive, sensory, or physical disability; sexual orientation or gender identity; geographic location; or other exclusion categories (Carter-Pokras & Baquet, 2002). Using this definition, the authors refer to populations with these disadvantages linked to health disparities as *vulnerable*. This chapter uses a health disparities lens to examine CenteringPregnancy® (CP), a midwifery innovation with evidence of improved perinatal outcomes for low-income, psychosocially at-risk women. We also provide an example of an enhanced Centering model that includes integrated mental health and social services.

## VULNERABLE POPULATIONS AND PERINATAL OUTCOMES

The maternal and child disparities faced by vulnerable pregnant women in the United States are staggering. In a recent review examining the intergenerational transmission of inequality, the authors calculate that the most economically disadvantaged U.S. women (defined as African American, unmarried, and less than a high school education) are three times more likely to deliver low-birth-weight infants when compared to those women with the most advantage (defined as non-Hispanic White, married, college educated; Aizer & Currie, 2014). In addition to higher risk for delivering low-birth-weight and preterm infants, women from vulnerable populations have higher rates of maternal mortality, prepregnancy obesity, postpartum weight retention, and postpartum depression compared to their more privileged counterparts (Alio et al., 2010; Braveman et al., 2015; Bryant, Worjoloh, Caughey, & Washington, 2010; Hauck, Tanabe, & Moon, 2011; Spong, Iams, Goldenberg, Hauck, & Willinger, 2011). The individual, family, and public cost of these disparities are far-reaching, as adverse birth outcomes are associated with a host of negative health trajectories, including greater risk of obesity and mental illness throughout life (Abel et al., 2010; Barker, 2006; Boney, Verma, Tucker, & Vohr, 2005; Gillman, 2005). Recently, the United States has been designated as the most unequal country among all developed countries, this inequality starting at birth (Central Intelligence Agency, 2013).

## Psychosocial Stressors

The underlying causes for the U.S. maternal and birth outcome disparities are multifactorial, linked to a variety of social and psychological determinants. Vulnerable women, those who are poor, younger, with less social capital, and from minority groups, are more likely to experience psychosocial risk and cumulative stress compared with more privileged women. Evidence suggests that stress over the life course, especially early life stress and experiences of discrimination and racism, negatively impacts general and reproductive health (Cox, 2009; Dayan et al., 2010; Dominguez, 2011; Love, David, Rankin, & Collins, 2010; Lu & Halfon, 2003; Rosenthal & Lobel, 2011). In addition to the significance of cumulative stress, stress and anxiety during pregnancy can impact maternal–child health outcomes as well (Dunkel Schetter & Tanner, 2012; Entringer, Buss, & Wadhwa, 2010; Giscombe & Lobel, 2005; Vrekoussis et al., 2010; Wadhwa, 2005). A recent national survey documents that women with social disadvantage (e.g., younger, unmarried, and minorities) are more likely to have experienced a stressful life event in the year before giving birth (Burns, Farr, & Howards, 2015). Experiences with perceived stress, racism, low self-esteem, negative perceptions of pregnancy, and significant stressful life events during pregnancy have all been independently associated with adverse birth outcomes (Carty et al., 2011; Collins et al., 2000; Hogue et al., 2013; Jesse & Alligood, 2002; Seravalli, Patterson, & Nelson, 2014). Although outside the scope of this chapter, recent literature reviews highlight the well-established associations between negative psychological processes (chronic stress, anxiety, and depression) and adverse birth outcomes (Dunkel Schetter & Tanner, 2012; Latendresse, 2009).

Given its high prevalence and strong association with adverse maternal–child health outcomes, depression is worth special consideration. For low-income and minority women, perinatal depression often occurs within a context of adversity across the life course (Davis, Stange, & Horwitz, 2012; Ertel, Rich-Edwards, & Koenen, 2011; Lu & Halfon, 2003). Approximately 17% of women in the United States will experience major depression during their lifetime (Hasin, Goodwin, Stinson, & Grant, 2005), but vulnerable women experience significantly higher rates than women in the general population. In community-based samples, pregnant Black women have higher rates of depression and posttraumatic stress disorder than White women (Gavin et al., 2011; Seng, Kohn-Wood, McPherson, & Sperlich, 2011). However, Black women are more likely to keep their depression secret and less likely to seek mental health treatment (O'Mahen, Henshaw, Jones, & Flynn, 2011; Seng et al., 2011). Depressed Black and Hispanic women are more likely to report multiple social adversities compared to depressed White women

(Ertel et al., 2011). Women from underserved populations are also more likely to live in violent neighborhoods and to have experienced intimate partner violence. This exposure to violence confers risks for pregnant women and their children, including an association with the development of perinatal depression (Alvarez-Segura et al., 2014; Barrios et al., 2015).

Despite effective treatment options, most pregnant women experiencing emotional distress do not get help. There are many individual and systemic barriers to accessing appropriate treatment among childbearing women. Recent data illustrate that only one of eight pregnant women in a representative U.S. sample who reported symptoms consistent with clinical depression had received any mental health care within the past year (Byatt, Xiao, Dinh, & Waring, 2016). Women may not seek mental health care for themselves because of competing priorities, stigma, or they do not recognize their distress as treatable (Freed, Chan, Boger, & Tompson, 2012). Furthermore, the risk factors for depression, the cultural experience of stress and mental illness, and provider sensitivity for screening differ across racial/ethnic minority groups and other vulnerable populations of women (Liu & Tronick, 2013).

Pregnancy during adolescence is a risk for adverse birth outcomes, with a substantial overlap with other vulnerabilities such as poverty, minority group status, and depression. Black and Latino adolescents in the United States are more likely to get pregnant than their White peers. Black teens have three times and Latino teens have four times the birth rate of their White counterparts (Basch, 2011). Teens who become pregnant are at risk for a variety of adverse maternal–child health outcomes and were more likely to have had adverse childhood experiences themselves (Bellis, Lowey, Leckenby, Hughes, & Harrison, 2014), again harkening to the intergenerational transmission of inequality. In one study of pregnant teens, nearly half of the sample met the criteria for moderate to severe depression, with African American adolescents as well as those exposed to prior verbal or physical abuse, community violence, family criticism, and less partner and general support reporting more symptoms of depression than others (Buzi, Smith, Kozinetz, Peskin, & Wiemann, 2015).

## Vulnerable Populations and Midwifery Efficacy

Historically, restrictive practice laws and the commitment of the profession to serving the poor characterized the rich history of midwifery's care for vulnerable and underserved women and their families. In 1925, Mary Breckinridge and the Frontier Nursing Service began work with impoverished rural Appalachians in Kentucky. Other early midwifery practices worked among equally economically depressed groups such as the tenement dwellers in New York City, the Hispanic poor of New Mexico, and indigent Black families in Alabama. The entry point for midwives into hospital-based practice was again with the underserved. In the 1970s, midwives were invited into busy publicly funded hospitals that trained medical students and obstetricians (Rooks, 1997). Today midwives work at all socioeconomic levels in diverse practice settings, although the strong professional commitment to public health continues.

Research on the efficacy of midwifery care for vulnerable populations began with the early modern midwifery practices. In their 2005 review article, Raisler and Kennedy observe that midwifery care of the poor supported excellent outcomes in access to prenatal care, physiologic care, and better neonatal and adolescent outcomes compared to reference statistics across the nation (Raisler & Kennedy, 2005). Further research is needed but the evidence suggests that the relationship-based, low-intervention, and high-touch care of midwifery leads to excellent outcomes for vulnerable women.

## THE CP MODEL

CP, first piloted in 1993, is a well-known group prenatal care model developed by Sharon Rising, CNM. Although its philosophical underpinnings are directly drawn from midwifery, the principles are now used by maternity care providers of all disciplines. The development and spread of CP are supported by the non-profit Centering Healthcare Institute (CHI) and there are active Centering sites in most of the 50 states and in numerous other countries (CHI, 2015).

CP is an empowerment-based care model that takes women out of exam rooms and into a group space for prenatal visits. Eight to 12 women with pregnancies at a similar gestational age become a cohort that attends group prenatal visits together. Group sessions mirror the frequency of individual visits but are much longer, with ten 2-hour sessions over the course of pregnancy co-led by a health care provider and a second group leader, typically another staff member with expertise in perinatal issues (e.g., registered nurses, medical assistants, social workers, or health educators). During each session, women engage in self-care activities, receive a physical assessment by the provider, build community, and participate in facilitated interactive discussions about issues important to pregnant and parenting women and families.

CP must include certain characteristics of a group care model. These characteristics, Essential Elements (see Table 11.1), pertain to the process of care rather than to content, a reflection of the belief that the transformative power of the

---

**TABLE 11.1   Essential Elements of CenteringPregnancy®**

Health assessment happens in the group space
Patients engage in self-care activities
Each session has a plan, but emphasis may vary
Groups are facilitated to be interactive
There is time for socializing
Groups are conducted in a circle
Group members, including facilitators and support people, are consistent
Group size is optimal for interaction
There is ongoing evaluation

*Source:* Centering Healthcare Institute (2015).

model lies in its ability to unseat the hierarchical expert-to-patient model of health care delivery (CHI, 2015). In 2013, support for the process over content premise was documented in a study that showed no relationship between health education content and preterm birth rates for CP, but a significant association between increased levels of group facilitation and decreased preterm birth rate (Novick et al., 2013).

## Evidence for Improved Outcomes

CP is an evidence-based midwifery-designed model that has been shown to improve maternal and birth outcomes when compared to individual prenatal care (Hale, Picklesimer, Billings, & Covington-Kolb, 2014; Ickovics et al., 2007, 2011; Picklesimer, Billings, Hale, Blackhurst, & Covington-Kolb, 2012; Tilden, Hersh, Emeis, Weinstein, & Caughey, 2014). Since its inception, CP has grown substantially in its evidence base, establishing efficacy and effectiveness, as well as programmatic reach. Although some dissenting studies exist, the majority of CP data show positive impact on birth outcomes, breastfeeding, and levels of patient satisfaction (Benediktsson et al., 2013; Devitt, 2013; Hale et al., 2014; Ickovics et al., 2007, 2011; Manant & Dodgson, 2011; Summers, 2014; Tanner-Smith, Steinka-Fry, & Lipsey, 2013, 2014; Tilden et al., 2014). This model of care was recently highlighted by the Agency for Healthcare Research and Quality website as a promising, innovative model with strong evidence for positive effects on birth outcomes, patient satisfaction, and provider efficiency (Briggs-Gowan, Carter, Skuban, & Horwitz, 2001). Several studies examining the effectiveness of CP have been conducted in vulnerable populations of women, specifically adolescents, women of color, and women in poverty who are served by public health systems. In the following section, we present the evidence compared with individual care, suggesting that CP is a more effective means of addressing health disparities and remediating health inequities for vulnerable women.

### Birth Outcomes

The strongest study documenting the positive impact of CP on birth outcomes comes from Ickovics et al. (2007), a randomized controlled trial (RCT) among a population of young (ages 15–24) women in two university-affiliated hospital prenatal clinics (New Haven, CT, and Atlanta, GA). Among this sample ($n = 1,047$) comprising 80% Black women, using intent-to-treat analyses, those randomized to group prenatal care were 33% less likely to have a preterm birth than those randomized to individual care. There were no differences in age, parity, education, or income between study conditions. The reduction in preterm birth was even more significant (41%) when the data were analyzed by African American status only. Picklesimer et al. (2012) provided additional evidence supporting CP as an intervention to reduce birth outcome disparities, especially for African American women. In this retrospective cohort study conducted among a diverse sample of low-income pregnant women in South Carolina, those who chose to participate in CP were less likely to deliver a preterm infant compared to those who chose traditional prenatal care. Given the finding that CP appears to close the gap in the Black–White disparity in preterm birth, this study earned a "race to press for benefit of scientific community" designation from the *American Journal of Obstetrics and Gynecology*.

Although less rigorous in design, other studies have demonstrated that CP reduces adverse birth outcomes across diverse populations, including Hispanic women. One study comparing Hispanic women in Palm Beach County, Florida (*n* = 176), found that those who chose CP over traditional prenatal care models were less likely than their individual care counterparts to have a preterm birth (Tandon, Colon, Vega, Murphy, & Alonso, 2012).

### Depression and Emotional Distress

A growing base of evidence shows that CP may also have the potential to positively influence psychological outcomes for vulnerable pregnant women. An RCT study examined a population of young, mostly African American women experiencing high levels of stress at baseline. The women were assigned to either group care or individual care. The group care population had decreased levels of depression and reduced reporting of social conflict at 12 months postpartum compared to those in individual care (Ickovics et al., 2011). These same highly stressed women, after group care interventions, also experienced a decrease in perceived stress and an increase in self-esteem between the second and third trimesters (Ickovics et al., 2011).

Other authors have documented improvements in postpartum depression for women enrolled in CP compared to those receiving individual care, including a study focused on adolescents, a group with high depression risk (Trotman et al., 2015). One group in Canada showed that CP participants had improvements in depression and anxiety compared to women who had both individual care and prenatal education classes (Benediktsson et al., 2013). This study is unusual in that it compares group care to individual care augmented by prenatal classes, suggesting that the efficacy of CP lies more in process than in content.

### Patient Engagement

Addressing the overall well-being of the pregnant woman, considering the mother–infant dyad, and adapting the curriculum for culturally specific needs of the group are important tenets of CP. These approaches may be especially meaningful for engaging underserved populations, including recent immigrants who are at risk for depression as a result of social isolation and acculturation-specific stress (D'Anna-Hernandez, Aleman, & Flores, 2015).

One study comparing Latina women in Palm Beach County, Florida (*n* = 176), found that those who chose CP over traditional prenatal care were both more satisfied and engaged in their prenatal care and more likely to establish a medical home for the newborn (Tandon, Cluxton-Keller, Colon, Vega, & Alonso, 2013). Other studies comparing Latinas in CP care and individual care have more mixed results. One study with a small sample size (*n* = 49) showed equivalent birth and psychosocial outcomes between CP care and individual care for Hispanic women (Robertson, Aycock, & Darnell, 2009). A larger study among Hispanic women found that women who selected CP had higher health care utilization but no differences in birth outcomes (Trudnak, Arboleda, Kirby, & Perrin, 2013). A limitation in each of these studies examining CP intervention for Hispanic women is the self-selection of women into CP versus individual care, with no randomized trials specifically for this patient population.

### Health Indicators

When compared to individual prenatal care, CP shows improvement across a variety of health indicators, including gestational weight gain, postpartum weight trajectory, utilization of family-planning services, and breastfeeding. Although often considered secondary outcomes in relation to the primary birth outcomes, these indicators have significant individual and public health ramifications and are often issues of inequities for vulnerable women and families. In an RCT study in young women (aged 14–21) in New York City, those randomized to CP showed more favorable patterns of gestational weight gain and postpartum weight trajectories compared to individual care. In addition, women with higher levels of prenatal distress and depression had the most benefit from CP on weight-gain outcomes (Magriples et al., 2015).

A recent retrospective chart study conducted among adolescents reported superior outcomes for appropriate gestational weight gain as well as initiation of breastfeeding and long-term contraception among teens enrolled in CP compared to those in individual care (Trotman et al., 2015). Another group reported that women who participated in CP were more likely than those who chose to enroll in individual care to utilize postpartum family-planning services, with the most dramatic increase in utilization of these services among African American women (Hale et al., 2014).

## Implementation of CP

Although the evidence presented previously supports the assertion that CP can reduce health inequities for vulnerable women, successful implementation of the CP model requires substantial systemic and paradigm shifts. These shifts can be more difficult in underresourced systems. Barriers to successful implementation may include lack of uptake and adherence at the individual patient level; provider resistance to philosophical and pragmatic change; and broader systemic issues with space, billing, institutional or policy obstacles. In their article, describing the introduction of CP into a busy public health system serving low-income, mostly African American, women, Klima, Norr, Vonderheid, and Handler (2009) describe that patients in CP had higher satisfaction with care, increased rates of breastfeeding, and attended more prenatal care visits compared to women in individual care, in spite of implementation challenges (Klima et al., 2009). Novick et al. (2015) state, "Thriving sites had organizational cultures that supported innovation, champions who advocated for [CP], and staff who viewed logistical demands as manageable hurdles. Struggling sites had bureaucratic organizational structures and lacked buy-in and financial resources, and staff were overwhelmed by the model's challenges" (Novick et al., 2015, p. 462).

Two recent reviews summarized challenges associated with implementing CP in various settings and offer practical recommendations for those considering adopting the CP model (DeCesare & Jackson, 2015; Tilden et al., 2014). In addition, qualitative studies provide rich data from patients and providers about their empowering experiences as a result of CP implementation (Baldwin & Phillips, 2011; Herrman, Rogers, & Ehrenthal, 2012). A recent study by Earnshaw et al. (2016) documents increased satisfaction and engagement in women enrolled in CP groups with participants who are more diverse in age, highlighting that group composition may also influence successful implementation.

## A Template for Integrated Care With Vulnerable Populations

Although Centering has been widely used and accepted by women of diverse socioeconomic backgrounds, a growing body of literature supports its efficacy especially with women from vulnerable populations. Within traditional health care models, psychosocial risk is often addressed in isolation from other health and social services, which results in limited uptake and adherence (Dennis, 2014). In contrast, interventions that integrate mental health care with primary care, partner with community-based organizations, and address the underlying social determinants of health show more favorable results (Jesse et al., 2015). Specific examples of promising interventions include a protocol to evaluate the effects of housing support for pregnant women (Allen, Feinberg, & Mitchell, 2014), use of community health workers to refer high-risk mothers to a parenting skills group (Muzik et al., 2015), and the integration of a culturally tailored, cognitive based therapy group into a prenatal setting (Jesse & Alligood, 2002). One recent report highlights two examples of community-based programs in Milwaukee, Wisconsin, designed to reduce maternal–child health disparities. These examples describe two tenets critical to success, also essential to the CP model: engagement and empowerment (Willis, McManus, Magallanes, Johnson, & Majnik, 2014).

## BEST PRACTICES

This evidence for community partnerships and client engagement provides support for best practices in the development of an augmented, integrated model described here. One of the first author's primary clinical practice sites is San Francisco General Hospital (SFGH), the safety net facility for the City and County of San Francisco, California. In 1999, the midwifery practice piloted CP in an effort to respond to the observed increasing social isolation of immigrant Latina clients and the limitations of the individual care model to address psychosocial needs adequately in a culturally sensitive manner. The observed isolation mirrored immigration shifts of the 1980s and 1990s: Increasingly, women were migrating from Mexico and Central America to the United States without family or a partner, in contrast to the historical trends of migration first by men, followed later by their families. Thus, CP seemed to be a way to provide social support as well as to address high rates of trauma, depression, anxiety, housing insecurity, intimate partner violence, and poverty.

There was almost immediate success following implementation of CP. Language and cultural concordance (group leadership by a Spanish-speaking midwife and a bilingual/bicultural staff person) was one of the many benefits of the group care model for a recent immigrant population. Aggregated concepts extrapolated from comments were as follows:

- I felt different in my Centering group than I did in the clinic, or in the hospital, or in the street.
- In those places, everyone acts like I'm stupid, or like I can't hear, since I don't speak English.
- Here people really listen.

In 2007, the SFGH Spanish-language groups became "opt-out," with roughly 50% of eligible midwifery clients in Centering. Other developments included Teen Centering (2003–2008) and English-speaking adult Centering (2008). All groups comprised publicly insured women who had incomes at less than 200% of the federal poverty level. Implementing the teen groups presented an opportunity. Because of space limitations at SFGH, leadership began to think about alternative sites. The clinic had a longstanding relationship with a nearby social service agency for pregnant teens, the Teenage Pregnancy and Parenting Program (TAPP). Given the limitations of traditional hospitals and clinics to address social needs, the Teen Centering program was established at TAPP, with groups co-led by a midwife from SFGH and a case manager from TAPP. The young women were patients of the SFGH who entered care at the hospital's clinic, but then had most prenatal visits off site at TAPP, thereby providing access to TAPP's population-specific social services. Observed successes went beyond the empowerment and community-building aspects of CP by increasing linkage to needed social services made accessible by the co-location model. Having care on-site at TAPP opened doors to services in a way that could not have happened otherwise.

This integrated model is exemplified in the case of Shivaun, a 16-year-old with a suspicion of social services borne of a long history in the foster care system. She begrudgingly agreed to participate in Centering at the TAPP site but by the second session became an active group participant. At first resistant to TAPP services, by 28 weeks of pregnancy, she began receiving case management services. At 6 months postpartum, she became a TAPP peer counselor. She now has the goal of finishing school and becoming a midwife.

The most longstanding relationship between the SFGH Centering program and a community-based social service agency began in 2007, when all adult groups moved to an agency for low-income pregnant and parenting families in San Francisco called the Homeless Prenatal Program (HPP). No longer exclusively for homeless families, this agency has case management services, groups, child care, community health worker training, housing assistance, and countless other offerings. This ongoing, highly collegial partnership is supported by a memorandum of understanding between the hospital and the social service agency. Most Centering participants begin as patients of SFGH and are not HPP clients prior to initiating Centering. Once care begins at the HPP, visits are billed to SFGH and are co-led by a midwife and an HPP staff person. These HPP staff are former HPP (and some Centering) clients, which provides an added cultural and experiential concordance between the Centering participants and group leadership. Since 2008, co-located groups have been conducted in Spanish and English.

A primary goal of the community collaborative model is to enhance the beneficial effects of Centering with vulnerable women by providing access to the services and support that these social service agencies can offer. Care providers know the feeling of powerlessness of being unable to fix another person's social challenges. Early analysis of participant experience in the HPP/SFGH Centering model revealed that 90% of women—very few of whom were HPP clients prior to initiation of Centering—had become HPP clients and made use of their services by the end of pregnancy, thus fixing their own problems to a certain extent.

More recent, a third partner has become a part of this care model, the SFGH-based Infant–Parent Program (IPP). This mental health agency provides services to at-risk parents of young children, with a focus on the parental–infant (or young child) bond. Together, these three agencies (SFGH, HPP, and IPP) provide integrated medical, social, and psychological care, with CP at its core. The IPP was first brought into the collaboration in 2008, with support of funding by a local foundation. Because of early successes, further funding has been procured to support ongoing mental health support and involvement.

The rationale for bringing in a mental health partner lies in the perceived need for greater competency among front-line staff in both the identification of mental health issues and successful referral to needed mental health services. A rough survey of all patients seen by the SFGH nurse-midwifery service revealed that greater than 50% suffer from some constellation of past and/or current depression, anxiety, and trauma. Centering embedded in the HPP was a step toward improving care for women with these and other mental health challenges; incorporation of the IPP took these efforts further. Activities since 2008 have included half-day workshops for a broad array of perinatal staff led by IPP psychologists in the areas of:

- Mental health and perinatal care for immigrant women
- Perinatal care for women with substance use disorders
- Mental health consultation support by IPP psychologists for midwives and HPP Centering staff

This has included on-site support for HPP staff, and monthly 1-hour consultation meetings with midwives and HPP staff. The latter has provided an opportunity to discuss and problem-solve regarding difficult cases related to mental health and the dynamics that emerge in multiple interfaces: 1·1 visits, Centering sessions, and inpatient care. Training and support for use of the Edinburgh Postnatal Depression Scale in Centering groups was introduced as a way to open discussion about mental health in pregnancy. These strategies have helped to improve integration of mental health services within all parts of the perinatal care system.

---

**USING THE EVIDENCE FOR BEST PRACTICE**

**Case Study 11.1    Centering at HPP: "My Bridge to This Culture"**

Stephanie had been in the United States for 2 years when she entered prenatal care at SFGH Women's Health Center. She and her husband had made plans to return to Mexico. Her time was spent at work, school, and at home with her husband, but she missed her family and her home, feeling out of place in this strange city. With the pregnancy, their plans changed and the couple made a decision to stay in the United States until after the baby was born, followed by a return to Mexico.

On initial presentation to the clinic, Stephanie refused group prenatal care. Looking back, she attributes this refusal to her depression. The last thing she wanted to do was talk to a group of other women. The nurse persisted in suggesting that she at least give Centering a try, and she finally agreed. In the first few sessions, she mostly observed, but eventually came out of her shell and became a leader for her group. She developed close relationships with other group members and with the HPP Centering leader, who is an immigrant Latina, a former HPP client, and is now HPP trained. This co-leader, with the help of the midwife, facilitated a rich discussion in the group about depression, and skillfully connected Stephanie to mental health services at SFGH.

As Stephanie gained confidence, she accessed the services at HPP before and after having the baby; Stephanie now describes her Centering experience at HPP as "my bridge to this culture." Because of the environment of care, she was finally able to acculturate. Stephanie became a peer health worker at HPP, volunteering as a Centering co-leader, and is working toward becoming a nurse.

---

# REFERENCES

Abel, K. M., Wicks, S., Susser, E. S., Dalman, C., Pedersen, M. G., Mortensen, P. B., & Webb, R. T. (2010). Birth weight, schizophrenia, and adult mental disorder: Is risk confined to the smallest babies? *Archives of General Psychiatry, 67*(9), 923–930. doi:10.1001/archgen psychiatry.2010.100

Aizer, A., & Currie, J. (2014). The intergenerational transmission of inequality: Maternal disadvantage and health at birth. *Science, 344*(6186), 856–861. doi:10.1126/science.1251872

Alio, A. P., Richman, A. R., Clayton, H. B., Jeffers, D. F., Wathington, D. J., & Salihu, H. M. (2010). An ecological approach to understanding Black–White disparities in perinatal mortality. *Maternal and Child Health Journal, 14*(4), 557–566. doi:10.1007/s10995-009-0495-9

Allen, D., Feinberg, E., & Mitchell, H. (2014). Bringing life course home: A pilot to reduce pregnancy risk through housing access and family support. *Maternal and Child Health Journal, 18*(2), 405–412. doi:10.1007/s10995-013-1327-5

Alvarez-Segura, M., Garcia-Esteve, L., Torres, A., Plaza, A., Imaz, M. L., Hermida-Barros, L., . . . Burtchen, N. (2014). Are women with a history of abuse more vulnerable to perinatal depressive symptoms? A systematic review. *Archives of Women's Mental Health, 17*(5), 343–357. doi:10.1007/s00737-014-0440-9

Baldwin, K., & Phillips, G. (2011). Voices along the journey: Midwives' perceptions of implementing the CenteringPregnancy model of prenatal care. *Journal of Perinatal Education, 20*(4), 210–217. doi:10.1891/1058-1243.20.4.210

Barker, D. J. (2006). Adult consequences of fetal growth restriction. *Clinical Obstetrics and Gynecology, 49*(2), 270–283.

Barrios, Y. V., Gelaye, B., Zhong, Q., Nicolaidis, C., Rondon, M. B., Garcia, P. J., . . . Williams, M. A. (2015). Association of childhood physical and sexual abuse with intimate partner violence, poor general health and depressive symptoms among pregnant women. *PLoS One, 10*(1), e0116609. doi:10.1371/journal.pone.0116609

Basch, C. E. (2011). Teen pregnancy and the achievement gap among urban minority youth. *Journal of School Health, 81*(10), 614–618. doi:10.1111/j.1746-1561.2011.00635.x

Bellis, M. A., Lowey, H., Leckenby, N., Hughes, K., & Harrison, D. (2014). Adverse childhood experiences: Retrospective study to determine their impact on adult health behaviours and health outcomes in a UK population. *Journal of Public Health, 36*(1), 81–91. doi:10.1093/pubmed/fdt038

Benediktsson, I., McDonald, S. W., Vekved, M., McNeil, D. A., Dolan, S. M., & Tough, S. C. (2013). Comparing CenteringPregnancy® to standard prenatal care plus prenatal education. *BMC Pregnancy Childbirth, 13*(Suppl. 1), S5. doi:10.1186/1471-2393-13-s1-s5

Boney, C. M., Verma, A., Tucker, R., & Vohr, B. R. (2005). Metabolic syndrome in childhood: Association with birth weight, maternal obesity, and gestational diabetes mellitus. *Pediatrics, 115*(3), e290–e296. doi:10.1542/peds.2004–1808

Braveman, P. A., Heck, K., Egerter, S., Marchi, K. S., Dominguez, T. P., Cubbin, C., . . . Curtis, M. (2015). The role of socioeconomic factors in Black–White disparities in preterm birth. *American Journal of Public Health, 105*(4), 694–702. doi:10.2105/AJPH.2014.302008

Briggs-Gowan, M. J., Carter, A. S., Skuban, E. M., & Horwitz, S. M. (2001). Prevalence of social–emotional and behavioral problems in a community sample of 1- and 2-year-old children. *Journal of the American Academy of Child and Adolescent Psychiatry, 40*(7), 811–819. doi:10.1097/00004583-200107000-00016

Bryant, A. S., Worjoloh, A., Caughey, A. B., & Washington, A. E. (2010). Racial/ethnic disparities in obstetric outcomes and care: Prevalence and determinants. *American Journal of Obstetrics and Gynecology, 202*(4), 335–343. doi:10.1016/j.ajog.2009.10.864

Burns, E. R., Farr, S. L., & Howards, P. P. (2015). Stressful life events experienced by women in the year before their infants' births—United States, 2000–2010. *Morbidity and Mortality Weekly Report, 64*(9), 247–251.

Buzi, R. S., Smith, P. B., Kozinetz, C. A., Peskin, M. F., & Wiemann, C. M. (2015). A socio-ecological framework to assessing depression among pregnant teens. *Maternal and Child Health Journal, 19*(10), 2187–2194. doi:10.1007/s10995-015-1733-y

Byatt, N., Xiao, R. S., Dinh, K. H., & Waring, M. E. (2016). Mental health care use in relation to depressive symptoms among pregnant women in the USA. *Archives of Women's Mental Health, 19*(1), 187–191. doi:10.1007/s00737-015-0524-1

Carter-Pokras, O., & Baquet, C. (2002). What is a "health disparity"? *Public Health Reports, 117*(5), 426–434.

Carty, D. C., Kruger, D. J., Turner, T. M., Campbell, B., DeLoney, E. H., & Lewis, E. Y. (2011). Racism, health status, and birth outcomes: Results of a participatory community-based intervention and health survey. *Journal of Urban Health, 88*(1), 84–97. doi:10.1007/s11524-010-9530-9

Centering Healthcare Institute (CHI). (2015). The Centering Model. Retrieved from http://centeringhealthcare.org/pages/centering-model/model-overview.php

Central Intelligence Agency. (2013). *The world factbook 2013–2014.* Washington, DC: Author.

Collins, J. W., Jr., David, R. J., Symons, R., Handler, A., Wall, S. N., & Dwyer, L. (2000). Low-income African-American mothers' perception of exposure to racial discrimination and infant birth weight. *Epidemiology, 11*(3), 337–339.

Cox, K. J. (2009). Midwifery and health disparities: Theories and intersections. *Journal of Midwifery and Women's Health, 54*(1), 57–64. doi:10.1016/j.jmwh.2008.08.004

D'Anna-Hernandez, K. L., Aleman, B., & Flores, A. M. (2015). Acculturative stress negatively impacts maternal depressive symptoms in Mexican-American women during pregnancy. *Journal of Affective Disorders, 176*, 35–42. doi:10.1016/j.jad.2015.01.036

Davis, E. M., Stange, K. C., & Horwitz, R. I. (2012). Childbearing, stress and obesity disparities in women. A public health perspective. *Maternal and Child Health Journal, 16*(1), 109–118. doi:10.1007/s10995-010-0712-6

Dayan, J., Creveuil, C., Dreyfus, M., Herlicoviez, M., Baleyte, J. M., & O'Keane, V. (2010). Developmental model of depression applied to prenatal depression: Role of present and past life events, past emotional disorders and pregnancy stress. *PLoS One, 5*(9), e12942. doi:10.1371/journal.pone.0012942

DeCesare, J. Z., & Jackson, J. R. (2015). CenteringPregnancy: Practical tips for your practice. *Archives of Gynecology and Obstetrics, 291*(3), 499–507. doi:10.1007/s00404-014-3467-2

Dennis, C. L. (2014). Psychosocial interventions for the treatment of perinatal depression. *Best Practice and Research: Clinical Obstetrics and Gynaecology, 28*(1), 97–111. doi:10.1016/j.bpobgyn.2013.08.008

Devitt, N. F. (2013). Does the CenteringPregnancy group prenatal care program reduce preterm birth? The conclusions are premature. *Birth, 40*(1), 67–69. doi:10.1111/birt.12034

Dominguez, T. P. (2011). Adverse birth outcomes in African American women: The social context of persistent reproductive disadvantage. *Social Work in Public Health, 26*(1), 3–16. doi:10.1080/10911350902986880

Dunkel Schetter, C., & Tanner, L. (2012). Anxiety, depression and stress in pregnancy: Implications for mothers, children, research, and practice. *Current Opinion in Psychiatry, 25*(2), 141–148. doi:10.1097/YCO.0b013e3283503680

Earnshaw, V. A., Rosenthal, L., Cunningham, S. D., Kershaw, T., Lewis, J., Rising, S. S., . . . Ickovics, J. R. (2016). Exploring group composition among young, urban women of color in prenatal care: Implications for satisfaction, engagement, and group attendance. *Women's Health Issues, 26*(1), 110–115. doi:10.1016/j.whi.2015.09.011

Entringer, S., Buss, C., & Wadhwa, P. D. (2010). Prenatal stress and developmental programming of human health and disease risk: Concepts and integration of empirical findings.

*Current Opinion in Endocrinology, Diabetes and Obesity, 17*(6), 507–516. doi:10.1097/MED.0b013e3283405921

Ertel, K. A., Rich-Edwards, J. W., & Koenen, K. C. (2011). Maternal depression in the United States: Nationally representative rates and risks. *Journal of Women's Health, 20*(11), 1609–1617. doi:10.1089/jwh.2010.2657

Freed, R. D., Chan, P. T., Boger, K. D., & Tompson, M. C. (2012). Enhancing maternal depression recognition in health care settings: A review of strategies to improve detection, reduce barriers, and reach mothers in need. *Families, Systems, & Health, 30*(1), 1–18. doi:10.1037/a0027602

Gavin, A. R., Melville, J. L., Rue, T., Guo, Y., Dina, K. T., & Katon, W. J. (2011). Racial differences in the prevalence of antenatal depression. *General Hospital Psychiatry, 33*(2), 87–93. doi:10.1016/j.genhosppsych.2010.11.012

Gillman, M. W. (2005). Developmental origins of health and disease. *New England Journal of Medicine, 353*(17), 1848–1850. doi:10.1056/NEJMe058187

Giscombe, C. L., & Lobel, M. (2005). Explaining disproportionately high rates of adverse birth outcomes among African Americans: The impact of stress, racism, and related factors in pregnancy. *Psychology Bulletin, 131*(5), 662–683. doi:10.1037/0033-2909.131.5.662

Hale, N., Picklesimer, A. H., Billings, D. L., & Covington-Kolb, S. (2014). The impact of Centering Pregnancy group prenatal care on postpartum family planning. *American Journal of Obstetrics and Gynecology, 210*(1), 50.e51–50.e57. doi:10.1016/j.ajog.2013.09.001

Hasin, D. S., Goodwin, R. D., Stinson, F. S., & Grant, B. F. (2005). Epidemiology of major depressive disorder: Results from the National Epidemiologic Survey on Alcoholism and Related Conditions. *Archives of General Psychiatry, 62*(10), 1097–1106. doi:10.1001/archpsyc.62.10.1097

Hauck, F. R., Tanabe, K. O., & Moon, R. Y. (2011). Racial and ethnic disparities in infant mortality. *Seminars in Perinatology, 35*(4), 209–220. doi:10.1053/j.semperi.2011.02.018

Herrman, J. W., Rogers, S., & Ehrenthal, D. B. (2012). Women's perceptions of Centering Pregnancy: A focus group study. *MCN American Journal of Maternal/Child Nursing, 37*(1), 19–26. doi:10.1097/NMC.0b013e3182385204

Hogue, C. J., Parker, C. B., Willinger, M., Temple, J. R., Bann, C. M., Silver, R. M., . . . Human Development Stillbirth Collaborative Research Network Writing Group. (2013). A population-based case-control study of stillbirth: The relationship of significant life events to the racial disparity for African Americans. *American Journal of Epidemiology, 177*(8), 755–767. doi:10.1093/aje/kws381

Ickovics, J. R., Kershaw, T. S., Westdahl, C., Magriples, U., Massey, Z., Reynolds, H., & Rising, S. S. (2007). Group prenatal care and perinatal outcomes: A randomized controlled trial. *Obstetrics and Gynecology, 110*(2, Pt. 1), 330–339. doi:10.1097/01.aog.0000275284.24298.23

Ickovics, J. R., Reed, E., Magriples, U., Westdahl, C., Schindler Rising, S., & Kershaw, T. S. (2011). Effects of group prenatal care on psychosocial risk in pregnancy: Results from a randomised controlled trial. *Psychological Health, 26*(2), 235–250. doi:10.1080/08870446.2011.531577

Jesse, D. E., & Alligood, M. R. (2002). Holistic obstetrical problem evaluation (HOPE): Testing a theory to predict birth outcomes in a group of women from Appalachia. *Health Care of Women International, 23*(6–7), 587–599. doi:10.1080/07399330290107359

Jesse, D. E., Gaynes, B. N., Feldhousen, E. B., Newton, E. R., Bunch, S., & Hollon, S. D. (2015). Performance of a culturally tailored cognitive-behavioral intervention integrated in a public health setting to reduce risk of antepartum depression: A randomized controlled trial. *Journal of Midwifery and Women's Health, 60*(5), 578–592. doi:10.1111/jmwh.12308

Klima, C., Norr, K., Vonderheid, S., & Handler, A. (2009). Introduction of CenteringPregnancy in a public health clinic. *Journal of Midwifery and Women's Health, 54*(1), 27–34. doi:10.1016/j .jmwh.2008.05.008

Latendresse, G. (2009). The interaction between chronic stress and pregnancy: Preterm birth from a biobehavioral perspective. *Journal of Midwifery and Women's Health, 54*(1), 8–17. doi:10.1016/j.jmwh.2008.08.001

Liu, C. H., & Tronick, E. (2013). Rates and predictors of postpartum depression by race and ethnicity: Results from the 2004 to 2007 New York City PRAMS survey (Pregnancy Risk Assessment Monitoring System). *Maternal and Child Health Journal, 17*(9), 1599–1610. doi:10.1007/s10995-012-1171-z

Love, C., David, R. J., Rankin, K. M., & Collins, J. W., Jr. (2010). Exploring weathering: Effects of lifelong economic environment and maternal age on low birth weight, small for gestational age, and preterm birth in African-American and white women. *American Journal of Epidemiology, 172*(2), 127–134. doi:10.1093/aje/kwq109

Lu, M. C., & Halfon, N. (2003). Racial and ethnic disparities in birth outcomes: A life-course perspective. *Maternal and Child Health Journal, 7*(1), 13–30.

Magriples, U., Boynton, M. H., Kershaw, T. S., Lewis, J., Rising, S. S., Tobin, J. N., . . . Ickovics, J. R. (2015). The impact of group prenatal care on pregnancy and postpartum weight trajectories. *American Journal of Obstetrics and Gynecology, 213*(5), 688.e681–688.e689. doi:10.1016/j.ajog.2015.06.066

Manant, A., & Dodgson, J. E. (2011). CenteringPregnancy: An integrative literature review. *Journal of Midwifery and Women's Health, 56*(2), 94–102. doi:10.1111/j.1542-2011.2010 .00021.x

Muzik, M., Rosenblum, K. L., Alfafara, E. A., Schuster, M. M., Miller, N. M., Waddell, R. M., & Kohler, E. S. (2015). Mom power: Preliminary outcomes of a group intervention to improve mental health and parenting among high-risk mothers. *Archives of Women's Mental Health, 18*(3), 507–521. doi:10.1007/s00737-014-0490-z

Novick, G., Reid, A. E., Lewis, J., Kershaw, T. S., Rising, S. S., & Ickovics, J. R. (2013). Group prenatal care: Model fidelity and outcomes. *American Journal of Obstetrics and Gynecology, 209*(2), 112.e111–112.e116. doi:10.1016/j.ajog.2013.03.026

Novick, G., Womack, J. A., Lewis, J., Stasko, E. C., Rising, S. S., Sadler, L. S., . . . Ickovics, J. R. (2015). Perceptions of barriers and facilitators during implementation of a complex model of group prenatal care in six urban sites. *Research in Nursing and Health, 38*(6), 462–474. doi:10.1002/nur.21681

O'Mahen, H. A., Henshaw, E., Jones, J. M., & Flynn, H. A. (2011). Stigma and depression during pregnancy: Does race matter? *Journal of Nervous and Mental Disease, 199*(4), 257–262. doi:10.1097/NMD.0b013e3182125b82

Picklesimer, A. H., Billings, D., Hale, N., Blackhurst, D., & Covington-Kolb, S. (2012). The effect of CenteringPregnancy group prenatal care on preterm birth in a low-income population. *American Journal of Obstetrics and Gynecology, 206*(5), 415.e411–415.e417. doi: 10.1016/j.ajog.2012.01.040

Raisler, J., & Kennedy, H. (2005). Midwifery care of poor and vulnerable women, 1925–2003. *Journal of Midwifery and Women's Health, 50*(2), 113–121. doi:10.1016/j.jmwh.2004.12.010

Robertson, B., Aycock, D. M., & Darnell, L. A. (2009). Comparison of centering pregnancy to traditional care in Hispanic mothers. *Maternal and Child Health Journal, 13*(3), 407–414. doi:10.1007/s10995-008-0353-1

Rooks, J. (1997). *Midwifery and childbirth in America.* Philadelphia, PA: Temple University Press.

Rosenthal, L., & Lobel, M. (2011). Explaining racial disparities in adverse birth outcomes: Unique sources of stress for Black American women. *Social Science and Medicine, 72*(6), 977–983. doi:10.1016/j.socscimed.2011.01.013

Seng, J. S., Kohn-Wood, L. P., McPherson, M. D., & Sperlich, M. (2011). Disparity in post-traumatic stress disorder diagnosis among African American pregnant women. *Archives of Women's Mental Health, 14*(4), 295–306. doi:10.1007/s00737-011-0218-2

Seravalli, L., Patterson, F., & Nelson, D. B. (2014). Role of perceived stress in the occurrence of preterm labor and preterm birth among urban women. *Journal of Midwifery and Women's Health, 59*(4), 374–379. doi:10.1111/jmwh.12088

Spong, C. Y., Iams, J., Goldenberg, R., Hauck, F. R., & Willinger, M. (2011). Disparities in perinatal medicine: Preterm birth, stillbirth, and infant mortality. *Obstetrics and Gynecology, 117*(4), 948–955. doi:10.1097/AOG.0b013e318211726f

Summers, L. (2014). Outcomes of Latina women in CenteringPregnancy group prenatal care compared with individual prenatal care. *Journal of Midwifery and Women's Health, 59*(1), 106. doi:10.1111/jmwh.12163

Tandon, S. D., Cluxton-Keller, F., Colon, L., Vega, P., & Alonso, A. (2013). Improved adequacy of prenatal care and healthcare utilization among low-income Latinas receiving group prenatal care. *Journal of Women's Health, 22*(12), 1056–1061. doi:10.1089/jwh.2013.4352

Tandon, S. D., Colon, L., Vega, P., Murphy, J., & Alonso, A. (2012). Birth outcomes associated with receipt of group prenatal care among low-income Hispanic women. *Journal of Midwifery and Women's Health, 57*(5), 476–481. doi:10.1111/j.1542-2011.2012.00184.x

Tanner-Smith, E. E., Steinka-Fry, K. T., & Lipsey, M. W. (2013). Effects of CenteringPregnancy group prenatal care on breastfeeding outcomes. *Journal of Midwifery and Women's Health, 58*(4), 389–395. doi:10.1111/jmwh.12008

Tanner-Smith, E. E., Steinka-Fry, K. T., & Lipsey, M. W. (2014). The effects of Centering-Pregnancy group prenatal care on gestational age, birth weight, and fetal demise. *Maternal and Child Health Journal, 18*(4), 801–809. doi:10.1007/s10995-013-1304-z

Tilden, E. L., Hersh, S. R., Emeis, C. L., Weinstein, S. R., & Caughey, A. B. (2014). Group prenatal care: Review of outcomes and recommendations for model implementation. *Obstetrical and Gynecological Survey, 69*(1), 46–55. doi:10.1097/ogx.0000000000000025

Trotman, G., Chhatre, G., Darolia, R., Tefera, E., Damle, L., & Gomez-Lobo, V. (2015). The effect of Centering Pregnancy versus traditional prenatal care models on improved adolescent health behaviors in the perinatal period. *Journal of Pediatric and Adolescent Gynecology, 28*(5), 395–401. doi:10.1016/j.jpag.2014.12.003

Trudnak, T. E., Arboleda, E., Kirby, R. S., & Perrin, K. (2013). Outcomes of Latina women in CenteringPregnancy group prenatal care compared with individual prenatal care. *Journal of Midwifery and Women's Health, 58*(4), 396–403. doi:10.1111/jmwh.12000

Vrekoussis, T., Kalantaridou, S. N., Mastorakos, G., Zoumakis, E., Makrigiannakis, A., Syrrou, M., . . . Chrousos, G. P. (2010). The role of stress in female reproduction and pregnancy: An update. *Annals of the New York Academy of Science, 1205,* 69–75. doi:10.1111/j.1749 -6632.2010.05686.x

Wadhwa, P. D. (2005). Psychoneuroendocrine processes in human pregnancy influence fetal development and health. *Psychoneuroendocrinology, 30*(8), 724–743. doi:10.1016/j .psyneuen.2005.02.004

Willis, E., McManus, P., Magallanes, N., Johnson, S., & Majnik, A. (2014). Conquering racial disparities in perinatal outcomes. *Clinical Perinatology, 41*(4), 847–875. doi:10.1016/j .clp.2014.08.008

# CHAPTER TWELVE

# POSTPARTUM MOOD AND ANXIETY DISORDERS: MAXIMIZING MIDWIFERY CARE

Cheryl Tatano Beck

## POSTPARTUM MOOD DISORDERS

In this chapter, the available evidence related to postpartum mood and anxiety disorders is presented. First, the three postpartum mood disorders—postpartum psychosis, bipolar II disorder, and postpartum depression—are addressed. The second half of the chapter concentrates on the postpartum anxiety disorders: postpartum onset of panic disorder, postpartum obsessive-compulsive disorder (OCD), and traumatic childbirth and the posttraumatic stress disorder (PTSD) it causes.

### Postpartum Psychosis

Postpartum psychosis is a psychiatric emergency that requires immediate intervention and hospitalization. The incidence of postpartum psychosis is one to two per 1,000 births (Kendell, Chalmers, & Platz, 1987). This dangerous mood disorder presents rapidly after birth. Symptoms can include rapid mood fluctuations, delusions, hallucinations, marked confusion, extreme agitation, severe insomnia, bizarre behavior, and disorganized speech. Children may become part of a mother's delusional thinking in which she believes she and her baby have to die. "The disorder is remarkable for is mercurial changeability, and lucid intervals may give a false impression of recovery" (Hamilton, Harberger, & Parry, 1992, p. 35). A risk factor for postpartum psychosis is a history of bipolar disorder.

A systematic review of interventions for prevention and treatment of postpartum psychosis was conducted by Doucet, Jones, Letourneau, Dennis, and Blackmore (2011). Twenty-six studies were reviewed with 10 of the studies focusing on prevention and 17 on treatment (one study included both prevention and treatment). Mood stabilizers, antipsychotics, and hormone therapy were examined in the prevention studies. Treatment studies for postpartum psychosis examined the use of electroconvulsive therapy, mood stabilizers, antipsychotics, hormones, and the beta-blocker propranolol. Because of weaknesses in these studies' methodology, such as small samples and retrospective designs, the authors concluded that extensive, firm recommendations on effective preventive and treatment interventions are limited at this time.

## Bipolar II Disorder: The Postpartum Depression Imposter

Another postpartum mood disorder that can plague mothers is bipolar II disorder. Sichel and Driscoll (1999) first labeled that disorder the "postpartum depression imposter." The American Psychiatric Association (APA) describes bipolar II disorder as a

> clinical course of recurring mood episodes consisting of one or more major depressive episodes and at least one hypomanic episode. The major depressive episode must last at least 2 weeks, and the hypomanic episode must last at least 4 days to meet the diagnostic criteria. (2013, p. 135)

Bipolar II depression after birth is often misdiagnosed as unipolar major depression (Beck & Driscoll, 2006). Munk-Olsen, Laursen, Pedersen, Mors, and Mortensen (2006) reported that women with bipolar disorder are especially at risk of a psychotic episode. During the first 4 weeks postpartum, mothers with bipolar disorders are at a 23.2% relative risk of being admitted to a psychiatric facility compared to women at any other time period after birth.

## Postpartum Depression

Major depressive disorder with peripartum onset is the specifier that the *Diagnostic and Statistical Manual of Mental Disorders*, 5th edition (*DSM-5*; APA, 2013) applies to a major depressive disorder whose most recent episode occurs if the onset of symptoms happens either during pregnancy or within the first 4 weeks after birth. The *DSM-5* reports that between 3% and 6% of women experience the onset of a major depressive episode during the prenatal period or in the weeks or months following birth. Peripartum onset of major depressive episode can be present with or without psychotic feature and can occur in one in 500 to one in 1,000 births. The *DSM-5* warns that infanticide most often occurs with postpartum psychotic episodes. Postpartum mood disorder with psychotic symptoms is most common in primiparous women. Once a mother has experienced a postpartum episode with psychotic features, she is at a 30% to 50% risk of a recurrence after another birth.

Postpartum depression not only negatively affects mothers' quality of life but it extends to negative consequences for their children. A meta-analysis of 19 studies revealed that postpartum depression had a moderate to large adverse effect on maternal–infant interaction during the first year of life. Consensus from systematic reviews also found that children of mothers with postpartum depression had poor language and IQ development (Grace, Evindar, & Stewart, 2003).

### Risk Factors

Yim, Tanner Stapleton, Guardino, Hahn-Holbrook, and Dunkel Schetter (2015) conducted a systematic review of psychosocial predictors of postpartum depression. Their search yielded 151 studies between 2000 and 2013. Yim and colleagues' systematic review confirmed earlier findings of Beck's (2001) and O'Hara and Swain's (1996) meta-analyses of risk factors for postpartum depression. Results of these meta-analyses on predictors of postpartum depression converge to identify a number of moderate to strong risk factors. These include prenatal depression, prenatal anxiety, history of depression, life stress, low self-esteem, poor marital relationship, maternity blues, and poor social support (O'Hara & McCabe, 2013). These meta-analyses provide the highest level of evidence on which to base our midwifery practice.

Midwives have clearly identifiable predictors that allow clinicians to screen and monitor these high-risk women for early intervention and help to prevent the development of postpartum depression. In a meta-analysis of 67 studies of domestic violence in the perinatal period, Howard, Oram, Galley, Trevillion, and Feder (2013) identified another risk factor. They found a threefold increase in the odds of elevated levels of postpartum depressive symptoms if women had experienced partner violence during their pregnancy.

The Postpartum Depression Predictors Inventory–Revised (PDPI–R; Beck, Records, & Rice, 2006; Records, Rice, & Beck, 2007) can be used to screen women for risk factors for postpartum depression. The PDPI–R was developed from Beck's (2001) meta-analysis of predictors of postpartum depression.

### Meta-Synthesis

A meta-synthesis of 18 qualitative studies of postpartum depression revealed four overarching themes: incongruity between expectations and the reality of motherhood, spiraling downward, pervasive loss, and making gains (Beck, 2002). Mothers faced a rude awakening when the dangerous myths of motherhood equating total joy and fulfillment were impossible to attain. Unrealistic expectations of women were shattered by the reality of motherhood. Spiraling downward encompassed a range of distressing emotions women experienced with postpartum depression, such as guilt, anger, anxiety, loneliness, contemplating harming themselves, obsessive thoughts, and cognitive impairment. Loss of self was pervasive as women suffered loss of control of their thoughts and emotion, loss of self, loss or relationships, and loss of their voice.

The fourth overarching theme revealed in this meta-synthesis focused on making gains as women began to recover from postpartum depression. First, women had to overcome the tremendous hurdle of seeking help as they surrendered to the reality that they needed treatment. The road to recovery was not easy. It involved a tortuous road to finally finding appropriate treatment. Women needed to readjust unrealistic expectations of motherhood and free themselves from these constraints. As women shifted expectations, they started to rebuild themselves and the healing process began in earnest.

### Cochrane Reviews on Preventing Postpartum Depression

Three Cochrane Reviews have been conducted on interventions designed to prevent postpartum depression. Dennis and Dowswell (2013a) reviewed psychosocial and psychological interventions for preventing postpartum depression. Twenty-eight trials were included in this meta-analysis, which involved promising interventions such as individualized home visits after the birth provided by midwives or public health nurses, lay (peer)-based telephone support, and interpersonal psychotherapy. The researchers concluded that these psychological and psychosocial interventions significantly decreased the number of mothers who developed postpartum depression.

Data from 27 randomized controlled trials assessing telephone support for women during pregnancy and the first 6 weeks postpartum were included in Lavender, Richens, Milan, Smyth, and Dowswell's (2013) Cochrane Review. These researchers concluded that, even though results were encouraging, there was insufficient evidence to recommend telephone support. The evidence from these trials was neither consistent nor strong.

Dietary supplements for preventing postpartum depression were the focus of another Cochrane Review (Miller, Murray, Beckmann, Kent, & MacFarlane, 2013). Only two randomized controlled trials were found and results indicated there was insufficient evidence to recommend dietary supplements for preventing postpartum depression.

### Cochrane Reviews for Treating Postpartum Depression

Dennis and Dowswell (2013b) conducted a Cochrane Review that focused on interventions other than those that offered psychosocial, psychological, or pharmacological help for treating prenatal depression. Six trials met the inclusion criteria for this review. The authors concluded that the evidence was inconclusive to permit any recommendations for treatment of prenatal depression. In 2014, Molyneaux, Howard, McGeown, Karia, and Trevillion conducted a Cochrane Review of antidepressant treatment for postpartum depression. Six trials were included and the authors concluded that there was limited evidence to make any recommendations.

### Paternal Postpartum Depression

Across the globe, the prevalence of paternal postpartum depression ranges from 1.8% (Serhan, Ege, Ayranci, & Kosgeroglu, 2012) to 17.8% (Tran, Tran, & Fischer, 2012). In a meta-analysis of 43 studies, the prevalence of paternal depression between the first trimester of pregnancy and 1 year postpartum was 10.4%. During the first 3 to 6 months after birth, the highest prevalence rate was 25.1% at 3 to 6 months after birth, and the lowest rate was 7.7% during the first 2 months postpartum. The U.S. mean prevalence rate for paternal postpartum depression was reported as 14.1%, compared to the international mean rate of 8.2%.

In their systematic review of 25 studies of correlates of antepartum and postpartum depression in fathers, Wee, Skouteris, Pier, Richardson, and Milgrom (2011) reported that partners being depressed was the most common correlate of fathers with postpartum depression. In addition, other risk factors for paternal postpartum depression included poor marital relationship and low social support.

Kane and Garber (2004) reported in their meta-analysis of 21 studies that fathers' depression had a moderate adverse effect size on children's internalizing and externalizing symptoms or diagnosis.

### Effects of Postpartum Depression on Child Development

Postpartum depression's disabling effects extend beyond the mother to her infant, especially if the maternal depression is chronic or recurrent without risk factors, such as low socioeconomic status. Negative patterns of mother–infant interaction related to postpartum depression can play a major role in poor child outcomes. Longitudinal studies of community samples have investigated the effects of postpartum depression on children's cognitive and emotional development. Murray et al. (2010) reported that boys at 16 years of age whose mothers had postpartum depression had significantly poorer school results than boys whose mothers did not struggle with postpartum depression.

Bagner, Petit, Lewinsohn, Seeley, and Jaccard (2013) found that, after controlling for later depression in mothers, postpartum depression predicted children's internalizing problems. Murray et al. (2011) also reported that children at age 16 whose mothers had postpartum depression were four times as likely as controls to experience an episode of depression. There is a definite need for future research on the effects of postpartum depression on children's behavioral and socioemotional development. Murray, Fearon, and Cooper (2015) call for the importance of examining parents' "emotional scaffolding sensitivity" (p. 150), which is the ability to be affectively attuned to their child's behaviors.

### Screening for Postpartum Depression

As evidenced by the research on the negative effects of postpartum depression not only on mothers but also on their children and significant others, screening for this devastating mood disorder is essential. Bowen, Bowen, Butt, Rahman, and Muhajarine (2012) reported that only 12% to 30% of mothers with perinatal depression receive treatment. Why is this? Difficulties exist at each stage of identifying, referring, and treating postpartum depression. Accessibility, links between screening and treatment, access to care, costs for treatment, and child care are some of these difficulties (Buist, O'Mahen, & Rooney, 2015). Compounding these difficulties is the heightened stigma attached to postpartum depression as women fear being labeled a "bad mother." Universal screening is the first step that must happen.

There are two instruments readily available to screening patients specifically for postpartum depression: the Edinburgh Postnatal Depression Scale (EPDS; Cox, Holden, & Sagovsky, 1987) and the Postpartum Depression Screening Scale (PDSS; Beck & Gable, 2002). The EPDS is a 10-item self-report scale that assesses symptoms such as inability to laugh, blaming oneself unnecessarily, being anxious or worried, having difficulty sleeping, feeling sad and crying, and thoughts of harming oneself. With a cut score of 12/13, Cox et al. reported the EPDS as having 86% sensitivity and 78% specificity. The items on the EPDS are written as symptoms of general depression.

The PDSS is a 35-item Likert scale that measures seven dimensions of post-partum depression: sleeping/eating disturbances, anxiety/insecurity, emotional lability, cognitive impairment, loss of self, guilt/shame, and contemplating harming oneself. The items are written in the context of new motherhood. For example, "Even when my baby is asleep, I cannot sleep." All the items on the PDSS come from Beck's series of qualitative studies on postpartum depression. Total score for the PDSS can range from 35 to 175. A cut score of 80 or more indicates a positive screen for postpartum depression with a sensitivity of 94% and specificity of 98% (Beck & Gable, 2002).

## BEST PRACTICES FOR MAXIMIZING MIDWIFERY CARE WITH POSTPARTUM DEPRESSION

Postpartum depression is a major public health problem. It is a thief who steals the dream of motherhood. Evidence from multiple meta-analyses provides midwives with predictors of this crippling mood disorder. These risk factors can be used as red flags that a mother may be at risk. Specific interventions can be put in place that fit the predictor profile for each individual mother. Meta-analyses have highlighted the most effective treatments for postpartum depression. To receive the benefits of these treatments, however, women must first be identified as suffering from postpartum depression. Early recognition is one of the disorder's most challenging aspects. This devastating mood disorder is often covertly suffered. Because of the stigma of depression after childbirth, mothers may be ashamed or fearful of sharing these negative feelings with clinicians.

Barriers to women seeking treatment need to be broken down. Women need to know that they are neither weak nor that they have done anything wrong because they have postpartum depression. It is a very treatable disorder. Routine screening of all mothers is necessary to identify, as early as possible, women who may be experiencing postpartum depression. Early treatment will not only help the women themselves, but also can have a beneficial effect on these vulnerable mother–infant dyads and the larger family. Midwives can share some informative websites regarding postpartum depression with mothers, such as the website of Postpartum Support International (2016).

## POSTPARTUM ANXIETY DISORDERS

There are three postpartum anxiety disorders that women can experience. These disorders include postpartum onset panic disorder, postpartum OCD, and PTSD following traumatic childbirth.

### Postpartum Onset Panic Disorder

This anxiety disorder in new mothers is characterized by panic attacks, acute onset of anxiety, rapid breathing, heart palpitations, dizziness, chest pain, sweating, numbness, and fear of dying (APA, 2013). Wenzel (2011) reported that the prevalence of postpartum panic disorder in community samples of mothers was from 0.5% to 2.9%, 6 to 10 weeks after birth. Panic disorder during pregnancy was a significant predictor of postpartum depression (Rambelli et al., 2010).

## Postpartum OCD

New mothers struggling with OCD can experience either obsessions or compulsions or both. The APA (2013) defines *obsessions* as recurring, persistent intrusive thoughts or impulses, or images that can lead to distress. Women may have repetitive thoughts of hearing their infants. Compulsions are repetitive behaviors or mental acts that a woman performs according to rigid rules. Examples of compulsions can include changing the baby's diaper or washing hands.

Russell, Fawcett, and Mazmanian (2013) conducted a meta-analysis of 12 studies on the prevalence and risk of OCD in pregnant and postpartum women. These authors reported an elevated prevalence of OCD in pregnancy and postpartum. The lowest prevalence was in the general female population (1.08%), greater during pregnancy (2.07%) and greatest during the postpartum period (2.43%). Wenzel (2011) identified the range of prevalence in OCD at 6 to 8 weeks after birth as 0.7% to 4.0%; at 6 months postpartum, 4.0%; and then, at 1 year after birth, less than 1%. Many times, mothers with OCD are fearful of being alone with their infants. These mothers may be hypervigilant in protecting their infants. Mothers with OCD are aware of their obsessions of harming their infants and know these are unreasonable. Unlike women with postpartum psychosis, mothers with OCD do not act on these terrifying thoughts of intentionally harming their infants.

## PTSD Following Childbirth

### Prevalence

The APA (2013) *DSM-5* diagnostic criteria for PTSD include:

- Being exposed to actual or threatened death, serious injury, or sexual violence
- Experiencing one or more intrusive symptoms or dreams related to the traumatic event such as recurring distressing thoughts of the traumatic event, flashbacks
- Psychological distress or physiological reaction to cues of the trauma
- Experiencing persistent avoidance of reminders of the traumatic event
- Experiencing negative alterations in thoughts and mood related to the trauma, such as being unable to remember aspects of the trauma
- Experiencing changes in arousal and reactivity related to the trauma, such as irritability, hypervigilance, reckless behavior, difficulty in concentrating, exaggerated startle response, and sleep disturbance

PTSD can occur following childbirth. In a meta-analysis of 78 studies published between 1980 and 2013, Grekin and O'Hara (2014) reported the prevalence of postpartum PTSD to be 3.1% and 15.7% in at-risk community samples. For community samples, the strongest risk factor for postpartum PTSD was postpartum depressive symptoms. Risk factors with a medium effect size included perceived quality of interactions with medical staff during labor and birth, pregnancy psychopathology, and a history of psychopathology. Predictors of postpartum PTSD in community samples that had small effect sizes were obstetric complications in pregnancy or during birth, a history of trauma, perceived postpartum support, and level of perceived control during labor and birth. When focusing on the at-risk samples in Grekin and O'Hara's meta-analysis, large effect sizes for the following risk factors were reported: postpartum depressive symptoms and maternal and infant complications. Social support during the postpartum period showed a medium association.

Anderson, Melvaer, Videbech, Lamont, and Joergensen (2012) conducted a systematic review of 31 observational studies published between 2003 and 2010 regarding risk factors for developing PTSD after childbirth. Studies with the highest quality reported a prevalence range of 1.3% to 2.4% between 1 and 2 months postpartum and 0.9% to 4.6% for the period of 3 to 12 months after birth. Strongest risk factors included subjective distress in labor and obstetrical emergencies. Moderately rated risk factors were infant complications, low support in labor and birth, psychological problems in pregnancy, and prior traumatic experiences. In a U.S. national survey of PTSD in new mothers ($n = 903$), 9% of the sample screened positive for meeting the *DSM-IV* (*Diagnostic and Statistical Manual of Mental Disorders*, 4th ed.; APA, 1994) criteria for a diagnosis of PTSD due to childbirth (Beck, Gable, Sakala, & Declercq, 2011). The strongest predictor of PTSD in this study was elevated postpartum depressive symptoms.

### Preterm Birth/NICU Admission and Posttraumatic Stress Response

Research findings are confirming that mothers of preterm infants and of infants in the neonatal intensive care unit (NICU) are at increased risk of elevated posttraumatic stress response and PTSD compared to mothers of full-term, healthy infants. Regarding the level of evidence, no systematic reviews or meta-analyses were found. However, individual studies are confirming this elevated risk. In Canada, Feeley et al. (2011) reported that 23% of their sample of 21 mothers of very-low-birth-weight infants scored in the clinical range on the Perinatal PTSD Questionnaire (PPQ; DeMier, Hynan, Harris, & Manniello, 1996) 6 months after discharge from the NICU. Shaw, Bernard, Storfer-Isser, Rhine, and Horwitz (2013) measured PTSD symptoms in 50 mothers of preterm infants at 1 month after birth using the Davidson Trauma Scale (Davidson et al., 1997). Thirty percent of the sample met the criteria for PTSD. In Norway, Misund, Nerdrum, and Diseth (2014) used the Impact of Event Scale (IES; Horowitz, Wilner, & Alvarez, 1979) to assess posttraumatic stress response in 35 mothers within 2 weeks after giving birth to preterm infants. In this sample, 52% ($n = 29$) of the mothers reported elevated posttraumatic stress response.

In a retrospective cohort study of 16,334 births, 3,049 (19%) involved women who had been diagnosed with PTSD; and, of those, 1,921 (12%) had unresolved

PTSD (Shaw, Asch, et al., 2014). Spontaneous premature birth was significantly higher in those mothers with unresolved PTSD than those with no PTSD or past PTSD.

### Termination of Pregnancy/Reproductive Loss

Daugirdaité, van den Akker, and Purewal (2015) conducted a systematic review of 48 studies on posttraumatic stress and PTSD after termination of pregnancy and reproductive loss. Most of the studies were conducted in either Europe (n = 24) or the United States (n = 18) with most participants being White. Persistent posttraumatic stress was measured with either the IES or its revised version (IES–R) or the Perinatal Event Scale, which was adapted from the IES.

Termination of pregnancy was categorized as nonmedical (usually for social reasons) or medical (evidence of fetal abnormality). Reproductive loss included miscarriage, perinatal death, stillbirth, neonatal death, and failed in vitro fertilization. The researchers classified the quality of studies as "mostly good." Following nonmedical termination of pregnancy, 12.6% of women met PTSD criteria. For medical termination of pregnancy, prevalence of posttraumatic stress was much higher, 64.5% with the prevalence decreasing to 41% at 12 months (Daugirdaité et al., 2015).

When considering all types of reproductive loss and termination of pregnancy, the prevalence of posttraumatic stress was greater than for PTSD. Women with longer gestational age reported higher levels of posttraumatic stress and PTSD. Risk factors for posttraumatic stress/PTSD after termination of pregnancy and reproductive loss included younger age, lower educational level, and history of prior traumas or mental health issues (Daugirdaité et al., 2015).

### Traumatic Childbirth

Just like beauty, birth trauma is in the eye of the beholder (Beck, 2004). What a woman perceives as a traumatic childbirth may be viewed quite differently as a routine birth by obstetric clinicians. What matters is the mother's perception. Evidence is accruing of the long-term, chronic negative impact of traumatic childbirth on women. For clinicians, the focus needs to be on preventing a traumatic birth in the first place. Beck's (2004) phenomenological study on the experience of women's traumatic birth provides an insider's view to guide evidence-based practice. The image women used most often to describe their traumatic births was that they felt like they were being raped on the delivery table with everyone watching and no one offering to help them. Four themes emerged from the mothers' descriptions:

- To care for me: Was that too much to ask?
- To communicate with me: Why was this neglected?
- To provide safe care: You betrayed my trust and I felt powerless.
- The end justifies the means: At whose expense? At what price?

Bohren et al. (2015) conducted a mixed-methods systematic review of 65 studies from 34 countries on the mistreatment of women during childbirth in health facilities. The following typology of this mistreatment was developed from synthesizing both the qualitative and quantitative evidence:

● Physical abuse
● Sexual abuse
● Verbal abuse
● Stigma and discrimination
● Failure to meet professional standards of care
● Poor rapport between women and providers
● Health system conditions and constraints

### Meta-Syntheses

Two meta-syntheses have been published regarding traumatic childbirth. In 2010, Elmir, Schmied, Wilkes, and Jackson reviewed 10 qualitative studies on women's perceptions of birth trauma. Using Noblit and Hare's (1988) method, six themes were identified:

● Feeling invisible and out of control
● Desire for humane treatment
● Feeling trapped: the reoccurring nightmare of my childbirth experience
● A rollercoaster of emotions
● Disrupted relationships
● Strength of purpose—a way to succeed as a mother

Fenech and Thomson (2014) included 13 qualitative studies in their meta-synthesis of traumatic childbirth. Using Noblit and Hare's (1988) meta-ethnographic method, three major themes evolved. *Consumed by demons* was the first theme that revealed the intense negative emotions women experienced such as violent flashbacks and drowning in darkness. Subsequent dysfunctional coping strategies were employed by mothers. The second theme focused on an *embodied sense of loss* through mothers' loss of self and of family ideals. *Shattered relationships* was the third theme, which described the difficult relationships women had with their infants and partners.

The second type of meta-synthesis is much less common and involves synthesizing qualitative studies on the same topic with all the studies having been conducted by the same researcher. There has been one meta-synthesis of this type published that focused on traumatic childbirth and the aftermath of PTSD. Beck (2011) integrated the findings from six qualitative studies on birth trauma and its resulting PTSD, all from her own research program. This meta-ethnography extended beyond mothers' experiences of traumatic childbirth to its aftermath in their lives. Three overarching themes evolved from using Noblit and Hare's (1988) method: stripped of protective layers, invisible wounds, and insidious repercussions.

Beck (2011) also discovered that in the aftermath of traumatic childbirth with all of its domino effects on motherhood amplifying causal looping was occurring. In amplifying causal looping, "as consequences become continually causes and causes continually consequences, one sees either worsening or improving progressions or escalating severity" (Glaser, 2005, p. 9). These causal loops center on feedback in which effects of a change can lead to either intensifying or opposing the original change. Feedback loops can be either balancing when feedback decreases the impact of change or reinforcing when feedback increases the impact of change. Causal looping can occur in either a positive or negative direction. Positive means the changes are reinforced, whereas negative indicates changes are resisted.

In Beck's (2011) meta-ethnography, the original trigger of birth trauma led to six amplifying feedback loops (Figure 12.1). Four feedback loops were reinforcing (positive direction) and two were balancing (negative direction). In reinforcing loop #1, the detrimental effects that PTSD can have on women's breastfeeding experiences are seen. Balancing loop #1 shows that breastfeeding for some mothers helped oppose the effects of their posttraumatic stress from birth trauma and led to a decrease in these distressing symptoms.

In Beck and Watson's (2008) phenomenological study of the impact of birth trauma on breastfeeding, a tale of two pathways was discovered. Three factors promoted breastfeeding: women proving themselves as mothers, women making atonement to their infants, and women mentally healing. Five factors, however, impeded breastfeeding: intruding flashbacks, disturbing detachment from their infants, enduring physical pain, feeling violated, and insufficient milk supply.

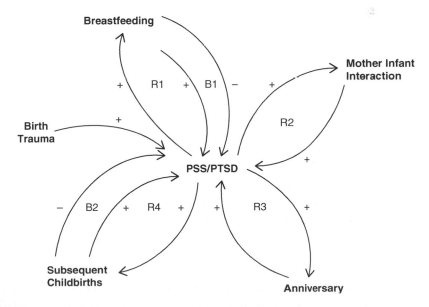

**Figure 12.1**  Amplifying causal loop diagram illustrating traumatic childbirth and its aftermath.

PSS, posttraumatic stress symptoms; PTSD, posttraumatic stress disorder.

*Source:* Beck (2011, p. 307). Reprinted with permission.

Reinforcing loop #2 focuses on the feedback between posttraumatic stress and mother–infant interaction. Infants tended to act as triggers to increase mothers' posttraumatic stress symptoms and distance women from their infants. The anniversary of birth trauma took center stage in reinforcing loop #3. Each year at anniversary time women experienced increased posttraumatic stress symptoms (Beck, 2006). Not only was the actual day of the anniversary of birth trauma difficult for mothers as they struggled with that day being either a celebration of their child's birthday or the torment of their traumatic childbirth, but the anniversary also encompasses so much more. There was a prologue, which was an agonizing time as women were plagued by distressing emotions and thoughts in the weeks and months leading up to the anniversary. Once the actual anniversary day passed, surviving the anniversary of their traumatic childbirth took a heavy toll on mothers as they were in a fragile state as a result of a feeling that their wounds were freshly reopened.

Reinforcing loop #4 highlights the distressing emotions women had to endure during the long 9 months of a subsequent pregnancy. Women revealed the strategies they used in attempting to reclaim their bodies and complete the journey to motherhood, such as practicing hypnosis for labor and interviewing potential obstetricians and midwives (Beck & Watson, 2010). Lastly, in balancing loop #2, some women experienced a healing birth and decrease in posttraumatic stress symptoms. Reverence was brought to the birthing process, which empowered women and helped them to reclaim their bodies. Women described being treated with respect and being engaged in communication during the subsequent labor and birth.

### Management of PTSD Caused by Childbirth

A Cochrane Review of debriefing interventions for the prevention of psychological trauma in women following childbirth was recently conducted (Bastos, Furuta, Small, McKenzie-McHarg, & Bick, 2015). Seven trials from three countries (United Kingdom, Australia, and Sweden) met the inclusion criteria of being either a randomized controlled trial or quasi-randomized trial. The researchers concluded that high-quality evidence that can inform clinical practice was not found in this review. Little or no evidence was available to support either a positive or negative effect of debriefing for the purpose of preventing psychological trauma in mothers after giving birth.

A systematic review of current treatment strategies for PTSD following childbirth involved eight randomized controlled trials published between 1995 and 2011 (Peeler, Chung, Stedmon, & Skirton, 2013). The interventions assessed individual and group counseling, debriefing, and expressive writing. The interventions led to a significant decrease in PTSD symptoms in only three of the eight studies. These three studies, however, used differing interventions such as expressive writing, face-to-face counseling, and listening and discussion. Another limitation involved the time of the interventions, namely, how many weeks after giving birth the interventions took place.

A third systematic review focused on midwife-led interventions to address postpartum posttraumatic stress (Cunen, McNeill, & Murray, 2014). Six primary studies and eight reviews were included. Five of the randomized controlled trials and one quasi-experimental study measured effects of debriefing and counseling interventions. Limitations included various interventions from structured debriefing to unstructured debriefing, group counseling, and structured counseling. Results of the systematic reviews were inconsistent as a result of significant variation in the quality of their methodology and use of dissimilar interventions. Cunen and colleagues concluded that there is no specific evidence-based midwifery intervention that can be recommended.

One meta-synthesis was located that synthesized 20 qualitative papers on the perceptions of women regarding debriefing during the postpartum period (Baxter, McCourt, & Jarrett, 2014). Ten studies were conducted in the United Kingdom, seven in Australia, and three in Sweden. These studies reported that mothers found value in talking about their birth experiences and being listened to by midwives. Debriefing after birth provides mothers with information and an increased understanding of their birth experiences. Debriefing resulted in a sense of relief as women understood what happened during their childbirth and reassurance was provided.

In one qualitative study, 10 mothers described their positive experiences of eye movement desensitization and reprocessing (EMDR) treatment for posttraumatic stress symptoms caused by traumatic childbirth (Beck, Driscoll, & Watson, 2013). Some women had experienced both talk therapy and EMDR treatment, and the women shared that the EMDR therapy provided much faster and lasting relief from their posttraumatic stress symptoms. EMDR treatment helped women process their birth trauma in a way that gave them a new understanding of what was so distressing to them and put these memories in a place within their minds where it was manageable (Beck et al., 2013).

Shaw, St. John, et al. (2013) developed a treatment manual for postpartum posttraumatic stress in mothers of preterm infants. The components of the intervention include six sessions over a 3-week period:

- Introduction to the NICU
- Cognitive restructuring
- Progressive muscle relaxation
- Introduction and education on trauma-focused cognitive behavioral therapy (CBT)
- Trauma narrative
- Infant redefinition

Shaw, St. John, et al. (2013) conducted a randomized controlled trial of their CBT intervention with 105 mothers of preterm infants. Mothers in the intervention group received six or nine sessions based on trauma-focused CBT with infant redefinition. The comparison group received one session on NICU education and parenting a preterm infant. Mothers completed the Davidson Trauma Scale at baseline, and 4 to 5 weeks after birth. Mothers in the intervention group reported a significantly greater decrease in their trauma symptoms as compared to the control group. Six months after birth, Shaw, St. John, et al. (2014) conducted a follow-up of these mothers to determine whether there was a long-term impact of their intervention. At this 6-month assessment, when comparing the intervention and control groups, the differences in scores on the Davidson Trauma Scale were even more pronounced with the intervention group reporting lower trauma symptoms ($p < .001$).

Three interventions for PTSD in mothers of preterm infants have been reported. Bernard et al. (2011), in a pilot study, tested a brief cognitive behavioral intervention to decrease mothers' symptoms of posttraumatic stress related to their infant's hospitalization in the NICU. Fifty-six mothers were randomly assigned to either the control or experimental group. The intervention group perceived three CBT sessions (45–55 minutes in length) over a 2-week period during their infants' NICU stay. Each session concentrated on a different CBT-based skill: (a) education about NICU and preterm infants, (b) cognitive restructuring to change negative thoughts of the infant's hospitalization, and (c) relaxation techniques. One month after the infant's hospital discharge, mothers were mailed the Davidson Trauma Scale (Davidson et al., 1997). At 1-month postdischarge, levels of posttraumatic stress symptoms in the intervention and control groups did not differ significantly. The hypothesis was not supported.

### Posttraumatic Stress Screening

The Posttraumatic Stress Disorder Symptom Scale-Self Report (PSS-SR; Foa, Riggs, Dancu, & Rothbaum, 1993) is a survey that can be used to screen mothers. PSS-SR is a 17-item Likert scale whose items correspond with the *DSM-IV* (APA, 1994) diagnostic criteria for PTSD. Each item is rated on 4 point scale from 0 = not at all to 3 = very much. Foa et al. (1993) designed an algorithm for the PSS-SR to detect a positive screen for meeting all the *DSM-IV* (APA, 1994) diagnostic criteria for PTSD. The symptoms assessed by the PSS-SR are grouped into three clusters: intrusion, avoidance, and arousal.

Ayers and Pickering (2001) adapted the PSS-SR to make its items specific to childbirth. An example of one of these adapted items is as follows: "In the past few weeks have you had upsetting thoughts or images about childbirth that come into your head when you do not want them to?" Total scores on the PSS-SR range from 0 to 51. A total score of 12 or more indicates a mother is experiencing some posttraumatic stress symptoms.

## Secondary Traumatic Stress Among Providers

Evidence is accumulating that the effects of traumatic birth may go beyond the mother and her family to obstetric health care providers. Secondary traumatic stress is "the natural consequent behaviors and emotions resulting from knowledge about a traumatizing event experienced by a significant other. This stress results from helping or wanting to help a traumatized or suffering person" (Figley, 1995, p. 10). Figley (1995) asks whether there is a cost for caring for patients.

Two mixed-methods studies have revealed that the answer to Figley's question is yes. Beck and Gable (2012) conducted a mixed-methods study of secondary traumatic stress in 464 maternity care nurses. In this sample, 35% of the nurses reported moderate to severe levels of secondary traumatic stress and 26% of the sample met all the diagnostic criteria for screening positive for PTSD resulting from their exposure to their laboring patients who were traumatized. Content analysis of the qualitative stand of the mixed-methods study revealed six themes:

- Magnifying the exposure to traumatic births occurred if mothers were adolescents, had abusive births, or a language barrier, and if nurses were new to labor and birth
- Struggling to maintain a professional role while with the traumatized patients
- Agonizing over what should have been
- Mitigating the aftermath of exposure to traumatic births through debriefing and prayer
- Haunted by secondary traumatic stress symptoms
- Considering foregoing careers in maternity care to survive

Secondary traumatic stress in 473 certified nurse-midwives (CNMs) was investigated in the second mixed-methods study (Beck, LoGiudice, & Gable, 2015). In this sample, 36% of the CNMs screened positive for PTSD caused by attending traumatic births. Forty-two percent of the CNMs reported moderate to severe posttraumatic stress symptoms. Content analysis of the qualitative strand identified six themes:

- Protecting my patients—Agonizing sense of powerlessness and helplessness
- Wreaking havoc—Trio of posttraumatic stress symptoms
- Circling the wagons—It takes a team to provide support . . . or not
- Litigation—Nowhere to go to unburden our souls
- Shaken belief in the birth process—Impacting midwifery practice
- Moving on—Where do I go from here?

## BEST PRACTICES: MIDWIFERY CARE AFTER TRAUMATIC CHILDBIRTH

Middle range theory can also be a valuable source for evidence-based practice. Using Morse's method of theoretical coalescence, Beck (2015) developed a middle range theory of traumatic childbirth. In theoretical coalescence, a series of studies on the same topic is integrated into a whole to increase the scope of qualitative theory by formalizing the connections among these separate studies. Beck formalized the connections among 14 individual studies she had conducted

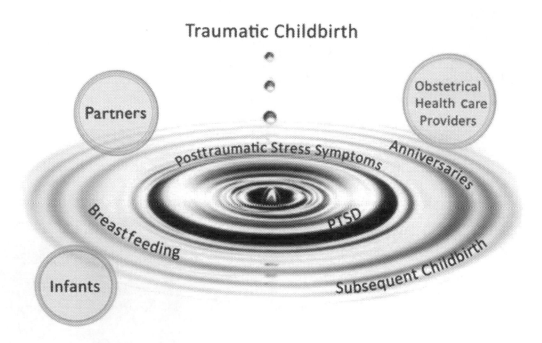

**Figure 12.2** Ever-widening ripple effect of traumatic childbirth.
PTSD, posttraumatic stress disorder.
*Source:* Beck (2015, p. 9). Reprinted with permission.

on traumatic childbirth and its aftermath. Beck titled her middle range theory of traumatic childbirth the "Ever-Widening Ripple Effect," which addresses the long-term chronic effects of birth trauma (Figure 12.2). The ripple effect of birth trauma widens out beyond the mothers to fathers or partners and clinicians present at the traumatic births who experience secondary traumatic stress. Ripples also touch the infants—a fact revealed as troubling insights into difficulties in mother–infant bonding are being discovered.

The evidence reported in this chapter can inform the practice of midwifery around these issues. The quantitative research findings provide prevalence rates, risk factors, and interventions, whereas the compelling evidence from qualitative research helps to bring visibility to the mostly invisible phenomenon of traumatic childbirth and provide guidance for best practices for midwives (Table 12.1).

The World Health Organization (WHO, 2014) issued the following statement on the prevention and elimination of disrespect and abuse during childbirth:

> Many women experience disrespectful and abusive treatment during childbirth in facilities worldwide. Such treatment not only violates the rights of women to respectful care, but can also threaten their rights to life, health, bodily integrity, and freedom from discrimination. This statement calls for greater action, dialogue, research and advocacy on this important public health and human rights issue. (p. 1)

---

**TABLE 12.1    Evidence-Based Best Practices for PTSD Caused by Traumatic Childbirth**

---

- Because reported prevalence of PTSD after childbirth is 3.1% to 15.7% routine screening should be initiated.
- Because there is a high comorbidity of postpartum depression and PTSD after traumatic births, if a mother screens positive for one of these postpartum disorders, she should be screened for the other disorder.
- Because mothers of preterm infants and infants in the NICU, and women who have experienced reproductive loss, are at high risk for perceiving their births to be traumatic, midwives need to be vigilant for symptoms of PTSD and to refer clients to mental health professionals as needed.
- Midwives cannot assume that a birth they perceive to be routine is free of trauma for a mother.
- During childbirth, women need to feel cared for, respected, communicated with, and treated with dignity to avoid birth trauma.
- Knowledge of risk factors for PTSD after childbirth, such as high levels of medical intervention and a history of prior trauma, is crucial for midwives to identify women at risk for birth trauma.
- Traumatic birth can impact a mother's breastfeeding experiences. Traumatized women may need intensive one-on-one support as they try to establish breastfeeding. Observing whether the mother seems distanced or detached from her infant during feeding can be a symptom of PTSD. Letting mothers know that it is their right to decide not to breastfeed without guilt or judgment is equally important for traumatized women.
- Each year as the anniversary of their birth trauma nears, women struggle because that day is also a day of celebration (the child's birthday). At anniversary time, midwives can ask mothers how they are doing. Anniversary time may be the first time midwives realize that a woman has been suffering in silence since the birth of her baby. It may be an opportunity for mental health referral.
- When caring for multiparous women during the antepartum period, midwives need to explore with women their perceptions of their previous births. Midwives have the professional responsibility to guide traumatized mothers through pregnancy, labor, and birth in order to help them reclaim their bodies and fulfill their journey to motherhood.
- When mothers experience a traumatic birth, it has the potential to disrupt the developing mother–infant bond. PTSD can isolate women from the world of motherhood leaving them detached from their infants.
- Midwives need to expand their circle of concern beyond the mother–infant dyad to also include the mothers' partners who have witnessed the traumatic birth. Partners too may be struggling with posttraumatic stress symptoms.
- Evidence is accruing that there is an ever-widening ripple effect of traumatic childbirth. Midwives are susceptible to this trauma, and continuing education regarding their risk for secondary traumatic stress and self-care is essential.

---

NICU, neonatal intensive care unit; PTSD, posttraumatic stress disorder.

*Source:* Beck (2015).

---

### USING THE EVIDENCE FOR BEST PRACTICE

**Case Study 12.1    The Ripple Effect: Impact on the Midwife**

The most traumatic birth that Lisa ever attended in her 24 years of midwifery practice was a shoulder dystocia. It occurred 14 years ago and it still haunts her. Every year, as the month of September approaches, she remembers the horror as if it happened a week ago.

*(continued)*

## USING THE EVIDENCE FOR BEST PRACTICE (continued)

The patient was nulliparous. Her labor was uneventful and went fairly quickly until she was fully dilated. The patient had no known risk factors for shoulder dystocia. Her pushing was difficult and progressed slowly but steadily without indication of any impending problems. The head was crowning and all seemed to be normal. Then the obstetric nightmare occurred—turtle sign. The midwife experienced a harrowing shoulder dystocia in which she did everything that she could using the standard maneuvers. After 7 minutes, the baby was born, sustaining a broken humerus and needing resuscitation, but she did not suffer any long-term adverse effects.

Lisa recalled that during that 7-minute period time stood still. The fear was overpowering. Her legs were shaking and folding under her. After making sure the mother was stabilized, Lisa went into the call room, crouched down in the corner, and sobbed. For days she could not sleep, reliving the scene over and over again.

### Exemplar of Best Practice

A few days after the event, there was a debriefing session with the chaplain, one of the physicians, and the nurses. Lisa perceived this session as helpful. She felt fortunate to work with such amazing colleagues. It took her months to get past fear as a woman approached the point of birth. She would start shaking as the head began to crown. She also began to feel panic when she was on call, feeling sick as her call day got closer. Lisa sought help from a counselor for her panic and depression, and gradually improved with the support of her family and colleagues.

Lisa did, however, make the decision to leave full-scope midwifery practice. She now works mostly with GYN patients. The experience of this birth scarred Lisa to this day. Her trust in the normal labor and birth process is forever shaken. Lisa experienced the ripple effect of secondary traumatic stress.

# REFERENCES

American Psychiatric Association (APA). (1994). *Diagnostic and statistical manual of mental disorders* (4th ed.). Washington, DC: Author.

American Psychiatric Association (APA). (2013). *Diagnostic and statistical manual of mental disorders* (5th ed.). Arlington, VA: American Psychiatric Press.

Anderson, L. B., Melvaer, L. B., Videbech, P., Lamont, R. F., & Joergensen, J. S. (2012). Risk factors for developing post-traumatic stress disorder following childbirth: A systematic review. *Acta Obstetricia et Gynecologica Scandinavica, 91*(11), 1261–1272. doi:10.1111/j.1600-0412.2012.01476.x

Ayers, S., & Pickering, A. D. (2001). Do women get post-traumatic stress disorder as a result of childbirth? A prospective study of incidence. *Birth, 28*(2), 111–118. doi:10.1046/j.1523-536X.2001.00111.x

Bagner, D. M., Petit, J. W., Lewinsohn, P. M., Seeley, J. R., & Jaccard, J. (2013). Disentangling the temporal relationship between parental depressive symptoms and early child behavior problems: A transactional framework. *Journal of Clinical Child & Adolescent Psychology, 42*(1), 78–90. doi:10.1080/15374416.2012.715368

Bastos, M. H., Furuta, M., Small, R., McKenzie-McHarg, K., & Bick, D. (2015). Debriefing interventions for the prevention of psychological trauma in women following childbirth *Cochrane Database of Systematic Reviews*, 2015(4). doi:10.1002/14651858.CD007194.pub2

Baxter, J. D., McCourt, C., & Jarrett, P. M. (2014). What is current practice in offering debriefing services to postpartum women and what are the perceptions of women in accessing these services: A critical review of the literature. *Midwifery*, 30(2), 194–219. doi:10.1016/j.midw.2013.12.013

Beck, C. T. (2001). Predictors of postpartum depression: An update. *Nursing Research*, 50(5), 275–285. doi:10.1097/00006199-200109000-00004

Beck, C. T. (2002). Postpartum depression: A metasynthesis. *Qualitative Health Research*, 12(4), 453–472. doi:10.1177/104973202129120016

Beck, C. T. (2004). Birth trauma: In the eye of the beholder. *Nursing Research*, 53(1), 28–35. doi:10.1097/00006199-200401000-00005

Beck, C. T. (2006). The anniversary of birth trauma: Failure to rescue. *Nursing Research*, 55(6), 381–390. doi:10.1097/00006199-200611000-00002

Beck, C. T. (2011). A metaethnography of traumatic childbirth and its aftermath: Amplifying causal looping. *Qualitative Health Research*, 21(3), 301–311. doi:10.1177/1049732310390698

Beck, C. T. (2015). Middle range theory of traumatic childbirth: The ever-widening ripple effect. *Global Qualitative Nursing Research*, 2, 1–13. doi: 10.1177/2333393615575313

Beck, C. T., & Driscoll, J. W. (2006). *Postpartum mood and anxiety disorders: A clinician's guide.* Sudbury, MA: Jones & Bartlett.

Beck, C. T., Driscoll, J. W., & Watson, S. (2013). *Traumatic childbirth.* New York, NY: Routledge.

Beck, C. T., & Gable, R. K. (2002). *The Postpartum Depression Screening Scale manual.* Los Angeles, CA: Western Psychological Services.

Beck, C. T., & Gable, R. K. (2012). A mixed methods study of secondary traumatic stress in labor and delivery nurses. *Journal of Obstetric, Gynecologic, and Neonatal Nursing*, 41(6), 747–760. doi:10.1111/j.1552-6909.2012.01386.x

Beck, C. T., Gable, R. K., Sakala, C., & Declercq, E. R. (2011). Posttraumatic stress disorder in new mothers: Results from a two-stage U.S. national survey. *Birth*, 38(3), 216–227. doi:10.1111/j.1523-536X.2011.00475.x

Beck, C. T., LoGiudice, J., & Gable, R. K. (2015). A mixed methods study of secondary traumatic stress in certified nurse-midwives: Shaken belief in the birth process. *Journal of Midwifery & Women's Health*, 60(1), 16–23. doi:10.1111/jmwh.12221

Beck, C. T., Records, K., & Rice, M. (2006). Further development of the Postpartum Depression Predictors Inventory—Revised. *Journal of Obstetric, Gynecologic, and Neonatal Nursing*, 35(6), 735–745. doi:10.1111/j.1552-6909.2006.00094.x

Beck, C. T., & Watson, S. (2008). Impact of birth trauma on breastfeeding: A tale of two pathways. *Nursing Research*, 57(4), 228–236. doi:10.1097/01.NNR.0000313494.87282.90

Beck, C.T., & Watson, S. (2010). Subsequent childbirth after a previous traumatic birth. *Nursing Research*, 59(4), 241–249. doi:10.1097/NNR.0b013e3181e501fd

Bernard, R. S., Williams, S. E., Storfer-Isser, A., Rhine, W., Horwitz, S. M., Koopman, C., & Shaw, R. J. (2011). Brief cognitive-behavioral intervention for maternal depression and trauma in the neonatal intensive care unit: A pilot study. *Journal of Traumatic Stress*, 24(2), 230–234. doi:10.1002/jts.20626

Bohren, M. A., Vogel, J. P., Hunter, E. C., Lutsiv, O., Makh, S. K., Souza, J. B., . . . Gülmezoglu, A. M. (2015). The mistreatment of women during childbirth in health faculties globally: A mixed-methods systematic review. *PLoS Medicine, 12*(6), e1001847. doi:10.1371/journal .pmed.1001847

Bowen, A., Bowen, R., Butt, P., Rahman, K., & Muhajarine, N. (2012). Patterns of depression and treatment in pregnant and postpartum women. *Canadian Journal of Psychiatry, 57*(3), 161–167.

Buist, A., O'Mahen, H., & Rooney, R. (2015). Acceptability, attitudes, and overcoming stigma. In J. Milgrom & A. W. Gemmill (Eds.). *Identifying perinatal depression and anxiety* (pp. 51–62). West Sussex, UK: John Wiley & Sons.

Cox, J. L., Holden, J. M., & Sagovsky, R. (1987). Detection of postnatal depression: Development of the 10-item Edinburgh Postnatal Depression Scale. *British Journal of Psychiatry, 150*(6), 782–786. doi:10.1192/bjp.150.6.782

Cunen, N. B., McNeill, J., & Murray, K. (2014). A systematic review of midwife-led interventions to address postpartum post-traumatic stress. *Midwifery, 30*(2), 170–184. doi:10.1016/j .midw.2013.09.003

Daugirdaité, V., van den Akker, O., & Purewal, S. (2015). Posttraumatic stress and PTSD after termination of pregnancy and reproductive loss: A systematic review. *Journal of Pregnancy.* Advance online publication. doi:10.1155/2015/646345

Davidson, J. R., Book, S. W., Colket, J. T., Tupler, L. A., Roth, S., David, D., . . . Davidson, R. M. (1997). Assessment of a new self-rating scale for posttraumatic stress disorder. *Psychological Medicine, 27*(1), 153–160.

DeMier, R. L., Hynan, M. T., Harris, H. B., & Manniello, R. L. (1996). Perinatal stressors as predictors of symptoms of posttraumatic stress in mothers of infants at high risk. *Journal of Perinatology, 16,* 276–280.

Dennis, C. L., & Dowswell, T. (2013a). Psychosocial and psychological interventions for preventing postpartum depression. *Cochrane Database of Systematic Reviews, 2013*(2). doi:10.1002/14651858.CD001134.pub3

Dennis, C. L., & Dowswell, T. (2013b). Interventions (other than pharmacological, psychosocial or psychosocial) for treating antenatal depression. *Cochrane Database of Systematic Reviews, 2013*(7). doi:10.1002/14651858.CD006795.pub3

Doucet, S., Jones, I., Letourneau, N., Dennis, C.L., & Blackmore, E. R. (2011). Interventions for the prevention and treatment of postpartum psychosis: A systematic review. *Archives of Women's Mental Health, 14*(2), 89–98. doi:10.1007/s00737-010-0199-6

Elmir, R., Schmied, V., Wilkes, L., & Jackson, D. (2010). Women's perceptions and experiences of a traumatic birth: A meta-ethnography. *Journal of Advanced Nursing, 66*(10), 2142–2153. doi:10.1111/j.1365-2648.2010.05391.x

Feeley, N., Zelkowitz, P., Cormier, C., Charbonneau, L., Lacroix, A., & Papageorgiou, A. (2011). Posttraumatic stress among mothers of very low birthweight infants at 6 months after discharge from the neonatal intensive care unit. *Applied Nursing Research, 24*(2), 114–117. doi:10.1016/j.apnr.2009.04.004

Fenech, G., & Thomson, G. (2014). Tormented by ghosts from their past: A meta-synthesis to explore the psychosocial implications of a traumatic birth on maternal well-being. *Midwifery, 30*(2), 185–193. doi:10.1016/j.midw.2013.12.004

Figley, C. R. (1995). Compassion fatigue: Toward a new understanding of the costs of caring. In B. H. Stamm (Ed.). *Secondary traumatic stress: Self-care issues for clinicians, researchers, and educators* (pp. 3–28). Lutherville, MD: Sidran Press.

Foa, E. B., Riggs, D. S., Dancu, C. V., & Rothbaum, B. O. (1993). Reliability and validity of a brief instrument for assessing posttraumatic stress disorder (PSS-SR). *Journal of Traumatic Stress*, 6(4), 459–473. doi:10.1007/BF00974317

Glaser, B. G. (2005). *The grounded theory perspective III: Theoretical coding.* Mill Valley, CA: Sociology Press.

Grace, S. L., Evindar, A., & Stewart, D. E. (2003). The effect of postpartum depression on child cognitive development and behavior: A review and critical analysis of the literature. *Archives of Women's Mental Health*, 6(4), 263–274. doi:10.1007/s00737-003-0024-6

Grekin, R., & O'Hara, M.W. (2014). Prevalence and risk factors of postpartum posttraumatic stress disorder: A meta-analysis. *Clinical Psychology Review*, 34(5), 389–401. doi:10.1016/j.cpr.2014.05.003

Hamilton, J. A., Harberger, P. N., & Parry, B. L. (1992). The problem of terminology. In J. A. Hamilton & P. N. Harberger (Eds.). *Postpartum psychiatric illness: A picture puzzle* (pp. 33–40). Philadelphia, PA: University of Pennsylvania Press.

Horowitz, M. J., Wilner, N., & Alvarez, W. (1979). Impact of Event Scale: A measure of subjective stress. *Psychosomatic Medicine*, 41(3), 209–218. doi:10.1097/00006842-197905000-00004

Howard, L. M., Oram, S., Galley, H., Trevillion, K., & Feder, G. (2013). Domestic violence and perinatal mental disorders: A systematic review and meta-analysis. *PLoS Medicine*, 10(5), e1001452. doi:10.1371/journal.pmed.1001452

Kane, P., & Garber, J. (2004). The relations among depression in fathers, children's psychopathology and father–child conflict: A meta-analysis. *Clinical Psychology Review*, 24(3), 339–360. doi:10.1016/j.cpr.2004.03.004

Kendell, R. E. Chalmers, J. C., & Platz, C. (1987). Epidemiology of puerperal psychosis. *British Journal of Psychiatry*, 150(5), 662–673.

Lavender, T., Richens, Y., Milan, S. J., Smyth, R. M., & Dowswell, T. (2013). Telephone support for women during pregnancy and the first six weeks postpartum. *Cochrane Database of Systematic Reviews*, 2013(7). doi:10.1002/14651858.CD009338.pub2

Miller, B. J., Murray, L., Beckmann, M. M., Kent, T., & MacFarlane, B. (2013). Dietary supplements for preventing postnatal depression. *Cochrane Database of Systematic Reviews*, 2013(10). doi:10.1002/14651858.CD009104.pub2

Misund, A. R., Nerdrum, P., & Diseth, T. H. (2014). Mental health in women experiencing preterm birth. *BMC Pregnancy and Childbirth*, 14(1), 263. doi:10.1186/1471-2393-14-263

Molyneaux, E., Howard, L. M., McGeown, H. R., Karia, A. M., & Trevillion., K. (2014). Antidepressant treatment for postnatal depression [Review]. *Cochrane Database of Systematic Reviews*, 2014(9). doi:10.1002/14651858.CD002018.pub2

Munk-Olsen, T., Laursen, T. M., Pedersen, C. B., Mors, O., & Mortensen, P. B. (2006). New parents and mental disorders: A population-based register study. *Journal of the American Medical Association*, 296(21), 2582–2589. doi:10.1001/jama.296.21.2582

Murray, L., Arteche, A., Fearon, P., Halligan, S., Croudace, T., & Cooper, P. (2010). The effects of maternal postnatal depression and child sex on academic performance at age 16 years:

A developmental approach. *Journal of Child Psychology and Psychiatry, 51*(10), 1150–1159. doi: 10.1111/j.1469-7610.2010.02259.x

Murray, L., Arteche, A., Fearon, P., Halligan, S., Goodyer, I., & Cooper, P. (2011). Maternal postnatal depression and the development of depression in offspring up to 16 years of age. *Journal of the American Academy of Child & Adolescent Psychiatry, 50*(5), 460–470. doi:10.1016/j.jaac.2011.02.001

Murray, L., Fearon, P., & Cooper, P. (2015). Postnatal depression, mother–infant interactions, and child development: Prospects for screening and treatment. In J. Milgrom & A. W. Gemmill (Eds.). *Identifying perinatal depression and anxiety* (pp. 139–164). West Sussex, UK: John Wiley & Sons.

Noblit, G. W., & Hare, R. D. (1988). *Metaethnography: Synthesizing qualitative studies.* Newbury Park, CA: Sage.

O'Hara, M. W., & McCabe, J. E. (2013). Postpartum depression: Current status and future directions. *Annual Review of Clinical Psychology, 9*(1), 379–407. doi:10.1146/annurev-clinpsy -050212-185612

O'Hara, M. W., & Swain, A. M. (1996). Rates and risk of postpartum depression-a meta-analysis. *International Review of Psychiatry, 8*(1), 37–54. doi:10.3109/09540269609037816

Peeler, S., Chung, M. C., Stedmon, J., & Skirton, H. (2013). A review assessing the current treatment strategies for postnatal psychological morbidity with a focus on post-traumatic stress disorder. *Midwifery, 29*(4), 377–388. doi:10.1016/j.midw.2012.03.004

Postpartum Support International. (2016). Homepage. Retrieved from http://www.postpartum .net

Rambelli, C., Montagnani, M. S., Oppo, A., Banti, S., Borri, C., Cortopassi, C., . . . Mauri, M. (2010). Panic disorder as a risk factor for post-partum depression. Results from the Perinatal Depression Research & Screening Unit (PND-ReScU) study. *Journal of Affective Disorders, 122*(1–2), 139–143. doi:10.1016/j.jad.2009.07.002

Records, K., Rice, M., & Beck, C. T. (2007). Psychometric assessment of the Postpartum Depression Predictors Inventory-Revised. *Journal of Nursing Measurement, 15*(3), 189-202. doi:10.1891/106137407783095775

Russell, E. J., Fawcett, J. M., & Mazmanian, D. (2013). Risk of obsessive-compulsive disorder in pregnant and postpartum women: A meta-analysis. *Journal of Clinical Psychiatry, 74*(4), 377–385. doi:10.4088/JCP.12r07917

Serhan, N., Ege, E., Ayranci, U., & Kosgeroglu, N. (2012). Prevalence of postpartum depression in mothers and fathers and its correlates. *Journal of Clinical Nursing, 22*(1–2), 279–284. doi:10.1111/j.1365-2702.2012.04281.x

Shaw, J. G., Asch, S. M., Kimerling, R., Frayne, S. M., Shaw, K. A., & Phibbs, C. S. (2014). Posttraumatic stress disorder and risk of spontaneous preterm birth. *Obstetrics & Gynecology, 124*(6), 1111–1119. doi:10.1097/AOG.0000000000000542

Shaw, R. J., Bernard, R. S., Storfer-Isser, A., Rhine, W., & Horwitz, S. M. (2013). Parental coping in the neonatal intensive care unit. *Journal of Clinical Psychology in Medical Settings, 20*(2), 135–142. doi:10.1007/s10880-012-9328-x

Shaw, R. J., St. John, N., Lilo, E. A., Jo, B., Benitz, W., Stevenson, D. K., & Horwitz, S. M. (2013). Prevention of traumatic stress in mothers with preterm infants: A randomized controlled trial. *Pediatrics, 132*(4), e886–e894. doi:10.1542/peds.2013-1331

Shaw, R. J., St. John, N., Lilo, E.A., Jo, B., Benitz, W., Stevenson, D. K., & Horwitz, S. M. (2014). Prevention of traumatic stress in mothers of preterms: 6-month outcomes. *Pediatrics, 134,* e481–e488. doi:10.1542/peds.2014–0529

Sichel, D., & Driscoll, J. W. (1999). *Women's moods: What every woman must know about hormones, the brain, and emotional health.* New York, NY: William Morrow.

Tran, T. D., Tran, T., & Fisher, J. (2012). Validation of three psychometric instruments for screening for perinatal common mental disorders in men in the north of Vietnam. *Journal of Affective Disorders, 136*(1–2), 104–109. doi:10.1016/j.jad.2011.08.012

Wee, K. Y., Skouteris, H., Pier, C., Richardson, B., & Milgrom, J. (2011). Correlates of ante- and postnatal depression in fathers: A systematic review. *Journal of Affective Disorders, 130*(3), 358–377. doi:10.1016/j.jad.2010.06.019

Wenzel, A. (2011). *Anxiety in childbearing women: Diagnosis and treatment.* Washington, DC: American Psychological Association.

World Health Organization (WHO). (2014). The prevention and elimination of disrespect and abuse during facility-based childbirth. Retrieved from http://www.who.int/reproductive health/topics/maternal_perinatal/statement-childbirth-data/en

Yim, I. S., Tanner Stapleton, L. R., Guardino, C. M., Hahn-Holbrook, J., & Dunkel Schetter, C. (2015). Biological and psychosocial predictors of postpartum depression: Systematic review and call for integration. *Annual Review of Clinical Psychology, 11,* 99–137. doi:10.1146/ annurev-clinpsy-101414-020426

# CHAPTER THIRTEEN

# MIND–BODY PRACTICES: INTEGRATION IN THE MIDWIFERY MODEL OF CARE

Kathleen A. Moriarty

## THE MIND IN HEALTH AND ILLNESS

The concept of the mind as being important in both health and illness dates back to ancient times. Virtually every system of medicine throughout the world treated the mind and body as a whole. However, in the Western world, the mind and body were seen as two distinct entities: in Greek philosophy, in early Christianity with St. Paul, during the Renaissance, and during the Age of Enlightenment. The body was seen as a machine with independent parts without connection. In the 20th century, mind–body connection and its link to health and illness emerged in Western health care thinking. This change was spurred by research investigating pain control, the placebo effect, and the effects of stress on health. Today, there is increasing demand for stress management therapies and training in mind–body practices.

As part of the National Institutes of Health, the National Center for Complementary and Integrative Health (NCCIH) is the federal government's lead agency for scientific research on complementary and integrative health approaches. The NCCIH defines mind–body practices as including a large and diverse group of procedures or techniques administered or taught by a trained practitioner or teacher (NCCIH, 2015c). The practices employ a variety of techniques designed to facilitate the mind's capacity to affect bodily function and symptoms. Examples include acupuncture, massage therapy, meditation, relaxation techniques, spinal manipulation, and yoga (NCCIH, 2015c). Relaxation techniques include a number of practices, such as progressive relaxation, guided imagery, biofeedback, self-hypnosis, and deep-breathing exercises (NCCIH, 2015d). All these techniques share a similar goal, which is to produce the body's natural relaxation response characterized by slower breathing, lower blood pressure, and a feeling of increased well-being. Meditation and practices that include meditation with movement, such as yoga and tai chi, can also promote relaxation (NCCIH, 2015b).

The latest National Health Interview Survey (Clarke, Black, Stussman, Barnes, & Nahin, 2015) was conducted and published in 2012. It is the most current, comprehensive, and reliable source of information on the use of complementary health approaches by adults and children in the United States. This nationwide survey revealed widespread use of mind and body practices with 33.2% of U.S. adults using complementary health approaches. The mind and body approaches most commonly used by adults include deep breathing (10.9%), yoga (9.5%, 21 million adults), chiropractic or osteopathic manipulation (8.4%), meditation (8%, 18 million adults), and massage therapy (6.9%; Clarke, Black, Stussman, Barnes, & Nahin, 2015). This chapter reviews key concepts related to stress and mind–body connection, evidence-based practices, and best mind–body practices for the practicing midwife.

## STRESS AND RELAXATION

### Stressors, Stress System, and Stress

In 1929, Cannon discovered that when individuals were subjected to a number of physically and mentally stressful events, they secreted a large amount of epinephrine. This prepared the person for action (Cannon, 1929). This phenomenon was later termed the "fight-or-flight response" and now is expanded to fight–flight–freeze.

In the 1930s, Walter Hess found that when he stimulated certain areas of the brain in laboratory animals, a physical reaction that was opposite to the fight–flight–freeze response occurred. This stimulation produced a reduction in muscle tone, breathing, and heart rate. This early work informed the definition of *stress* as a state of disharmony or of threatened homeostasis (Chrousos & Gold, 1992). In everyday language, the term *stress* is usually used to describe negative stress or distress, whereas mild stress, events, or thoughts that stimulate, excite, or motivate an individual are positive stress or *eustress*. The three components of negative stress include:

- Stimuli or events that are the cause of the stress (stressor)
- Appraisal, perception, or interpretation of the affected individual
- Undesirable response of the individual as a result of his or her perception of the stress (Conduit, 1995)

The stress response is an automatic protective mechanism that occurs in reaction to a threatening situation. The stress system is composed of elements of the central nervous system, the hypothalamic–pituitary–adrenal axis, autonomic nervous system, and immune system. In today's world, the pace of life and the rate of change can be a major contributor to chronic stress and an increased perception of stress (Seaward, 2011). Successful coping requires the ability to adapt appropriately to changing demands (Lazarus & Folkman, 1984).

The role of stress in exacerbating illness is well documented and long-term exposure predisposes one to cardiovascular risk, weakened immune functioning with inflammation, and a host of illnesses. Studies have begun to demonstrate how stress can even alter genomic structures (Damjanovic et al., 2007; Epel et al., 2004;

Humpheys et al., 2012). During the perinatal period, maternal distress can create an environment for the developing fetus, and later for the very young child, that will have negative developmental and educational impacts over the course of the child's life (Bergman, Sarkar, O'Connor, Modi, & Glover, 2007). Exposure to toxic and chronic stress, early in development when the brain is most vulnerable, can leave a long-term imprint as the nervous system is growing and the brain is being constructed. When the stress response has prolonged activation and there is no protective buffering, long-term changes in the brain's structure can occur (Gunnar & Quevedo, 2007). These changes may also lead to emotional problems and a negative effect on working memory, attention, and inhibitory control (Shonkoff, Boyce, & McEwen, 2009). Mind–body practices encourage one to become mindful of the stress response and to develop skills for self-care and wellness.

## Relaxation Response

At Harvard Medical School where Cannon had earlier described the fight-or-flight response, Benson, in 2000, described a physiological response known as the *relaxation response*. This refers to the physiological state that occurs while meditating, characterized by decreased response of the sympathetic nervous system (decreased metabolism, heart rate, blood pressure, rate of breathing, and increased alpha and theta brainwaves). The relaxation response is the opposite of the stress response. Although the stress response occurs automatically, the relaxation response can be elicited voluntarily (Benson, 2000). Stress management and relaxation training are nonpharmacological, noninvasive ways to approach chronic stress and rapid changes in one's environment. A number of relaxation techniques and various complementary therapies have been demonstrated to induce the relaxation response.

## Theoretical Mechanisms of Action

All stress reduction is centered within the mind–body connection. Neuroscientists, psychoneuroendocrinologists, and immunological research all validate the interconnection of our thoughts and emotions to biological, psychological, and physiological responses (Eisenberger & Cole, 2012; Fredrickson et al., 2013; McDonald, O'Connell, & Lutgendorf, 2013). With the stress response, *fight* or *flight* is initiated, resulting in the production of stress hormones (cortisol) and neurotransmitters such as epinephrine and norepinephrine. The autonomic nervous system and the two neural pathways of the sympathetic (accelerator) and parasympathetic (brake) nervous systems have opposing functions that serve to balance each other. Mind–body practices and focus on eliciting the relaxation response help to turn off the sympathetic nervous system and turn on the parasympathetic nervous system. Although chronic stressors and exposure to toxins are part of the environment, the meaning attached to the stressful event can influence response (Siegal, 2001). Lazarus and Folkman (1984) state that successful coping is the ability to adapt appropriately to changing demands. According to the stress and coping theory proposed by Folkman (1997), some individuals perceive an event as threatening or harmful, whereas others may appraise the same event as a challenge. Changing behaviors, thoughts, and emotions can promote resilience, coping, and the ability to overcome incredible obstacles. An individual can build resilience by enhancing connections with support systems and resources, and by developing goals and individualizing strategies to address the mind, body, and spirit, including mind–body modalities (Folkman, 1997). This approach promotes health and prevents disease (Antonovsky, 1996).

## STRESS IN CHILDBEARING: THE EVIDENCE

Pregnancy is a transformative time that brings both joy and tribulation. Although the impact of stress on pregnancy is not completely understood, it can have serious negative effects on the health of the pregnant woman and the child during the fetal period, infancy, and childhood (Lupien, McEwan, Gunner, & Heim, 2009). Physiological and psychological stress has been implicated in adverse outcomes, along with other etiologies. These adverse outcomes can include:

- Premature birth (Hogue & Bremner, 2005; Holzman & Paneth, 1998; Lederman et al. 2004; Livingston, Otado, & Warren, 2003; Lockwood, 1999; Misra, Strobino, & Trabert, 2010; Rich-Edwards & Grizzard, 2005; Schulkin, 1999; Stein, Lu, & Gelberg, 2000; Wadhwa, Sandman, & Garite, 2001)
- Low birth weight (Huizik, Robles de Medina, Mulder, Visser, & Buitelaar, 2003)
- Reduced fetal movement, postpartum depression, the quality of mother–infant attachment, and infant mortality (Austin & Leader, 2000; Ruiz & Avant, 2005)

Stress in parenting that escalates to maladaptive parenting has been implicated in long-term adverse health outcomes for children (Deater-Deckard, 2004; March of Dimes, 2012; Talge, Neal, & Glover, 2007). With over 3.93 million births in 2012 in the United States (Centers for Disease Control and Prevention [CDC], 2013), innovative and accessible interventions for addressing stress during pregnancy, childbirth, and parenting are critically needed.

## MIND–BODY PRACTICES

Mind–body practices are nonpharmacologic and emphasize how interactions among the mind, body, and behavior influence health. These practices focus on how an individual can utilize various techniques to facilitate the mind's capacity to affect bodily function, improve symptoms, and foster health. Mind–body practices are self-care modalities for stress and anxiety or increasing relaxation. Techniques can be used for common discomforts of pregnancy period, to cope with discomfort or pain during labor and birth, during the postpartum period, and with early parenting. Table 13.1 outlines examples of a multitude of common mind–body practices.

**TABLE 13.1   Description of Common Mind–Body Techniques**

| | |
|---|---|
| Acupuncture and acupressure | Practitioner stimulates specific points (acupoints) on the body—most often by inserting thin needles through the skin (acupuncture) or applying pressure with the fingers (acupressure) to achieve balance or homeostasis. |
| Autogenics | Trains one to concentrate on physical sensations of warmth, heaviness, and relaxation in different parts of the body. |
| Biofeedback-assisted relaxation | Measures and gives information about body functions to teach conscious regulation. Uses electronic devices to teach how to produce changes associated with relaxation, breathing, heart rate, blood pressure, and muscle tension. |
| Chiropractic manipulation | Manipulation that focuses on structures in the body, primarily the spine |
| Deep breathing | Conscious control and focus on slow, deep, even breaths |
| Expressive writing | Frequent journaling about thoughts, feelings, and meanings regarding symptoms and health events |
| Guided imagery | A technique that focuses on pleasant images to replace negative or stressful feelings; guided imagery may be self-directed or led by a practitioner or a recording. |
| Healing arts | Techniques used to stimulate awareness; relaxation; mood alteration; tension release; and resolution of thoughts, feelings, emotions, or conflicts. Examples are art, dance, and music therapy. |
| Massage therapy | The therapist presses, rubs, and otherwise manipulates muscles and soft tissues of the body using hands, fingers, and sometimes forearms, elbows, or feet. |
| Meditation | Originating from Eastern religious or spiritual traditions, most types of meditation have four elements in common: a quiet location with as few distractions as possible; a specific, comfortable posture (sitting, lying down, walking, etc.); a focus of attention (through a specially chosen word or set of words, an object, or the sensations of the breath); and an open attitude (letting distractions come and go naturally without judging them). Popular forms are transcendental meditation, Mindfulness-Based Stress Reduction (MBSR), mindfulness-based cognitive therapy (MBCT), loving kindness, and Zen. Mindfulness-Based Childbirth and Parenting (MBCP) is an adaptation of MBSR used during pregnancy, childbirth, and through parenting. It addresses stress, fear, and pain during childbirth, and enhancing parenting skills through mindfulness-based antenatal preparation. |
| Movement-related meditations | Yoga, tai chi, and qigong; yoga, a mind and body practice with historical origins in ancient Indian philosophy, combines physical postures, breathing techniques, and meditation or relaxation. Tai chi originated in China as a martial art. Slow and gentle movements are combined with deep breathing and meditation. It can be practiced alone or in a group and the movements make up what are called forms or routines. Qigong is an ancient Chinese discipline combining the use of gentle physical movements, mental focus, and deep breathing directed toward specific parts of the body. Performed in repetitions, the exercises are normally performed two times or more a week for 30 minutes at a time. |

*(continued)*

| TABLE 13.1 Description of Common Mind–Body Techniques (*continued*) | |
|---|---|
| Progressive relaxation | Also called progressive muscle relaxation; involves tightening and relaxing various muscle groups. Often combined with guided imagery and breathing exercises. |
| Self-hypnosis | Production of the relaxation response or an altered state of consciousness when prompted by a phrase or nonverbal cue (called a suggestion). |
| | Hypnobirthing is a program employing the principles and techniques of hypnosis and self-relaxation. |

*Source:* Adapted from NCCIH (2015f) and Clarke et al. (2015).

## Mindfulness-Based Meditation

Meditation is defined as mind and body practices that increase calmness and physical relaxation, improve psychological balance, aid in coping with illness, and enhance overall health and well-being (see description in Table 13.1). Mindfulness-based meditation approaches in health care began in the United States in 1979 with Jon Kabat-Zinn's pioneering Mindfulness-Based Stress Reduction (MBSR) program at the University of Massachusetts Medical Center. The hospital-based program took the form of an eight-session intervention that demonstrated benefits for patients with chronic pain, hypertension, heart disease, anxiety, and stress (Kabat-Zinn, 1982, 2013; Kabat-Zinn et al., 1992). Kabat-Zinn defined *mindfulness* as the awareness that emerges through purposeful attention in the present moment, and nonjudgmental unfolding of experience moment by moment (Kabat-Zinn, 2003). The fostering and development of mindfulness is thought to enhance the state of awareness by increasing one's ability to notice and pay attention to thoughts, feelings, and sensations. Through the practice of mindfulness, one seeks to promote a healthy state of well-being by truly being with whatever is happening in the present moment and recognizing that it will pass and be replaced by a new experience in the next moment (Kabat-Zinn, 2003; Wallace & Shapiro, 2006).

Mindfulness practice increases awareness of what is happening in that moment as well as fostering greater acceptance and less reactivity to whatever is taking place on a bodily/somatic, thinking/cognitive, feeling/affective, or acting/behavioral level. Mindfulness can be practiced informally and formally. Formal mindfulness practice involves taking time each day to intentionally sit, stand, or lie down and focus on the breath, bodily sensations, sounds, other senses, or thoughts and emotions. Informal practice involves bringing mindful awareness to daily activities. Those activities can be eating, exercising, relating to others, or engaging in any action.

## Foundational Attitudes for MBSR

There are seven foundational attitudes of MBSR. Holding these seven qualities in mind, cultivating and reflecting upon them strengthens the practice of mindfulness. Part of the training within mindfulness is keeping these attitudes in mind and channeling them into a process for growth and increased capacity for happiness, health, and well-being. These foundational attitudes are inter-dependent. The seven foundational attitudes or qualities are:

- Beginner's mind—approaching an experience without preconceived ideas based on past, present, or future expectations
- Nonjudgment—entering an experience without deciding what is good or bad but to just be with what is occurring while being gentle and kind
- Patience—awareness that events unfold at their own pace and allowing them to unfold
- Nonstriving—not straining or forcing a specific result
- Trust—trusting one's own experience, learning, and intuition
- Acknowledgment that moves toward acceptance—avoiding being reactive or judgmental and accepting things with clarity and kindness
- Letting go—avoiding control while turning toward the difficult and let-ting it be (Kabat-Zinn et al., 1992)

There are several adaptations of the MBSR program. One is mindfulness-based cognitive therapy. This program is designed to help those suffering from repeated bouts of depression and chronic unhappiness. It combines cognitive therapy with meditative practices that cultivate mindfulness (Teasdale et al., 2000). Another adaptation of the MBSR program is Mindfulness-Based Childbirth and Parenting (MBCP) developed by Nancy Bardacke, CNM (Bardacke, 2012). This adaptation is discussed in the Best Practices section.

## EFFECTIVENESS OF MINDFULNESS PRACTICES: THE EVIDENCE

Data on mind–body interventions for alleviating prenatal stress and anxiety or targeting perinatal outcomes are limited. There is, however, evidence on the effec-tiveness of meditation and mindfulness. This body of knowledge helps to estab-lish scientific value and facilitates integration into mainstream health care. The practice of mindfulness decreases mental and physical symptoms across a wide variety of conditions involving cardiac, endocrine, and immune function and increases a sense of well-being (Kabat-Zinn, 2013). Research findings suggest that mindfulness-based interventions targeting pregnant women and their partners may be expected to enhance participants' ability to cope with the stress of tran-sition to parenthood. Positive adaptation may, in turn, influence stress responses that can impact long-term physical and mental health outcomes for parents and their children (Beddoe & Lee, 2008).

### Impact of Meditation

Many studies have investigated the use of meditation as a therapy. There is evi-dence-based research supporting the efficacy of medication in preventing, treat-ing, and managing various conditions (Table 13.2).

**TABLE 13.2   Literature Review: Efficacy of Meditation**

| Condition | Research on Efficacy |
|---|---|
| Reduction in blood pressure | Brook et al. (2013)<br>Goldstein, Josephson, Xie, and Hughes (2012) |
| Decrease in symptoms of irritable bowel syndrome | Gaylord et al. (2011) |
| Reduction in exacerbations of ulcerative colitis | Jedel et al. (2014) |
| Decrease in the incidence, duration, and the severity of acute respiratory illnesses | Barrett et al. (2012) |
| Improvement in immune function | Lerner, Kibler, and Zeichner (2013)<br>Morgan, Irwin, Chung, and Wang (2014) |
| Reduction in symptoms of anxiety | Chen et al. (2012)<br>Hoge et al. (2013) |
| Reduction in symptoms of depression | Teasdale et al. (2000) |
| Alleviation of insomnia | Ong et al. (2014) |
| Management of substance abuse | Bowen et al. (2006) |
| Management of eating disorders | Tapper et al. (2009) |
| Management of chronic pain | Kabat-Zinn, Lipworth, and Burney (1985)<br>Kabat-Zinn (2004) |
| Improvement in sense of well-being and quality of life | Carmoday and Baer (2008) |
| Measurable changes in the brain regions involved in memory, learning, and emotion | Holzel et al. (2011)<br>Lovibond et al. (2011)<br>Luders et al. (2012) |
| Modifiable changes in neural structure | Vargo and Silbersweig (2012) |

## Impact of Mindfulness-Based Intervention on Childbearing/Childrearing

Research findings suggest that mindfulness-based interventions targeting pregnant women and their partners may be expected to enhance participants' ability to cope with the stress of transition to pregnancy and parenthood (Duncan, Coatsworth, & Greenberg, 2009; Dunn, Hanieh, Roberts, & Powrie, 2012; Hughes et al., 2009; Nierop, Wirtz, Bratsikas, Zimmermann, & Ehlert, 2008). Positive adaptation may, in turn, influence stress responses that can impact long-term physical and mental health outcomes for parents and their children (Beddoe & Lee, 2008). Duncan and Bardacke (2009) conducted a pilot study of a mindfulness-based prenatal intervention and demonstrated significant increases in positive affect along with decreases in anxiety and depression. Byrne and colleagues published results of their pilot study of 18 pregnant women, which investigated the feasibility of using mindfulness-based childbirth education, which integrates mindfulness meditation along with a skills-based childbirth education program (Byrne, Hauck, Fisher, Bayes, & Schutze, 2014). They reported that a blended mindfulness- and skills-based prenatal education intervention were both acceptable and feasible. The intervention was associated with statistically significant improvements, and large effect sizes were observed for childbirth self-efficacy and fear of childbirth. However, improvements in depression, mindfulness, and birth outcome expectations were underpowered.

During the postpartum follow-up with this study, significant improvements were found in anxiety. They conducted focus groups at 4 months post-participation with 12 mothers and seven birth-support partners. The mothers and their support partners described a sense of empowerment and community along with themes of "awakening my existing potential" and being in a community of like-minded parents. Participants stated that mindfulness techniques learned during the study facilitated their sense of control during birth, with both the content and the approach enabling them to be involved in decision making during birth (Fisher, Hauck, Bayes, & Byrne, 2012).

Many relaxation techniques, such as guided imagery, progressive muscle relaxation, and breathing techniques, are utilized in childbirth and may be useful in managing labor discomfort. Research has shown that women who were taught self-hypnosis have a decreased need for pain medicine during labor (Smith, Levett, Collins, & Crowther, 2011). Jorm and colleagues evaluated 15 studies and concluded that relaxation techniques are better than no treatment in reducing symptoms of depression but are not as beneficial as cognitive behavioral therapy (Jorm, Morgan, & Hetrick, 2008). Cognitive behavioral therapy may be useful for women with ongoing anxiety disorders (Cuijpers et al., 2014). Some selected uses for relaxation therapies for general health care needs have been insomnia (Morin et al., 2006), posttraumatic stress disorder (Wahbeh, Senders, Neuendorf, & Cayton, 2014), and menopausal symptoms (Innes, Selfe, & Vishnu, 2010).

# BEST PRACTICES FOR MIDWIVES: USING MIND–BODY MODALITIES

## Mindfulness-Based Childbirth and Parenting

MBCP, developed by Nancy Bardacke, CNM, utilizes Kabat-Zinn's work to modify the program to address stress, fear, and pain during childbirth and to enhance parenting skills through mindfulness-based antenatal preparation (Bardacke, 2012). MBCP can cultivate lifelong skills for healthy living and wise parenting. Engaging in MBCP invites participants to develop a life perspective on how to thrive in the face of unknowns and to cultivate greater kindness and caring for self, child, and partner (Bardacke, 2012).

The course consists of ten 3-hour sessions for 9 weeks and then an all-day silent retreat on a weekend between class 6 and 7. A reunion class is hosted between postpartum weeks 4 to 12. The recommended class size is eight to 12 pregnant women along with their support persons. There is formal mindfulness meditation instruction along with practicing at home using guided meditation CDs. The recommended practice time is 30 minutes per day, 6 days per week. The course includes current evidence-based information and an array of mind–body pain coping skills along with awareness skills for coping with daily stresses. Participants are given class materials that include the book *Full Catastrophe Living: How to Cope with Stress, Pain and Illness Using Mindfulness Meditation* (Kabat-Zinn, 2004), guided meditation CDs, and a workbook with readings and resources. A sense of community is also fostered with snack breaks to allow for mingling and engagement.

Meditation is generally considered to be safe for healthy people, including pregnant women. However, participation could be limited by certain physical or psychiatric conditions (NCCIH, 2015e). Individuals with physical limitations may be impacted especially if the meditative practice includes movement. Psychiatric problems, such as anxiety and depression, should be monitored as individuals with these disorders can experience a worsening of their symptoms. Any previous psychiatric diagnosis of psychosis or dissociative states may be particularly at risk for adverse reactions to meditation (Perez-De-Albeniz & Homes, 2000). Monitoring of medications and stress-related physiologic responses should be ongoing with collaboration among meditative instructors and various care providers as needed.

## Steps to Incorporating Mind–Body Practices in Midwifery Care

### Self-Care

So as to be credible to clients, the midwife who wishes to introduce mind–body practices needs to begin by personally practicing some of these techniques. Taking a deep breath and clearing thoughts before seeing a client may help the midwife to be fully present when engaged in clinical care. Another example is to practice being positive and compassionate.

### Assessment for Mind–Body Practices

The midwife needs to complete an integrative assessment that focuses on the strengths of the woman and where she is in her journey. The assessment should address the mind, body, spirit, emotions, and beliefs about health and pregnancy. It is important to include interests, hobbies, physical activity, major sources of stress, coping strategies to manage stress, current use of relaxation techniques or how this individual recharges, past and present religious affiliations, and past and current experiences with complementary therapies. This process aims to increase awareness of values, behaviors, and goals. It is most effective if the midwife elicits what the client's goals are and assists with goal setting, realizing that she is the expert on her own desires and choices.

### Matching the Client With Resources and Options

It is important to assist the client with the selection of the practice(s) that fits with her personality, culture, belief system, and lifestyle. In helping the client select a method (or methods), the midwife can offer resources for the client to explore. The NCCIH website has links for assistance with how to choose a provider (NCCIH, 2015e) and how to find and evaluate online resources on complementary health approaches (NCCIH, 2015a). Table 13.3 identifies computer applications, websites, and print media that may help the client and her support people.

### Overcoming Barriers to Implementing Mind–Body Practices

Barriers for the midwife in using evidence-based mind–body modalities can include differences in philosophy of care with colleagues who adhere to the medical model, finding a qualified practitioner, locating resources, and collaboration with the health care team. The midwife can work with the health care team in promoting collaboration and establishing client goals in mind–body practices.

## CONCLUSION

Exploring the literature is an initial way to assist the client. Making an informed choice entails guidance on options and resources and, if necessary, finding practitioners. It involves learning how to incorporate mind–body practices based upon individualized care, lifestyle, and personality. Stress is part of life but it can adversely impact health and well-being of both the mother and her child, born or unborn. Midwives can mitigate symptoms of stress and enhance mental and physical health by using mind–body practices. The current state of the science demonstrates that there is sufficient evidence to recommend mind–body practices for health promotion and disease prevention.

---

**TABLE 13.3   Mindfulness Resources**

**Websites**
Center for Mindfulness in Medicine, Healthcare and Society: University of Massachusetts http://www.umassmed.edu/cfm/research

Mind and Life Institute: https://www.mindandlife.org

Mindfulness-Based Cognitive Therapy: http://mbct.com

Mindfulness-Based Childbirth and Parenting: http://mbpti.org/mbcp-mindfulness-based-childbirth-and-parenting

National Center for Complementary and Integrative Healthcare: https://nccih.nih.gov

University of Wisconsin School of Medicine and Public Health: https://www.fammed.wisc.edu/integrative http://www.fammed.wisc.edu/our-department/media/mindfulness http://www.fammed.wisc.edu/files/webfm-uploads/documents/outreach/mindfulness/solar-ties-meditation-tables.doc http://www.fammed.wisc.edu/integrative/modules

---

*(continued)*

---

**TABLE 13.3  Mindfulness Resources (*continued*)**

**Computer Applications**

Buddhify: http://buddhify.com

Calm: http://www.calm.com

Headspace: https://www.headspace.com/headspace-meditation-app

Mindful Birthing: http://www.mindfulbirthing.org/products

Mindful Meditation: http://www.mentalworkout.com/store/programs/mindfulness-meditation

Mindful Meditation™: https://itunes.apple.com/ca/app/the-mindfulness-training-app/id687853790?mt=8

Omvana: http://www.omvana.com

Smiling Mind: http://smilingmind.com.au

Stop, Breathe, Think: http://stopbreathethink.org

Take a Break: https://itunes.apple.com/us/app/take-break!-guided-meditations/id453857236?mt=8

**Magazines**

*Mindful*

*Inquiring Mind*

**Books**

Bardacke, N. *Mindful birthing*: *Training the mind, body and heart for childbirth and beyond*. HarperCollins Publishers.

Baer, R. *Mindfulness-based treatment approaches: Clinicians guide to evidence base and applications* (2nd ed.). Wiley-Blackwell, BMJI Books.

Kabat-Zinn, J. *Wherever you go—There you are: Mindfulness meditation in everyday life.* Hyperion Books.

Kabat-Zinn, J. *Full catastrophe living: Using the wisdom of your body and mind to face stress, pain, and illness* (Rev. ed.). Bantam Books.

Maizes, V., & Low Dog, T. *Integrative women's health* (2nd ed.). Oxford University Press.

Rakel, D. *Integrative medicine* (3rd ed.). Elsevier.

Segal, Z. V., Williams, J. M. G., Teasdale, J. D. *Mindfulness-based cognitive therapy for depression* (2nd ed.). Guilford Press.

Stahl, B., & Goldstein, E. *A mindfulness-based stress reduction workbook*. New Harbinger Publications.

Teasdale, J., Williams, M., & Segal, Z. *The mindful way workbook: An 8-week program to free yourself from depression and emotional distress*. Guilford Press.

Vieten, C. *Mindful motherhood*. New Harbinger Publications and Noetic Books.

Willimas, M., Teasdale, J., Segal, Z., & Kabat-Zinn, J. *The mindful way through depression: Freeing yourself from chronic unhappiness* (with CD). Guilford Press.

---

**USING THE EVIDENCE FOR BEST PRACTICE**

**Case Study 13.1   Learning Mindfulness in Pregnancy**

Jasmine, a 20-year-old gravida 1 para 0000, presents at 18 weeks gestation with several challenges, including an unplanned pregnancy, living on her own, and financial stress. She also has many strengths, including a supportive and engaged partner who is accepting of this unplanned pregnancy, a supportive family that lives nearby, employment with a part-time job, and being a student at a local university. She also has a maternal–infant visiting nurse coming to see her. She is healthy and without medical risks for her pregnancy. She voiced frustration with several recent episodes of anxiety, feelings of frustration, and feelings of anger. She stated there were several incidents during which she let her temper escalate and she felt that these episodes were projections of the stress occurring in her current life. She also stated she felt overwhelmed and worse after these incidents.

The midwife listened carefully and asked Jasmine to tell her what she currently does for stress management, coping, and recharging herself. She also asked her whether she would like to explore some options to help her deal with her stress, including mindfulness. Jasmine had never heard of mindfulness. Jasmine stated she was interested in learning more.

The midwife explained stress response; health in the context of mind, body, and spirit; and how pregnancy is a stressor. She offered to listen with her to a quick segment on mindfulness on the midwife's phone app. Jasmine agreed. The segment she listened to explained that events around one's thoughts, feelings, and body sensations can trigger old habits. If we are finding these thoughts and actions unhelpful, we can learn how to become more aware in the moment. This gives the possibility of choice rather than automatic response.

Under her midwife's guidance, Jasmine did an initial practice of a body scan exercise, which deliberately focuses attention on physical sensations and helps to anchor awareness in the moment. She voiced interest in learning mindfulness practices and she and the midwife developed a plan. The midwife gave her handouts with tips for stress reduction, resources, and a reading list.

After a few weeks of practice using the app on her phone, Jasmine noticed a new level of awareness and a decrease in mood fluctuation. She told the midwife she felt more capable of coping with stress and that she and her partner were practicing mindfulness together. Jasmine experienced a healthy pregnancy and gave birth vaginally to a healthy baby boy. She continued her mindfulness exercises during the postpartum and while breastfeeding her baby.

**Exemplar of Best Practice**

This case study exemplifies evidence-based best practice through incorporation of the mind–body modality of mindfulness. It exemplifies the effect that mindfulness training in pregnancy can have on the woman, her partner, and her baby, extending beyond pregnancy into childrearing.

# REFERENCES

Antonovsky, A. (1996). The salutogenic model as a theory to guide health promotion. *Health Promotion International, 11*(1), 11–18.

Austin, M. P., & Leader, L. (2000). Maternal stress and obstetric and infant outcomes: Epidemiological findings and neuroendocrine mechanisms. *Australian and New Zealand Journal of Obstetrics & Gynecology, 40*(3), 331–337.

Bardacke, N. (2012). *Mindful birthing: Training the mind, body and heart for childbirth and beyond.* New York, NY: HarperCollins Publishers.

Barrett, B., Hayney, M. S., Muller, D., Rakel, D., Ward, A., Obasi, C. N., Brown, R., . . . Coe, C.L. (2012). Meditation or exercise for preventing acute respiratory infection: A randomized controlled trial. *Annals of Family Medicine, 10*(4), 337–346.

Beddoe, A. E., & Lee, K. A. (2008). Mind–body interventions during pregnancy. *Journal of Obstetric, Gynecologic, & Neonatal Nursing, 37*(2), 165–175. doi:10.1111/j.1552-6909 .2008.00218.x

Benson, H. (2000). *The relaxation response.* New York, NY: Avon Books.

Bergman, K., Sarkar, P., O'Connor, T. G., Modi, N., & Glover, V. (2007). Maternal stress during pregnancy predicts cognitive ability and fearfulness in infancy. *Journal of the American Academy of Child & Adolescent Psychiatry, 46*(11), 1454–1463.

Bowen, S., Witkiewitz, K., Dillworth, T. M., Chawla, N., Simpson, T. L., Ostafin, B. D., . . . Marlatt, G. A. (2006). Mindfulness meditation and substance use in an incarcerated population. *Psychology of Addictive Behaviors, 20*(3), 343–347.

Brook, R. D., Appel, R. J., Rubenfire, M., Ogedegbe, G., Bisognano, J. D., Elliott, W. J., . . . Rajagopalan, S. (2013). Beyond medications and diet: Alternative approaches to lowering blood pressure: A scientific statement from the American Heart Association. *Hypertension, 61*(6), 1360–1383.

Byrne, J., Hauck, Y., Fisher, C., Bayes, S., & Schutze, R. (2014). Effectiveness of a mindfulness-based childbirth education pilot study on maternal self-efficacy and fear of childbirth. *Journal of Midwifery & Women's Health, 59*(2), 192–197.

Cannon, W. (1929). *Bodily changes in pain, hunger, fear, and rage.* New York, NY: Appleton.

Carmody, J., & Baer, R. A. (2008). Relationships between mindfulness practice and levels of mindfulness, medical and psychological symptoms and well-being in a mindfulness-based stress reduction program. *Journal of Behavioral Medicine, 31*(1), 23–33.

Centers for Disease Control and Prevention (CDC). (2013). Vital statistics. Retrieved from http://www.cdc.gov/nchs/data_access/vitalstats/vitalstats_births.htm

Chen, K. W., Berger, C. C., Manheimer, E., Forde, D., Magidson, J., Dachman, L., & Lejuez, C. W. (2012). Meditative therapies for reducing anxiety: A systematic review and meta-analysis of randomized controlled trials. *Depression and Anxiety, 29*(7), 545–562.

Chrousos, G. P., & Gold, P. W. (1992). The concepts of stress and stress system disorders: Overview of physical and behavioral homeostasis. *Journal of the American Medical Association, 267*(9), 1244–1252.

Clarke, T. C., Black, L. I., Stussman, B. J., Barnes, P. M., & Nahin, R. L. (2015). *Trends in the use of complementary health approaches among adults: United States, 2002–2012* (National

Health Statistics Reports, No. 79). Hyattsville, MD: National Center for Health Statistics. Retrieved from http://www.cdc.gov/nchs/data/nhsr/nhsr079.pdf

Conduit, E. (1995). *The body under stress: Developing skills for keeping healthy*. East Sussex, UK: Lawrence Erlbaum Associates.

Cuijpers, P., Sijbrandij, M., Koole, S., Huibers, M., Berking, M., & Andersson, G. (2014). Psychological treatment of generalized anxiety disorder: A meta-analysis. *Clinical Psychology Review, 34*(2), 130–140.

Damjanovic, A. K., Yang, Y., Glaser, R., Kiecolt-Glaser, J. K., Nguyen, H., Laskowski, B., . . . Weng, N. P. (2007). Accelerated telomere erosion is associated with a declining immune function of caregivers of Alzheimer's disease patients. *Journal of Immunology, 179*(6), 4249–4254.

Deater-Deckard, K. (2004). *Parenting stress*. New Haven, CT: Yale University Press. Retrieved from http://www.jstor.org/stable/j.ctt1nq6k2

Duncan, L. G., & Bardacke, N. (2009). Mindfulness-based childbirth and parenting education: Promoting family mindfulness during the perinatal period. *Journal of Child and Family Studies, 19*(2), 190–202. doi:10.1007/s10826-009-9313-7

Duncan, L. G., Coatworth, J. D., & Greenberg, M. T. (2009). A model of mindful parenting: Implications for parent–child relationships and prevention research. *Clinical Child and Family Psychology Review, 12,* 255–270. doi:10.1007/s10567-009-0046-3

Dunn, C., Hanieh, E., Roberts, R., & Powrie, R. (2012). Mindful pregnancy and childbirth: Effects of a mindfulness-based intervention on women's psychological distress and well-being in the perinatal period. *Archives of Women's Mental Health, 15*(2), 139–143. doi:10.1007/s00737-012-0264-4

Eisenberger, N. I., & Cole, S. W. (2012). Social neuroscience and health: Neurophysiological mechanisms linking social ties with physical health. *Nature Neuroscience, 15,* 669–674.

Epel, E. S., Blackburn, E. H., Lin, J., Dhabhar, F. S., Adler, N. E., Morrow, J. D., & Cawthon, R. M. (2004). Accelerated telomere shortening in response to life stress. *Proceedings of the National Academy of Sciences of the United States of America, 101*(49), 17312–17315.

Fisher, C., Hauck, Y., Bayes, S., & Byrne, J. (2012). Participant experiences of mindfulness-based childbirth education: A qualitative study. *BMC Pregnancy & Childbirth, 12,* 126.

Folkman, S. (1997). Positive psychological states and coping with severe stress. *Social Science & Medicine, 45,* 1207–1221.

Fredrickson, B. L., Grewen, K. M., Coffey, K. A., Algoe, S. B., Finestine, A. M., Arevalo, J. M. G., . . . Cole, S. W. (2013). A functional genomic perspective on human well-being. *Proceedings of the National Academy of Sciences of the United States of America, 33,* 13684–13689.

Gaylord, S. A., Palsson, O. S., Garland, E. L., Faurot, K. R., Coble, R. S., Mann, J. D., . . . Whitehead, W. E. (2011). Mindfulness training reduces the severity of irritable bowel syndrome in women: Results of a randomized controlled trial. *American Journal of Gastroenterology, 106*(9), 1678–1688.

Goldstein, C. M., Josephson, R., Xie, S., & Hughes, J. W. (2012). Current perspectives on the use of meditation to reduce blood pressure. *International Journal of Hypertension, 2012.* doi:10.1155/2012/578397

Gunnar, M., & Quevedo, K. (2007). The neurobiology of stress and development. *Annual Review of Psychology, 58,* 145–173. doi:10.1146/annurev.psych.58.110405.085605

Hoge, E. A., Bui, E., Marques, L., Metcalf, C. A., Morris, L. K., Robinaugh, D. J., Worthington, J. J., . . . Simon, N. M. (2013). Randomized controlled trial of mindfulness meditation for generalized anxiety disorder: Effects on anxiety and stress reactivity. *Journal of Clinical Psychology, 74*(8), 786–792. doi:10.4088/JCP.12m08083

Hogue, C. J., & Bremner, J. D. (2005). Stress model for research into preterm delivery among black women. *American Journal of Obstetrics & Gynecology, 192*(Suppl. 5), S47–S55.

Holzel, B. K., Carmody, J., Vangel, M., Congleton, C., Yerramsetti, S. M., Gard, T., & Lazar, S. W. (2011). Mindfulness practice leads to increases in regional brain gray matter density. *Psychiatry Research: Neuroimaging, 191*(1), 36–43.

Holzman, C., & Paneth, N. (1998). Preterm birth from prediction to prevention. *American Journal of Public Health, 88*(2), 183–184.

Hughes, A., Williams, M., Bardacke, N., Duncan, L. G., Dimidjian, S., & Goodman, S. H. (2009). Mindfulness approaches to childbirth and parenting. *British Journal of Midwifery, 17*(10), 630–635.

Huizik, A. C., Robles de Medina, P. G., Mulder, E. J., Visser, G. H., & Buitelaar, J. K. (2003). Stress during pregnancy is associated with developmental outcome in infancy. *Journal of Child Psychology and Psychiatry, 44*(6), 810–818.

Humpheys, J., Epel, E. S., Cooper, B. A., Lin, J., Blackburn, E. H., & Lee, K. A. (2012). Telomere shortening in formerly abused and never abused women. *Biological Research for Nursing, 14*(2), 115–123. doi:10.1177/1099800411398479

Innes, K. E., Selfe, T. K., & Vishnu, A. (2010). Mind-body therapies for menopausal symptoms: A systematic review. *Maturitas, 66*(2), 135–149.

Jedel, S., Hoffman, A., Merriman, P., Swanson, B., Voigt, R., Rajan, K. B., . . . Keshavarzian, A. (2014). A randomized controlled trial of mindfulness-based stress reduction to prevent flare-up in patients with inactive ulcerative colitis. *Digestion, 89*(2), 142–155.

Jorm, A. F., Morgan, A. J., & Hetrick, S. E. (2008). Relaxation for depression. *Cochrane Database of Systematic Reviews, 4,* CD007142.

Kabat-Zinn, J. (1982). An outpatient program in behavioral medicine for chronic pain patients based on the practice of mindfulness meditation: Theoretical considerations and preliminary results. *General Hospital Psychiatry, 4,* 33–47. doi:10.1016/0163-8343(82)90026-3

Kabat-Zinn, J. (2003). Mindfulness-based interventions in context: Past, present, and future. *Clinical Psychology: Science and Practice, 10,* 144–156. doi:10.1093/clipsy/bpg016

Kabat-Zinn, J. (2004). *Full catastrophe living: How to cope with stress, pain and illness using mindfulness meditation.* London, UK: Piatkus.

Kabat-Zinn, J. (2013). *Full catastrophe living: Using the wisdom of your body and mind to face stress, pain, and illness.* New York, NY: Bantam Books. Original work published 1990.

Kabat-Zinn, J., Lipworth, L., & Burney, R. (1985). The clinical use of mindfulness meditation for the self-regulation of chronic pain. *Journal of Behavioral Medicine, 8*(2), 163–190.

Kabat-Zinn, J., Massion, A.O., Kristeller, J., Peterson, L. G., Fletcher, K.E., Pbert, L., . . . Santorelli, S. F. (1992). Effectiveness of a meditation-based stress reduction program in the treatment of anxiety disorders. *American Journal of Psychiatry, 149*(7), 936–943.

Lazarus, R. S., & Folkman, S. (1984). *Stress, appraisal and coping.* New York, NY: Springer Publishing Company.

Lederman, S. A., Rauh, V., Weiss, L., Stein, J. J., Hoepner, L. A., Becker, M., & Perera, F. P. (2004). The effects of the World Trade Center event on birth outcomes among term deliveries at three lower Manhattan hospitals. *Environmental Health Perspective*, *112*(17), 1772–1778.

Lerner, R., Kibler, J. L., & Zeichner, S. B. (2013). Relationship between mindfulness-based stress reduction and immune function in cancer and HIV/AIDS. *Cancer and Clinical Oncology*, *2*(1), 62–72.

Livingston, I. L., Otado, J. A., & Warren, C. (2003). Stress, adverse pregnancy outcomes, and African-American females. *Journal of the National Medical Society*, *95*(11), 1103–2209.

Lockwood, C. J. (1999). Stress-associated preterm delivery: The role of corticotropin-releasing hormone. *American Journal of Obstetrics & Gynecology*, *180*(1, Pt. 3), S264–S266.

Lovibond, P. F., Lovibond, S. H., Hölzel, B. K., Carmody, J., Vangel, M., Congleton, C., . . . Lazar, S. W. (2011). Mindfulness practice leads to increases in regional brain gray matter density. *Psychiatry Research: Neuroimaging*, *191*(1), 36–43. doi:10.1016/j.pscychresns.2010.08.006

Luders, E., Kurth, F., Mayer, E. A., Toga, A. W., Narr, K. L., & Gaser, C. (2012). The unique brain anatomy of meditation practitioners: Alterations in cortical gyrification. *Frontiers in Human Neuroscience*, *6*, 1–9. doi:10.3389/fnhum.2012.00034

Lupien, S. J., McEwen, B. S., Gunnar, M. R., & Heim, C. (2009). Effects of stress throughout the lifespan on the brain, behaviour and cognition. *National Review Neuroscience*, *10*(6), 434–445. doi:10.1038/nrn2639

March of Dimes. (2012). Stress and pregnancy. Retrieved from http://www.marchofdimes.org/pregnancy/stress-and-pregnancy.aspx

McDonald, P. G., O'Connell, M., & Lutgendorf, S. K. (2013). Psychoneuroimmunology and cancer: A decade of discovery, paradigm shifts, and methodological innovations. *Brain, Behavior, & Immunity*, *30*(0), S1–S9. Retrieved from https://nccih.nih.gov/health/meditation/overview.htm

Misra, D., Strobino, O., & Trabert, B. (2010). Effects of social and psychosocial factors on risk of preterm birth in black women. *Paediatric Perinatal Epidemiology*, *24*(6), 546–554.

Morgan, N., Irwin, M. R., Chung, M., & Wang, C. (2014). The effects of mind-body therapies on the immune system: Meta-analysis. *PLoS One*, *9*(7), 1–14.

Morin, C. M., Bootzin, R. R., Buysse, D. J., Edinger, J. D., Espie, C. A., & Lichstein, K. L. (2006). Psychological and behavioral treatment of insomnia: Update of the recent evidence (1998–2004). *Sleep*, *29*(11), 1398–1414.

National Center for Complementary and Integrative Health (NCCIH). (2015a). Finding and evaluating online resources on complementary health approaches. Retrieved from https://nccih.nih.gov/health/webresources

National Center for Complementary and Integrative Health (NCCIH). (2015b). Meditation: What you need to know. Retrieved from https://nccih.nih.gov/health/meditation/overview.htm

National Center for Complementary and Integrative Health (NCCIH). (2015c). Mind–body practices. Retrieved from https://nccih.nih.gov/health/mindbody

National Center for Complementary and Integrative Health (NCCIH). (2015d). Relaxation techniques for health: What you need to know. Retrieved from https://nccih.nih.gov/health/stress/relaxation.htm

National Center for Complementary and Integrative Health (NCCIH). (2015e). Six things to know when selecting a complementary health practitioner. Retrieved from https://nccih.nih.gov/health/tips/selecting

National Center for Complementary and Integrative Health (NCCIH). (2015f). Stress and relaxation techniques. Retrieved from https://nccih.nih.gov/health/providers/digest/relaxation

Nierop, A., Wirtz, P. H., Bratsikas, A. Zimmermann, R., & Ehlert, U. (2008). Stress-buffering effects of psychosocial resources on physiological and psychological stress response in pregnant women. *Biological Psychology, 78*(3), 261–268.

Ong, J. C., Manber, R., Segal, Z., Xia, Y., Shapiro, S., & Wyatt, J. K. (2014). A randomized controlled trial of mindfulness meditation for chronic insomnia. *Sleep, 37*(9), 1553–1563.

Perez-De-Albeniz, A., & Holmes, J. (2000). Meditation: Concepts, effects and uses in therapy. *International Journal of Psychotherapy, 5*(1), 49–58.

Rich-Edwards, J. W., & Grizzard, T. A. (2005). Psychosocial stress and neuroendocrine mechanisms in preterm delivery. *American Journal of Obstetrics & Gynecology, 192*(Suppl. 5), S30–S35.

Ruiz, R. J., & Avant, K. C. (2005). Effects of maternal prenatal stress on infant outcomes: A synthesis of the literature. *Advanced Nursing Science, 28*(4), 345–355.

Schulkin, J. (1999). Corticotropin-releasing hormone signals adversity in both the placenta and the brain: Regulation by glucocorticoids and allostatic overload. *Journal of Endocrinology, 161*(3), 349–356.

Seaward, B. L. (2011). *Essentials of managing stress* (2nd ed.). Burlington, MA: Jones & Bartlett Learning.

Shonkoff, J. P., Boyce, T., & McEwen, B. S. (2009). Neuroscience, molecular biology, and the childhood roots of health disparities: Building a new framework for health promotion and disease prevention. *Journal of the American Medical Association, 301*(21), 2252–2259. doi:10.1001/jama.2009.754

Siegal, D. J. (2001). *The developing mind: How relationships and the brain interact to shape who we are.* New York, NY: W. W. Norton.

Smith, C. A., Levett, K. M., Collins, C. T., & Crowther, C. A. (2011). Relaxation techniques for pain management in labour. *Cochrane Database of Systematic Reviews, 12.* doi:10.1002/14651858.CD009514

Stein, J. A., Lu, M. C., & Gelberg, L. (2000). Severity of homelessness and adverse birth outcomes. *Health Psychology, 19*(6), 524–534.

Talge, N. M., Neal, C., & Glover, V. (2007). Antenatal maternal stress and long-term effects on child neurodevelopment: How and why? *Journal of Child Psychology and Psychiatry, 48*(3–4), 245–261.

Tapper, K., Shaw, C., Ilsley, J., Hill, A. J., Bond, F. W., & Moore, L. (2009). Exploratory randomised controlled trial of a mindfulness-based weight loss intervention for women. *Appetite, 52*(2), 396–404.

Teasdale, J. D., Segal, Z. V., Williams, J. M. G., Ridgeway, V., Soulsby, J., & Lau, M. (2000). Prevention of relapse/recurrence in major depression by mindfulness-based cognitive therapy. *Journal of Consulting and Clinical Psychology, 68*, 615–623.

Vargo, D. R., & Silbersweig, D. A. (2012). Self-awareness, self-regulation, and self-transcendence (S-ART): A framework for understanding the neurobiological mechanisms of mindfulness. *Frontiers in Human Neuroscience, 6,* 296. doi:10.3389/fnhum.2012.00296

Wadhwa, P. D., Sandman, C. A., & Garite, T. J. (2001). The neurobiology of stress in human pregnancy: Implications for prematurity and development of the fetal central nervous system. *Progressive Brain Research, 133,* 131–142.

Wahbeh, H., Senders, A., Neuendorf, R., & Cayton, J. (2014). Complementary and alternative medicine for posttraumatic stress disorder symptoms: A systematic review. *Journal of Evidence-Based Complementary & Alternative Medicine, 19*(3), 161–175.

Wallace, B. A., & Shapiro, S. L. (2006). Mental balance and well-being: Building bridges between Buddhism and Western psychology. *American Psychologist, 61*(7), 690–701.

# CHAPTER FOURTEEN

# THE FREESTANDING BIRTH CENTER: EVIDENCE FOR CHANGE IN THE DELIVERY OF HEALTH CARE TO CHILDBEARING FAMILIES

Susan E. Stone, Eunice K. M. Ernst, and Susan R. Stapleton

Pioneers of freestanding birth centers have worked to provide evidence for best midwifery practice as an alternative to hospital care for childbearing women and their families. This chapter provides historical background on why and how the shift to hospitalization for all childbearing women occurred in the United States. We describe why and how the Maternity Center Association (MCA) decided to launch and evaluate their demonstration of freestanding birth centers as a safe place for the practice of midwifery, what has been achieved by birth centers to date, and the remaining work to be done to overcome the barriers to replication and growth of birth centers. As part of its organizational evolution and growth, in 2005, MCA changed its name to Childbirth Connection; its mission is to promote safe, effective, evidence-based maternity care in all settings and to provide a voice for the needs and interests of childbearing families (MCA, 1994).

## BACKGROUND

In the early 20th century, the care of childbearing women in the United States was focused on saving the lives of mothers and infants through public health measures, in part, through improvements in safe water, sewage disposal, and working and living conditions. Enormous public health gains occurred with the development of prenatal care and education, family planning, improvements in and access to medical education, hospital care for childbirth complications, attention to asepsis, availability of blood transfusions and antibiotics, and safer surgery and anesthesia (Centers for Disease Control and Prevention [CDC], 2011).

Concurrent with these public health and maternal–infant health improvements was a major paradigm shift from care provided mostly by midwives in the mothers' homes to care by obstetric/surgical specialists in acute care hospitals. As a result of the trend of not triaging the care of those women who needed the care of an obstetric specialist and hospital confinement, over a period of a few decades more than 99% of all childbearing women were hospitalized for birth (MCA, 1994). During this time, little attention was given to identifying the educational, physical, or emotional needs of healthy pregnant women or to changing hospital routines (designed for the care of mothers and neonates with complications) to accommodate the majority of women who anticipated uncomplicated births. Despite parallel development of midwifery and obstetrics in most other industrialized countries, and contrary to the evidence for safe care, midwifery in the United States was almost eliminated, led by obstetrics professors who publicly debated "the midwife problem" and made authoritative pronouncements describing childbirth as a pathological process for most women (Rooks, 1997). A leading obstetrician asserted that, "If the profession would realize that parturition viewed with modern eyes is no longer a normal function, but that it has imposing pathological dignity, the midwife would be impossible to even mention" (DeLee, 1915, para. 2).

As the shift of births from home to hospital proceeded, obstetricians/surgeons became the dominant authorities in the care of all childbearing women. Routine medical intervention in hospital care for normal births escalated. Women were often heavily sedated, anesthetized, and delivered with forceps. Laboring women who became agitated under the influence of drugs were restrained by a camisole (straight-jacket) or wrist-to-bed restraints. Newborns, drugged by medications given to the mothers during labor, were separated from their mothers to recover under observation in newborn nurseries. Once there, the newborns were fed sugar water. At that juncture in the history of maternity and newborn care, the importance of maternal–newborn attachment and breastfeeding, obvious to farmers in the care of animals, had yet to be researched in the care of human mothers and their babies (Ernst, 1994).

The second author (Ernst) recounts her exposure as a nursing student in the 1940s attending hospital births during which women were heavily drugged in labor and placed flat on their backs with legs spread, raised, and strapped to stirrups "to be delivered" with episiotomies and low forceps. Alternately, Ms. Ernst observed a strong Appalachian mountain woman in her one-room cabin, sitting in her own bed giving birth. This mother was surrounded by her sleeping children and attended by nurse-midwives from Frontier Nursing Service (FNS). That was the moment of epiphany when the author first understood the fundamental differences between midwifery and obstetrical approaches to childbirth. Ms. Ernst realized that although the knowledge and skills of the obstetrician were needed at times, midwifery knowledge and skills were sorely missing in maternity care in the United States (E. K. M. Ernst, personal communication, August 22, 2015). At that point in time, three institution-based exceptions to the hospital medical model of care were:

- Home birth services provided to poor women by nurse-midwives trained in public health in collaboration with physicians at the FNS in the remote, rural mountains of Kentucky (established in 1925)
- The MCA's care of disadvantaged women in New York City (established in 1930)

● Care provided by the Catholic Maternity Institute serving the Hispanic population surrounding Santa Fe, New Mexico (established 1944; Cockerham & Keeling, 2010)

These services, with nurse-midwives and physicians working collaboratively, achieved significantly improved maternal and infant outcomes by supporting the natural process of birth unless medical intervention was warranted. These initial nurse-midwife services helped to establish the practice of professional midwives and to develop the beginning of nurse-midwifery practice and education in the United States (Cockerham & Keeling, 2010; Cockerham & King, 2014; Laird, 1955).

The cultural shift in births from home to hospital, and midwife to obstetrician, for all women gained momentum after World War II. Factors influencing this shift were:

● Growth of employer-based health insurance that paid only for physicians and hospitals
● Doubling of the number of medical schools
● The GI Bill paying for medical education
● The Hill–Burton Act for building community hospitals
● Medicaid coverage for uninsured, disadvantaged families (Relman, 1991)

These social and political changes, along with the advancement of anesthesia specialization, pharmaceuticals, and medical technologies, spawned the growth of multiple medical equipment and supply industries that supported routine interventions during labor and birth. Often without sufficient evidence weighing the benefits and hazards, medical interventions, such as labor induction, use of Pitocin to augment labor, intravenous fluids, continuous electronic fetal monitoring, and epidural anesthesia, became almost routine, and the cesarean delivery rate increased (Relman, 1991).

In the mid-1950s, a sociologist and a nurse-midwife at New York Cornell Medical Center asked women what they needed from nurses during pregnancy and childbirth. In addition to physical care, the women wanted information during pregnancy, a sustaining presence during labor, and to be united with the newborn after the birth (Lesser & Keane, 1956). From the 1950s to the present, insufficient attention to these basic needs has created vacuums in care that—with support from enlightened physicians, nurses, and midwives—generated many consumer-driven movements (E. K. Ernst, personal communication, August 22, 2015). Bookstore shelves went from one or two publications on childbirth to hundreds. Today, the Internet provides free access to a wealth of such information.

As technology played an increasing role in maternity care, the use of continuous electronic fetal monitoring and epidurals for pain relief in labor became routine. Systematic reviews of research on trained, continuous support in labor, first published in *Effective Care in Pregnancy and Childbirth* (Chalmers, Enkin, & Keirse, 1989), helped to launch the consumer-driven doula movement. This review has been updated several times, most recently in 2013, when it summarized findings from 21 randomized controlled trials (RCTs) involving more than 15,000 women (Hodnett, Gates, Hofmeyr, & Sakala, 2013).

As the evidence for change mounted, hospitals offered childbirth education classes, allowed fathers and others to support the laboring mother, created more comfortable environments, and allowed mothers to keep and breastfeed their babies after birth. Demonstration projects of rooming-in units were followed by labor, delivery, recovery, and postpartum (LDRP) single-room maternity care and time for maternal–infant bonding. However, a growing number of well-informed women still felt restricted in their ability to control their birth experience and gave birth at home unattended or under the care of an apprentice-trained, unlicensed midwife (E. K. Ernst, personal communication, August 22, 2015).

## BIRTH CENTERS AS A SOLUTION

### The MCA Demonstration

In the late 1960s and early 1970s, media attention focused on the increase in professionally unattended home birth by informed, educated, insured women seeking more control over their birth experience. There was concern at public health and policy levels over this growing trend. The MCA framed the problem as a failure to include midwifery in a collaborative team approach in the care of mothers and families. MCA had operated a successful home birth service for disadvantaged or socially at-risk women in underserved areas of New York City for three decades (1930–1960). MCA's leadership now considered whether it would be better to re-establish that service or to create a homelike environment where women could have more control over their experience and give birth safely within the health care system (Lubic, 1979).

In 1971, the American College of Obstetricians and Gynecologists (ACOG) and the American College of Nurse-Midwives (ACNM) collaborated on the first joint statement on nurse-midwifery practice. This effort was an important step toward a collaborative team approach to care to reduce the marginalization of midwifery in the United States (ACNM, 2011).

At that time, MCA was also providing consultation to the Salvation Army's Booth Maternity Center in Philadelphia, where an obstetrician, nurse-midwife, and childbirth educator were converting a small, underutilized modern hospital and home for single pregnant teens into a family-centered maternity hospital, with nurse-midwives as the primary care providers (Baruffi et al., 1984).

Although this innovation promised great potential for the women of Philadelphia, no similar facility was available in New York. The MCA leadership decided that home births would not be cost-effective unless properly organized and staffed, and that being in a hospital would compromise the freedom needed to develop and sustain the midwifery care women were seeking. Thus, planning began for the Childbearing Center (CbC) to be located within MCA's headquarters in a spacious, Upper East Side Manhattan townhouse (Lubic, 1979).

The idea behind the CbC was not new to health care in the United States. Maternity centers, clinics, and doctor's offices had provided complete maternity services over many years—unregulated, and usually in response to a local need for a birthplace in communities faced with few care providers for underserved populations, rural distances too great for home births, families unable to pay for hospital care, or religious/cultural preferences. Two such centers were established in Santa Fe, New Mexico, by Sister M. Theophane Shoemaker and Sister M. Patrick Shean of the Medical Mission Sisters (1946), and Su Clinica Familiar in Raymondsville, Texas, by Sr. Angela Murdaugh of the San Franciscan Sisters of Mary (1972; Cockerham & Keeling, 2010; Texas Woman's University, 2010).

Developing a proposal for a freestanding birth center with smooth access to hospital services within the complex regulatory system of New York City presented a series of daunting tasks requiring a different approach from previous birth center demonstrations (Lubic, 1979). The birth center had to be presented as care on a continuum within the existing health care system, providing legitimate, recognizable, accountable, and reimbursable services as part of a team approach to nurse-midwifery-led primary care. The first challenge was convincing the Certificate of Need board of a compelling need for such a service, and that all applicable regulations and requirements for construction, licensure, accreditation, liability coverage, and reimbursement would be met (Lubic, 1979). Experienced obstetric, pediatric, midwifery, and nursing consultants were recruited to plan the program on a continuum of care that included access and triage to hospitals' obstetric and pediatric specialists as indicated. Based on the existing evidence, a multidisciplinary Research Advisory Committee drafted criteria for defining the low-risk childbearing women eligible to use the service (Lubic, 1979). Remodeling a historic building, obtaining multiple permits and licenses, negotiating reimbursement, and securing accreditation and funding for the project all presented complex problems to be resolved—starting with the educational process required to respond to strong resistance (Lubic, 1979).

Most of the negotiations to establish the CbC were conducted in a largely hostile environment with a culture of fear that all out-of-hospital (OOH) births are unsafe and that, with few exceptions, midwifery care was neither necessary nor desirable in the delivery of obstetrical services (Lubic, 1979). The most common response to the word "midwife" was "I didn't know we had them anymore." To gain support, it was essential that negotiations with multiple agencies began with the available scientific evidence on the benefits of nurse-midwifery care and the safety of organized OOH births. After more than 3 years of intensive planning and sometimes tense negotiations, the CbC opened in December 1975 as the first modern, urban, and licensed birth center in the United States with charges reimbursed by BlueCross BlueShield (Lubic, 1979).

### Mission and Goals of the MCA Demonstration

MCA's mission was to respond to educated women activists who were seeking more control over their childbirth experience and rejecting the routine policies and medical practices interfering with birth in busy hospital maternity services.

CbC's primary goals were to demonstrate and evaluate an alternative setting with a program of care that would meet the unmet needs of low-risk childbearing women. It sought to address safety, satisfaction, and savings as the major concerns of the project (Lubic, 1979).

### Safety

Safety for mother and baby is a way for low-risk women to enter a continuum of care with referral and transfer to obstetric and neonatal specialists in acute-care hospitals when indicated. Safety begins with qualified care providers functioning as a team and using evidence-based risk criteria for eligible program enrollment. Safety further requires a secure environment, comprehensive policies and procedures for operations, staff drills for rare emergencies, and transfer as needed to obstetric and neonatal care.

### Satisfaction

Satisfaction for the mother and family is enhanced by meeting needs for evidence-based information, fully informed consent, emotional support, and shared decision making.

### Cost Savings

Cost savings for families and insurers are promoted by creating a program of time- and education-intensive care to nurture self-reliance and self-responsibility for subsequent personal and family health. The short-term savings are obvious for the use of a low-cost, primary-care facility that relies on the more expensive hospital acute-care services only as needed. However, as more is learned about the benefits of physiologic birth to mother and infant and the health risks related to unnecessary medical and surgical interventions, the long-term savings may prove to be the most significant (E. K. Ernst, personal communication, August 22, 2015).

## The Birth Center Model in Urban, Impoverished Areas: The Work of Ruth Lubic

In 1988, replicating the CbC model, which primarily reached middle-class women, Dr. Lubic and the MCA established a birth center in the most impoverished neighborhood of the southwest Bronx in New York City. Birth outcomes were comparable to other birth centers, in spite of economic and ethnic differences. The word *empowerment* began to surface in descriptions of the birth experience by both mother and family members (R. W. Lubic, personal communication, 2011). The film, *Hope Reborn: Empowering Families in the South Bronx*, captures this sense of empowerment (MCA, 1994).

Dr. Lubic then established the Family Health and Birth Center (FHBC) in Washington, DC's fifth and sixth wards, a low-income neighborhood with one of the highest infant mortality rates in the country, offering an integrated model of education and services aiming to reduce health disparities. Within 7 years, the FHBC; the Healthy Babies Project (HBP); and the Nation's Capital Child and

Family Development (NCCFD), an education-oriented day care, entered into partnership under the umbrella of the District of Columbia, Developing Families Center (DCDFC; R. W. Lubic, personal communication, 2011). Health disparities were reduced and perinatal outcomes improved (Lubic & Flynn, 2010). The DCDFC is acknowledged in the landmark Institute of Medicine (IOM) report, *The Future of Nursing: Leading Change, Advancing Health* (IOM, 2011).

## Definition and Licensure of Birth Centers

Entrepreneurial nurse-midwives, responding to the need for an alternative to hospital birth in their communities, quickly replicated the CbC model. In 1979, MCA brought directors of 14 birth centers to New York to discuss their needs. The major issues identified were the need for national standards; licensure regulations; reimbursement for services; and evaluation of the safety, satisfaction, and cost of the services provided. In 1981, the Cooperative Birth Center Network (CBCN) was established to develop the national infrastructure to ensure quality care, conduct research, and lay a foundation to support future replication. MCA sought help from the largest and most knowledgeable organization of public health professionals in the United States, the American Public Health Association (APHA). In 1982, an APHA multidisciplinary team published a policy statement supporting the innovation and guidelines for regulation and licensure based on a core definition of a birth center as an OOH place where low-risk births are planned; it did not include home birth (APHA, 1983).

### Definition

In 1983, the CBCN became the National Association of Childbearing Centers (NACC) with the goal of ensuring quality of care by promoting licensure and national standards for accreditation. In 2005, NACC became the American Association of Birth Centers (AABC). In 2008, AABC provided a detailed, descriptive definition of the birth center, including who it serves, place, program of care, practice of midwifery, and interface with the system (AABC, 2008).

### Licensure

By 2015, birth centers were licensed under regulations adopted by 41 states (82%) and the District of Columbia (AABC, 2015b) (see Figure 14.1).

## National Standards and Accreditation

Accreditation is usually a voluntary process by which a facility evaluates and demonstrates compliance with evidence-based national standards and guidelines for quality care. The CbC demonstration set the bar for quality assurance by including the National League for Nursing (NLN)/APHA program for accreditation of home health agencies and community nursing services. In 1985, when MCA's efforts to negotiate re-accreditation through the Joint Commission for

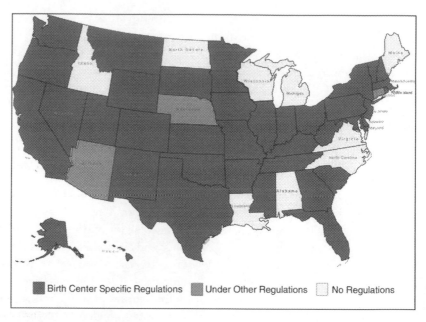

**Figure 14.1** Birth centers regulations map.
*Source:* AABC (2015b). Reprinted with permission.

Accreditation of Hospitals and the American Association for Accreditation of Ambulatory Health Care failed, AABC developed the *National Standards for Birth Centers* and established the Commission for the Accreditation of Birth Centers (CABC; AABC, 2015b). CABC's commissioners were volunteers representing obstetrics, neonatology, midwifery, nursing, and consumers. Members of the site visit teams were professionals with experience in birth centers and training to conduct surveys for the CABC (CABC, 2015a). Although birth centers were initially slow to seek accreditation, the impetus to become accredited began to increase in 1988 when the office of Civilian Health and Medical Program of the Uniformed Health Services (CHAMPUS) required CABC accreditation for birth center reimbursement (AABC, 2015c). In 2008, the ACOG, which had previously opposed all OOH births, modified their stance, stating, "Unless a woman is in a hospital, an accredited freestanding birthing center, or birthing center within a hospital complex, with physicians ready to intervene quickly if necessary, she puts herself and her baby's health and life at unnecessary risk" (ACOG, 2008, p. 1).

As of 2015, three states required CABC accreditation for licensure; others are considering it. A growing number of health care insurers, requiring evidence for safety and quality, now mandate CABC accreditation for contracting with and reimbursing birth centers. As of September 2015, one third of U.S. birth centers known to AABC were CABC accredited or in the process of becoming accredited. This degree of participation in the accreditation process is a significant increase over prior years, and the number of birth centers seeking accreditation is expected to continue to rise as both consumers and payers demand that birth centers demonstrate that they are providing high-quality care (CABC, 2014, 2015b).

## Costs, Charges, and Reimbursement

Birth centers began as single-service units. Unlike hospitals that provide many services that may allow maternity care to serve as a loss leader in the total revenue stream, birth center charges closely reflect the actual cost of delivering the services. Hospitals usually provide information on charges rather than actual costs. Initially, CbC users were insured, economically secure women who paid out of pocket when insurance coverage was denied. The first analysis of birth center cost benefits, from a study of MCA's CbC by BlueCross BlueShield of Greater New York, reported savings of up to 40% over hospital charges for an uncomplicated vaginal birth. Savings from 30% to 40% have been consistent over the years (Cannoodt, Sieverts, & Schachter, 1982).

Data from AABC Perinatal Data Registry™ (PDR) practice profile for 2012 to 2015 show a mean charge of $6,688 for total professional and facility charges for 90 birth centers (AABC, 2015d). National statistics on normal pregnancy and/or delivery from the Health Care Cost and Utilization Project (HCUP) reported a mean charge of $12,387 for 202,960 hospital births in 2012 (U.S. Department of Health and Human Services, 2013). On average, the hospital charge alone for an uncomplicated vaginal birth is about five times the average birth center charge for a vaginal birth (Childbirth Connection, 2015).

When MCA opened a second birth center in collaboration with Morris Heights Health Center to serve mainly Puerto Rican and African American low-income families in the southwest Bronx, Medicaid was the primary payer. Although most Medicaid programs have paid the nurse-midwife provider, centers continue to struggle to receive a separate facility fee. In 2015, 129 birth centers responded to an AABC survey on Medicaid reimbursement. Among the responding centers, 78 accepted Medicaid clients. Among those centers not accepting Medicaid clients, the primary reason was lack of reimbursement (AABC, 2015e).

The Affordable Care Act (ACA) mandates that Medicaid pays facility service fees for birth centers and increases payment for services provided by nurse-midwives from 65% to 100% of physician reimbursement for comparable services (Patient Protection and Affordable Care Act, 2010). However, Medicaid payment is administered at the state level and many states have delayed or declined to follow the ACA directives. Most private health care insurers now reimburse both birth center facility and care provider charges, thus removing a major barrier not only for birth centers but also for hospitals and physician practices wanting to include midwifery-led units or birth centers to their services (AABC, 2015e).

## Liability Insurance

The purpose of liability insurance is to protect the public in the event of provider negligence or malpractice. In the mid-1980s, the rising number of legal claims and high amounts of court awards against maternity care providers created a nationwide crisis when insurance companies dropped their coverage of obstetricians, nurse-midwives, and birth centers. This singular event caused the immediate closure of 25% of all operating birth centers and resulted in the loss of interest by more than 100 parties who had been exploring opening a birth center. Obtaining affordable liability insurance continues to be a challenge for all maternity care providers. Although expensive, AABC continues to seek and negotiate affordable coverage. Three national and several regional liability insurers now offer liability insurance for qualified midwives and birth centers, but many issues surrounding the availability and affordability of liability insurance for all maternity care providers have yet to be resolved (AABC, 2015f).

## Membership Organization

AABC is a membership organization that provides advocacy and a national voice for birth centers. It is governed by a multidisciplinary board of directors and offers membership to all established and developing birth centers as well as birth center supporters (AABC, 2015g, 2015h). AABC's regional "How to Start a Birth Center" workshops educate individuals and groups on the birth center concept and the business aspects of operating an independent practice and small health care facility. The workshops, offered quarterly at accredited birth centers, provide a birth center tour for the on-site demonstration of birth center operations as well as discussions with experienced birth center professionals. The staff role-plays care for normal births and how to manage a hospital transfer. The workshops are designed to help interested parties determine their readiness, market, and resources for embarking on a birth center in their community. The workshop manual guides the process of developing a birth center (AABC, 2015i). AABC also provides education and networking for members and supporters through the annual AABC Birth Institute, a quarterly newsletter, an online LISTSERVE, telephone assistance to members encountering problems, and linkage to consultants (AABC, 2015j).

## THE EVIDENCE ON BIRTH CENTER CARE

Ideas for innovation must first prove worthy of replication with positive outcomes demonstrated by research findings. The most reliable research method, the RCT, requires random assignment of pregnant women to care, not necessarily of their own choosing. This research methodology poses an ethical dilemma. As a result, most reports of outcomes of freestanding birth centers are retrospective, descriptive, comparative studies.

## Early Studies and Reports on Birth Centers

The first birth center study was conducted by BlueCross BlueShield of Greater New York, as reported previously (Cannoodt et al., 1982). The conclusion of the study's authors was that women who gave birth at the CbC site received excellent care at lower cost (Cannoodt et al., 1982). Also in 1982, IOM commissioned a committee of experts to review knowledge on the safety of different birth settings.

The experts determined that birth settings had not been studied sufficiently and they offered a number of appropriate research designs (IOM, 1982).

In the 1980s, several key publications reported findings supportive of freestanding birth centers. In an issue of *Lancet*, Bennetts and Lubic (1982) reported a neonatal mortality rate of 4.6/1,000 births among 1,938 births in 11 nurse-midwifery-run birth centers from 1972 to 1979. NACC (now AABC) reported a neonatal mortality rate of 2.5/1,000 births in a survey of 102 birth centers (NACC, 1983). Eakins and Richwald (1986) analyzed neonatal mortality in 1984 and reported a neonatal mortality rate of 4/1,000 births in 16 birth centers in California.

A study conducted from May 1984 through April 1985 evaluated the safety and effectiveness of birth center care for mothers assigned to a birth center in Miami compared with mothers who voluntarily chose birth center care. The birth center had been established in association with a tertiary care hospital in Miami that served a primarily indigent population. Initially, all women chose where to give birth, but when it became necessary to reduce overcrowding in the hospital's obstetric unit, the hospital assigned low-risk women to the birth center for care (Scupholme & Kamons, 1987).

This study was designed to determine whether there was a difference in outcomes between the group of women assigned to the birth center versus the group who chose birth center care. From each group, 148 women were matched for parity and demographic variables. There were no differences between the two groups in cervical dilatation on admission, the length of labor timed from the mother's report of the onset of regular contractions, use of pharmacological analgesia, meconium-stained amniotic fluid, intrapartum transfers to the hospital, reasons for intrapartum transfers, the rate of normal spontaneous vaginal births, or reasons for neonatal transfers. Concerns about women in the assigned group missing prenatal appointments or not returning to the birth center for follow-up within 36 hours after discharge did not materialize. Among the women assigned to the birth center, the rate of prenatal appointments that were kept, and follow-up appointments was 100%. Although satisfaction was not evaluated, many mothers in the assigned birth center group returned for subsequent pregnancies and referred friends and family to the birth center. The cost of care in the birth center for labor and birth was 30% less than care of comparable in-hospital (IH) patients (Scupholme & Kamons, 1987).

## The First National Birth Center Study

AABC responded to the need for the large study recommended by the BlueCross BlueShield of Greater New York study by conducting a 2-year prospective, descriptive study of 11,814 women who were admitted in labor to 84 freestanding birth centers in 35 states. This landmark study, published in *The New England Journal of Medicine* in 1989, occurred between 1985 and 1987. The primary objective was to address the safety of birth center care under the care of a variety of providers, including physicians and midwives. Satisfaction with birth center care was high. In this study, 76% of the women completed an evaluation. Among the respondents,

99% were satisfied with the care and would recommend the birth center to friends and 94% would use the same birth center again. Among transferred women who completed the evaluation, 97% stated they would recommend birth center care and 83% would return to the same birth center (Rooks et al., 1989).

During labor, 16% of the women were transferred to hospitals and 4.4% had cesarean births. There were no maternal deaths. The combined intrapartum fetal–neonatal mortality rate was 1.3/1,000 births but dropped to 0.7/1,000 births when deaths associated with fetal anomalies were excluded. This finding was comparable to outcomes of low-risk births in hospitals and lower than rates in earlier studies of care in birth centers. The authors attributed these findings to enhanced safety, including birth center regulation and licensure, peer review, accreditation, and education (Rooks et al., 1989).

The authors concluded:

> Few innovations in health care service promise lower cost, greater avail-ability, and a high degree of satisfaction with a comparable degree of safety. The results of this study suggest that modern birth centers can identify women who are low risk for obstetrical complications and can care for them in a way that provides these benefits. (Rooks et al., 1989, p. 1810)

Detailed reports from the study were also published in a three-part series in the *Journal of Nurse-Midwifery* (Rooks, Weatherby, & Ernst, 1992a, 1992b, 1992c).

Between 1985 and 1987, using the National Birth Center Study (NBCS) instrument, NAAC (now AACB) collected data on 2,256 births in 15 hospital-based nurse-midwifery practice sites. Outcomes were comparable; however, IH births were associated with more medical intervention. There was no maternal mortality, and neonatal mortality rates could not be determined with accuracy. The authors noted that hospital care offered no advantage for low-risk women (Fullerton & Severino, 1992).

## National Study of Vaginal Birth After Cesarean in Birth Centers

In the 1980s, research on trial of labor after cesarean delivery (TOLAC) chal-lenged the long-held opinion in obstetrics that vaginal birth after cesarean (VBAC) was too dangerous (NACC, 1989). In 1999, based on new evidence on surgical techniques, ACOG published a modified position on VBAC (ACOG, 2010). Still, some women were unable to find physicians or midwives willing to attend a VBAC birth and they turned to birth centers. Because of the risk that a scarred uterus could rupture during labor, these women were not eligible for birth center care. Some of these women chose unattended home births or births attended by unlicensed midwives. In response, the AABC Standards Committee developed evidence-based criteria and approved a 10-year study of TOLAC in birth centers after documentation of a single low-transverse cesarean section (AABC, 2015a). From 1990 to 2000, the study (*n* = 1,453 postcesarean women) was conducted in 41 birth centers. There were six documented uterine ruptures and seven peri-natal deaths, two of the deaths related to uterine rupture. There was a higher rate of perinatal mortality compared to the findings of the NBCS. There were no maternal deaths; 24% of the women were transferred to the hospital and 87% of study participants were able to give birth vaginally. When the data were compared to a similar group in an acute hospital setting, the rate of uterine rupture and the rate of maternal adverse outcomes was 1.4%, the same as the rate for the birth center group. The hospital group had no fetal deaths. The authors cited other studies that showed low rates of perinatal mortality in a hospital setting and concluded that because adverse outcomes are somewhat increased, women undergoing TOLAC are best cared for in a hospital setting (Lieberman, Ernst, Rooks, Stapleton, & Flamm, 2004).

## The San Diego Birth Center Study

The San Diego Birth Center Study (1994–1996) examined outcomes, safety, and use of resources among low-risk, low-income women, comparing a collaborative management/birth center option and traditional physician-based perinatal care. Collaborative management included the birth center, private medical offices, and neighborhood health centers, as well as community and tertiary hospitals. This study enrolled 1,808 women who had the option to use the birth center. Women who had traditional care but met birth center eligibility criteria ($n = 1,149$) were also enrolled in the study. Although 30% of the collaborative management participants saw only nurse-midwives throughout their pregnancies and births, 65% were managed collaboratively through consultation or necessary visits with an obstetrician, and 5% required exclusive prenatal management by an obstetrician. More than 65% of the participants chose a birth center; and 45% of them remained low risk, giving birth at the birth center. Although both scenarios resulted in safe outcomes for mothers and babies, the collaborative care/birth center option resulted in fewer operative deliveries and less use of medical resources (Jackson et al., 2003).

## The AABC PDR

The web-based data registry, the AABC PDR, (formerly known as the Uniform Data Set [UDS]), collects prospective data on the process and outcomes of midwifery care (AABC, 2015k). This registry was developed in 2002 and now uses guidelines published by the Agency for Healthcare Research and Quality (AHRQ; Gliklich & Dreyer, 2007). The purposes of the registry are to improve the quality of care for childbearing families, to provide for the ongoing and systematic collection of data on physiologic birth, and to facilitate research about normal birth. The AABC strives to ensure that this data use remains both ethical and purposeful. It encourages use by facilities and individuals who have contributed the data as well as by outside researchers. AABC has a defined process for researchers to apply in using the PDR (AABC, 2015l). As of June 2015, the UDS included approximately 65,000 records and the second registry, the PDR, includes 38,300 records from 115 birth center practices (S. Stapleton, personal communication, August 16, 2015).

## The National Birth Center Study II

The second National Birth Center Study (NBCS II; Stapleton, Osborne, & Illuzzi, 2013) was conducted between 2007 and 2010, using data collected in the American Association of Birth Centers Perinatal Data Registry (AABC PDR). As a prospective cohort study, the NBCS II examined the outcomes of 15,574 women who gave birth in 79 midwifery-led birth centers in 33 states. The authors concluded that the results of NBCS I and NBCS II were strikingly similar. Outcomes and intrapartum emergency transfer rates were nearly the same. Mortality, transfer, complication, and operative birth rates were similar despite differences in the two study populations. The second study had a higher proportion of women aged 35 or older, African American, unmarried, and nulliparous. Although cost was not examined, it was projected that the 79 birth centers saved more than $30 million in health care expenses during the 4-year study period. The authors noted that all of the birth centers in the study held AABC membership. Findings cannot be generalized to all birth centers (Stapleton et al., 2013).

## The Planned OOH Birth and Birth Outcomes Study

A recently published study by Snowden et al. (2015) addressed a serious methodological flaw in many previous studies comparing all OOH births with all IH births. The research usually did not differentiate between planned or unplanned OOH birth, so that a precipitous unplanned birth in an automobile was not disaggregated from a carefully planned birth in a birth center (Snowden et al., 2015). Parallel to this flaw has been counting all IH births as if they were planned hospital births, regardless of transfer from home, birth center, or unplanned place of birth.

This current study addresses one aspect of this issue, that is, outcomes by planned place of birth. Inclusion criteria in this retrospective cohort study were cephalic, singleton term, normal neonates born in Oregon between 2012 and 2013 (n = 79,727 births). Births were classified as *planned* IH births or *planned* OOH births, even if the planned OOH birth mother was transferred and delivered at a hospital. The data used the revised Oregon birth certificate, which captures data on planned place of birth and outcomes (Snowden et al., 2015).

Overall, this study found few serious adverse outcomes for mothers, regardless of birth setting, with lower rates of obstetrical intervention in the OOH setting. Admission of infants to the NICU was lower in the OOH group and there was no significant increase in the odds ratio for infant death by planned place of birth. The study notes an increase in the odds ratio (2.43) for perinatal death as well as depressed 5-minute Apgar scores, neonatal seizures, and increased rate of maternal blood transfusion with planned OOH births. Although fetal death was higher in planned OOH birth, the rate did not reach the level of statistical significance. In summary, the absolute risk of perinatal death was low in both planned OOH and planned IH settings (Snowden et al., 2015).

A major issue in evaluating planned OOH birth is that few studies, with the exception of the National Birth Center I and II studies, address planned OOH outcomes disaggregating data *exclusive* to birth centers. Although not addressing this specific issue, this current study still adds to existing knowledge about planned OOH birth (Snowden et al., 2015).

Further, in examining outcomes in planned OOH birth in the United States, there are significant differences in birth centers and the qualifications of midwives practicing in birth centers. Not all birth centers are accredited. When considering birth outcomes, it is imperative to determine birth center accreditation status. There is marked heterogeneity in birth centers across the nation, many of which are unaccredited (Dekker, 2015). Not all midwives meet the International Confederation of Midwives (ICM) standard (ICM, 2011). Snowden and colleagues (2015) spoke to these issues in comparing the safety of planned OOH birth in economically comparable developed European nations with that of the United States. The authors noted that these nations have excellent outcomes with planned OOH birth, midwives are trained to ICM standards (ICM, 2011), and they are well integrated into health care systems, as opposed to the United States where midwifery credentialing and a well-coordinated system of collaboration are sporadic (Snowden et al., 2015).

## The Evidence From Comparable High-Resource Countries

While freestanding birth centers were still developing in the United States, freestanding birth centers and IH alternative birth settings were developed and studied in England, Scotland, Sweden, Australia, New Zealand, and Denmark (Borquez & Wiegers, 2006; Davis et al., 2011; Gottvall, Grunewald, & Waldenstrom, 2004; Laws, Lim, Tracy, & Sullivan, 2009; Overgaard, Moller, Frenger-Gron, Knudsen, & Sandall, 2011; Rogers, Harman, & Selo-Ojeme, 2011; Thorgen & Crang-Svalenius, 2009; Waldenstrom & Nilsson, 1997).

Interest was prompted by the work of the National Perinatal Epidemiology Unit in Oxford, England, which was formed to assemble a registry of controlled trials in perinatal medicine. The results of that review were reported for general readership in the first of three editions of *A Guide to Effective Care in Pregnancy and Childbirth* (Enkin et al., 2013). In 1993, the National Perinatal Epidemiology Unit became the Cochrane Collaboration, which usually limits reviews to RCTs. In 2012, despite no RCTs of freestanding birth center care, it published a review of eight quasi-controlled trials of nearly 11,000 births comparing outcomes in environments with *bedroom-like settings* to those in conventional labor wards (Hodnett, Downe, & Walsh, 2012).

Recently, Alliman and Phillippi (2016) published an integrative review of the literature on birth center outcomes from multiple countries. They reviewed only studies published in English. This review included 23 quantitative and nine qualitative studies involving 84,300 births. Alliman and Phillippi reported that birth center care is associated with greater rates of spontaneous vaginal birth and lower rates of assisted vaginal and cesarean birth compared with hospital care. In the review, severe morbidity was rare and there was no mortality. The authors concluded that birth centers are an option for low-risk women when integrated within a system capable of providing higher level care as needed (Alliman & Phillippi, 2016).

## BEST PRACTICES: SCALING UP BIRTH CENTER CARE IN THE UNITED STATES

### Strong Start for Mothers and Newborns Initiative

In 2012, the Center for Medicare & Medicaid Innovation (CMMI) acknowledged the need to improve maternity care with the Strong Start for Mothers and Newborns Initiative (SSI; Centers for Medicare & Medicaid Services [CMS], 2015). CMMI embraced projects with potential to achieve better outcomes, cost savings, and patient satisfaction (Berwick, Nolan, & Whittington, 2008).

In 2013, the CMS awarded 27 SSI grants to study the costs and outcomes of three models of enhanced prenatal care: centering/group prenatal visits, maternity care homes, and birth centers. AABC received the largest award ($5.35 million for over 4 years; AABC, 2013). AABC convened 45 birth centers from 19 states in a project to enroll 10,000 women in birth center care during 3 years and to collect data analyzing processes and outcomes related to women's experience of care, preterm births, and other perinatal outcomes. Birth centers participating in this project provide prenatal care to women enrolled in Medicaid or the Children's Health Insurance Program (CHIP). The women in the project also have peer support throughout pregnancy and the immediate postpartum period. AABC's involvement in the SSI provides an opportunity to demonstrate birth center outcomes for underserved women, with potential to change federal policies and increase access to birth center care for a more diverse population (AABC, 2013; Alliman, Jolles, & Summers, 2015).

### Education of Midwifery Students

A critical barrier to making the midwifery/birth center model of care more available has been an inability to educate enough midwives with experience to establish and staff birth centers. The major restriction on increasing enrollment in midwifery education has been the denial of access to hospital clinical training sites. In the early 1980s, NACC (now AABC), MCA, the Frontier School of Midwifery and Family Nursing (FSMFN; now Frontier Nursing University [FNU]), and the Frances Payne Bolton School of Nursing at Case Western Reserve University partnered to address this need. The goals were to increase enrollment in nurse-midwifery education using an innovative distance learning program and to prepare nurse-midwifery students for practice in birth centers and rural and underserved areas. Although the distance learning model in midwifery education has been replicated, FNU is the only nurse-midwifery education program offering a course in setting up a clinical practice, including attendance at an AABC "How to Start a Birth Center" workshop with a required follow-up assignment of developing a business plan.

# REFERENCES

Alliman, J., Jolles, D., & Summers, L. (2015). The innovation imperative: Scaling freestanding birth centers, CenteringPregnancy, and midwifery-led maternity health homes. *Journal of Midwifery and Women's Health, 60*(3), 244–249. doi:10.1111/jmwh.12320

Alliman, J., & Phillippi, J. (2016). Maternal outcomes in birth centers: An integrative review of the literature. *Journal of Midwifery and Women's Health, 61*(1), 21–51. Retrieved from http://onlinelibrary.wiley.com/doi/10.1111/jmwh.12356/abstract. doi:10.1111/jmwh.12356

American Association of Birth Centers (AABC). (2008). What is a birth center? Retrieved from http://www.birthcenters.org/?page=bce_what_is_a_bc&hh

American Association of Birth Centers (AABC). (2013). AABC leads successful national grant award with 48 local birth center sites [Press release March 1, 2013]. Retrieved from http://www.birthcenters.org/news/news.asp?id=229197&terms=%22strong+and+start+and+m others%22

American Association of Birth Centers (AABC). (2015a). National standards for birth centers. Retrieved from www.birthcenters.org/?page=Standards

American Association of Birth Centers (AABC). (2015b). Birth centers regulations. Retrieved from http://www.birthcenters.org/?page=bc_regulations

American Association of Birth Centers (AABC). (2015c). A historical timeline: Highlights of 35 years of developing the birth center concept in the US. Retrieved from http://www.birthcenters.org/?page=history

American Association of Birth Centers (AABC). (2015d). *Practice profile data from AABC Perinatal Data Registry* (Unpublished data). Perkiomenville, PA.

American Association of Birth Centers (AABC). (2015e). *Update on AABC Medicaid survey of birth centers.* Retrieved from http://www.birthcenters.org/news

American Association of Birth Centers (AABC). (2015f). Liability insurance. Retrieved from http://www.birthcenters.org/?page=liability_insurance

American Association of Birth Centers (AABC). (2015g). Join now. Retrieved from http://www.birthcenters.org/?page=JoinNow

American Association of Birth Centers (AABC). (2015h). Who's who at AABC. Retrieved from http://www.birthcenters.org/?page=whos_who

American Association of Birth Centers (AABC). (2015i). How to start a birth center: Bringing midwifery to main street. Retrieved from http://www.birthcenters.org/?page=hsbc_work shops

American Association of Birth Centers (AABC). (2015j). Access your member benefits. Retrieved from http://www.birthcenters.org/?page=Access_Benefits

American Association of Birth Centers (AABC). (2015k). What is the AABC perinatal data registry? Retrieved from https://aabc.site-ym.com/general/custom.asp?page=PDR

American Association of Birth Centers (AABC). (2015l). What is the AABC Perinatal Data Registry™? Retrieved from http://www.birthcenters.org/?PDR

American College of Nurse-Midwives (ACNM). (2011). Joint statement of practice relations between obstetrician-gynecologists and certified nurse midwives/certified midwives. Retrieved from http://www.midwife.org/ACNM/files/ACNMLibraryData/UPLOADFILENAME/000000000224/ACNM.ACOG%20Joint%20Statement%203.30.11.pdf

American College of Obstetricians and Gynecologists (ACOG). (2008). ACOG statement on home births [Press release]. Retrieved from http://www.cfmidwifery.org/pdf/ACOGPR nr0206082cfm.pdf

American College of Obstetricians and Gynecologists (ACOG). (2010). Vaginal birth after previous cesarean (ACOG Practice Bulletin no. 115). Retrieved from http://www.acog.org/ Resources-And-Publications/Practice-Bulletins/Committee-on-Practice-Bulletins-Obste trics/Vaginal-Birth-After-Previous-Cesarean-Delivery

American Public Health Association (APHA). (1983). Guidelines for licensing and regulating birth centers [Policy Number 8209(PP)]. *American Journal of Public Health, 73*(3), 331–334.

Baruffi, G., Dellinger, W. S., Jr., Stobino, D. M., Rudolph, A., Timmons, R. Y., & Ross, A. (1984). A study of pregnancy outcomes in a maternity center and tertiary care hospital. *American Journal of Public Health, 74*(9), 973–978. doi:10.2105/AJPH.74.9.973

Bennetts, A. B., & Lubic, R. W. (1982). The free-standing birth centre. *Lancet, 319*(8268), 378–380. doi:10/1016/S0140-6736(82)9401–5

Berwick, D. M., Nolan, T. W., & Whittington, J. (2008). The triple aim: Care, health, and cost. *Health Affairs, 27*(3), 759–769. doi:10.1377/hlthaff.27.3.759

Borquez, H. A., & Wiegers, T. A. (2006). A comparison of labour and birth experiences of women delivering in a birthing centre and at home in the Netherlands. *Midwifery, 22*(4), 339–347. doi:10.1016/j.midw.2005.12.004

Cannoodt, L., Sieverts, S., & Schachter, M. (1982). Alternatives to the conventional in-hospital delivery: The childbearing center experience. *Acta Hospitalia, 22*(4), 324–339.

Centers for Disease Control and Prevention (CDC). (2011). Public health then and now: Celebrating 50 years of MMWR at CDC. *Morbidity and Mortality Weekly Report, 60*(Suppl.). Retrieved from http://www.cdc.gov/mmwr/pdf/other/su6004.pdf

Centers for Medicare & Medicaid Services (CMS). (2015). Strong start for mothers and newborns initiative: General information. Retrieved from https://innovation.cms.gov/ initiatives/strong-start

Chalmers, I., Enkin, M., & Keirse, M. (1989). *Effective care in pregnancy and childbirth*. Oxford, UK: Oxford University Press.

Childbirth Connection. (2015). Average charges for giving birth: State charts (Transforming Maternity Care blog). Retrieved from http://transform.childbirthconnection.org/resources/ datacenter/chargeschart/statecharges

Cockerham, A. Z., & Keeling, A. W. (2010). Finance and faith at the Catholic Maternity Institute, Santa Fe, New Mexico, 1944–1969. *Nursing History Review, 18*(1), 151–166. doi:10.1891/1062–8061.18.151

Cockerham, A. Z., & King, T. L. (2014). One hundred years of progress in nurse-midwifery: With women, then and now. *Journal of Nurse-Midwifery and Women's Health, 59*(1), 3–7. doi:10.1111/jmwh.12161

Commission for the Accreditation of Birth Centers (CABC). (2014). 2014 annual report. Retrieved from https://www.birthcenteraccreditation.org/wp-content/uploads/2015/04/2 CABCAnnualReport2014.pdf

Commission for the Accreditation of Birth Centers (CABC). (2015a). In the pursuit of excellence. Retrieved from https://www.birthcenteraccreditation.org

Commission for the Accreditation of Birth Centers (CABC). (2015b). Accredited birth centers. Retrieved from https://www.birthcenteraccreditation.org/find-accredited-birth-centers

Davis, D., Baddock, S., Pairman, S., Hunter, M., Benn, C., Wilson, D., . . . Herbison, P. (2011). Planned place of birth in New Zealand: Does it affect mode of birth and intervention rates among low-risk women? *Birth, 38*(2), 111–119. doi:10.1111/j.1523-536X.2010.00458.x

Dekker, R. (2015). Evidence confirms birth centers provide top-notch care. AABC National Birth Center Study II. Retrieved from http://www.birthcenters.org/?page=NBCSII

DeLee, J. F. (1915). Progress towards ideal obstetrics. In *1915 Campaign to eliminate the midwife*. Retrieved from http://www.theunnecesarean.com/blog/2009/12/9/joseph-delees-1915-campaign-to-eliminate-the-midwife.html

Eakins, P. S., & Richwald, G. A. (1986). Free-standing birth centers in California: Structure, cost, medical outcome and issues. In *The California Birth Center study*. Berkeley, CA: UCLA Department of Public Health and Stanford University Institute for Research on Women and Gender. Retrieved from https://pamelaeakins.net/CA_Birth_Center_Study.html

Enkin, M., Keirse, M. C., Neilson, J., Crowther, C., Duley, L., Hodnett, E., & Hofmeyr, J. (2013). *Guide to effective care in pregnancy and childbirth* (3rd ed.). Oxford, UK: Oxford University Press. doi:10.1093/med/9780192631732.001.0001

Ernst, E. K. (1994). Health care reform as an ongoing process. *Journal of Obstetric, Gynecologic, and Neonatal Nursing, 23*(2), 129–138. doi:10.1111/j.1552–6909.1994.tb01862.x

Fullerton, J. T., & Severino, R. (1992). In-hospital care for low-risk childbirth: Comparison with results from the National Birth Center Study. *Journal of Nurse-Midwifery, 37*(5), 331–340. doi:10.1016/0091-2182(92)90240-4

Gliklich, R., & Dreyer, N. (2007). *Registries for evaluating patient outcomes: A user's guide* (AHRQ Publication No. 07-EHC001-1). Rockville, MD: Agency for Healthcare Research and Quality. Retrieved from http://www.effectivehealthcare.ahrq.gov/index.cfm/search-for-guides-reviews-and-reports/?pageaction=displayProduct&productID=12

Gottvall, K., Grunewald, C., & Waldenstrom, U. (2004). Safety of birth centre care: Perinatal mortality over a 10-year period. *International Journal of Obstetrics and Gynecology, 111*(1), 71–78. doi:10.1046/j.1471-0528.2003.00017.x

Hodnett, E. D., Downe, S., & Walsh, D. (2012). Alternative versus conventional institutional settings for birth. *Cochrane Database of Systematic Reviews, 2012*(9), 1–31. doi:10.1002/14651858.CD000012.pub3

Hodnett, E. D., Gates, S., Hofmeyr, G. J., & Sakala, C. (2013). Continuous support for women during childbirth. *Cochrane Database of Systematic Reviews, 2013*(7). doi:10.1002/14651858.CD003766.pub5

Institute of Medicine (IOM). (1982). *Research issues in the assessment of birth settings*. Washington, DC: National Academies Press. doi:10.17226.18297

Institute of Medicine (IOM). (2011). *The future of nursing: Leading change, advancing health*. (Committee on the Robert Wood Johnson Foundation Initiative on the Future of Nursing). Washington, DC: National Academies Press.

International Confederation of Midwives (ICM). (2011). ICM international definition of the midwife. Retrieved from http://internationalmidwives.org/who-we-are/policy-and-practice/icm-international-definition-of-the-midwife

Jackson, D. J., Lang, J. M., Swartz, W. H., Ganiats, T. G., Fullerton, J., Ecker, J., & Nguyen, U. (2003). Outcomes, safety, and resource utilization in a collaborative care birth center program compared with traditional physician-based perinatal care. *American Journal of Public Health*, 93(6), 999–1006. doi:10.2105/AJPH.93.6.999

Laird, M. D. (1955). Report of the Maternity Center Association Clinic, New York, 1931-1951. *American Journal of Obstetrics and Gynecology*, 69(1), 178–184.

Laws, P. J., Lim, C., Tracy, S., & Sullivan, E. A. (2009). Characteristics and practices of birth centres in Australia. *Australian and New Zealand Journal of Obstetrics and Gynaecology*, 49(3), 290–295. doi:10.1111/j.1479-828X.2009.01002.x

Lesser, M. S., & Keane, V. R. (1956). *Nurse-patient relationships in a hospital maternity service*. St. Louis, MO: Mosby.

Lieberman, E., Ernst, E. K., Rooks, J. P., Stapleton, S., & Flamm, B. (2004). Results of the national study of vaginal birth after cesarean in birth centers. *Obstetrics and Gynecology*, 104(5, Pt. 1), 933–942. doi:10.1097/01.AOG.0000143257.29471.82

Lubic, R. W. (1979). *Barriers and conflict in maternity care innovation* (Unpublished doctoral dissertation). Teachers College, Columbia University, New York, NY. Retrieved from https://aabc.site-ym.com/store/ViewProduct.aspx?id=4153536&hhSearchTerms=%2522Ba rriers+and+conflict+in+maternity+care+innovation%2522

Lubic, R. W., & Flynn, C. (2010). The Family Health and Birth Center—A nurse-midwife managed center in Washington, DC. *Alternative Therapies in Health and Medicine*, 16(5), 58–60.

Maternity Center Association (MCA). (1994). Hope reborn: Empowering families in the South Bronx [Video]. Retrieved from http://www.birthcenters.org

National Association of Childbearing Centers (NACC). (1983). AABC birth center update: 1983 survey. *NACC News*, 12(3–4), 4–18.

National Association of Childbearing Centers (NACC). (1989). Committee opinion: Vaginal birth after cesarean section (Standards Committee; Unpublished document). American Association of Birth Centers, Perkiomenville, PA.

Overgaard, C., Moller, A. M., Frenger-Gron, M., Knudsen, L. B., & Sandall, J. (2011). Freestanding midwifery unit versus obstetric unit: A matched cohort study of outcomes in low-risk women. *BMJ Open*, 1(2), 1–11. doi:10.1136/bmjopen-2011-000262

Patient Protection and Affordable Care Act, 42 U.S.C. § 18001 et seq. (2010). Retrieved from http://www.govtrack.us/congress/bill.xpd?bill=h111-3590

Relman, A. S. (1991). Shattuck lecture—The health care industry: Where is it taking us? *New England Journal of Medicine*, 325(12), 854–859. doi:10.1056/NEJM199109193251205

Rogers, C., Harman, J., & Selo-Ojeme, D. (2011). Perceptions of birth in a stand-alone centre compared to other options. *British Journal of Midwifery*, 19(4), 237–244. doi:10.12968/bjom.2011.19.4.237

Rooks, J. P. (1997). *Midwifery & childbirth in America*. Philadelphia, PA: Temple University Press.

Rooks, J. P., Weatherby, N. L., & Ernst, E. K. (1992a). The National Birth Center Study Part I—Methodology and prenatal care and referrals. *Journal of Nurse-Midwifery*, 37(4), 222–253. doi:10.1016/0091-2182(92)90128-P

Rooks, J. P., Weatherby, N. L., & Ernst, E. K. (1992b). The National Birth Center Study Part II—Intrapartum and immediate postpartum and neonatal care. *Journal of Nurse-Midwifery*, 37(5), 301–313. doi:10.1016/0091-2182(92)90239-Y

Rooks, J. P., Weatherby, N. L., & Ernst, E. K. (1992c). The National Birth Center Study Part III—Intrapartum and immediate postpartum and neonatal complications and transfers, postpartum and neonatal care, outcomes, and client satisfaction. *Journal of Nurse-Midwifery, 37*(6), 361–397. doi:10.1016/0091-2182(92)90122-J

Rooks, J. P., Weatherby, N. L., Ernst, E. K., Stapleton, S., Rosen, D., & Rosenfield, A. (1989). Outcomes of care in birth centers: National birth center study. *New England Journal of Medicine, 321*(26), 1804–1811. doi:10.1056/NEJM198912283212606

Scupholme, A., & Kamons, A. (1987). Are outcomes compromised when mothers are assigned to birth centers for care? *Journal of Nurse-Midwifery, 32*(4), 211–215. doi:10.1016/0091-2182(87)90112-1

Snowden, J. M., Tilden, E. L., Synder, J., Quigley, B., Caughey, A. B. & Cheng, Y. W. (2015). Planned out-of-hospital birth and birth outcomes. *New England Journal of Medicine, 2015*(373), 2642–2653. doi:10.1056/NEJMsa501738

Stapleton, S., Osborne, C., & Illuzzi, J. (2013). Outcomes of care in birth centers: Demonstration of a durable model. *Journal of Midwifery and Women's Health, 58*(1), 3–14. doi:10.1111/jmwh.12003

Texas Woman's University. (2010). Texas Women's Hall of Fame: Murdaugh, Sister Angela. Retrieved from http://www.twu.edu/twhf/tw-amurdaugh.asp

Thorgen, A., & Crang-Svalenius, E. (2009). Birth centres in the East Midlands: Views and experiences of midwives. *British Journal of Midwifery, 17*(3), 144–151. doi:10.12968/bjom.2009.17.3.40076

U.S. Department of Health and Human Services. (2013). *HCUPnet, Healthcare Cost and Utilization Project.* Rockville, MD: Agency for Healthcare Research and Quality. Retrieved from http://hcupnet.ahrq.gov

Waldenstrom, U., & Nilsson, C. (1997). A randomized controlled study of birth center care versus standard maternity care: Effects on women's health. *Birth, 24*(1), 17–26. doi:10.1111/j.1523-536X.1997.00017.pp.x

# CHAPTER FIFTEEN

# CREATING A BIRTH CENTER: ENTREPRENEURIAL MIDWIFERY

Kathryn Schrag and Barbara A. Anderson

## CREATING A BIRTH CENTER: THE BACKGROUND

Although birth centers have existed in the United States for over four decades, they are not normative in American culture. Opening a birth center in a community may be met with positive and negative reactions, including enthusiastic support, resistance from vested interests, fear of safety for birth outside of the hospital, and fear of pain in a low-intervention setting. The National Birth Center Study II (NBCS II; Stapleton, Osborne, & Illuzi, 2013), a Cochrane Review on site of birth (Hodnett, Downe, & Walsh, 2012), and the research by the Birthplace in England Collaborative Group (Brocklehurst et al., 2011) have all demonstrated safety and consumer satisfaction with birth center care.

The birth center model has been a practice site primarily for midwifery rather than medicine. The birth center has a strong history of innovation (Ernst & Stone, 2013) and the endeavor requires a spirit of entrepreneurship as described by Frakes and Harrison (2010). Establishing a successful birth center is contingent upon expertise in the triad of physiologic birth in the community setting (birth center or home), the business of midwifery, and the politics of implementing change. This chapter focuses on principles in establishing a birth center. The American Association of Birth Centers (AABC) core document, *National Standards for Birth Centers* (AABC, 2015a), should be the primary resource in guiding this process. A key companion document, available at no cost, is the more detailed indicators for meeting those standards that have been published by the Commission for the Accreditation of Birth Centers (CABC; 2015a). The lead author is the founder of a successful birth center and is faculty for the national-level course, "How to Start a Birth Center," provided by the AABC. The second author founded a successful community-based education program for preparing women, their partners, and doulas for childbirth.

## Developing the Philosophical Framework for the Birth Center

In exploring the feasibility of starting a birth center, it is essential for midwives and their teams to discuss their vision, beliefs, and knowledge about birth centers. Some initial brain-storming questions are:

- What is their belief about the doctor/hospital model as the safest place for normal birth, and what is their personal experience with birth outside the hospital?
- Does the power and shared decision making of pregnancy and birth lie with the woman or the health care provider, or both?
- What is a realistic profit margin goal for a birth center?

## Examining History and Trends

The United States spends more money and engages in more intervention in perinatal care than any country in the world while having poorer outcomes in comparison to other developed nations. Sponsored by Childbirth Connection, the Reforming States Group, and the Milbank Memorial Fund, Sakala and Corry (2008) published a well-disseminated report describing the U.S. situation as the "perinatal paradox": while spending and intervening more in pregnancy than most affluent countries, the U.S. clinical outcomes are worse. The outcome of this report was the initiation of the Transforming Maternity Care project. This project began a public–private partnership for national action toward creating a high-quality, high-value maternity care system, with midwifery and birth center care as important components of this vision (Childbirth Connection, 2015).

Midwifery care in the birth center setting is now recognized by other health care policy and planning entities as part of the solution to the perinatal paradox. In 2013, the Institute of Medicine (IOM) convened a national-level workshop to examine birth settings (IOM, 2013) and recent articles by Romano (2013, 2015) and Alliman, Jolles, and Summers (2015) address system-level solutions that birth centers offer. In 2015, the American College of Obstetricians and Gynecologists (ACOG) and the Society for Maternal–Fetal Medicine (SMFM) recognized birth centers in the consensus document *Levels of Maternity Care* (ACOG, 2015).

## DETERMINING THE NEED

Although the image of the birth center is a place for labor and birth, the setting also provides prenatal and well-woman office visits, programs for education and support, and newborn care (Ernst & Stone, 2013). The birth center becomes the *maternity health home* for women, in the context of an integrated system of community services (Alliman et al., 2015). Evaluating the local community and assessing the need for additional clinical services will impact the direction the entrepreneurs will take in creating the birth center.

## Community Assessment

A key preliminary step in creating a birth center is performing an in-depth community assessment (Table 15.1). These questions examine the demographics and health status of the community, review the current providers of maternal health care, assess the demand for midwifery services, and identify the target market of the proposed birth center. Of particular use in assessing consumer interest are the findings from the *Listening to Women III: New Mothers Speak Out* survey (Declercq, Sakala, Corry, Applebaum, & Herrlich, 2013). This survey of 744 women who had given birth in a hospital examined openness to out-of-hospital birth. In response to openness to a birth center as place of birth, 25% reported "definitely"; 39% "would consider"; 27% "definitely would not"; and 5% "unsure." The same line of questioning was used for openness to home birth as place of birth with 11% reporting "definitely" and 64% reporting "definitely would not." These data support growing interest in out-of-hospital birth, with a preference for birth center rather than home birth (Declercq et al., 2013).

## Service Provision

### Clinical Services

The unique core expertise of the birth center is the provision of time- and education-intensive care of the healthy mother in labor and of the mother–baby dyad in the hours following birth and transition to home (Table 15.2). Many birth centers offer nonmaternity services such as gynecologic and primary care, support groups, complementary health services, and retail. The provision of each service will generate expense, revenue, quality issues, and marketing opportunities and needs to be considered carefully.

### Birth Attendant

The category of "birth attendant" is important to consider, as a number of clinicians use the midwifery model of care: nurse-midwives; direct-entry midwives, including certified professional midwives (CPMs) who could be licensed midwives (LMs); family physicians; obstetricians; and naturopathic physicians. Of the 16,913 birth center births operating in 2013, 53% were attended by certified nurse-midwives (CNMs) or certified midwives (CMs), 39% by "other midwives," 4% by physicians, and 4% by "other" (unspecified; Martin, Hamilton, Osterman, Curtin, & Matthews, 2015). Of the 318 birth centers known to AABC, 30% are staffed with CNMs only, 44% with direct-entry midwives only, 26% with a combination of birth attendants, and 5% with physicians (K. Bauer, personal communication, November 20, 2015). The CABC (2015b) reports that the midwifery staffing of the 95 CABC-accredited birth centers consists of 62% of the birth centers being staffed by only CNMs/CMs, 11% by only CPMs/LMs, and 27% staffed by a combination of midwives with both types of credentials. Fourteen percent of CABC-accredited birth centers' staff includes physicians as well as midwives and other staff (R. Senjem, personal communication, November 23, 2015).

**TABLE 15.1 Determining the Need for a Birth Center: Community-Assessment Questions**

| Assessment Parameters | Questions | Potential Resources |
|---|---|---|
| Demographics | What are the age, income, and education pyramids of the community?<br><br>How many births occur in this community annually?<br><br>How many of these births occur among women who reside in the community?<br><br>What are the pregnancy outcomes (maternal and infant mortality, preterm birth, teen pregnancy, cesarean section, breastfeeding) in this community compared to regional, state, and national data? | National Center for Health Statistics www.cdc.gov/nchs<br><br>Healthy People 2020 Goals http://www.healthypeople .gov/2020/topics-objectives/topic/ maternal-infant-and-child-health<br><br>State Health Department March of Dimes Peri-Stats www .marchofdimes.org<br><br>Private foundations such as: Kaiser Family Foundation http://kff.org/statedata<br><br>Robert Wood Johnson Foundation http://www.rwjf.org |
| Existing care | Who currently provides care, including prenatal, intrapartal, postpartum, and newborn care, as well as education, ultrasound, and genetic testing?<br><br>Who pays for the care?<br><br>Who are the largest employers of pregnant women, which insurance companies are provided as benefits, and with which hospitals do those commercial insurers contract?<br><br>How much is lack of access to care an issue? | Birth certificate data on Centers for Disease Control and state health department website<br><br>Local networking and inquiry |
| Demand | Does the community want a birth center? | Focus groups about current place of birth and acceptance and choice of midwives<br><br>Market surveys<br><br>Comparison to Listening to Women III (see Declercq et al., 2013) |
| Target audience | Who are the women the birth center would serve (all those within 1–2 hours of the birth center site, high or low income or both, a specific religious community, alternative health care group, and/or cultural group desiring physiologic birth)? | Focus groups about current place of birth and acceptance and choice of midwives |

### Open Versus Closed Model

Another important consideration is whether the birth center will follow a closed or open staffing model. The closed staffing model employs the birth attendants, and is analogous to an outpatient center owned by a private practice medical group. In contrast, an open staff model is similar to a small community hospital with a process for credentialing licensed health care providers. Historically, the first birth centers were all closed staff, and, although this continues to be the model of the majority of current birth centers, there is increasing interest in the more inclusive open model (K. Bauer, personal communication, November 18, 2015).

### Collaboration

The birth center has long been a model of successful interagency and interdisciplinary health care. Within each community, important relationships must be cultivated to support the core services of the birth center. Many birth centers include nurse practitioners as members of the clinical team. Collaborating physicians may include obstetricians, family medicine physicians, hospitalists, maternal medicine specialists, pediatricians, and neonatologists. The birth center may affiliate with a single hospital for all transfers, or several hospitals depending on distance, reason for transfer, patient insurance, and admitting privileges. Mutually understood relationships and expectations with local emergency medical services (EMS) for emergency transfers/transports are another key component of an integrated system of patient care.

## PLANNING FOR IMPLEMENTATION

## Compliance With Regulations

Exploring regulatory issues for birth centers at the state health department is the first step in legal compliance (Ernst & Stone, 2013). The lack of birth-center-specific licensing in a minority of states does not prohibit opening a birth center, but may bring challenges of credibility, insurance reimbursement, and compliance with birth-specific maternity requirements. Although the number of states that still require a certificate of need (CON) to open a new health care facility is decreasing, the majority of states have a CON program that may include birth centers (National Conference of State Legislatures [NCSL], 2015). The birth center must also operate within national health care regulations, that is, Americans with Disabilities Act (ADA), Occupational Safety and Health Administration (OSHA), and Clinical Laboratory Improvement Amendments (CLIA). Local regulations can include business licenses, zoning, fire codes, parking, and construction.

## Deciding Upon Organizational Structure

Historically, most birth centers were *bottom-up* projects, started by passionate midwives and many today continue to be small independent midwife-owned

**TABLE 15.2  Determining Service Provision**

| Clinical Service Provision | Questions |
|---|---|
| Core services | What are the resources and the mechanism by which the birth center can provide the following services?<br>● Time-intensive prenatal care<br>● Information and education<br>● Care during birth and to the mother–baby dyad immediately after birth<br>● Discharge to home<br>● Follow-up care to the mother–baby dyad in time-specified intervals at home or in office |
| Birth attendants | What categories of provider will attend the births?<br>Will the attendants reflect the practice of midwifery? |
| Closed versus open staffing model | Will the birth center be an "open-staff" or "closed-staff" model? |
| Collaborative care | How will the birth center reflect interagency and interdisciplinary collaboration?<br><br>What categories of physicians will provide collaboration; how will authority and resources be shared; what are the benefits to the collaborating physicians?<br><br>How will the birth center collaborate with admitting hospitals in terms of emergent and nonemergent transfers? Are there admitting privileges for midwives? Do admitting hospitals accept client insurance? What is the impact of the birth center and collaborative affiliation on the hospital? How will relationships with emergency medical services be cultivated for hospital transfers?<br><br>What are the resources and the mechanism by which the birth center can provide the following services, internally or with referral within the community?<br>● Diagnostic testing (laboratory, ultrasound, fetal surveillance)<br>● Maternal–fetal medicine and perinatology consultation<br>● Genetic counseling and testing<br>● Primary care and mental health services<br>● Childbirth education, support groups<br>● Doula services<br>● Lactation services |

practices. Increasingly, there are also *top-down* centers, begun by larger institutions or corporations as a value-added service. In addition, birth center corporations have more than one location under a parent organization. Some birth centers are incorporated as a for-profit organization, whereas others are nonprofit or a combination of both. This decision has far-reaching implications and should be determined after consultation with attorneys, other birth centers, and local for-profit and not-for-profit organizations.

For those birth centers that are part of a larger organization, efforts must be made to maintain visibility and appropriate autonomy, with the delegation of authority to maintain standards and quality of care. Examples of the latter include access to financial information; participation in annual budgeting; creation of clinical guidelines and birth-center-specific policies; authority to hire, evaluate, and terminate employees; clinical data collection and analysis; participation in outreach and marketing; and direct reporting to the senior leadership of the organization. As exemplars, hospital-owned birth centers in the United Kingdom report cost savings, patient satisfaction, and excellent clinical outcomes (McCourt, Rance, Rayment, & Sandall, 2011).

## Resource Management

### Financial Management

Writing a business plan is the first step in planning for financial management. The implementation plan needs to include a start-up budget, cash-flow analysis, and a 3-year projection of operational income and expenses with a profit-and-loss statement. The most challenging part of these projections is the revenue side, as both utilization of the services and reimbursement are initially unpredictable.

The concept of utilization is driven not only by how many women begin prenatal care intending to give birth at that site but also the rate of transfers out of the practice. The transfer rates in NBCS II can be used as a guide for transfer rates (Stapleton et al., 2013). Although Medicaid and Medicare reimbursement amounts for medical services are publicly available (Centers for Medicare & Medicaid Services [CMS], 2015), networking with other birth centers and midwives is key in assessing reasonable potential revenue. A valuable resource for creating start-up and operating budgets is the set of birth-center-specific budget templates and reviews offered in the AABC's "How to Start a Birth Center" workshop (AABC, 2015b).

Beginning a new business may take more time than money. Applying for a small grant for a feasibility study can help to defray costs related to time. Existing organizations that plan to add a birth center need to recognize the planning time involved and to allocate sufficient time in the workload of the staff charged with developing the business plan. A particular challenge in maternity care is that payment generally occurs only after the birth of the baby, meaning the clinician is providing months of prenatal care without income. Many independent start-up birth centers create a women's health care practice (without birth, or with birth at the hospital or home), and later add the birth center facility services.

The classic small-business model is for entrepreneurs to provide their own time (sweat equity) and to self-fund through savings and home equity loans budgeting for a return on investment within 3 to 5 years. Private equity investors may be a source of capital, although clear expectations regarding return on investment are critical. Nonprofit centers may be able to secure grant funding for a start-up, especially if it meets a local need for economic development or serves a vulnerable population. Birth centers can obtain lines of credit or loans with lending institutions, but likely will need to provide collateral. Cash flow may be enhanced by leasing the facility and equipment rather than purchasing, it as well as and the judicious use of a line of credit.

Understanding charges, billing, and coding is essential to financial management. An important start-up question is whether to create a single tax identification number for billing services rendered, or to have separate ones for the professional and facility services. Another consideration is whether to do in-house billing or to outsource to a billing service. It is vital that staff at the birth center have a basic understanding of the principles of medical billing, and work closely with a billing expert. A key concept in working within the current managed care system is that the cost of a service is not necessarily what gets charged (billed) and, furthermore, what is billed will vary significantly from what is paid (reimbursed). Because the majority of births are paid for by managed care insurance companies, contracts need to be negotiated and secured with each company.

All members of the leadership team of the birth center need to be educated about the business of midwifery (Table 15.3). AABC (see www.birthcenters.org) offers the widest number of resources targeted to birth center management, but national midwifery, obstetrical, medical, and business organizations provide professional development in business.

### Facility, Equipment, and Supplies

As in all aspects of opening a birth center, the leadership team is advised to review the AABC standards (AABC, 2015a) and the CABC indicators (CABC, 2015a) for guidance on choosing a site and purchasing furnishings, equipment, and supplies.

When assessing potential sites for a birth center, the midwives may need to work with a realtor, an architect, an interior designer, and some consumers as advisors. The location needs to be accessible to the clients, financially realistic, and within zoning regulations. If serving low-income women, it is crucial to consider proximity to public transportation. The distance from an admitting hospital(s) for routine and emergency transfers must also be considered. Another major decision is whether to lease or buy the building. If purchasing property, the midwives should consider the building as a real estate investment, with or without the birth center occupying the space. Rent and mortgage are fixed expenses so it may be practical to rent out unused portions of a building or office suite, or to secure a small site that can be expanded as growth happens. Although historically a birth center was opened in a personal residence, commercial building space opens new opportunities. Most birth centers are housed under one roof, but often with separate entrances. Some have more than one building for the facility services, office visits, administration, and education and meeting.

The business needs to invest in medical, residential, and office furnishings, equipment, and supplies. The signature mark of a birth center is an environment that is designed to encourage physiologic birth. Walking through the door should not feel like entering a medical office or a hospital. There is, however, remarkably little research exploring architectural features enhancing physiologic birth. Hospital delivery rooms were initially designed to serve physicians and nurses

---

**TABLE 15.3   Birth Center Resources and Links**

**American Association of Birth Centers** (www.birthcenters.org)
- "How to Start a Birth Center" workshop and manual: 2-day workshop; national locations with case study and tour of an accredited birth center; manual available only to attendees
- LISTSERVE
- Webinars on business topics
- Birth Institute annual meeting: administrative tract (business topics)
- Publications: *Policies and Procedures; Continuous Quality Improvement Manual*
- Newsletter, website samples, and articles

**American College of Nurse-Midwives** (www.midwives.org)
- Annual meeting
- Business LISTSERVE
- Midwifery Works: annual 3-day meeting on administrative topics for midwifery
- Webinars on business topics
- Publications: *Getting Paid, Professional Liability Resource Kit*

**Other midwifery and medical professional organization's resources**
- Midwives Alliance of North America: www.mana.org: annual meetings and publications
- American College of Obstetrics & Gynecology: www.acog.org: meetings; *Business of Medicine Manual*
- American Academy of Family Practice: www.aafp.org: meetings; *Family Practice Management*
- Medical Group Management Association: http://www.mgma.com
  Publications and conferences specific to administration of women's health practices

**Other business of health care web-based resources**
- Nurse Practitioner Business Owner: http://npbusiness.org. E-mail LISTSERVE, articles, lectures by nurse practitioners
- Building a Practice website: http://learn.gwnursing.org/Education/practice/index.htm. *Guide for Health Care Professionals'* articles, forms, and templates
- Medscape Business of Medicine: e-mail LISTSERVE
- Carolyn Buppert, NP, JD: http://buppert.com/articles; author of training module: *Safe Smart Billing and Coding*; free articles on practice management

**Small Business Association** (www.SBA.gov)
- Learning-center webinars
- E-mail alerts
- Writing a Business Plan template
- Starting and Managing a Business article series

**Books**
- *Nurse Practitioner's Business Practice and Legal Guide* (5th ed.), (2015), Carolyn Buppert, NP, JD
- *Business Concepts for Health Professionals* (2004), Joan Slager, CNM
- *An Administrative Manual for Midwifery Services* (4th ed.) (in press), Joan Slager, CNM

---

and to handle emergencies. Many hospital birth rooms have now been redesigned to include space for families but still they are equipped with electronic fetal monitors, wall oxygen and suction, visible newborn resuscitation equipment, and birthing beds, implying that the bed for birth is different than one's family bed at home. The hospital delivery suite rarely addresses the needs of women with physiologic birth.

Qualities of a physiologic birth environment include privacy, space to move, calming color and lighting, subdued sound, good air quality, absence of noxious smells, furniture and bars that facilitate the woman leaning and pulling, birthing stools and balls, tubs for labor and birth, and the family bed (Fahy, Foureur, & Hastie, 2008; Walsh & Gutteridge, 2011).

Nonetheless, Dopplers, birth kits, emergency equipment, supplies, and medications for both the mother and the baby need to be purchased while not losing sight that equipment for higher acuity labor and birth, prohibited by AABC standards, include electronic fetal monitoring and vacuum extractors. A significant expense is electronic equipment (telephones, computers, printers) and the accompanying software for scheduling appointments, managing finances and billing, and using the electronic health record (EHR). The transition to EHRs as the standard makes it prudent for a new birth center to invest in the necessary equipment. Although most EHRs are based on the medical model of care, midwifery-focused systems are being developed. Medicare and Medicaid providers using EHRs are required to demonstrate meaningful use of this technology. CMS (2015) has established a financial incentive program to assist in the implementation.

### Human Resources

As in most person-centered businesses, approximately 50% of a birth center budget is usually invested in the staff. With extraordinary service being a defining characteristic of the birth center experience, satisfied personnel at all levels, from the front desk to the health care providers, are critical to success. The midwives need to give careful consideration to what expertise and functions are needed (clinical and administrative) and what functions can be outsourced. In addition to the birth attendants (CNM, CPM, physician), consideration must be given to the type of birth assistants used. Some state licensing requires that function to be filled by an RN. Where the RN credential is not required, some birth centers use nonlicensed birth assistants trained by the birth center or elsewhere, or midwifery students.

In addition to clinical care, other functions in the birth center include reception, office management, billing, housekeeping, client education, home visiting, marketing, and human resources (Ernst & Stone, 2013). Human resources include job descriptions, orientation, payroll, verifying and tracking credentialing, obtaining and tracking malpractice insurance, and organizing performance evaluations. Small independent birth centers often start with a core group of several midwives, an RN, and an office person, all of whom perform many functions as they learn the business.

### Networking and Marketing

Strategic networking is vital to assuring community acceptance. The midwives need to establish ongoing communication with agencies and professionals working with pregnancy and birth, including collaborating physicians, admitting hospitals, diagnostics sites, childbirth education services, and lactation resources. The networking circle should also extend to complementary health providers, mothers' groups, university departments of business or women's studies, local small business or the nonprofit community, fitness centers, health-related retail stores, and secondary schools. The birth center staff should integrate into the community via social media, community events, and local news sources. Forming a birth center advisory group from the community and a more formal "Friends of the Birth Center" network are examples of strategic networking.

The opening of the birth center should be preceded by significant levels of social media networking and direct marketing. The women using the birth center are prime users of social media and word will spread quickly. Expectations will be high for compassionate care, client-centered care, and efficiency. Equally fast moving will be reports from women who utilize the birth center. The entire start-up team needs to be highly sensitive to community opinion and use every opportunity to speak to and live the mission of the birth center.

## MONITORING FOR QUALITY

As an innovation is still questioned by some, the birth center will need to prove its value. The first step is providing evidence of monitoring for quality in clinical outcomes, client satisfaction, and cost savings. The web-based data-collection and reporting tool created specifically for birth centers is AABC's Perinatal Data Registry™ and its use is highly recommended for all birth centers (AABC, 2015c). Although the safety of birth centers has been demonstrated in the United States and abroad, these impressive outcomes are a result of adherence to defined standards of care. A robust quality-assurance and quality-improvement program must be in place to ensure the best care and to safeguard the reputation of all birth centers. In addition to resources from AABC (see Table 15.3), the national Quality Improvement Tools & Resources kit (U.S. Department of Health and Human Services, Health Resources and Services Administration [HRSA], 2015) provides guidance in developing a program.

A key quality issue in a birth center setting is ensuring that the birth center serves healthy women within clearly defined parameters of clinical eligibility. From the first prenatal contact through postpartum visits, the assessment of appropriateness for birth center care is ongoing. When indicated, transfers should be made to a higher level of acuity. The transfer rates reported in the recent NBCS II have remained similar to the first study conducted decades earlier: 13.7% of women enrolled in a birth center caseload were transferred during pregnancy, 4.5% were transferred at the onset of labor but before admission to the birth center; 12.4% of women admitted in active labor were transferred before birth; and 2.4% of postpartum mothers and 2.6% of newborns born in the birth centers were transferred (Stapleton et al., 2013).

Emergency transfers from high-quality birth centers are rare, but do occur. According to Stapleton et al. (2013), most transfers were nonemergent with an emergency maternal and newborn transfer rate after admission to the birth center of 1.9%. The standard of care is 30 minutes for transfer; therefore, it is recommended that the birth center has access to a higher acuity facility within that time frame. In a large, cross-sectional study, Thomas, Paranjothy, and James (2004) examined critical intervals for maternal or fetal distress to cesarean section concluding that, in most cases, an interval of 15 to 75 minutes resulted in good fetal and maternal outcomes.

It is essential to design a well-articulated emergency plan regarding transfers, emergent or otherwise. All staff must be prepared to identify, stabilize, and efficiently move those patients into a hospital setting. The continuous quality-improvement processes within the birth center assure this preparedness. The program should include clinical guidelines, eligibility criteria, staff in-service education, equipment and supply monitoring, collection and analysis of outcome data, critical-incident review, and peer chart reviews.

Since early in the history of the birth center movement in this country, a need for national accreditation has been recognized. In 2014, AABC issued a position paper on birth center quality supporting accreditation (AABC, 2014). For a developing birth center, planning for CABC accreditation from the start will provide the blueprint for excellence. In addition to internal quality, accreditation is increasingly required by commercial and governmental payers, and provides a proven mark of excellence for consumers and collaborating providers.

The American Association of Birth Centers Foundation (AABCF) raises funds to support the advancement of the AABC birth center model as the standard to improve maternity and women's health care (AABCF, 2014). The foundation provides grants that assist birth centers with AABC membership, CABC accreditation and scholarships to attend the annual AABC Birth Institute, and the AABC "How to Start a Birth Center" workshop. AABCF also provides research grants for birth centers, fiscal sponsorship for developing birth centers, and projects that fulfill the mission of the foundation (K. Bauer, personal communication, November 20, 2015).

## CONCLUSION

Entrepreneurs need to have a passion to start a birth center, the ability to inspire and empower others, and the planning skills and organizational capabilities to create a new organization. The literature on servant leadership focuses on the well-being of people and their communities rather than the autocratic accumulation of power and wealth (Greenleaf Center for Servant Leadership, 2015). This is a particularly appropriate model of leadership for midwives creating a birth center. Strategic planning and analysis in the process of creating and sustaining a new business can be facilitated using SWOT analysis (strengths, weaknesses, opportunities, and threats) in which the participants acknowledge internal strengths and weaknesses as well as external opportunities and threats (Helms & Nixon, 2010).

The rapidly changing environment of our health care system provides opportunities for midwifery-led innovation. The triple aim of health care reform—improving the client experience, decreasing cost, and improving health (Berwick, Nolan, & Whittington, 2008)—has been demonstrated in the birth center model. The call for disruptive innovation in health care (Christensen,

Bohmer, & Kenagy, 2000) can be met by midwives and their colleagues who recognize the birth center model as a solution to the perinatal quality crisis in the United States (Alliman, Jolles, & Summers, 2015; Romano, 2013).

---

**USING THE EVIDENCE FOR BEST PRACTICE**

**Case Study 15.1 Creating a Birth Center**

Diana, CNM, worked at a hospital-owned collaborative CNM-OB practice in which three CNMs attend about 300 births annually at one of two local hospitals. Diana became a CNM because of her belief in physiologic birth but is now under pressure to medicalize her practice. Jennifer was a CPM in a private home birth practice for two decades who attended about 60 births annually. Jennifer transfers nonemergent clients to a university hospital 45 minutes away because of resistance to home birth by the local OB community. After years as the sole home birth provider, Jennifer was seeking professional camaraderie and greater efficiency in her practice. Diana was aware that the university hospital was planning a new labor, delivery, recovery, and postpartum (LDRP) unit and there was talk that only one of the local hospitals would survive.

Diana and Jennifer are friends. Their clients were asking for a birth center and the two midwives dream of creating a birth center together. Initially, they met with local birth activists and the director of a birth center in the state who encouraged them to study opening a local birth center.

The midwives joined AABC as developing birth center members, and Jennifer used the complimentary registration to go to the "How to Start a Birth Center" workshop. After the workshop, the two midwives wrote a business plan with a projected opening date of 1 to 2 years. Their projected goal was to attend 70 births in the first year. The midwives used the AABC standards and the CABC Attributes for Accreditation to guide their planning.

The two midwives decided to approach Diana's practice group with a request to be collaborating partners. After several meetings with hospital administration and the physicians in Diana's practice, they secured support for collaboration. The hospital realized the future loss of a few births to the birth center, but the gain of referrals and transfers from the birth center. The hospital was happy about the marketing edge this would provide and hoped it would ensure their survival.

With collaboration in place, Jennifer and Diana went public with their plans, following a sequence of steps in creating their birth center:

- They signed a 3-year lease on a 1,800-square-foot residential house 3 miles from the hospital and renovated it to provide two birth rooms and two exam rooms. A third room would be subleased to offset costs.
- They formed a "Friends of the Birth Center" Facebook page to keep connected and created an advisory group, mostly comprising their previous clients, to provide targeted support (lawyer, real estate broker, architect, family physician, public health nurse, doula).
- They incorporated as a for-profit professional corporation and developed a relationship with a local banker. The financial plan involved both Diana and Jennifer contributing savings, obtaining a second mortgage on their two homes, and securing a line of credit. The midwives projected 30% of their

*(continued)*

> **USING THE EVIDENCE FOR BEST PRACTICE (continued)**
>
> clients would be covered by Medicaid and the others by private insurance or cash pay.
> - Jennifer stopped doing home births when they started seeing clients at the birth center to be able to focus full time on administrative and clinical services, whereas Diana continued working half time with her original hospital practice.
> - Starting small, the midwives hired only an office receptionist/manager, and a nurse with responsibility in the office as a birth assistant, a home visitor, and an educator. The midwives chose national billing services familiar with birth centers.
> - The midwives obtained a license from the state, a business license from the city, and scheduled their first site visit from the CABC.
> - The midwives were active on the AABC LISTSERVE, and through the advice of other birth center directors, purchased malpractice and general liability insurance, a practice management software system, and a basic EHR system.
>
> Within 18 months of planning, they opened their doors with extensive coverage by the local press. A year later, they were enrolling 15 women per month for planned birth center births. Diana left her previous practice, and they began discussing hiring another midwife and another nurse.

# REFERENCES

Alliman, J., Jolles, D., & Summers, L. (2015). The innovation imperative: Scaling freestanding birth centers, centering pregnancy and midwifery led-maternity homes. *Journal of Midwifery and Women's Health, 60*(3), 244–249. doi:10.1111/jmwh.12320

American Association of Birth Centers (AABC). (2014). Position statement on birth center quality. Retrieved from http://www.birthcenters.org/news/news.asp?id=229205

American Association of Birth Centers (AABC). (2015a). National standards for birth centers. Retrieved from www.birthcenters.org/?page=Standards

American Association of Birth Centers (AABC). (2015b). How to start a birth center workshop. Retrieved from http://www.birthcenters.org/?page=hsbc_workshops

American Association of Birth Centers (AABC). (2015c). What is the AABC Perinatal Data Registry™? Retrieved from http://www.birthcenters.org/?PDR

American Association of Birth Centers Foundation (AABCF). (2014). Homepage. Retrieved from http://www.aabcfoundation.org

American College of Obstetricians and Gynecologists (ACOG). (2015). Levels of maternity care: ACOG/SMFM obstetric care consensus. Retrieved from http://www.acog.org/Resources-And-Publications/Obstetric-Care-Consensus-Series/Levels-of-Maternal-Care

Berwick, D. M., Nolan, T. W., & Whittington, J. (2008). The triple aim: Care, health and cost. *Health Affairs, 27*(3), 759–769. doi:10.1377/hlthaff.27.3.759

Brocklehurst, P., Hardy, P., Hollowell, J., Linsell, L. Macfarlane, A., McCourt, C., . . . Stewart, M. (2011). Perinatal and maternal outcomes by planned place of birth for healthy women with low risk pregnancies: The Birthplace in England national prospective cohort study. *British Medical Journal, 343*(7840), d7400. doi:10.1136/bmj.d7400

Centers for Medicare & Medicaid Services (CMS). (2015). Physician fee schedule look-up tool. Retrieved from https://www.cms.gov/Medicare/Medicare-Fee-for-Service-Payment/PFSLookup/index.html?redirect=/pfslookup

Childbirth Connection. (2015). 2020 Vision for a high-quality, high-value maternity care system. Retrieved from http://transform.childbirthconnection.org/vision

Christensen, C. M., Bohmer, R., & Kenagy, K. (2000). Will disruptive innovation cure health care? *Harvard Business Review, 78*(5), 102–112.

Commission for the Accreditation of Birth Centers (CABC). (2015a). The CABC indicators for compliance with standards for birth centers, reference edition 1.0. Retrieved from https://www.birthcenteraccreditation.org/go/get-cabc-indicators

Commission for the Accreditation of Birth Centers (CABC). (2015b). Accredited birth centers. Retrieved from https://www.birthcenteraccreditation.org/find-accredited-birth-centers

Declercq, E. R, Sakala, C., Corry, M. P., Applebaum, S., & Herrlich, A. (2013). Listening to Mothers III: New mothers speak out. Retrieved from Childbirth Connection website: http://transform.childbirthconnection.org/wp-content/uploads/2013/06/LTM-III_NMSO.pdf

Ernst, E., & Stone, S. (2013). The birth center: Innovation in evidence-based maternity care. In B. A. Anderson & S. E. Stone (Eds.). *Best practices in midwifery: Using the evidence to implement change.* New York, NY: Springer Publishing Company.

Fahy, K., Foureur, M., & Hastie, C. (2008). *Birth territory and midwifery guardianship: Theory for practice, education and research.* Sydney, Australia: Elsevier.

Frakes, M., & Harrison, T. (2010). Measure your entrepreneurial instinct. Retrieved from Forbes website: http://www.forbes.com/2010/08/02/entrepreneurs-personality-quiz-methodology -thomas-harrison-entrepreneurs-management-serial-startups-10.html

Greenleaf Center for Servant Leadership. (2015). What is servant leadership? Retrieved from https://www.greenleaf.org/what-is-servant-leadership

Helms, M. M., & Nixon, J. (2010). Exploring SWOT analysis—Where are we now?: A review of academic research from the last decade. *Journal of Strategy and Management, 3*(3), 215–251. doi:10.1108/17554251011064837

Hodnett, E. D., Downe, S., & Walsh, D. (2012). Alternative versus conventional institutional settings for birth. *Cochrane Database of Systematic Reviews, 2012*(8). doi:10.1002/14651858 .CD000012.pub4

Institute of Medicine (IOM). (2013). An update on research issues in the assessment of birth settings—Workshop summary. Retrieved from http://iom.nationalacademies.org/Reports/2013/An-Update-on-Research-Issues-in-the-Assessment-of-Birth-Settings.aspx

Martin, J. A., Hamilton, B. E., Osterman, M. J., Curtin, S. C., & Matthews, T. J. M. (2015). Births: Final data for 2013. *National Vital Statistics Reports, 64*(1), 1–65.

McCourt, C., Rance, S., Rayment, J., & Sandall, J. (2011). Birthplace qualitative organisational case studies: How maternity care systems may affect the provision of care in different birth settings (Birthplace in England research programme. Final report part 6). Retrieved from http://www.nets.nihr.ac.uk/__data/assets/pdf_file/0008/84950/FR6-08 -1604-140.pdf

National Conference of State Legislatures (NCSL). (2015). Certificate of need: State health laws and programs. Retrieved from http://www.ncsl.org/research/health/con-certificate-of-need -state-laws.aspx

Romano, A. (2013). New opportunities for birth centers in a transforming health care system. *Journal of Midwifery & Women's Health, 58*(5), 492–493. doi:10.1111/jmwh.12095

Romano, A. (2015, April). Why invest in maternity care innovation? Retrieved from http://maternityneighborhood.com/whitepapers/why-invest-in-maternity-care-innovation

Sakala, C., & Corry, M. P. (2008). Evidence-based maternity care: What is it and what can it achieve. Retrieved from http://www.milbank.org/uploads/documents/0809MaternityCare/0809MaternityCare.html

Stapleton, S., Osborne, C., & Illuzi, J. (2013). Outcomes of care in birth centers: Demonstration of a durable model. *Journal of Midwifery and Women's Health, 58*(1), 3–14. doi:10.1111/jmwh.12003

Thomas, J., Paranjothy, S., & James, D. (2004). National cross-sectional survey to determine whether the decision to delivery interval is critical in emergency caesarean. *British Medical Journal, 328*(7441), 665. doi:http://dx.doi.org/10.1136/bmj.38031.775845.7C

U.S. Department of Health and Human Services, Health Resources and Services Administration. (2015). Quality improvement tools & resources. Retrieved from http://www.hrsa.gov/quality/toolsresources.html

Walsh, D., & Gutteridge, K. (2011). Using the birth environment to increase women's potential in labour. *MIDIRS Midwifery Digest, 21*(2), 143–147.

# CHAPTER SIXTEEN

# HOME AS THE PLACE OF BIRTH: THE EVIDENCE FOR SAFETY

Judith P. Rooks and Suzan Ulrich

The Cochrane Collaboration is an independent international network of researchers and health professionals dedicated to using the best possible evidence as the basis for evaluating health care. In 2012, Cochrane published a report on the benefits and harms of planned hospital births compared with planned home births for low-risk women (Olsen & Clausen, 2012). Although there have been virtually no randomized controlled trials (RCTs) to compare outcomes of planned hospital births versus planned home births for low-risk pregnant women, the quality of observational study evidence in favor of home birth has been steadily increasing. Nevertheless, nothing but a randomized trial can overcome bias caused by self-selection of women who choose home births and selection by midwives who, prioritizing safety, must limit out-of-hospital (OOH) births to low-risk women. This chapter summarizes the best available evidence to compare the safety, risks, and benefits of planned home births with the safety, risks, and benefits of births planned to occur in hospitals. It is limited to findings from studies of home births attended by midwives in developed countries during or after 2000 and published in English.

Birthplace is a profoundly important aspect of the childbirth experience for both women and midwives. Midwifery care provided during home births is different from midwifery care during births in hospitals. A mother's home is *her domain*; she is used to making major decisions in her own home. In contrast, hospitals are the domain of health providers who attend births in hospitals. That difference changes the relationship between a midwife and a laboring woman during home births compared with births in hospitals. No matter how committed a midwife is to serving the mother, a midwife attending hospital births works within the hospital's culture and must follow its rules. Using intermittent auscultation (IA) to monitor the fetal heart rate (FHR) instead of an electronic fetal monitor that produces a paper record is a very demanding work. The midwife must listen intensely while focusing her attention on any audible change in the rate over a period of time or intervals during and after contractions throughout labor (American College of Nurse-Midwives [ACNM], 2015). Midwives attending home births also lack quick, easy access to additional equipment, advice, and professional assistance in case of an emergency, including direct care provided by a physician and a cesarean birth, if needed.

## HOME BIRTH IN THE UNITED STATES

Following a gradual decrease over the course of five decades, after 1990 the percentage of OOH births in the United States began to increase: from 0.87% of all births in 2004 to 1.4% in 2013 (MacDorman, Mathews, & Declercq, 2014; Martin, Hamilton, Osterman, Curtin, & Matthews, 2015). Nearly two thirds of all OOH births in 2013 were home births; 30% were in birth centers. The increasing proportion of OOH births in the United States is entirely due to non-Hispanic White women, who began to have more OOH births in 1994, whereas OOH births were declining among all other major racial and ethnic groups of American women. Non-Hispanic White women accounted for more than 80% of all OOH births in the United States in 2013, when slightly more than 2% of their births were OOH. In comparison, only 0.5% of births to both non-Hispanic Black women and Hispanic women were OOH (Martin et al., 2015).

### Who Attends Home Births in the United States?

Midwives attended two thirds of all home births in the United States in 2013, including 71% of those by non-Hispanic White women, 54% of those by Hispanic women, and 24% of those by non-Hispanic Black women. Physicians attended less than 4% of all home births, but 17% of those were home births by non-Hispanic Black women (Martin et al., 2015). Certified nurse-midwives (CNMs) attended 23% of all home births, a third of all home births attended by midwives. Other midwives attended 44% of all home births and two thirds of those attended by midwives. Someone else attended 27% of all home births (Martin et al., 2015). Naturopaths attended 14% of all home births in Oregon in 2014 (Oregon Health Authority, 2015).

### How Are They Educated?

As described in Chapter 1, CNMs and certified midwives (CMs) in the United States meet the educational standards of the International Confederation of Midwives (ICM) and are certified by the American Midwifery Certification Board. They can practice in hospitals, birth centers, or home settings (see Chapter 1). Direct-entry midwives, who attend a large proportion of home births, have no degree requirements and most learn midwifery skills through apprenticeship and self-study. As of December 2015, direct-entry midwives were legally authorized to practice in 28 states in the United States (Midwives Alliance of North America, 2015).

Oregon is an exemplar of a state that has many direct-entry midwives. The Oregon Health Licensing Agency (2015) requires certification in cardiopulmonary resuscitation (CPR) for adults and newborns and completion of a specified number of supervised births and management visits. As of 2015, a direct-entry midwife in Oregon must also pass the North American Registry of Midwives (NARM) examination and become a certified professional midwife (CPM; Oregon Health Licensing Agency, 2015). Traditional midwives, also known as community midwives or lay midwives, are neither certified, licensed, nor formally educated. In Oregon, traditional midwives are required by law to provide full disclosure to clients (Oregon Laws, 2015). Naturopathic physicians (naturopaths), who are not medical doctors and do not practice in hospitals, are allowed to attend births in OOH settings in Oregon if they complete four didactic courses at the National College of Naturopathic Medicine, located in Portland, Oregon. Students must make their own arrangements for clinical supervision (National College of Natural Medicine, 2016). As described in Chapter 1, the US MERA (Midwifery Education, Regulation, and Association) coalition is currently working to achieve uniformity in education in line with the standards of the ICM (see Chapter 1).

## The Availability and Accuracy of Data on Outcomes of Planned Home Births in the United States

Lacking national or state health care systems that provide care to all pregnant women in specific jurisdictions, it is impossible to conduct prospective population-based studies of home births in the entire United States or specific states similar to studies that have been conducted in many other countries (Brocklehurst et al., 2011; Davis et al., 2011; de Jonge et al., 2015; Li et al., 2015). Studies based on voluntary participation by midwives do not include all births by midwives and have the potential to be biased because midwives who participate may be different from those who do not.

Important birth outcomes are maternal deaths, fetal deaths during labor, 5-minute Apgar scores, neonatal (NN) seizures, NN deaths, cesarean births, breastfeeding, damage to the mother while giving birth, and her satisfaction with her birth. Most studies of home births in the United States are based on data from birth certificates and NN death reports. An item that asks whether a home birth was planned or accidental was added to the 2003 revision of the U.S. Standard Certificate of Live Birth. Individual states adopted use of the revised form over time. By 2010, that information was available from 27 states, which represented 65% of all home births in the United States (Cheng, Snowden, King, & Caughey, 2013); by 2015, all 50 states and the District of Columbia were using the 2003 revision of the Standard Birth Certificate (Centers for Disease Control and Prevention [CDC], 2014). A study that compared the accuracy of information from selected items on the 2003 birth certificate with data from medical records for a representative sample of births in New York City and Vermont in 2009 found that birth certificate data were more than 90% accurate for almost all items (Dietz et al., 2015).

The U.S. Standard Fetal Death Report did not have an item to distinguish antepartum (AP) fetal deaths *before the onset* of labor from intrapartal (IP) fetal deaths *during* labor until a question that asks whether the fetus died before labor, during labor, or the timing was unknown was added when the form was revised in 2003. By 2014, 41 states, the District of Columbia, and New York City were using the revised fetal death report (MacDorman & Gregory, 2015). However, it is new and the timing-of-fetal-death item is often not completed or is coded as "unknown" in part because the timing of fetal deaths relative to the onset of labor is in fact not known in many cases. Some state-level vital statisticians consider many unknowns to reflect poor quality and do not use the data. As a result, the United States lacks complete and reliable data on fetal deaths during labor for births in hospitals as well as OOH births.

Fetal deaths during labor have long been accepted as an epidemiologic indicator of the quality of care provided during labor (Kiely, Paneth, & Susser, 1985). The United States has inadequate data on fetal deaths, including whether they occurred before or during labor.

## Studies of Home Births in the United States

### Two Studies of Home Births Attended Entirely or Primarily by CPMs

The first study reported prospectively collected data on 5,418 women who expected to give birth at home in 2000 with care provided by 409 CPMs. Ninety-eight percent of the births were in the United States; 2% were in Canada. Participation in the study was mandatory for CPM recertification, so participation was high. The report emphasized that most CPMs are trained through apprenticeship and are not well integrated into the U.S. health care system (Johnson & Daviss, 2005).

Twelve percent of the mothers were transferred to hospitals during labor, half for failure to progress, exhaustion, or need for pain relief. After the births, 1.3% of the mothers and 0.7% of the newborns were transferred to hospitals, usually because of maternal hemorrhage, retained placenta, or respiratory problems of the newborn; more than 3% of the transfers were urgent. Transfers were four times more frequent among nulliparous than parous women, although urgent transfers were only twice as common among nulliparous women. The IP fetal plus NN mortality rate was 1.7/1,000 among women with planned home births who were assessed to be at low risk at the beginning of labor. This figure excluded babies with life-threatening congenital anomalies, and rose to 2.03/1,000 births when high-risk births were included. The high-risk births included planned twin and planned breech births. Thirteen percent of the babies were born under water. Five-minute Apgar scores were less than 7 for 1.3% of the babies; less than 4 for 0.6%. Table 16.1 summarizes data on rates of fetal and NN deaths and low 5-minute Apgar scores found during home birth studies described in this chapter (see Table 16.1). The cesarean birth rate was 3.7%. Ninety percent of the women would choose the same midwife for a future birth; 9% would choose another CPM (Johnson & Daviss, 2005).

**TABLE 16.1** Intrapartum, Neonatal Mortality, and 5-Minute Apgar Scores From Planned Home Birth Studies Discussed in This Chapter

| Country, First Author (Year Published) | Year(s) of Data | Number of Planned Home Births | Deaths/1,000 Nonanomalous Births | | | 5-Minute Apgar Scores (%) | |
| --- | --- | --- | --- | --- | --- | --- | --- |
| | | | Intrapartum (IP) | Neonatal (NN) or Early Neonatal | IP + NN | < 7 | < 4 |
| Canada, Janssen (2009) | 2000 2004 | 2,889 | 0.00 | 0.35 | 0.34 | 0.9 | NA* |
| Canada, Hutton (2009) | 2003 2006 | 6,692 | 0.45 | 0.9 | 1.34 | 0.7 | 0.1 |
| England, Brocklehurst et al. (2011) | 2008 2010 | 16,839 | 0.36 | 0.30 | 0.65 | NA* | NA* |
| Australia, Catling-Paull (2013) | 2005 2010 | 1,807 | NA* | NA* | 1.7 | 0.7 | NA* |
| Netherlands, de Jonge (2015) | 2000 2009 | Nulliparous 198,469 | 0.57 | 0.50 | 1.07 | 0.8 | 0.1 |
| | | Parous 267,526 | 0.33 | 0.28 | 0.61 | 0.3 | 0.06 |
| United States, 98%; Canada, 2%; Johnson and Daviss (2005) | 2000 | 5,418 | 0.92 | 1.11 | 2.03 | 1.3 | 0.6 |
| United States, Cheyney (2014) | 2004 2009 | 16,924 | 1.3 | 0.77 | 2.10 | 1.5 | 0.6 |

*Information not in the study report.

Adapted by Rooks and Ulrich (2015).

The second study was based on prospectively collected data on 16,924 planned home births attended by 432 midwives, 79% of whom were CPMs, from 2004 through 2009 (Cheyney et al., 2014). Twenty-two percent of the mothers were nulliparous; 8% of the parous mothers had a prior cesarean birth. Sixty women were carrying twins, 222 babies were breech. Two percent had chronic or pregnancy-induced hypertension or preeclampsia; 10 women had eclampsia with seizures during labor. Ninety-two percent were full term, 2.5% were preterm (< 1% low birth weight), and 5% were postterm (23% macrosomic). Eleven percent of the mothers were transferred to hospitals during labor; 1.5% of the mothers and 0.9% of the newborns were transferred after the birth. Ninety-four percent of the women had spontaneous vaginal births, 5.2% had cesarean births, and 1.2% had assisted vaginal births. Excluding deaths associated with lethal congenital anomalies, the IP fetal death rate was 1.3/1,000 births, the rate of early neonatal (ENN) deaths was 0.9/1,000, the total NN death rate was 1.3/1,000, and the IP fetal plus ENN death rate was 2.2/1,000. Although the IP fetal death rate was more than three times higher for nulliparous women (2.92/1,000 vs. 0.84 for parous women; $p < .01$), live newborns of women having their first births were not at increased risk. Similarly, although parous women undergoing a trial of labor after cesarean (TOLAC) had an increased rate of IP fetal deaths (2.85/1,000 vs. 0.66/1,000; $p = .05$), they did not have an increased risk of NN deaths. The IP fetal plus NN death rate was 22.67/1,000 for babies in breech presentation compared with 1.75/1,000 for babies presenting vertex.

When births by women with twins, breech presentation, gestational diabetes, or preeclampsia were removed from the data set, the IP fetal death rate was 0.85/1,000 (Cheyney et al., 2014). Nulliparous women had more IP deaths than parous women (2.92/1,000 vs. 0.84/1,000), but no increased risk of NN deaths. Although most of the deaths in Cheyney et al.'s large study of home births occurred during labor attended by direct-entry midwives, the United States lacks routinely collected data on IP fetal deaths during labor.

### Studies Comparing NN Outcomes of Planned Home Versus Planned Hospital Births

Because of the lack of data on IP fetal deaths, studies based on birth certificate and infant mortality data are limited to NN outcomes. A study of all term, singleton live births in the United States during 2008 compared the incidence of NN outcomes associated with long-term neurological impairment among 12,039 planned home births with those of more than two million births in U.S. hospitals (Cheng et al., 2013). The study was based on birth certificate data from the 27 states that had adopted the 2003 revision of the U.S. Standard Certificate of Live Birth, which collects data on whether home births were planned or accidental. Sixty-five percent of all births in the United States in 2008 were included. The data are based on the actual place of birth, not the intended place of birth. The study did not report on NN deaths but focused on 5-minute Apgar scores of less than 4 and NN seizures (as per the American Academy of Pediatrics [AAP]), each of which is associated with hypoxic-ischemic encephalopathy and increased risk of serious long-term neurological impairment.

Those outcomes were reported separately for home births attended by CNMs and those attended by other midwives. Twenty-six percent of the home births were attended by CNMs, 51% by other midwives. Five-minute Apgar scores of less than 4 were significantly more common among planned home births (0.37%) compared with hospital births (0.24%; adjusted odds ratio [aOR] = 1.87; 95% confidence interval [CI; 1.36–2.58]); and the incidence of NN seizures was three times higher, 0.06% compared with 0.02% among hospital births (aOR = 3.08; 95% CI [1.44–6.58]). However, there were no statistically significant differences in the rates of low Apgar scores or NN seizures when home births attended by CNMs were compared to rates for births in hospitals. Women having planned home births had fewer interventions, including induction and augmentation of labor, and operative vaginal births (Cheng et al., 2013).

A study based on birth and infant death files for births from 2000 to 2004 compared NN outcomes of 13,529 home births attended by CNMs and 42,375 home births attended by other midwives with outcomes of more than a million hospital births attended by CNMs (Malloy, 2010). The data were based on the actual place of birth; births by women transferred from homes to hospitals during labor were included with hospital births. The study was limited to term, singleton, vaginal births. Breech presentation was approximately as likely among CNM-attended home births (5.4/1,000) as among births attended by CNMs in hospitals (5.0/1,000). The rate of NN seizures was the same (0.3/1,000 births) for newborns in both settings, but births attended by CNMs at home were almost eight times more likely to have 5-minute Apgar scores of less than 4 (5.5/1,000 for CNM home births vs. 0.7/1,000 CNM births in hospitals), and higher than for home births attended by other midwives (2.3/1,000). However, the incidence of seizures among babies whose home births were attended by other midwives was 1.1/10,00 births, compared with 0.3/1,000 for babies whose home births were attended by CNMs. Low Apgar scores unaccompanied by NN seizures do not predict subtle developmental dysfunction evident at school-entry age (Blackman, 1988). Seizures are a much more ominous sign for significant early and late developmental sequelae (Pisani & Spagnoli, 2015). The NN mortality rate for home births attended by CNMs was 1.0/1,000 compared with 1.8/1,000 for home births attended by other midwives. The NN mortality rate for CNM-attended births in hospitals was 0.5/1,000. Twenty-one percent of NN deaths among home births attended by CNMs were attributed to birth asphyxia, compared with 6% of NN deaths following in-hospital births attended by CNMs (Malloy, 2010).

A series of studies related to home births in the United States was published by Grünebaum et al. in 2013, 2014, and 2015. The first one used birth certificate data on singleton term births with birth weights greater than or equal to 2,500 g to compare the occurrence of 5-minute Apgar scores of 0 and of seizures or serious neurologic dysfunction in more than 12 million physician-attended births in hospitals compared with 67,429 home births attended by midwives in the United States from 2007 to 2010 (Grünebaum et al., 2013). Apgar scores are well reported on birth certificates (DiGiuseppe et al., 2002). Stratified analyses were conducted for babies born to nulliparous and parous women. The relative risk for hospital births attended by physicians was set as 1.00. Babies born at home attended by midwives were more than 10 times more likely to have 5-minute Apgar scores of 0 compared with babies born in hospitals attended by physicians. The rate of 5-minute Apgar scores of 0 among babies born at home to nulliparous women was more than 14 times higher than for nulliparous women giving birth in hospitals. Home births were also associated with an almost fourfold higher rate of NN seizures and/or serious neurologic dysfunction, 0.86/1,000 home births vs. 0.22/1,000 hospital births (Grünebaum et al., 2013). Although the differences in the rates were substantially greater for women having their first babies, the rates were statistically significant regardless of parity. The study did not collect data on NN mortality. The lack of systematically collected data on fetal deaths during labor is presumably why obstetricians who wanted to know how common fetal deaths are during home births resorted to using data on 5-minute Apgar scores of 0 (Grünebaum et al., 2013).

A study published in 2014 by many of the same obstetricians used a linked birth-and-infant-death data set for the United States from 2006 through 2009 (almost 14 million births) to compare NN mortality for singleton, vertex term births with birth weight greater than or equal to 2,500 g and no documented congenital malformations to compare NN mortality for babies born in hospitals compared with home births attended by CNMs (Grünebaum et al., 2014). The NN mortality rate associated with home births attended by all kinds of midwives was nearly four times higher than the rate for births attended by CNMs in hospitals (1.26 NN deaths/1,000 home births attended by midwives vs. 0.32/1,000 for hospital births attended by CNMs or nurse-midwifery students under the supervision of a CNM). The risk difference was nearly sevenfold for first babies born at home (2.19 NN deaths/1,000 home births attended by midwives vs. 0.33/1,000 first births attended by CNMs in hospitals) and for home births attended by midwives at greater than or equal to 41 weeks gestation (1.84 NN deaths/1,000 births for home births vs. 0.27/1,000 for births at 41 weeks attended by CNMs in hospitals; Grünebaum et al., 2014).

A third study by many of the same authors compared risks associated with 736,070 hospital births attended by CNMs, 19,263 home births attended by CNMs, and 36,877 home births attended by other midwives from 2010 through 2012 with the American College of Obstetricians and Gynecologists (ACOG) and the AAP recommendations regarding risk factors and home births (Grünebaum et al., 2015). More than 28% of women having planned home births attended by midwives during those 3 years were at greater than or equal to 41 completed weeks of gestation, 4.4% had a history of prior cesarean birth, 0.74% of the babies were in breech presentation, and 0.64% of the mothers were carrying twins. Each of those risk factors was significantly higher among midwife-attended planned home births than among hospital births attended by CNMs. Vaginal breech births, births by mothers with a prior cesarean birth, and births of twins were significantly more frequent among planned home births attended by midwives other than CNMs and CMs than among home births attended by

CNMs. At least 30% of midwife-attended planned home births did not conform to low risk as defined by ACOG and AAP (ACOG, 2011; Grünebaum et al., 2015; Watterberg, 2013).

## HOME BIRTH IN HIGH-RESOURCE COUNTRIES

Home births attended by midwives are part of state-sponsored health care in many high-resource countries. It is important to note that home births in those high-resource countries are attended by midwives educated to the ICM Global Standards for the Education of Midwives (ICM, 2013). Most of the studies summarized in this section of the chapter compare outcomes of planned home births with outcomes of planned births attended by either midwives or physicians in hospitals. Data on IP fetal and NN mortality, and on low Apgar scores were reported in almost every study, as shown in Table 16.1. Findings related to differences in the frequency of interventions during labor and maternal morbidity related to those interventions are only reported if the frequency of the intervention or morbidity among home-birth mothers was significantly different than the frequency among mothers in the control group. Although most studies reviewed report admission of newborns to neonatal intensive care units (NICUs) as an outcome, that information is not included in summaries of some of these studies. Many variables affect which newborns are admitted to NICUs. Babies born in hospitals that have NICUs may be more likely to be admitted than those born in homes because of proximity (de Jonge et al., 2015). When comparing across birth settings, NICU admission is not an accurate outcome measure for NN morbidity (Wiegerinck, Danhof, Van Kaam, Tamminga, & Mol, 2014).

## Canada

Home births attended by Canadian midwives educated to ICM standards are well integrated into the public-funded maternity care in four of the 10 Canadian provinces. Population-based studies of home births attended by midwives have been conducted in two of those provinces.

### A Study Conducted in Ontario

Hutton, Reitsma, and Kaufman (2009) used the Ontario Ministry of Health's database of midwife-attended births from April 2003 through March 2006 to compare outcomes of 6,692 planned home births with a matched group of hospital births attended by midwives. Midwives attended almost 7% of all births in Ontario during that period. All measures of serious maternal morbidity were lower in the planned home birth group as were rates of all interventions. Women who planned to give birth at home were almost 3% less likely to have a cesarean birth (5.2% vs. 8.1% RR [relative risk]; 95% CI: 0.63 [0.56–0.73]) and less likely to have perineal trauma or blood loss of more than 1,000 mL. IP fetal deaths and NN deaths through 27 days of life were 1.0 per 1,000 births for both the home and hospital birth groups, excluding deaths associated with fetal anomalies. NN morbidity including 5-minute Apgar scores of less than 4, need for resuscitation with cardiac compression, and 4 or more days in intensive care were similar for home and hospital births. The authors concluded that midwives who were integrated into the health care system with good access to emergency services, consultation, and transfer of care provided care that resulted in good outcomes for women planning both home and hospital births (Hutton et al., 2009).

### A Study Conducted in British Columbia

A study in British Columbia compared planned home births attended by midwives with planned hospital births attended by the same midwives and a matched group of women who gave birth with obstetricians in hospitals (Janssen et al., 2009). There were no IP fetal deaths in any of the three groups and one NN death in the home-birth group, a rate of 0.35/1,000 live births for planned home births. The NN mortality rate for the planned hospital births attended by midwives was 0.57/1,000 live births compared to 0.64/1,000 live births for planned hospital births attended by physicians. Differences in the rates were not statistically significant. Babies born at home had less birth trauma, needed less resuscitation, and fewer needed oxygen beyond 24 hours. Women giving birth at home were significantly less likely than those who planned a hospital birth with midwives or physicians to have augmentation of labor, electronic fetal monitoring, assisted vaginal births, cesarean births, perineal lacerations, postpartum hemorrhage, or elevated temperatures. Registered midwives in British Columbia are well educated and are an integral part of the provincial health care system (Janssen et al., 2009).

## England

The Royal College of Obstetricians and Gynaecologists and Royal College of Midwives both support offering place-of-birth options to women with low-risk pregnancies (McNutt, Thornton, Sizer, Curley, & Clarke, 2013; National Institute for Health and Care Excellence [NICE], 2014). About 92% of all births in England in 2007 were in hospital obstetric units, 3% percent were in midwifery units in hospitals, 2.8% were home births, and 2% were in freestanding (out-of-hospital) midwifery units (Brocklehurst et al., 2011).

### The Birthplace in England Study

A prospective cohort study of singleton term births in England from April 2008 through April 2010 compared perinatal and maternal outcomes and interventions during labor for 64,538 women with low-risk pregnancies and 15,236 women with risk factors who were booked to give birth in one of four different settings at the start of care during labor, a total of 79,774 births (Brocklehurst et al., 2011). The four settings included a stratified random sample of 36 hospital obstetrical units (OUs), 97% of all home birth services, 95% of all freestanding midwifery units (FMUs), and 84% of all alongside midwifery units (AMUs), which are midwifery units that are in hospitals but separate from the obstetric unit. Women who planned to give birth at home were of higher parity, older, and more likely to be White, economically advantaged, and understand English well compared with women choosing to give birth in OUs. Women choosing home births were also much less likely to be nulliparous (27%), compared with 46% of women laboring in FMUs, 50% of women laboring in AMUs, and 54% of those giving birth in an OU (Brocklehurst et al., 2011).

The primary outcome was a composite of perinatal mortality and specific NN morbidities designed to capture outcomes that may be related to the quality of IP care, including those associated with IP asphyxia and birth trauma. The individual components, "events" that comprised the primary outcome included IP fetal death after the start of care during labor, ENN death, NN encephalopathy, meconium aspiration syndrome, brachial plexus injury, fractured humerus, and fractured clavicle. There were 250 primary outcome events, an overall incidence of 4.3/1,000 births. IP fetal NN encephalopathy accounted for 46%; meconium aspiration syndrome for 30%. The outcomes for the fetus or newborn were determined by the number of noted "events," that is, components of the primary outcome per 1,000 births (Brocklehurst et al., 2011).

Almost 20% of women who planned to give birth in an OU had one or more complicating conditions when they were admitted for care during labor; 2.5% had two or more complications. Only 5% of women initiating care for home births had complicating conditions at the onset of labor, and only 0.3% had two or more complications. When the incidence of primary outcome events for all home births was compared to that for all obstetric unit births, there was virtually no difference. When women with complicating conditions noted at the start of care in labor were excluded from the analysis, home births were associated with a significantly higher rate of primary outcome events (4.0/1,000 births) compared with 3.1 for obstetric unit births (aOR = 1.59; 95% CI [1.01–2.52]; Brocklehurst et al., 2011).

The incidence of primary outcome events was higher for babies of nulliparous women having home births (9.3 primary outcome events/1,000) compared with 5.3/1,000 for babies of nulliparous women giving birth in hospital obstetric units (aOR = 1.75; 95% CI [1.07–2.86]). When women with complicating conditions noted at the start of labor were excluded from the analysis, the incidence of primary outcome events for babies of nulliparous home birth mothers was 9.5/1,000 births compared with 3.5/1,000 for nulliparous births in obstetric units (aOR = 2.80; 95% CI [1.59–4.92]). There were no statistically significant differences in the incidence of primary outcome events between OU births and home births by parous mothers (Brocklehurst et al., 2011).

Ninety-three percent of home-birth mothers had spontaneous vaginal births, compared with 74% of births planned to occur in obstetric units. The cesarean birth rate for home births (2.8% vs. 11.1% for OU births) and rates of vacuum-assisted birth (2.0% vs. 8.1%), forceps-assisted birth (2.1% vs. 6.8%), and third- or fourth-degree perineal trauma (1.9% vs. 3.2%) were all significantly lower for home-birth mothers. Normal births were defined as births without induction of labor, epidural or spinal analgesia, general anesthesia, forceps or vacuum-assisted birth, cesarean birth, or episiotomy. Eighty-eight percent of home-birth mothers had normal births compared with 58% of births in obstetric units, 83% of births in FMUs, and 76% of births in AMUs (Brocklehurst et al., 2011).

The authors concluded that the study results support a policy of offering healthy women with low-risk pregnancies a choice of birth settings. Women planning births in midwifery units that are separate from an OU and parous women planning home births experience fewer interventions than those who labor and give birth in the OU with no impact on perinatal outcomes. Nulliparous women having planned home births also have fewer interventions, but had poorer perinatal outcomes (Brocklehurst et al., 2011).

### Secondary Analysis of Data on High-Risk Births

After the main paper was published by Brocklehurst and colleagues in 2011, a secondary analysis of the data on 8,180 "higher risk" women in the Birthplace in England cohort was conducted to compare outcomes of births by higher risk women having hospital obstetric unit births with those of higher risk women having planned home births (Li et al., 2015). Higher risk women included those with postterm pregnancies or specific medical or obstetric risk factors known before the onset of labor. In nulliparous women, body mass index (BMI) of more than 35 kg/m$^2$ was a common risk factor in both settings; and postterm pregnancy was more common among planned home births. Among parous women, common risk factors in both settings included BMI greater than 35 kg/m$^2$, previous cesarean birth, postterm pregnancy, and known carriage of group B streptococcus (GBS). BMI greater than 35 kg/m$^2$ and postterm pregnancy were more common in planned home births.

Among higher risk women, planned home births were associated with a significantly reduced risk of IP-related mortality and morbidity or NN admission within 48 hours of birth for a hospitalization of greater than 48 hours (adjusted [aRR] = 0.50; 95% CI [0.31–0.81]). The difference was the result of a high rate of NICU admissions for babies born in hospitals, which has been observed in many studies that compare out-of-hospital births with births in hospitals, perhaps because it is much easier to admit a newborn to an NICU if the baby was born in a hospital with an NICU. When the measure of poor perinatal outcome was restricted to IP-related mortality and morbidity, the direction of the effect was reversed, with a higher proportion of adverse outcomes associated with planned home births by higher risk women, although the difference in risk was not statistically significant (Li et al., 2015).

In planned home births, the risk of a poor perinatal outcome was significantly higher among the higher risk women than in low-risk women (aRR = 1.89; 95% CI [1.23–2.90]). Adjusted relative risks did not differ significantly by parity. The authors questioned why higher risk women choose home births, positing that many may be motivated by a desire to avoid interventions during birth. Because many hospital midwifery units exclude women with risk factors, home births may be the only option for some higher risk women who want to avoid excessive interventions. Obstetric intervention rates were lower in higher risk women who planned home births compared with those who gave birth in the hospital OU (Li et al., 2015).

Overall, the risk of experiencing the main composite perinatal outcome in the home-birth group was significantly higher for women with risk factors compared with women at low risk (RR = 1.89; 95% CI [1.23–2.90]) and did not differ by parity. Higher risk women giving birth at home had significantly fewer obstetrical interventions and more vaginal births than higher risk women giving birth in obstetric units (Li et al., 2015).

## Japan

Japan's planned out-of-hospital birth rate of 1.1% in 2010 included births in both birth centers and homes. Independent midwives, who complete nursing school followed by formal midwifery education, based upon ICM standards, are well integrated into the health care system and provide care during home births that are supported by communication and cooperation between midwives and obstetricians and a secure transfer system (Kataoka, Eto, & Iida, 2013).

Two small retrospective cohort studies found similar outcomes of planned home births compared with hospital births attended by Japanese midwives (Hiraizumi & Suzuki, 2013; Kataoka et al., 2013). A study that compared outcomes of 168 home births attended by six independent midwives with 123 hospital births attended by midwives found no difference between the outcomes of the two groups except for more transfers to shared obstetric–midwifery care among the hospital births (34% vs. 21%, $p = .01$) including twice as many transfers for postpartum hemorrhage (11% vs. 5.4%, $p = .032$). The six independent midwives who cared for all the women in both birth settings adhered to strict exclusion criteria (Hiraizumi & Suzuki, 2013).

Kataoka et al. (2013) found similar results when they examined data on 5,477 home and birth-center births conducted by 19 of the 43 independent midwives in Tokyo from 2001 to 2006 (Kataoka et al., 2013). Nine midwives cared for 882 women who gave birth at home, whereas 10 midwives provided care to 4,592 women who gave birth in a birth center. Thirty-one percent of nulliparous women selected a birth center; 20% selected a home birth. Perinatal outcomes for the birth center and home-birth groups were similar, with fewer than 0.5% Apgar scores of less than 7 at 5 minutes for both nulliparous and parous mothers. The incidence of postpartum blood loss greater than 500 mL was significantly higher for both nulliparous and parous women who gave birth in birth centers than for those who gave birth at home. Among parous mothers, blood loss greater than 1,000 mL was also more frequent in birth centers than at home (4.2% vs. 2.4%; RR = 1.75; 95% CI [1.04–2.82]; Kataoka et al. 2013). Authors of both studies concluded that risk assessment with strict criteria for women eligible for midwifery home births and integration of independent midwives into overall maternity care contributed to the good outcomes (Hiraizumi & Suzuki, 2013; Kataoka et al., 2013).

## The Netherlands

Twenty percent of all births in the Netherlands were home births in 2010. Midwives in the Netherlands also provided care for low-risk women in midwifery units in hospitals. Well-integrated home-birth services and short transfer distances support home births (de Jonge et al., 2015). A national cohort study of women with low-risk pregnancies at the onset of labor from 2000 through 2009 compared outcomes of 466,041 planned home births with those of 276,958 planned hospital births (de Jonge et al., 2015).

Somewhat like the Birthplace in England study's use of a composite outcome, this important Dutch study created a severe adverse perinatal outcome that includes IP and NN death and admission to an NN intensive care unit within 28 days of birth. All of the women had spontaneous onset of labor at 37 to 42 weeks gestation. The IP plus fetal and NN death rates, 5-minute Apgar scores of less than 7, and NICU admissions were compared separately for births by nulliparous and parous women. ORs were adjusted for factors known to affect planned place of birth and perinatal outcomes, including gestational age, maternal age, ethnic background, and socioeconomic status (de Jonge et al., 2015).

There were no significant differences between the IP fetal plus NN death rates per 1,000 births up to 28 days for planned home births compared with planned hospital births for either nulliparous or parous women. Home births were associated with fewer 5-minute Apgar scores of less than 7 for babies of parous mothers compared with planned hospital births (aOR = 0.77; 95% CI [0.69–0.86]), but no significant difference for babies of nulliparous women. There were no significant differences based on planned place of birth for 5-minute Apgar scores of less than 4 or NICU admission within 7 days. Home births were associated with a significantly lower incidence of NICU admission within 28 days for babies of parous women (aOR 79; 95% CI [0.66–0.93]), but there was no significant difference for babies of nulliparous women. The study found no increased risk of adverse outcomes for planned home births among low-risk women. The authors noted that their results may only apply to regions where home births are well integrated into the maternity care system (de Jonge et al., 2015).

## Australia and New Zealand

### Australia

Although 80% of births in Australia are attended by midwives (Miller & Skinner, 2012), home birth is not endorsed by the Royal Australian and New Zealand College of Obstetricians and Gynaecologists; and home births accounted for less than 1% of all births in Australia in 2010 (Catling-Paull, Coddington, Foureur, & Homer, 2013). In a study of 1,807 planned home births from 2005 through 2010 (97% of all publicly funded home births in the country), 15 births (1% of the births) occurred before the midwife arrived at the mother's home, 16% of the mothers were transferred to hospitals during labor, 84% gave birth at home, and 1.6% of the mothers or babies were transferred to hospitals after the birth. More than 90% were normal vaginal births, 5.4% were cesarean births, and 0.6% were vaginal breech births. Fifty-six percent of the mothers had intact perinea, 34% had first- or second-degree perineal lacerations, 2.6% had episiotomies; 1.1% had third- or fourth-degree lacerations. Nearly three fourths of the women had expectant management of the third stage of labor; one fourth had active management; 2% had postpartum hemorrhage. There were two IP fetal deaths and four ENN deaths: three were the result of previously diagnosed fetal anomalies; all three of those mothers continued with their plan to give birth at home. Excluding deaths resulting from fetal anomalies, the rate of fetal deaths during labor plus ENN deaths was 1.7/1,000 births (Catling-Paull et al., 2013).

### New Zealand

Data on 16,453 births by low-risk women in New Zealand in 2006 and 2007 were used to study the effect of place of birth on the mode of birth and intervention rates among low-risk women (Davis et al., 2011). Four options for place of birth existed for these women: home births, births in primary care units, and in secondary and tertiary hospitals. Primary maternity care units provide in-hospital labor, birth, and immediate postnatal care for low-risk women but do not have on-site obstetric, pediatric, or anesthesia services. In the study, 11% of the women chose home births, 18% chose a primary care unit, 45% chose secondary hospitals, and 25% chose tertiary hospitals. Ninety-five percent of women who chose home births or birth in primary care units had normal vaginal births compared with 85% of those who chose secondary hospitals, and 73% of those who chose tertiary hospitals. The emergency cesarean birth rate was 2.6% for women planning home births, 3.2% for births in primary units, 8.5% for births in secondary hospitals, and 14.9% for births in tertiary hospitals (Davis et al., 2011).

Births in primary care units were used as the reference group for calculating aRRs for mode of birth by planned place of birth. There were no statistically significant differences between home births and births in primary units for vacuum assistance use of forceps or emergency cesareans; but there were highly statistically significant associations between higher use of each of those modes of birth and births in secondary and tertiary hospitals. Home births were significantly associated with decreased use of augmentation of labor, artificial rupture of membranes, pharmacological pain management, episiotomy, and perineal trauma (Davis et al., 2011).

Data on births by 16,210 women who had a documented planned place of birth at the onset of labor in 2006 and 2007, and were low risk for postpartum hemorrhage, were used for a retrospective study of severe postpartum hemorrhage (Davis et al., 2012). There was a significant difference in blood loss of less than 1,000 mL by place of birth. Relative risks were adjusted for maternal age, parity, ethnicity and smoking, augmentation of labor, type of birth, episiotomy, perineal trauma, babies weighing more than 4,000 g, and active versus physiologic third-stage management. Only 1.3% of women experienced severe blood loss; there was no difference by place of birth. There was a twofold relative risk of severe postpartum blood loss for women with active management of third-stage labor regardless of the setting (RR = 2.12; 95% CI [1.39–3.22]). Home birth mothers were least likely to have active third-stage management (26%), compared with 78% of mothers who gave birth in tertiary hospitals. The authors noted that their findings of increased blood loss with active management of third-stage labor contrast with other reports, recommended further study, and stressed the need for care that promotes physiologic birth (Davis et al., 2012).

A small retrospective study of 109 planned home births and 116 planned hospital births by nulliparous women attended by the same 12 experienced midwives from November 2006 through April 2007 found the usual fewer interventions in the home-birth group (Miller & Skinner, 2012). Gestational age at the onset of spontaneous labor and lengths of both the first and second stages of labor were similar for both groups. Twenty percent of women having planned hospital births had assisted or surgical births compared with 4.6% of women planning home births. Women having planned home births who had more than a 2-hour second stage of labor were significantly more likely to achieve a normal birth than women planning hospital births whose second stages were equally long. Active management of third-stage labor was more common in the hospital and was associated with significantly shorter third stages and significantly more postpartum hemorrhage than during home births. Apgar scores, birth weights, need for resuscitation, and NICU admission were similar in both groups, although babies with meconium were more likely to be suctioned (not evidence based) in the planned hospital group. Midwives spent significantly more time with the women during planned hospital births: 10 hours and 8 minutes versus 8 hours and 40 minutes, compared with the home birth group, a surprising finding. The authors concluded that midwives used evidence-based practice to support physiological birth at home but had more difficulty doing so in hospitals, except for management of the third stage of labor (Miller & Skinner, 2012).

## Nordic Countries

There is a strong midwifery tradition in Iceland, Denmark, Norway, and Sweden (Sjöblom, Idvall, & Lindgren, 2014). Home is an accepted option for birth: the percentage of home births ranges from 0.1% in Norway and Sweden to 2.2% in Iceland and Denmark (Halfdansdotter et al., 2015; Sjöblom et al., 2014).

A retrospective cohort study compared 307 planned home births with 921 planned hospital births matched for parity and age in Iceland from 2005 to 2009 (Halfdansdottir, Smarason, Olafsdottir, Hildingsson, & Sveinsdottir, 2015). There were no maternal deaths, stillbirths, or NN deaths. Ninety-four percent of women who had home births and 93% of those who gave birth in hospitals had spontaneous vaginal births. Four percent of the home births and 5% of the hospital births were operative vaginal births. Cesarean birth rates were low regardless of place of birth, 2% for home birth and 3% for births in hospitals. The authors credited one-on-one midwifery support for the high rate of spontaneous vaginal births. Oxytocin augmentation and epidural anesthesia were used more frequently during planned hospital births. The incidence of postpartum blood loss greater than 500 mL was 13% for home births and 20% for hospital births. First stages of labor were longer during hospital births and oxytocin augmentation was used more often, 26% versus 9% for women who had planned to give birth at home. The incidence of 5-minute Apgar scores of less than 7 was the same for both home and hospital births (Halfdansdottir et al., 2015).

## Conclusion

Population-based home-birth studies from high-resource countries with midwives educated to ICM standards generally apply standard low-risk criteria for home births. This criteria integrates home-birth services into the maternity care system. Consistently, these studies find less use of obstetrical interventions for women planning home births than for women planning hospital births with no increase in IP fetal deaths, NN death, or other adverse fetal or NN outcomes (with the possible exception of births by nulliparous women). Findings from these studies support the safety of home births for low-risk women, especially parous women, who desire physiologic birth with support provided by midwives. It is, however, misleading to use data from countries that have these characteristics as proof of the safety of home births in the United States.

Beyond safety, these studies found that women who planned home births are less likely to have many obstetric interventions common in many hospitals as well as fewer complications related to use of interventions. It is not clear, however, how much credit for those benefits should accrue to home births as compared to the women who chose to have them. Although subtle, there are likely to be differences between the women who plan birth at home and those who plan to give birth in hospitals (Hutton et al., 2009). Hutton and colleagues (2009) state that the women who seek midwifery care are self-selected and women who plan home birth may wish to avoid interventions, such as epidural analgesia, thus decreasing the likelihood of further intervention.

## WHY ARE OUTCOMES OF HOME BIRTHS WORSE IN THE UNITED STATES THAN IN OTHER HIGH-RESOURCE COUNTRIES?

The answer to the question posed is twofold. First, home births are not supported by physicians and the medical establishment in the United States, as they are in most other countries. That lack of support probably delays needed transfers to hospitals and works against the safety of home births in general. Second, two thirds of home births in the United States are attended by direct-entry midwives, many of whom have not completed a formal program of midwifery education and are not educated to ICM standards (see Chapter 1).

All midwives who attend home births in other highly resourced countries are educated to ICM standards, and those countries have better outcomes of planned home births. Table 16.1 describes the rates of IP fetal and NN mortality and low Apgar scores for two studies from the United States and five studies from other countries. The two studies from the United States had the highest rates of IP plus NN deaths per 1,000 births and much higher rates of low (< 7) and very low (< 4) 5-minute Apgar scores (see Table 16.1).

There were 36,080 home births in the United States in 2013 (Martin et al., 2015). Two thirds of them were attended by midwives. Only a third of home births attended by midwives were attended by CNMs; two thirds were attended by *other midwives*, including CPMs, less than half of whom have completed a formal midwifery education program (Cheyney et al., 2015). Malloy's study of nearly 56,000 home births in the United States from 2000 to 2004 found an NN mortality rate of 1.0/1,000 associated with home births attended by CNMs, compared with 1.8/1,000 home births attended by *other midwives* (Malloy, 2010). Although the demand for home births is increasing, the United States does not produce enough midwives educated to ICM standards to meet the need (Department of Health and Human Services, Health Resources and Services Administration, 2015).

In the study by Cheyney and colleagues (2014), of 17,000 planned home births in the United States from 2004 through 2009, most of these births were attended by midwives other than CNMs. The IP fetal plus NN death rate was 2.07/1,000 planned home births, almost identical to the rate in the other study of home births attended by CPMs in the United States (Johnson & Daviss, 2005), but higher than the rates reported in studies conducted in Canada, England, the Netherlands, and Australia. Cheyney et al. (2014) estimated that only 20% to 30% of actively practicing CPMs participated in their study, which was probably skewed toward more experienced CPMs, whereas all of the studies from other countries included data on all low-risk births in the countries or provinces where they were conducted. Less than half of 568 CPMs surveyed in 2011 had completed a midwifery education program (Cheyney et al., 2015).

Many high-risk women have home births in the United States, even women known to be carrying twins and babies in breech presentation. Two thirds of the women in the study by Cheyney et al. (2014) were postterm; 8% had previous cesarean births; 6% of the mothers had diabetes, 2% had hypertension, preeclampsia, or eclampsia; 1.3% of the babies presented breech; and there were 60 sets of twins (Cheyney et al., 2014). Informed decision making about the place of birth necessitates an accurate assessment of the woman's risk status. Women attempting a home birth should be truly low risk and have adequate counseling on risk.

Nulliparity is an important risk factor. Nulliparity is associated with five additional adverse NN outcomes per 1,000 planned home births by otherwise low-risk women, and nine adverse NN outcomes per 1,000 babies during home births versus 4/1,000 babies born in hospitals (ACNM, 2015b). Distance and time to reach the closest hospital that is able to initiate a cesarean birth quickly at any time is an important factor. Risk stratification for home births requires clear guidelines to identify women who are at higher risk for a poor outcome, and then advising them that it would be safer to give birth in a hospital. This recommendation does not include all nulliparous women. Conditions that suggest the need for a planned hospital birth include:

- Previous fetal or NN death related to an IP event
- History of previous postpartum hemorrhage, cesarean birth, or shoulder dystocia resulting in injury

- Medical conditions, including hypertension, insulin-dependent diabetes, active infection with hepatitis, HIV, genital herpes, syphilis, or tuberculosis; conditions that required acute medical supervision during pregnancy and could impact the birth; substance abuse or dependence; psychiatric conditions that could affect IP care or maternal or NN care after the birth
- Evidence of a congenital fetal anomaly that will require immediate assessment or management by a neonatologist, or fetal growth restriction
- Preterm labor
- Malpresentation (including breech), need for pharmacological induction of labor, postterm pregnancy, multiple gestations, oligohydramnios with or without other complicating factors, polyhydramnios, third-trimester placenta previa, hypertensive disorders of pregnancy, and Rh isoimmunization (ACNM, 2016)

## BEST PRACTICES FOR MIDWIVES ATTENDING HOME BIRTHS

### Risk Screening

During prenatal care, the midwife should screen out women with high-risk factors, and inform women thinking about or planning for a home birth to consider the possible need for transfer to a hospital, hospital care, and procedures that may be necessary (ACNM, 2016).

### Intermittent Auscultation

Fetal deaths during labor constitute a large part of all deaths during home births. Home-birth-based midwives must be proficient at IA of the FHR. The report by Sholapurkar (2015) points out that many unexpectedly asphyxiated babies have been born despite rigorously performed and documented IA. The author of that article reappraised current standards for IA and concluded that the standards may pose a risk of missing many pathological late FHR decelerations. Although all national standards recommend auscultation of the FHR for 60 seconds after a contraction, this author recommends auscultation just before and after contractions, using the FHR just before the contraction as the baseline, and interpreting the postcontraction FHR in relation to that baseline (Sholapurkar, 2015).

### Clinical Practice Guidelines

Midwives should establish comprehensive home-birth clinical practice guidelines and use them as part of shared decision making between the midwife and a woman considering a home birth as well as between the midwife and a physician, if necessary, to consult during a home birth (ACNM, 2016). The clinical guidelines should include ongoing clinical assessment to inform risk evaluation and clinical decision making, and the need for consultation, collaboration, referral, and transfer to a hospital, if necessary. Access to transportation, and the distance and time to travel from the woman's home to the nearest hospital with continuous access to emergency cesarean birth must be considered. Clear, transparent, ongoing, shared decision making between the midwife and the woman and her family is essential; and the responsibilities of the midwife and the pregnant women should be delineated clearly.

## Responsibilities of the Home-Birth Midwife

### Provision of Care

The midwife is responsible for:

- Providing accurate, evidence-based information to help the woman make informed decisions about her birth site and options for care
- Ongoing vigilance for potential or emergent complications
- Providing necessary equipment and medications
- Offering evidence-based interventions to maintain the health of the woman, fetus, or newborn
- Referring or transferring the woman or newborn to in-hospital care as needed
- Assuring physical presence at the birth of at least two health care professionals with current Neonatal Resuscitation Program (NRP) and CPR training, knowledge, and skills who can assess and implement interventions as needed (ACNM, 2016)

### Education and Collaboration With the Woman Planning a Home Birth

The midwife must also make sure that the pregnant woman understands and fulfills her responsibilities, which include:

- Arranging for personal support persons to support her throughout the pregnancy, labor, birth, and after the birth
- Acknowledging her responsibility for herself and her newborn related to her informed choice of birth site
- Studying and agreeing to the scope of care defined by the midwife's clinical practice guidelines
- Preparing all persons she requests to be present during the labor and birth
- Preparing the birthing environment and obtaining necessary supplies
- Assuring that the midwife and other members of the birth team have access to the home in terms of parking, weather conditions, the neighborhood, and safety
- Committing to open, honest, and clear communication and shared decision making with the midwife (ACNM, 2016)

### Contingency Plans for Transfer

Best practices related to transfer to a hospital include:

- Arranging for seamless consultation, referral, transportation, and transfer of care when necessary

- Informing the woman about hospital care and procedures that may become necessary and working with her to develop a plan for a hospital transfer if needed.
- Notifying the receiving caregiver or hospital of the incoming transfer, the reason for it, a brief clinical history, the planned mode of transport, and expected time of arrival
- Continuing to provide routine or urgent care during the transfer in coordination with any emergency services personnel while addressing the psychosocial needs of the woman
- Providing a verbal report, including details about the woman's or baby's current health status and need for urgent care, and a legible copy of relevant prenatal and labor medical records on arrival at the hospital
- Ensuring that the woman understands the hospital plan of care, and hospital personnel understand the woman's need for information regarding care options
- Offering to stay at the hospital to provide continuity and support to the woman if she wants the midwife to do so (Home Birth Summit, 2013)

This chapter summarizes the best available evidence to compare the safety, risks, and benefits of planned home births with the safety, risks, and benefits of births planned to occur in hospitals. The home-birth midwife needs to be fully informed in order to provide evidence-based care.

# REFERENCES

American College of Nurse-Midwives (ACNM). (2015). Intermittent auscultation for intrapartum fetal heart rate surveillance. *Journal of Midwifery and Women's Health*, 60(5), 626–632. doi:10.1111/jmwh.12372

American College of Nurse Midwives (ACNM). (2016). *Midwifery provision of home birth services* (Clinical Bulletin No. 14), 61(1), 127–133.

American College of Obstetricians and Gynecologists (ACOG). (2011). Planned home birth (Committee Opinion Number 476; reaffirmed 2015). Retrieved from http://www.acog.org/Resources-And-Publications/Committee-Opinions/Committee-on-Obstetric-Practice/Planned-Home-Birth

Blackman, J. A. (1988). The value of Apgar scores in predicting developmental outcome at age five. *Journal of Perinatology*, 8(3), 206–210.

Brocklehurst, P., Hardy, P., Hollowell, J., Linsell, L., Macfarlane, A., McCourt, C., . . . Stewart, M. (2011). Perinatal and maternal outcomes by planned place of birth for healthy women with low risk pregnancies: The Birthplace in England national prospective cohort study. *British Medical Journal*, 343(7840), d7400. doi:10.1136/bmj.d7400

Catling-Paull, C., Coddington, R. L., Foureur, M. J., & Homer, C. S. (2013). Publicly-funded homebirth in Australia: A review of maternal and neonatal outcomes over 6 years. *Medical Journal of Australia*, 198(11), 626–630.

Centers for Disease Control and Prevention (CDC). (2014). The birth certificate (finally) goes national. Retrieved from http://www.cdc.gov/nchs/features/birth_certificate_goes_final.htm

Cheng, Y. W., Snowden, J. M., King, T. L., & Caughey, A. B. (2013). Selected perinatal outcomes associated with planned home births in the United States. *American Journal of Obstetrics and Gynecology, 209*(4), 325.e1–325.e8. doi:10.1016/j.ajog.2013.06.022

Cheyney, M., Bovbjerg, M., Everson, C., Gordon, W., Hannibal, D., & Verdam, S. (2014). Outcomes of care for 16,924 planned home births in the United States: The Midwives Alliance of North America Statistics Project, 2004–2009. *Journal of Midwifery & Women's Health, 59*(1), 17–27. doi:10.1111/jmwh.12172

Cheyney, M., Olsen, C., Bovbjerg, M., Everson, C., Darragh, I., & Potter, B. (2015). Practitioner and practice characteristics of certified professional midwives in the United States: Results of the 2011 North American Registry of Midwives survey. *Journal of Midwifery & Women's Health, 60*(5), 534–45. doi:10.1111/jmwh.12367

Davis, D., Baddock, S., Pairman, S., Hunter, M., Benn, C., Wilson, D., . . . Herbison, P. (2011). Planned place of birth in New Zealand: Does it affect mode of birth and intervention rates among low-risk women? *Birth, 38*(2), 111–119. doi:10.1111/j.1523-536X.2010.00458.x

Davis, D., Baddock, S., Pairman, S., Hunter, M., Benn, C., Wilson, D., . . . Herbison, P. (2012). Risk of severe postpartum hemorrhage in low-risk childbearing women in New Zealand: Exploring the effect of place of birth and comparing third stage management of labor. *Birth, 39*(2), 98–105. doi:10.1111/j.1523-536X.2012.00531.x

de Jonge, A., Geerts, C. C., van der Goes, B. Y., Mol, B. W., Buitendijk, S. E., & Nijhuis, J. G. (2015). Perinatal mortality and morbidity up to 28 days after birth among 743 070 low-risk planned home and hospital births: A cohort study based on three merged national perinatal databases. *British Journal of Obstetrics and Gynaecology, 122*(5), 720–728. doi:10.1111/1471-0528.13084

Department of Health and Human Services, Health Resources and Services Administration. (2015). Sex, race, and ethnic diversity of U.S. health occupations (2010 -2012). Retrieved from http://bhpr.hrsa.gov/healthworkforce/supplydemand/usworkforce/diversityushealth occupations.pdf

Dietz, P., Bombard, J., Mulready-Ward, C., Gauthier, J., Sackoff, J., Brozicevic, P., & Farr, S. (2015). Validation of selected items on the 2003 U.S. standard certificate of live birth: New York City and Vermont. *Public Health Reports, 130*(1), 60–70.

DiGiuseppe, D. L., Aron, D. C., Ranbom, L., Harper, D. L., & Rosenthal, G. E. (2002). Reliability of birth certificate data: A multi-hospital comparison to medical records information. *Maternal and Child Health Journal, 6*(3), 169–179.

Grünebaum, A., McCullough, L. B., Brent, R. L., Arabin, B., Levene, M. I., & Chervenak, F. A. (2015). Perinatal risks of planned home births in the United States. *American Journal of Obstetrics & Gynecololography, 212*(3), 350.e1–350.e6. doi:10.1016/j.ajog.2014.10.021

Grünebaum, A., McCullough, L. B., Sapra, K. J., Brent, R. L., Levene, M. I., Arabin, B., & Chervenak, F. A. (2013). Apgar score of 0 at 5 minutes and neonatal seizures or serious neurologic dysfunction in relation to birth setting. *American Journal of Obstetrics and Gynecology, 209*(4), 323.e1–323.e6. doi:10.1016/j.ajog.2013.06.025

Grünebaum, A., McCullough, L. B., Sapra, K. J., Brent, R. L., Levene, M. I., Arabin, B., & Chervenak, F. A. (2014). Early and total neonatal mortality in relation to birth setting in the United States, 2006–2009. *American Journal of Obstetrics & Gynecololography, 211*(4), 390. e1–390.e7. doi:10.1016/j.ajog.2014.03.047

Halfdansdottir, B., Smarason, A. K., Olafsdottir, O. A., Hildingsson, I., & Sveinsdottir, H. (2015). Outcome of planned home and hospital births among low-risk women in Iceland in 2005–2009: A retrospective cohort study. *Birth*, 42(1), 16–26. doi:10.1111/birt.12150

Hiraizumi, Y., & Suzuki, S. (2013). Perinatal outcomes of low-risk planned home and hospital births under midwife-led care in Japan. *Journal of Obstetrics and Gynaecology Research*, 39(11), 1500–1504. doi:10.1111/jog.12094

Home Birth Summit. (2013). Best practice guidelines: Transfer from planned home birth to hospital. Retrieved from http://www.homebirthsummit.org/best-practice-transfer-guidelines

Hutton, E. K., Reitsma, A. H., & Kaufman, K. (2009). Outcomes associated with planned home and planned hospital births in low-risk women attended by midwives in Ontario, Canada, 2003–2006: A retrospective cohort study. *Birth*, 36(3), 180–189. doi:10.1111/j.1523-536X .2009.00322.x

International Confederation of Midwives (ICM). (2013). Global standards for midwifery education, with companion guidelines (ICM Core Document 2010, amended 2013). Retrieved from http://www.internationalmidwives.org/assets/uploads/documents/Global%20 Standards%20Comptencies%20Tools/English/MIDWIFERY%20EDUCATION%20 PREFACE%20&%20STANDARDS%20ENG.pdf

Janssen, P. A., Saxell, L., Page, L. A., Klein, M. C., Liston, R. M., & Lee, S. K. (2009). Outcomes of planned home birth with registered midwife versus planned hospital birth with midwife or physician. *Canadian Medical Association Journal*, 181(6–7), 377–383. doi:10.1503/ cmaj.081869

Johnson, K. C., & Daviss, B. A. (2005). Outcomes of planned home births with certified professional midwives: Large prospective study in North America. *British Medical Journal*, 330(7505), 1416. doi:10.1136/bmj.330.7505.1416

Kataoka, Y., Eto, H., & Iida, M. (2013). Outcomes of independent midwifery attended births in birth centres and home births: A retrospective cohort study in Japan. *Midwifery*, 29(8), 965–972.

Kiely, J. L., Paneth, N., & Susser, M. (1985). Fetal death during labor: An epidemiologic indicator of level of obstetric care. *American Journal of Obstetrics and Gynecology*, 153(7), 721–727. doi:10.1016/0002-9378(85)90331-X

Li, Y., Townend, J., Rowe, R., Brocklehurst, P., Knight, M., Linsell, L., . . . Hollowell, J. (2015). Perinatal and maternal outcomes in planned home and obstetric unit births in women at "higher risk" of complications: Secondary analysis of the Birthplace national prospective cohort study. *British Journal of Obstetrics and Gynaecology*, 122(5), 741–753. doi:10.1111/1471 -0528.13283

MacDorman, M. F., & Gregory, E. C. (2015). Fetal and perinatal mortality: United States, 2013. *National Vital Statistics Reports*, 64(8), 1–24.

MacDorman, M. F., Mathews, T. J., & Declercq, E. (2014). Trends in out-of-hospital births in the United States, 1990–2012. *NCHS Data Brief*, 2014(144), 1–8.

Malloy, M. H. (2010). Infant outcomes of certified nurse midwife attended home births: United States 2000 to 2004. *Journal of Perinatology*, 30(9), 622–627. doi:10.1038/jp.2010.12

Martin, J. A., Hamilton, B. E., Osterman, M. H. Curtin, S., & Matthews, M. S. (2015). Births: Final data for 2013. *National Vital Statistics Reports*, 64(1), 1–68. Retrieved from http:// www.cdc.gov/nchs/data/nvsr/nvsr64/nvsr64_01.pdf

McNutt, A., Thornton, T., Sizer, P., Curley, A., & Clarke, P. (2014). Opinions of UK perinatal health care professionals on home birth. *Midwifery, 30*(7), 839–846. doi:10.1016/j.midw .2013.08.007

Midwives Alliance of North America. (2015). Legal status of U.S. midwives. Retrieved from http://mana.org/about-midwives/legal-status-of-us-midwives

Miller, S., & Skinner, J. (2012). Are first-time mothers who plan home birth more likely to receive evidence based care? A comparative study of home and hospital care provided by the same midwives. *Birth, 39*(2), 135–144. doi:10.1111/j.1523-536X.2012.00534.x

National College of Natural Medicine. (2016). Course curricula. Retrieved from http://admissions .ncnm.edu/academics/course-curricula

National Institute for Health and Care Excellence (NICE). (2014). Intrapartum care: Care of healthy women and their babies during childbirth. Retrieved from http://www.nice.org.uk/ guidance/cg190/chapter/1-recommendations

North American Registry of Midwives (NARM). (2016). Written exam questions and scoring. Retrieved from http://narm.org/testing/written-exam-questions-and-scoring

Olsen, O., & Clausen, J. A. (2012). Planned hospital birth versus planned home birth. *Cochrane Database Systematic Reviews, 2012*(9). doi:10.1002/14651858.CD000352.pub2

Oregon Health Authority. (2015). Oregon vital statistics annual report: Planned attendant by planned place of birth, Oregon occurrence, 2014 (Table 2–28). Retrieved from https://public .health.oregon.gov/BirthDeathCertificates/VitalStatistics/annualreports/Volume1/Docu ments/2014/Table0238.pdf

Oregon Health Licensing Agency. (2015). Direct entry midwifery legend drugs and devices. Continuing education (renewal). Retrieved from http://www.oregon.gov/OHLA/DEM/docs/ DEM_continuing_education/Education_Curriculum_-_Continuing.pdf

Oregon Laws. (2015). Practice of direct entry midwifery without license prohibited (Vol. 15, §687.415). Retrieved from http://www.oregonlaws.org/ors/687.415

Pisani, F., & Spagnoli, C. (2015). Neonatal seizures: A review of outcomes and outcome pre-dictors. *Neuropediatrics.* Advance online publication. doi:10.1055/s-0035-1567873

Sholapurkar, S. L. (2015). Intermittent auscultation in labor: Could it be missing many path-ological (late) fetal heart rate decelerations? Analytical review and rationale for improve-ment supported by clinical cases. *Journal of Clinical and Medical Research, 7*(12), 919–925. doi:10.14740/jocmr2298w

Sjöblom, I., Idvall, E., & Lindgren, H. (2014). Creating a safe haven: Women's experiences of the midwife's professional skills during planned home birth in four Nordic countries. *Birth, 41*(1), 100–107. doi:10.1111/birt.12092

Watterberg, K. L. (2013). Policy statement on planned home birth: Upholding the best inter-ests of children and families. *Pediatrics, 132*(5), 924–926. doi:10.1542/peds.2013-2596

Wiegerinck, M. M., Danhof, N. A., Van Kaam, A. H., Tamminga, P., & Mol, B. W. (2014). The validity of the variable "NICU admission" as an outcome measure for neonatal morbidity: A retrospective study. *Acta Obstetricia et Gynecologica Scandinavica, 93*(6), 603–609. doi:10.1111/aogs.12384

# THE INTRAPARTAL PERIOD: USING THE EVIDENCE

Rebeca Barroso

*The place of birth is the mother's sacred space: a vulnerable place that the midwife strives to protect. Section III, "The Intrapartal Period: Using the Evidence," examines best practices in protecting the mother and infant. This section identifies critical issues in midwifery attendance of women in labor and birth. Chapter 17 addresses therapeutic presence and labor support, defining elements of midwifery care. Chapter 18 questions prevailing practices in maternity care in view of the need to advance physiologic birth as a best practice. Chapters 19 and 20 evaluate the responsibilities of the midwife in educating women and fostering informed choice about vaginal birth after cesarean (VBAC), elective induction of labor, and cesarean birth on maternal request. Chapters 21, 22, and 23 bring management controversies to the fore: Chapter 21 considers the evidence supporting "watchful waiting" (vs. induction of labor) with prelabor rupture of membranes at term; Chapter 22 describes the role of the midwife as a catalyst for change with hydrotherapy guidelines; and Chapter 23 addresses the efficacy of nitrous oxide use during labor and birth. Last, Chapter 24 reminds the reader that the midwife has always been the guardian, entrusted to "save (maternal) blood" through astute clinical management of the third and most dangerous stage of bringing forth new life.*

# CHAPTER SEVENTEEN

# THERAPEUTIC PRESENCE AND CONTINUOUS LABOR SUPPORT: HALLMARKS OF MIDWIFERY

Robin G. Jordan

## WOMAN-CENTERED CHILDBIRTH

Childbearing is a major transformative life event that is both physically and emotionally demanding. The emotional processes that start during pregnancy and continue during the childbearing event have a major impact on the evolving mother–child relationship (Buckley, 2015; Wiklund, Edman, Larsson, & Andolf, 2009). A woman-centered approach to childbirth services acknowledges and attends to the psychological and social components of childbearing. Attention to these components during labor and birth is essential to a woman's perception of mastery and satisfaction with this pivotal life experience. Research findings have repeatedly documented that attending to a woman's psychological and social needs via therapeutic presence and continuous labor support improves maternal and infant health outcomes (Gruber, Cupito, & Dobson, 2013; Hodnett, Gates, Hofmeyr, & Sakala, 2013; Kozhimannil, Hardeman, Attanasio, Blauer-Peterson, & O'Brien, 2013).

One of the defining hallmarks of midwifery practice within the philosophy of care of the American College of Nurse-Midwives (ACNM; 2012) is the therapeutic value of human presence. Therapeutic presence is a human-to-human interaction that embodies caring behaviors and a supportive demeanor to help others in need (Burgess, 2014; Folkman & Lazarus, 1988; Hodnett, 2002). Labor support embodies therapeutic presence (Amran et al., 2014; Barrett & Stark, 2010; Sauls, 2004) and is an intentional tool provided to laboring women to improve outcomes (Green & Hotelling, 2014). Current mainstream obstetrical practice often substitutes technology for physical and emotional care. In hospital birth settings, it is common for continuous labor support to be overshadowed by the focus on the biomechanics of labor and birth and its attendant technology (Deveraux & Sullivan, 2013; Hayes, 2010; McDonald, 2013). In most hospital settings, labor support is considered less important than the management of the biomechanics of birth. For example, use of continuous or near-continuous electronic fetal monitoring is accepted as the established norm within the hospital labor and birth setting despite recommendations for intermittent auscultation and years of evidence citing inconclusive usefulness (James, 2011; Riffle, 2014; Smith, Begley, Clarke, & Devane, 2012). The presence of a labor and birth support person is commonly viewed as a nice amenity rather than an essential evidence-based intervention to improve outcomes (Jansen, Gibson, Bowles, & Leach, 2013). Substituting routine application of technology in place of human support during physiologic birth has created high rates of medical intervention with adverse effects (Hotelling, 2007; McDonald, 2013; Rossignol, Chaillet, Bourghrassa, & Moutquin, 2014).

## Therapeutic Presence and Continuous Labor Support

Therapeutic presence includes three elements:

- Emotional support, including physical presence, encouragement, reassurance, and providing a sense of security
- Tangible assistance, including direct care and comfort measures
- Knowledge support, including explanation, advice, and information (Amran et al., 2014; Burgess, 2014; Folkman & Lazarus, 1988; Hodnett, 2002; Hodnett et al., 2013)

Lehrman (1988) developed a theoretical framework to describe relationships among midwifery care, psychosocial outcomes, and maternal psychosocial variables. Through her work, a construct for the concept of therapeutic presence was developed and summarized as "one on one personal attention and availability of the nurse-midwife for the woman in labor" (p. 44). Lehrman's research demonstrated that positive therapeutic presence by midwives increases a woman's self-esteem and satisfaction with the labor experience.

Labor support is the work of personal caring and sustaining behaviors provided to the laboring woman, and encompasses the dimensions of therapeutic presence. Continuous labor support is the third of six practices advocated to support normal birth as endorsed by Lamaze International (2016). These specific behaviors of labor support can be categorized into three areas that encompass the elements of therapeutic presence: emotional support, physical care and comfort, and advocacy for the laboring woman (Amran et al., 2014; Barrett & Stark, 2010; Lothian, 2014; Ross-Davie & Cheyne, 2014; Sauls, 2004).

*Emotional support behaviors* are defined as continuous human presence; exhibiting a caring attitude; providing reassurance, verbal support, and encouragement; attending to spiritual aspects of the experience; and providing care to the laboring woman's partner (Adams & Bianchi, 2008; Amran et al., 2014; Burgess, 2014; Ross-Davie & Cheyne, 2014). Verbal encouragement that fosters a sense of ability to cope with the challenge of labor pain enhances the woman's ability to overcome fears and self-doubt about coping, and leads to feelings of pride, elation, and empowerment after birth (Leap, Sandall, Buckland, & Huber, 2010).

Physical care behaviors are directed toward providing comfort during labor and birth. These specific behaviors include: repositioning and enhancing the woman's mobility; using therapeutic touch, massage, cold or hot compresses; providing warm-water therapy via tub or shower; facilitating fluid intake or other nourishment; helping the woman maintain an empty bladder; and modifying the environment by diminishing lighting and noise levels (McDonald, 2013; Payant, Davies, Graham, Peterson, & Clinch, 2008). Providing physical care that promotes comfort during labor can enhance a woman's sense of control and confidence in her labor experience (Ross-Davie & Cheyne, 2014; Schuiling & Sampselle, 1999). A woman's perspective of her control and mastery during childbirth has been demonstrated to be a key component in maternal satisfaction with the childbirth experience (Amran et al., 2014; Ford, Ayers, & Wright, 2009; Malacrida & Boulton, 2014).

*Advocacy for the laboring woman* is defined as providing a voice for the woman while she is focusing on the work of labor and protecting her from unwanted and/or unnecessary interventions (Burgess, 2014). Advocacy is achieved by the support person acting as the woman's voice for making her needs known when she has turned inward in performing the work of labor, and protecting her from unnecessary intrusions and interruptions (Deveraux & Sullivan, 2013). When advocating for the laboring woman, the support person must convey respect, acknowledge the mother's expectations, and resolve conflict (Adams & Bianchi, 2008; Amran et al., 2014). A large body of evidence consistently documents benefits of continuous therapeutic labor support among women worldwide and across socioeconomic strata (Hodnett et al., 2013; Steel, Frawley, Adams, & Diezel, 2015). Because continuous labor support is an evidence-based practice to improve maternal and infant outcomes, the question then becomes, Why is this support not the standard of care within all maternity units in U.S. hospitals?

## Barriers

Birth is unlike all other conditions that are dealt with in a hospital setting. Hospital-based birth is largely technology and provider driven (Bergman & Bergman, 2013; James, 2011; Sakala & Corry, 2008). Although there are changes in the direction of women having more positive hospital birth experiences, the hospital is not an environment that generally places the woman at the center of decision making or moves with her intrinsic timing during the labor process (McCourt, 2010; Miller & Schriver, 2012; Simkin, 2014). Because of institutional constraints in the hospital setting, the transfer of research findings validating evidence-based practice is frequently obstructed by multiple barriers unrelated to the defined best practice models (Glenn, Stocker-Schnieder, McCune, McClelland, & King, 2012; Graham, Logan, Davies, & Nimrod, 2004; James, 2011; Simkin, 2014).

### Institutional Barriers

Institutional policies are often directed toward meeting provider needs of efficiency, time management, and rapid outcome. Providers often attempt to control the timing of birth, obstetrical unit workflow, and their discomfort with the sounds of labor (McCourt, 2010; Miller & Schriver, 2012). Although efforts are being made to curtail the practice, elective induction of labor for improved physician lifestyle as well as productivity and reimbursement issues has become a common medical practice in the past two decades (Bonsack, Lathrop, & Blackburn, 2014; Kaplan & Ballard, 2011; Simpson, 2010). Anesthesia informed-consent procedures are inconsistent and department policies may include rounding on each laboring woman, even if uninvited, to offer epidural anesthesia services in order to generate income (Sakala & Corry, 2008; Trumble, Lee, Slater, Sellors, & Cyna, 2015). A dedicated support person providing therapeutic presence and continuous labor support may be viewed as interference in a well-oiled production line (Martin, 2001; McDonald, 2013). Hospital staffing may preclude one-to-one nursing care and support for each laboring woman. Remote monitoring systems allow nurses to observe the labor patterns of multiple women at one time (Anderson, Scerbo, Belfore, & Abuhamad, 2011; Glenn et al., 2012). Remote monitoring is an efficient method to care for several women at once, saving hospital dollars on nursing staff (Williams, Ivey, Benton, & Rhoads, 2010).

Each woman's labor is an unknown in terms of time, process, and maternal and fetal reaction (Buckley, 2015; Lamaze International, 2016; McCourt, 2010). Physiological variations make staffing needs and length-of-stay times difficult to predict. Hospital practices are often geared toward eliminating uncertainty by controlling labor timing and process (elective induction or cesarean birth) and eliminating unknown reactions from women (epidural anesthesia; Glenn et al., 2010; Levine & Lowe, 2014). This controlled scenario provides an operationally efficient unit, albeit at the expense of an individual woman's physiologic and emotional needs and desires.

### Barriers for Labor Nurses

Young labor nurses and nursing students often lack role models and mentoring in promoting the normalcy of physiologic birth and in advocating for continuous labor support (Jansen et al., 2013). These nurses and nursing students may seldom or never see a birth occur under a woman's own power and may lack skill in labor support (Simkin, 2014; Sleutel, Schultz, & Wyble, 2007). Although older and more experienced nurses are more likely to provide labor support (Barrett & Stark, 2010), they are often expected to do so with minimal guidelines or formal instruction on effective support measures (Curl & Lothian, 2013; Sauls, 2006). Nurses report being unable to provide labor support while caring for more than one woman (Barrett & Stark, 2010) and may perceive that women with epidural analgesia need minimal support (Payant et al., 2008). In addition, nurses may be unaware of the benefits of labor support (Burgess, 2014). As a measure to manage information overload, maternity care curricula in some nursing programs have been modified to cover primarily the procedural aspects of nursing responsibilities on the labor and birth unit (Forbes & Hickey, 2009). Unfortunately, the majority of nurses working within labor and birth units in the United States do not provide continuous labor support as a result of the multiple duties that demand the nurse's attention in addition to the laboring woman (Lennon & Seaver, 2014; Simkin, 2014). Thus, this labor support content may not be taught during the didactic portion or modeled during the clinical component of nursing education (Glenn et al., 2012). Assuming new nurses possess knowledge of the benefits and methods of continuous labor support, new graduates quickly modify care practices to conform to expected practice norms in order to feel competent within the group they are joining (Curl & Lothian, 2013; Mooney, 2007).

### Barriers for Childbearing Women

Birthing women face multiple barriers in receiving the therapeutic presence and continuous labor support needed for optimal childbearing. These barriers include the cost and accessibility of doulas, lack of institutional valuing of the benefits of therapeutic presence, and an environment of conflict that may punish deviance from institutional norms (Hunter, 2012; McCourt, 2010; Miller & Shriver, 2012). The lack of midwifery services in many areas of the United States also leaves women with fewer options for support during hospitalized labor and birth (Martin, Hamilton, Osterman, Curtin, & Matthews, 2015).

Regional and individual institutional practice variations are normal and expected within medical practice. However, in the area of childbearing, evidence-based practices that eliminate routine procedures are commonly not implemented because of perceived liability fears, institutional resistance to change, competing interests, and potential disruption to staff routines (Curl & Lothian, 2013; Kaplan & Ballard, 2011; Main et al., 2012; Simkin, 2014)

The Western concept of pain as a purely physiologic occurrence without purpose and the need to avoid pain at all costs affects how providers, women, their partners, and the general society perceive labor and birth (Stoll & Hall, 2013). The idea of pain in childbirth has eclipsed the event of giving birth itself as an experience with inherent meaning and significance, deserving of distinct treatment (Greer, Lazanbatt, & Dunne, 2014; Wolf, 2009). Significant cultural barriers and socialization of girls and young women create an environment of fear and avoidance on the topic of childbirth (Romano, 2010).

## Negative Outcomes With Lack of Continuous Labor Support

Overuse of childbirth technology for nontherapeutic reasons is wasteful of human resources and health care dollars as well as unethical (Lothian, 2014). However, the physical and emotional costs to women are even greater. Routine use of intervention, without valid indications, can transform childbirth from a normal physiologic process and family event into a medical or surgical procedure (Declercq, Sakala, Corry, Applebaum, & Herrlich, 2013). Concerns stemming from the common use of epidurals during normal labor, the escalating cesarean birth rate with its attendant placental problems in subsequent pregnancies, repeat operative deliveries, and widespread professional neglect of evidence regarding the safety of vaginal birth after cesarean (VBAC) are covered elsewhere in this book.

Less apparent are the psychosocial and emotional effects of highly interventive birth coupled with lack of therapeutic presence and continuous labor support. Recent research documents links among lack of support, negative birth experiences, and stress disorders (Corrigan, Kwasky, & Groh, 2015; Nelson, Freeman, Johnson, McIntire, & Leveno, 2013). A phenomenological descriptive study was conducted with women pregnant with their second child who reported intense fear of birth resulting from a prior negative birth experience. All participants cited lack of support during labor as a primary source of their prior negative experience (Nilsson, Bondas, & Lundgren, 2010).

Negative birth experiences have been associated with the development of perinatal mood disorders and posttraumatic stress disorder (PTSD; Nelson et al., 2013). Although complicated instrumental and operative birth can be associated with PTSD, many women with severe PTSD symptoms have had a physiologic vaginal birth (Ayers & Ford, 2009; Banker & LaCoursiere, 2014; Nelson et al., 2013). Ford and Ayers (2008) investigated how stressful labor events and support from hospital staff affect a woman's anxiety and perception of control. Study findings indicated that a woman's emotional and anxiety reactions are affected more by the level of support received during birth than by the level of complications or interventions during birth (Ford & Ayers, 2008).

Meeting a woman's innate social need for therapeutic presence and support is highly relevant to reducing emotional trauma and pathology after birth (Corrigan et al., 2015). Those providing care to childbearing women need to acknowledge the high prevalence of perinatal mood disorders and PTSD diagnoses among postpartum women, and examine how emotional trauma can be avoided by providing continuous labor support.

## THERAPEUTIC PRESENCE AND CONTINUOUS LABOR SUPPORT: EVIDENCE FOR BEST PRACTICE

### Birth Outcomes

A large body of evidence documents the positive influence of continuous labor support on maternal and fetal outcomes across socioeconomic strata and nations (Steel et al., 2015). A randomized controlled trial (RCT) done by McGrath and Kennell (2008) with 420 middle-class women in the United States demonstrated that continuous labor support significantly reduced the incidence of cesarean birth and the need for analgesia as well as increased positive feelings women had about their childbirth experience. Women with continuous labor support are more likely to report higher satisfaction with their birth experience than women who do not have this support (Hodnett et al., 2013). More recent, clinical projects utilizing doula care have demonstrated improved maternal and infant outcomes (Gruber et al., 2013; Kozhimannil et al., 2013; Lennon & Seaver, 2014).

The Cochrane Systematic Review titled "Continuous Support for Women During Childbirth" presents compelling evidence of the benefits of continuous labor support. This meta-analysis included 22 clinical trials from 15 countries examining more than 15,200 childbearing women in a variety of settings (Hodnett et al., 2013). Outcome benefits are consistent and significant. Women with continuous one-to-one labor support had:

- Shorter labors
- Fewer cesarean births
- Less need for analgesia and anesthesia
- Reduced use of synthetic oxytocin in labor
- Greater maternal satisfaction with the childbirth experience
- Enhanced coping skills during the experience (Hodnett et al., 2013)

Infant outcomes were also improved. Babies born to women with continuous labor support had higher Apgar scores. The Cochrane reviewers concluded that continuous labor support is a no-risk intervention that substantially improves outcomes and should be provided to all women throughout labor (Hodnett et al., 2013).

Unlike other interventions that are used routinely in childbirth, such as continuous electronic monitoring (level C evidence—a consensus opinion), the intervention of continuous labor support is level A evidence (consistent with science and highly reliable). Ordinary intuition informs us that human touch and supportive care during the profound experience of labor and birth can have powerful and positive effects on a woman in labor. Clinical research firmly supports this intuitive assertion.

## Positive Physiological Responses to Continuous Labor Support

The positive maternal outcomes of continuous labor support are likely the result of the physiologic response to this kind of support (Burgess, 2014). The fight-or-flight stress response is generated by the laboring woman's sympathetic nervous system in response to the stress of labor pain, anxiety, and fear (Buckley, 2015). This response increases production of the catecholamines epinephrine and norepinephrine. Increased epinephrine can negatively influence fetal heart rate (FHR) patterns, causing providers to interpret fetal distress and initiate a cascade of technological interventions (Buckley, 2015; Smith et al., 2012). Animal and human research indicates that when catecholamine levels increase in labor, release of oxytocin from the posterior pituitary is blocked, uterine contractions are decreased, and blood flow to the uterus and placenta is reduced (Heinricks, von Dawans, & Domes, 2009; Simkin & Ancheta, 2011). The decrease in uterine blood flow sets up a cascade of interlocking events: reduced uterine contractility and slower dilation of the cervix making for a longer labor (Kennell, Klaus, McGrath, Robertson, & Hinkley, 1991; Simkin & Ancheta, 2011). Increased catecholamine secretion also increases pain perception (Buckley, 2015; Simkin & O'Hara, 2002).

The laboring environment can influence this fight-or-flight response and increase in catecholamines and epinephrine. Individuals engaged in continuous labor support help to manage the birth environment as part of comfort and advocacy behaviors to reduce interruptions for the laboring woman and to promote labor progress (Amram, 2014; Deveraux & Sullivan, 2013; Gruber et al., 2013). Hospital rooms are generally perceived by patients and hospital staff to be a space that belongs to the staff not the patient, and therefore the staff enters and manages the environment at will (Hunter, 2012). Auditory, physical, and spatial intrusions by various unknown personnel for examinations, procedures, cleaning, and restocking supplies are common in a hospital setting (Jansen et al., 2013). Providing a measure of personal control over visual access, bodily exposure, family visitation, as well as meeting emotional and physical needs allows the woman to respond to labor unimpeded and focus on the work of laboring and birthing (Ross-Davie & Cheyne, 2014).

Mediating the birthing environment can also influence labor progress (Amram et al., 2014). For example, lighting may help or hinder a woman's physiologic labor processes. Humans increase the production of melatonin, the hormone responsible for inducing sleep, in darkness and, in most humans, melatonin levels peak in the early hours of the morning. Melatonin synergizes with oxytocin to promote uterine smooth muscle contractions and to facilitate the gap junction activity required for effective labor (Olcese, Lozier, & Paradise, 2013). It is reasonable to conclude that laboring women may benefit from lower light levels to enhance melatonin production.

Women who are well supported during labor and birth are more likely to have freedom of movement to assume positions that facilitate labor progress, avoiding the need for exogenous oxytocin (Romano & Lothian, 2008; Simkin, 2014). Endogenous oxytocin is referred to as "the hormone of love" because of its role in regulating emotion, sexual activity, orgasm, birth, and breastfeeding (Heinricks et al., 2009). Oxytocin is released from the hypothalamus gland to initiate the rhythmic uterine contractions of labor. At the end of labor, the stretch receptors in the lower vaginal vault give positive feedback to the pituitary to release large amounts of oxytocin to coordinate the final powerful uterine contractions, promoting rapid passage of the fetal head. This phenomenon is the fetal ejection reflex. Additional oxytocin is released postbirth in response to skin-to-skin contact with the infant and breast stimulation with breastfeeding. These physical events protect the mother against hemorrhage (Buckley, 2015).

Tethering the woman during labor is a key factor precipitating the cascade of events that results in a high level of intervention as well as dampening down the effects of naturally produced oxytocin (Simkin & Acheta, 2011). Continuous labor support promotes the natural production of oxytocin and helps inhibit stress response, thus promoting increased mobility, maternal relaxation, cervical muscle dilation rate, and increased pelvic capacity—variables in promoting fetal passage through the pelvis and soft tissues (Deveraux & Sullivan, 2013; Romano & Lothian, 2008).

Oxytocin has important roles beyond the birthing period. It is linked with establishing mothering behaviors, altruistic and adaptive behaviors, slowing heart rate, and reducing blood pressure (Buckley, 2015; Gutkowska, Jankowski, Mukaddem-Daher, & McCann, 2000). Behavioral cues in the newborn have been shown to be sensitive to synthetic oxytocin (Bell, White-Traut, & Rankin, 2013). Newborn suckling and feeding behaviors can be depressed after the administration of intrapartum oxytocin (Fernández et al., 2012). Research has suggested that malfunction in the production of oxytocin may play a role in autism spectrum disorders, drug-dependency behaviors, and schizophrenia (Bartz & Hollander, 2008; Heinrichs, von Dawans, & Domes, 2009). Science does not yet fully understand the significance of endogenous oxytocin. Until more is known, it may be prudent to favor physiologic care practices that facilitate a woman's own oxytocin production during labor.

## Birth Satisfaction

Women receiving continuous labor support report high levels of satisfaction and positive memories of the birth experience (Harvey, Rach, Stainton, Jarrell, & Brant, 2002; Hunter, 2012; McGrath & Kennell, 2008). A sustaining human presence during labor decreases pain, anxiety, and fear that detract significantly from positive memories and perceptions of birth (Briddon, Isaac, & Slade, 2015; Hodnett, 2002; Rouhe et al., 2013; Waldenström, 2004). Bryanton, Gagnon, Johnston, and Hatem (2008) examined factors that influence a woman's perceptions of her childbirth experience. Of the 20 predictors of a woman's childbirth perceptions, the two strongest were the type of birth and the degree of awareness, relaxation, and control she had during labor and birth. Receiving therapeutic presence from a knowledgeable person throughout labor and birth increases the woman's sense of control and self-confidence with the birth experience (Bryanton et al., 2008; Hayes, 2010; Hodnett et al., 2013; Ross-Davie & Cheyne, 2014).

A systematic review examined 137 studies of factors that influenced women's satisfaction with the childbirth experience (Hodnett, 2002). Three factors emerged from the data as influencing birth satisfaction more powerfully than pain experienced, analgesia or anesthesia used, or medical interventions:

- Personal expectations. Women who had high expectations of the birth experience that were met or exceeded expressed high satisfaction.
- Labor support and caregiver communication. Continuous labor support along with good communication was a strong predicator of satisfaction with childbirth.
- Personal control and involvement with decision making. Women who felt they had control over what happened to them during labor and birth reported high satisfaction (Hodnett, 2002).

Other studies since the time of that meta-analysis have confirmed the strong link between continuous labor support and satisfaction with the birth experience (Campbell, Lake, Falk, & Backstrand, 2006; Gruber et al., 2013; Kozhimannil et al., 2013; McDonald, 2013). An RCT of 420 middle- and upper-class women examined the influence of continuous labor support by a doula. All women in the doula group rated the doula's presence as positive to very positive during labor and birth and said it enhanced the birth experience (McGrath & Kennell, 2008). These findings have been confirmed more recently by both Hunter (2012), and Deveraux and Sullivan (2013).

In an effort to determine relationships among labor support from nurses, stress during childbirth, and perceptions of the childbirth experience, a questionnaire was administered to 122 new mothers 1 to 2 days after giving birth (Srisuthisak, 2009). Stress reduction resulting from support received from the nursing staff was a significant predictor of a positive childbirth experience. Childbirth is a significant event in a woman's life; indeed, many women characterize it as the most important event in their lives. Childbirth memories are vivid, poignant, and deeply felt even 15 to 20 years after the birth (Simkin, 1992). Attending to a woman's need for therapeutic support during labor has long-term positive effects on satisfaction with childbearing experiences (Malacrida & Boulton, 2014; Waldenström, 2004)

Although continuous therapeutic labor support can be provided by a variety of individuals, studies' results suggest that support provided by an experienced person, such as a birth doula or midwife, who is not in the woman's social support group or family, is most beneficial to women (Campbell et al., 2006; Gruber et al., 2013; Hodnett et al., 2013; Pascali-Bonaro & Kroeger, 2004). Although women have been serving as doulas throughout time, birth doulas have experienced a surge in popularity in the past two decades, providing emotional, physical, and informational support to a woman and her family during labor. Some hospitals in the United States have begun to sponsor doula services in an effort to reduce high rates of cesarean section and improve patient satisfaction (Maher, Crawford-Carr, & Neidigh, 2012).

The Cochrane Review examined the effect of support from those in a woman's social network, hospital nursing staff, and companions intentionally chosen by the woman to provide labor support, such as a doula or midwife (Hodnett et al., 2013). Labor support provided by a person from the woman's social network, such as a partner or friend, increased satisfaction with the birth experience but did not influence other factors such as length of labor or the use of medical interventions. Labor support provided by a nurse did not have any detected influence on maternal satisfaction with the birth experience or cesarean birth rates. However, women who received continuous labor support care provided by a knowledgeable companion for the purpose of labor support, such as a doula, were:

- 28% less likely to have a cesarean birth
- 31% less likely to use synthetic oxytocin to augment labor
- 9% less likely to use any intrapartum analgesia
- 34% less likely to rate their childbirth experience negatively (Hodnett et al., 2013)

Continuous support that begins earlier in labor appears to be more effective than support that begins later in labor (Green & Hotelling, 2014). Labor support from fathers or partners did not appear to confer the same outcome benefits as support from a doula or midwife (Hodnett et al., 2013; Scott, Klaus, & Klaus, 1999).

## Educating Students and Stakeholders

Exemplary midwives and midwifery educators consider continuous one-to-one labor support to be an expected behavior of midwives (Cox & King, 2015; Kennedy, 2000; King & Pinger, 2014; Rooks, 1999). Laboring women also highly value and expect this behavior (Bryanton et al., 2008; Hodnett et al, 2013). Despite commitment to supporting women with therapeutic presence and continuous labor support to achieve a normal birth, even midwives find it challenging in today's hospital-based childbearing culture to implement these practices (Ainsworth, 2013; Aune, Amundsen, & Skaget Aas, 2014; Jordan & Farley, 2008; Sakala & Corry, 2008). In actual practice, continuous labor support translates into using time-intensive physical and emotional energy to encourage, support, and comfort women during active labor, highly impacting staffing patterns. The daily life of a midwife is physically and emotionally demanding, and optimal scheduling to meet both personal life and client needs can be challenging. Scheduling call days separate from office days, and developing team caseloads in large practices can allow for more time-intensive, one-to-one labor care (Atsalos et al., 2014; McCourt, 2010; Page & McCandlish, 2006). Supporting midwives in their efforts to provide continuous labor support is crucial for successful implementation of this evidence-based practice.

Educators need to be cognizant of opportunities for midwifery students to learn and practice behaviors of therapeutic continuous labor support. Students may or may not experience providing continuous labor support when they are in their clinical rotations. Although it is well known that new labor nurses and nursing students often lack role models and mentoring in promoting the normalcy of birth (Simkin, 2014; Sleutel et al., 2007), the question arises whether midwife students observe and are mentored in exemplary midwifery practice, including therapeutic presence and continuous labor support. In a study examining U.S. midwifery student and preceptor behaviors (Lange & Kennedy, 2006), new midwifery graduates were asked to rate selected dimensions of midwifery practice on two items: the importance they personally placed on the selected dimensions of midwifery practice, and how much emphasis they observed their preceptors placing on that practice. "Support for the normal processes of birth" had the highest degree of incongruence between stated importance placed on this value and actual preceptor practice behaviors. Although supporting the normal processes of birth is idealized and espoused as an important part of midwifery philosophy of care, this concept is often not reflected in care practices among practicing midwives because of institutional constraints (Aune et al., 2014; Lange & Kennedy, 2006).

Best practices in midwifery education include didactic teaching of the outcome benefits of continuous labor support, how to perform continuous labor support, and designing clinical experiences for students to implement the specific continuous labor support behaviors. Adams and Bianchi (2008) identify the following curricular content:

- Positioning and movement
- Use of hot/cold therapy
- Relaxation techniques using breathing and focus
- Use of therapeutic touch
- Verbal support and encouragement
- Informational support
- Partner support
- Birth environment management

Adams and Bianchi (2008) discussed the need to teach continuous labor support behaviors as a best practice not only to students but also to practicing midwives. Midwives working within hospital settings can provide educational in-services to nursing and obstetrical staff on the benefits and methods of continuous labor support for all laboring women. In maternity care practices where continuous labor support is precluded by institutional restraints, midwives can assist pregnant women in finding doula services and supporting agencies that will provide funding for them. Some insurance companies now offer full or partial payment for doula services. Educating hospital administrators, obstetricians, childbirth educators, pregnant women, and other stakeholders on the multiple maternal outcomes afforded by continuous labor support can lead to collaborative efforts toward changing institutional practice. There is a growing movement for more humane and evidence-based childbirth care within the health care system and the public via groups such as Childbirth Connection, Lamaze International, Coalition for Improving Maternity Services, and BirthNetwork National. A best practice for midwives is to join these groups and provide a voice for these efforts.

## CONCLUSION

Women worldwide share a common need and desire for continuous therapeutic support in labor (Campero et al., 1998; Hodnett et al., 2013; Mahdi & Habib, 2010; Miller & Shriver, 2012; Price, Noseworthy, & Thornton, 2007; Ross-Davie & Cheyne, 2014; Steel et al., 2015). Continuous therapeutic labor support promotes improved maternal and fetal health outcomes without risk and should be provided as a routine for all laboring women (Deveraux & Sullivan, 2013; Gruber et al., 2013; Hunter, 2012; Kozhimannil et al., 2013; McDonald, 2013). One of the 16 hallmarks of the midwifery profession is the value of therapeutic presence in providing health care to women (ACNM 2012). Midwives are ideal leaders in educating nurses, obstetrical teams, and childbearing women on the benefits and implementation of continuous labor support for all women as a routine intervention in all birth settings.

**USING THE EVIDENCE FOR BEST PRACTICE**

**Case Study 17.1   Therapeutic Presence and Continuous Labor Support**

Two midwives joined a four-physician practice 2 years ago. They have their own case-loads, attending approximately 20 births per month in the local 400-bed regional referral hospital. Women in the community are signing up for midwifery services in ever-increasing numbers. The physicians are asking that they take on more clients; however, they remain dedicated to providing labor support. In an effort to bring their physician colleagues to a better understanding of their practice scheduling, the midwives presented the evidence on the outcome benefits of continuous labor support during a monthly staff meeting.

This presentation prompted discussion on maternal–newborn outcome markers and strategies to allow physician group clients to benefit from this support. A committee of one midwife, one physician, and one nurse from the labor and birth unit was formed to gather evidence and ideas to bring back to the group. The committee recommendations included using privately hired doulas, enlisting the support of the director of the school of nursing, who subsequently agreed to integrate labor support behaviors in the didactic and clinical maternity nursing courses.

A presentation to the labor and birth unit nursing staff on the benefits of continuous labor support was given by committee members. A local doula service was contacted to discuss services. It was decided that doulas would teach the childbirth education classes covering support in labor. Informational brochures about doula services would be provided during the class as well as at the midwife and physician offices.

**Exemplar of Best Practice**

In reviewing outcome markers at the 8-month period, data revealed a decrease in oxytocin use and operative birth, and an increase in client satisfaction scores.

Hospital administration was impressed by the efforts of the midwife and physician groups to improve outcomes. They noted a concomitant decrease in hospital length-of-stay, likely related to the decrease in operative birth. As a result, they became more involved in efforts to provide one-to-one care in the labor and birth unit. Hospital administrators also used funds from the childbirth education department to pay for doula services for women unable to afford the cost. Efforts are ongoing to enlist the involvement of all nurses on the unit to provide continuous labor support and to orient new nurses to labor support behaviors.

# REFERENCES

Adams, E. D., & Bianchi, A. L. (2008). A practical approach to labor support. *Journal of Obstetric, Gynecologic, and Neonatal Nursing, 37*(1), 106–115. doi:10.1111/j.1552-6909.2007.00213.x

Ainsworth, A. (2013). Changing childbirth practices—An impossible job? *Midwifery Matters, 136*, 8–10.

American College of Nurse-Midwives (ACNM). (2012). Core competencies for basic midwifery practice. Retrieved from http://www.midwife.org/ACNM/files/ACNMLibraryData/UPLOAD FILENAME/000000000050/Core%20Comptencies%20Dec%202012.pdf

Amran, N. L., Klein, M. C., Mok, H., Simkin, P., Lindstrom, K., & Grant, J. (2014). How birth doulas help clients adapt to changes in circumstances, clinical care, and client preferences during labor. *Journal of Perinatal Education, 23*(2), 96–103. doi:10.1891/1058-1243.23.2.96

Anderson, B. L., Scerbo, M. W., Belfore, L. A., & Abuhamad, A. Z. (2011). Time and number of displays impact critical signal detection in fetal heart rate tracings. *American Journal of Perinatology, 28*(6), 435–442. doi:10.1055/s-0030-1268718

Atsalos, C., Biggs, K., Boensch, S., Gavegan, F. L., Heath, S., Payk, M., & Trapolini, G. (2014). How clinical nurse and midwifery consultants optimize patient care in a tertiary referral hospital. *Journal of Clinical Nursing, 23*(19/20), 2874–2885. doi:10.1111/jocn.12567

Aune, I., Amundsen, H. H., & Skaget Aas, L. C. (2014). Is a midwife's continuous presence during childbirth a matter of course? Midwives' experiences and thoughts about factors that may influence their continuous support of women during labour. *Midwifery, 30*(1), 89–95. doi:10.1016/j.midw.2013.02.001

Ayers, S., & Ford, E. (2009). Birth trauma: Widening our knowledge of postnatal mental health. *European Health Psychologist, 11*(2), 16–19.

Banker, J. E., & LaCoursiere, D. Y. (2014). Postpartum depression: Risks, protective factors, and the couple's relationship. *Issues in Mental Health Nursing, 35*(7), 503–508. doi:10.310 9/01612840.2014.888603

Barrett, S. J., & Stark, M. A. (2010). Factors associated with labor support behaviors of nurses. *Journal of Perinatal Education, 19*(1), 12–18. doi:10.1624/105812410X481528

Bartz, J. A., & Hollander, E. (2008). Oxytocin and experimental therapeutics in autism spectrum disorder. *Progress in Brain Research, 170*(8), 451–462. doi:10.1016/S0079-6123(08)00435-4

Bell, A. F., White-Traut, R., & Rankin, K. (2013). Fetal exposure to synthetic oxytocin and the relationship with prefeeding cues within one hour postbirth. *Early Human Development, 89*(3), 137–143. doi:10.1016/j.earlhumdev.2012.09.017

Bergman, J., & Bergman, N. (2013). Whose choice? Advocating birth practices according to baby's biological needs. *Journal of Perinatal Education, 22*(1), 8–13. doi:10.1891/1058 -1243.22.1.8

Bonsack, C. F., Lathrop, A., & Blackburn, M. (2014). Induction of labor: Update and review. *Journal of Midwifery & Women's Health, 59*(6), 606–615. doi:10.1111/jmwh.12255

Briddon, E., Isaac, C., & Slade, P. (2015). The association between involuntary memory and emotional adjustment after childbirth. *British Journal of Health Psychology, 20*(4), 889–903. doi:10.1111/bjhp.12151

Bryanton, J., Gagnon, A. J., Johnston, C., & Hatem, M. (2008). Predictors of women's perceptions of the childbirth experience. *Journal of Obstetric, Gynecologic, and Neonatal Nursing, 37*(1), 24–34. doi:10.1111/j.1552-6909.2007.00203.x

Buckley, S. (2015). *Hormonal physiology of childbearing: Evidence and implications for women, babies, and maternity care.* New York, NY: Childbirth Connection.

Burgess, A. (2014). An evolutionary concept analysis of labor support. *International Journal of Childbirth Education, 29*(2), 64–72.

Campbell, D. A., Lake, M. F., Falk, M., & Backstrand, J. R. (2006). A randomized control trial of continuous support in labor by a lay doula. *Journal of Obstetric, Gynecologic, and Neonatal Nursing, 35*(4), 456–464. doi:10.1111/j.1552-6909.2006.00067.x

Campero, L., Garcia, C., Duaz, C., Ortiz, O., Reynoso, S., & Langer, A. (1998). "Alone, I wouldn't have known what to do": A qualitative study on social support during labor and delivery in Mexico. *Social Science & Medicine, 47*(3), 395–403. doi:10.1016/S0277-9536(98)00077-X

Corrigan, C. P., Kwasky, A. N., & Groh, C. J. (2015). Social support, postpartum depression, and professional assistance: A survey of mothers in the Midwestern United States. *Journal of Perinatal Education, 24*(1), 48–60. doi:10.1891/1058-1243.24.1.48

Cox, K. J., & King, T. L. (2015). Preventing primary cesarean births: Midwifery care. *Clinical Obstetrics and Gynecology, 58*(2), 282–293. doi:10.1097/GRF.0000000000000108

Curl, M., & Lothian, J. (2013). Evidence based maternity care: Can new dogs learn old tricks? *Journal of Perinatal Education, 22*(4), 234–240. doi:10.1891/1058-1243.22.4.234

Declercq, E. R., Sakala, C., Corry, M. P., Applebaum, S., & Herrlich, A. (2013). Listening to mothers III: Pregnancy and birth. Report of the Third National U.S. Survey of Women's Childbearing Experiences. Retrieved from http://transform.childbirthconnection.org/wp-content/uploads/2013/06/LTM-III_Pregnancy-and-Birth.pdf

Deveraux, Y., & Sullivan, H. (2013). Doula support while laboring: Does it help achieve a more natural birth? *International Journal of Childbirth Education, 28*(2), 54–61.

Fernández, O. I., Gabriel, M. M., Martínez, M. A., Fernández-Cañadas, M. A., López Sánchez, F., & Costarelli, V. (2012). Newborn feeding behaviour depressed by intrapartum oxytocin: A pilot study. *Acta Paediatrica, 101*(7), 749–754. doi:10.1111/j.1651-2227.2012.02668.x

Folkman, S., & Lazarus, R. S. (1988). The relationship between coping and emotion: Implications for theory and research. *Social Science & Medicine, 26*(3), 309–317. doi:10.1016/0277-9536(88)90395-4

Forbes, M. O., & Hickey, M. T. (2009). Curriculum reform in baccalaureate nursing education: Review of the literature. *International Journal of Nursing Education Scholarship, 6*(1). doi:10.2202/1548-923X.1797

Ford, E., & Ayers, S. (2008). Stressful events and support during birth: The effect on anxiety, mood and perceived control. *Journal of Anxiety Disorders, 23*(2), 260–268. doi:10.1016/j.janxdis.2008.07.009

Ford, E., Ayers, S., & Wright, D. B. (2009). Measurement of maternal perception of support and control in birth (SCIB). *Journal of Women's Health, 18*(2), 245–252. doi:10.1089/jwh.2008.0882

Glenn, L. A., Stocker-Schnieder, J., McCune, R., McClelland, M., & King, D. (2012). Caring nurse practice in the intrapartum setting: Nurses' perspectives on complexity, relationships and safety. *Journal of Advanced Nursing, 68*(1), 2019–2030. doi:10.1111/jan.12356

Graham, I. D., Logan, J., Davies, B., & Nimrod, C. (2004). Changing the use of electronic fetal monitoring and labor support: A case study of barriers and facilitators. *Birth, 31*(4), 293–301. doi:10.1111/j.0730-7659.2004.00322.x

Green, J., & Hotelling, B. A. (2014). Healthy birth practice #3: Bring a loved one, friend, or doula for continuous support. *Journal of Perinatal Education, 23*(4), 194–197. doi:10.1891/1058-1243.23.4.194

Greer, J., Lazanbatt, A., & Dunne, L. (2014). "Fear of childbirth" and ways of coping for pregnant women and their partners during the birthing process: A salutogenic analysis. *Evidence Based Midwifery, 12*(3), 95–100.

Gruber, K. J., Cupito, S. H., & Dobson, C. F. (2013). Impact of doulas on healthy birth outcomes. *Journal of Perinatal Education, 22*(1), 49–58. doi:10.1891/1058-1243.22.1.49

Gutkowska, J., Jankowski, M., Mukaddem-Daher, S., & McCann, S. M. (2000). Oxytocin is a cardiovascular hormone. *Brazilian Journal of Medical and Biological Research, 33*(6), 625–633. doi:10.1590/S0100-879X2000000600002

Harvey, S., Rach, D., Stainton, C., Jarrell, J., & Brant, R. (2002). Evaluation of satisfaction with midwifery care. *Midwifery, 18*(4), 260–267. doi:10.1054/midw.2002.0317

Hayes, T. (2010). Labour and birth: Self-control and the laboring woman. *MIDIRS Midwifery Digest, 20*(3), 335–341.

Heinrichs, M., von Dawans, B., & Domes, G. (2009). Oxytocin, vasopressin, and human social behavior. *Frontiers in Neuroendocrinology, 30*(4), 548–557. doi:10.1016/j.yfrne.2009.05.005

Hodnett, E. D. (2002). Pain and women's satisfaction with the experience of childbirth: A systematic review. *American Journal of Obstetrics and Gynecology, 186*(5), S160–S172.

Hodnett, E. D., Gates, S., Hofmeyr, G. J., & Sakala, C. (2013). Continuous support for women during childbirth. *Cochrane Database of Systematic Reviews, 2013*(7). doi:10.1002/14651858.CD003766.pub5

Hotelling, B. A. (2007). The Coalition for Improving Maternity Services: Evidence basis for the ten steps of mother-friendly care. *Journal of Perinatal Education, 16*(2), 38–43. doi:10.1624/105812407X197744

Hunter, C. (2012). Intimate space within institutionalized birth: Women's experiences birthing with doulas. *Anthropology & Medicine, 19*(3), 315–326. doi:10.1080/13648470.2012.692358

James, D. C. (2011). Routine obstetrical interventions: Research agenda for the next decade. *Journal of Perinatal and Neonatal Nursing, 25*(2), 148–152. doi:10.1097/JPN.0b013e3182116e69

Jansen, L., Gibson, M., Bowles, B. C., & Leach, J. (2013). First do no harm: Interventions during childbirth. *Journal of Perinatal Education, 22*(2), 83–92. doi:10.1891/1058-1243.22.2.83

Jordan, R., & Farley, C. L. (2008). The confidence to practice midwifery: Preceptor influence on student self-efficacy. *Journal of Midwifery & Women's Health, 53*(5), 413–420. doi:10.1016/j.jmwh.2008.05

Kaplan, H. D., & Ballard, J. (2011). Changing practice to improve patient safety and quality of care in perinatal medicine. *American Journal of Perinatology, 28*(9), 1–8. doi:10.1055/s-0031-1285826

Kennedy, H. P. (2000). A model of exemplary midwifery practice: Results of a Delphi study. *Journal of Midwifery & Women's Health, 45*(1), 4–19. doi:10.1016/S1526-9523(99)00018-5

Kennell, J., Klaus, M., McGrath, S., Robertson, S., & Hinkley, C. (1991). Continuous emotional support during labor is a US hospital. *Journal of the American Medical Association, 265*(17), 2197–2201. doi:10.1001/jama.1991.03460170051032

King, T. L., & Pinger, W. (2014). Evidence based practice for intrapartum care: The pearls of Midwifery. *Journal of Midwifery & Women's Health, 59*(6), 572–585. doi:10.1111/jmwh.12261

Kozhimannil, K. B., Hardeman, R. R., Attanasio, L. B., Blauer-Peterson, C., & O'Brien, M. (2013). Doula care, birth outcomes, and costs among Medicaid beneficiaries. *American Journal of Public Health, 103*(4), e113–e121. doi:10.2105/AJPH.2012.301201

Lamaze International. (2016). Lamaze healthy birth practices. Retrieved from http://www .lamazeinternational.org/p/cm/ld/fid=214

Lange, G., & Kennedy, H. P. (2006). Student perceptions of ideal and actual midwifery practice. *Journal of Midwifery & Women's Health, 51*(2), 71–77. doi:10.1016/j.jmwh.2005.10.003

Leap, N., Sandall, J., Buckland, S., & Huber, U. (2010). Journey to confidence: Women's experiences of pain in labour and relational continuity of care. *Journal of Midwifery & Women's Health, 55*(3), 234–242. doi:10.1016/j.jmwh.2010.02.001

Lehrman, E. (1988). A theoretical framework for nurse-midwifery practice. *Dissertation Abstracts International,* 49–173:5230. UMI No. 8905798.

Lennon, J., & Seaver, D. (2014). A collaborative practice initiative to reduce the rate of cesarean deliveries: The Vaginal Delivery Optimization Team. *Journal of Obstetric, Gynecologic and Neonatal Nursing, 43*(Suppl. 1), S20–S21. doi:10.1111/1552-6909.12413

Levine, M. S., & Lowe, N. K. (2014). Nurse attitudes toward childbirth: A concept clarification. *Nursing Forum, 49*(2), 88–99. doi:10.1111/nuf.12040

Lothian, J. A. (2014). Promoting optimal care in childbirth. *Journal of Perinatal Education, 23*(4), 174–177. doi:10.1891/1058-1243.23.4.174

Mahdi, S. S., & Habib, O. S. (2010). A study on preferences and practices of women regarding place of delivery. *Eastern Mediterranean Health Journal, 16*(8), 874–878.

Maher, S., Crawford-Carr, A., & Neidigh, K. (2012). The role of the interpreter/doula in the maternity setting. *Nursing for Women's Health, 16*(6), 472–481. doi:10.1111/j.1751-486X .2012.01775.x

Main, E. K., Morton, C. H., Melsop, K., Hopkins, D., Giuliani, G., & Gould, J. B. (2012). Creating a public agenda for maternity safety and quality in cesarean delivery. *Obstetrics & Gynecology, 120*(5), 1194–1198. doi:10.1097/AOG.0b013e31826fc13d

Malacrida, C., & Boulton, T. (2014). The best laid plans? Women's choices, expectations and experiences in childbirth. *Health, 18*(1), 41–59. doi:10.1177/1363476964

Martin, E. (2001). *The woman in the body: A cultural analysis of reproduction.* Boston, MA: Beacon Press.

Martin, J. A., Hamilton, B. E., Osterman, M. J., Curtin, S. C., & Mathews, T. J. (2015). Births: Final data for 2013. *National Vital Statistics Report, 64*(1), 1–65. Retrieved from http:// www.cdc.gov/nchs/data/nvsr/nvsr64/nvsr64_01.pdf

McCourt, C. (Ed.). (2010). *Childbirth, midwifery and concepts of time.* New York, NY: Berghahn Books.

McDonald, S. (2013). Women who receive continuous support during labour have reduced risk of caesarean, instrumental delivery or need for analgesia compared to usual care. *Evidence Based Nursing, 16*(2), 40–41. doi:10.1136/ebn.2011.100194

McGrath, S. K., & Kennell, J. H. (2008). A randomized controlled trial of continuous labor support for middle class couples: Effect on cesarean delivery rates. *Birth, 35*(2), 92–97. doi:10.1111/j.1523-536X.2008.00221.x

Miller, A. C., & Shriver, T. E. (2012). Women's childbirth preferences and practices in the United States. *Social Sciences & Medicine, 75*(4), 709–716. doi:10.1016/j.socscimed.2012.03.051

Mooney, M. (2007). Professional socialization: The key to survival as a newly qualified nurse. *International Journal of Nursing Practice, 13*(2), 75–80. doi:10.1111/j.1440-172X.2007.00617.x

Nelson, D. B., Freeman, M. P., Johnson, N. L., McIntire, D. D., & Leveno, K. J. (2013). A prospective study of postpartum depression in 17,648 parturients. *Journal of Maternal–Fetal and Neonatal Medicine, 26*(12), 1155–1161. doi:10.3109/14767058.2013.777698

Nilsson, C., Bondas, T., & Lundgren, I. (2010). Previous birth experience in women with intense fear of childbirth. *Journal of Obstetric, Gynecologic, and Neonatal Nursing, 39*(3), 290–309. doi:10.1111/j.1552-6909.2010.01139.x

Olcese, J., Lozier, S., & Paradise, C. (2013). Melatonin and the circadian timing of human parturition. *Reproductive Sciences, 20*(2), 168–174. doi:10.1177/1933719112442244

Page, L. A., & McCandlish, R. (2006). *The new midwifery: Science and sensitivity in practice* (2nd ed.). Philadelphia, PA: Churchill Livingstone.

Pascali-Bonaro, D., & Kroeger, M. (2004). Continuous female companion during childbirth: A crucial resource in times of stress or calm. *Journal of Midwifery & Women's Health, 49*(4, Suppl. 1), 19–27. doi:10.1016/j.jmwh.2004.04.017

Payant, L., Davies, B., Graham, I. D., Peterson, W. E., & Clinch, J. (2008). Nurses' intentions to provide continuous labor support to women. *Journal of Obstetric, Gynecologic, and Neonatal Nursing, 37*(4), 405–414. doi:10.1111/j.1552-6909.2008.00257.x

Price, S., Noseworthy, J., & Thornton, J. (2007). Women's experience with social presence during childbirth. *American Journal of Maternal/Child Nursing, 32*(3), 184–191. doi:10.1097/01.NMC.0000269569.94561.7c

Riffle, E. M. (2014). Fetal heart rate assessment best practice. *International Journal of Childbirth Education, 29*(4), 55–58.

Romano, A. M. (2010). Creating a culture of consumer engagement in maternity care. *Journal of Perinatal Education, 19*(2), 50–54. doi:10.1624/105812410X495550

Romano, A. M., & Lothian, J. A. (2008). Promoting, protecting, and supporting normal birth: A look at the evidence. *Journal of Obstetric, Gynecologic, and Neonatal Nursing, 37*(1), 94–104. doi:10.1111/j.1552-6909.2007.00210.x

Rooks, J. P. (1999). The midwifery model of care. *Journal of Nurse-Midwifery, 44*(4), 370–374. doi:10.1016/S0091-2182(99)00060-9

Ross-Davie, M., & Cheyne, H. (2014). Intrapartum support: What do women want? A literature review. *Evidence Based Midwifery, 12*(2), 52–58.

Rossignol, M., Chaillet, N., Bourghrassa, F., & Moutquin, J. (2014). Interrelations between four antepartum obstetric interventions and cesarean delivery in women at low risk: A systematic review and modeling of the cascade of interventions. *Birth, 41*(1), 70–78. doi:10.1111/birt.12088

Rouhe, H., Salmela-Aro, K., Toivanen, R., Tokola, M., Halmesmäki, E., & Saisto, T. (2013). Obstetric outcome after intervention for severe fear of childbirth in nulliparous women–randomised trial. *British Journal of Obstetrics and Gynaecology, 120*(1), 75–84. doi:10.1111/1471-0528.12011

Sakala, C., & Corry, M. P. (2008). Evidence–based maternity care: What it is and what it can achieve. Retrieved from http://www.milbank.org/reports/0809MaternityCare/0809Mater nityCare.html

Sauls, D. J. (2004). Adolescents' perception of support during labor. *Journal of Perinatal Education, 13*(4), 36–42. doi:10.1624/105812404X6216

Sauls, D. J. (2006). Dimensions of professional labor support for intrapartum practice. *Journal of Nursing Scholarship, 38*(1), 36–41. doi:10.1111/j.1547-5069.2006.00075.x

Schuiling, K. D., & Sampselle, C. M. (1999). Comfort in labor and midwifery art. *Journal of Nursing Scholarship, 31*(1), 77–81. doi:10.1111/j.1547-5069.1999.tb00425.x

Scott, K. D., Klaus, P. H., & Klaus, M. H. (1999). The obstetrical and postpartum benefits of continuous support during childbirth. *Journal of Women's Health & Gender-Based Medicine, 8*(10), 1257–1264. doi:10.1089/jwh.1.1999.8.1257

Simkin, P. (1992). Just another day in a woman's life? Part II: Nature and consistency of women's long-term memories of their first birth experiences. *Birth, 19*(2), 64–81. doi:10.1111/j.1523-536X.1992.tb00382.x

Simkin, P. (2014). Preventing primary cesareans: Implications for laboring women, their partners, nurses, educators, and doulas. *Birth, 41*(3), 220–222. doi: 10.1112/birt.12124

Simkin, P., & Ancheta, R. (2011). *Labor progress handbook: Early interventions to prevent and treat dystocia* (3rd ed.). Boston, MA: Wiley-Blackwell.

Simkin, P., & O'Hara, M. (2002). Nonpharmacologic relief of pain during labor: Systematic reviews of five methods. *American Journal of Obstetrics and Gynecology, 186*(5), S131–S159. doi:10.1016/S0002-9378(02)70188-9

Simpson, K. R. (2010). Reconsideration of the cost of convenience: Quality, operational, and fiscal strategies to minimize elective labor induction. *Journal of Perinatal & Neonatal Nursing, 24*(1), 43–52. doi:10.1097/JPN.0b013e3181c6abe3

Sleutel, M., Schultz, S., & Wyble, K. (2007). Nurses' views of factors that help and hinder their intrapartum care. *Journal of Obstetric, Gynecologic, and Neonatal Nursing, 36*(3), 203–211. doi:10.1111/j.1552-6909.2007.00146.x

Smith, V., Begley, C. M., Clarke, M., & Devane, D. (2012). Professionals' views of fetal monitoring during labour: A systematic review and thematic analysis. *BMC Pregnancy and Childbirth, 12*(1), 166–183. doi:10.1186/1471-2393-12-166

Srisuthisak, S. (2009). *Relationships among stress of labor, support and experience of childbirth in postpartum mothers* (Unpublished doctoral dissertation). Virginia Commonwealth University, Richmond, VA. Retrieved from http://hdl.handle.net/10156/2631

Steel, A., Frawley, J., Adams, J., & Diezel, H. (2015). Trained or professional doulas in the support and care of pregnant and birthing women: A critical integrative review. *Health and Social Care in the Community, 23*(3), 225–241. doi:10.1111/hsc.12112

Stoll, K., & Hall, W. A. (2013). Attitudes and preferences of young women with low and high fear of childbirth. *Qualitative Health Research, 23*(11), 1495–1505.

Trumble, J., Lee, J., Slater, P. M., Sellors, J., & Cyna, A. M. (2015). Consent for labor epidural analgesia: An observational study at a single institution. *Anaesthesia & Intensive Care, 43*(3), 323–327.

Waldenström, U. (2004). Why do some women change their opinion about childbirth over time? *Birth, 31*(2), 102–107. doi:10.1111/j.0730-7659.2004.00287.x

Wiklund, I., Edman, G., Larsson, C., & Andolf, E. (2009). First-time mothers and changes in personality in relation to mode of delivery. *Journal of Advanced Nursing, 65*(8), 1636–1644. doi:10.1111/j.1365-2648.2009.05018.x

Williams, D. Ivey, T., Benton, T., & Rhoads, S. (2010). Another set of eyes: Remote fetal monitoring surveillance aids the busy labor and delivery unit. *Journal of Obstetric, Gynecologic and Neonatal Nursing, 39*(Suppl. S1), S41. doi:10.1111/j.1552.6909.2010.0119_30.x

Wolf, J. H. (2009). *Deliver me from pain: Anesthesia & birth in America*. Baltimore, MD: Johns Hopkins University Press.

# CHAPTER EIGHTEEN

# UNTETHERING IN LABOR: USING THE EVIDENCE FOR BEST PRACTICE

Susan M. Yount, Meghan Garland, and Rebeca Barroso

## LIFE SATISFACTION WITH CHILDBIRTH EXPERIENCE

Historically, policy makers and clinicians have responded to public demands for the provision of services. Examples are the demand for birth center care and for less medicated birth in the 1960s and 1970s (Childbirth Connection, 2010, 2016). The term *birth center,* however, has been co-opted into highly medicalized birthing environments, creating an illusion of a culture of safety rather than actual increased safety (Cheng, Declercq, Belanoff, Stotland, & Iverson, 2015; Kozhimannil, Law, & Virnig, 2013; Moore & Low, 2012). This current culture of safety is as much about concerns overescalating costs, protection from litigation, and clinician convenience as it is about evidence-based safety for mother and child (Eggermont, 2015; Kachalia & Bates, 2014; Sakala, Yang, & Corry, 2013; Thompson et al., 2015; Wolk, Sine, & Paull, 2014). This illusion needs to be confronted in order to provide optimally safe and satisfying physiologic birth.

## Technology and Tethering

High-technology use in physiologic birth requires tethering women to cables and hoses, restricting freedom of movement. This tethering increases the likelihood for a cascade of medical interventions disrupting physiologic birth and affecting the woman's ability for decision making (Buckley, 2015; Van Teijlingen, Lowis, McCaffery, & Porter, 2011). Any intervention disrupting the physiologic process of birth, although at times necessary, has the potential of creating this cascade of escalating consequences and needs to be carefully evaluated (Goer & Romano, 2012). However, clinicians with a stake in high technology and convenience are likely to resist this assessment and the ensuing conversation (Smith, Begley, Clarke, & Devane, 2012).

This labor management conversation needs to change among all stakeholders, including clinicians, institutions, insurance carriers, childbearing women, and families (Kennedy et al., 2015; Lawrence et al., 2012). The discussion needs to center on optimal outcomes for the woman and her infant rather than convenience, prevention of litigation, or the apparent ease of immediate pharmacological intervention for pain (Moore & Low, 2012; Wassen et al., 2015; Zwecker, Azoulay, & Abenhaim, 2011). For example, a laboring woman's experience of pain may not necessitate an immediate movement to epidural placement. The solution to pain depends on the root of her pain (Rooks, 2012; Sanders, 2015). If her baby is malpositioned or the woman is anxious, a low-risk intervention, such as offering reassurance, changing positions in or out of bed, ambulating, the use of a birth ball, or helping the woman immerse in a warm bath or shower, may facilitate optimal fetal positioning, pain reduction, and labor progression (Makvandi, Larifnejad Roudsari, Sadeghi, & Karimi, 2015; Simkin, 2010; Stark, 2013). These evidence-based measures deserve an attempt, as the first line of therapy, before escalating to potentially risky interventions.

## Results of the Listening to Mothers Surveys

Many informants in both the Listening to Mothers II and Listening to Mothers III surveys provided favorable ratings for the use of drug-free measures of pain relief such as warm-water tubs, hot or cold applications, showers, or birthing balls (Declercq, Sakala, Corry, & Applebaum, 2007; Declercq, Sakala, Corry, Applebaum, & Herrlich, 2014). Informants in the Listening to Mothers III survey indicated an overwhelming desire to have risks and benefits, as well as the option of no treatment, discussed with them prior to interventions (Declercq et al., 2014). Among survey informants giving birth for the first time at term, those who had neither an epidural nor labor induction had a cesarean section rate of 5%. Informants who had either an epidural or labor induction had a cesarean rate of 19% to 20%. Those women who experienced a labor as well as an epidural induction had a cesarean birth rate of 31%, six times greater than those without either intervention (Brody & Sakala, 2013).

Among nearly 4 million births annually, the cesarean birth rate in the United States is high, averaging 32.2% (Centers for Disease Control and Prevention [CDC], 2015). Cesarean births carry morbidity and mortality risks for both mother and child. The CDC recommends promotion of physiologic birth to improve birth outcomes and to decrease cesarean births (CDC, 2015).

## EVIDENCE AND BEST PRACTICES FOR UNTETHERING IN LABOR

## Hydration and Nutrition in Labor

Food and fluid have both physical and psychological importance for the laboring woman. According to the American College of Nurse-Midwives (ACNM), nutritional deprivation (nutrition and hydration) is one factor that can disrupt the normal physiologic processes that occur during childbirth (ACNM, 2015a). Most women will drink to thirst and eat to appetite if provided a supportive environment. In the absence of an evidence-based reason, denying the laboring woman access to food and fluid of her choice can lead to increased stress and a decrease in sense of control (Buckley, 2015; Sharts-Hopko, 2010).

Although oral intake for laboring women in hospital settings has been largely restricted since the mid-1940s because of aspiration concerns, there is little research to support the origins of the practice, and current research refutes enforcing oral intake restrictions (Davies & Deery, 2014; Sharts-Hopko, 2010). Laboring women who are nauseous or vomiting will self-limit oral intake.

In seminal work exploring in-labor stressors, Simkin (1986) surveyed post-partum women about stressors associated with childbirth. Approximately 25% identified restriction of food in labor as stressful, whereas more than 50% described restriction of oral fluids as stressful. Vallejo, Cobb, Steen, Singh, and Phelps (2013) reported on a study in which women reported satisfaction with high-protein drinks in labor in contrast to the usual offerings of water and ice chips. The gastric-emptying rates with high-protein drinks and water/ice chips were measured and found to be comparable (Vallejo et al., 2013).

A Cochrane Collaboration meta-analysis found that poor nutrition during labor could be associated with longer labors and increased pain in labor (Singata, Tranmer, & Gyte, 2013). The authors reviewed research that included women with restricted food or fluids compared to women who ate freely and drank fluids during labor. In women at low risk for anesthesia use, no benefits were identified for the restriction of food or fluids during labor (Singata et al., 2013). No further studies have been published to support or challenge these findings.

The American College of Obstetricians and Gynecologists (ACOG), in a committee opinion reaffirmed in 2013 (ACOG, n.d.), offers support for maternal intake of "modest amounts of clear fluids" (ACOG, 2009a, para. 3). Other than expert opinion, no further current evidence is provided to support this recommendation (ACOG, 2009a).

In the absence of impending surgery and in view of what is known, supporting the low-risk woman in choosing how much and when to eat and drink respects her autonomy. Best practice is to eat light food and drink fluids low in acid, sugar, and salt (ACNM, 2015b). ACNM (2015b) concludes, "care decisions related to nutritional support should be individualized, and standard protocols do not apply to every woman in labor" (para. 1).

## Vital Signs in Labor

### Monitoring Maternal Vital Signs

It is difficult to ascertain the origin and evidence supporting the recommendations for the assessment of intrapartum maternal vital signs in labor. In *Varney's Midwifery* (King et al., 2015), this statement is found: "Unfortunately, the standards for the frequency of vital signs for low risk women in labor may be based in nursing and institutional traditions rather than on evidence of clinical relevance in laboring women" (p. 832).

*Williams Obstetrics* (Cunningham et al., 2014) provides a framework of at least every 4 hours for the assessment of intrapartum maternal vital signs in active labor (p. 450). The Commission for the Accreditation of Birth Centers (CABC) concurs with these recommendations and directs maternal vital signs assessment on admission and then at least every 4 hours in the absence of identified risk factors (CABC, 2015, p. 142). The U.K.'s National Institute for Health and Care Excellence (NICE) expert opinion guidelines state that maternal vital signs should be assessed when the woman first presents for intrapartum care with subsequent hourly evaluations of her pulse; and every-4-hour evaluations of blood pressure and temperature (NICE, 2014, Sections 1.4.2, 1.12.7). Deviations from the defined limits of normal warrant closer surveillance.

In contrast, *Varney*'s authors and the Association of Women's Health, Obstetric and Neonatal Nurses (AWHONN) recommend, beyond the initial assessment, maternal pulse, respirations, and blood pressure hourly; and temperature every 2 hours (King et al., 2015, pp. 832–833; Simpson & Creehan, 2014, p. 356). No sources are cited for these recommendations, and it is not stated, by either group of authors (King et al., 2015; Simpson & Creehan, 2014), whether the basis for the recommendations is expert opinion or "nursing and institutional traditions" (King et al., 2015 p. 832).

Until clinical trials are conducted and there is subsequent definitive evidence to guide clinical practice, a best practice to increase freedom of movement in labor for low-risk women without impaired mobility is to use the blood pressure equipment on the 4-hour regimen or as needed depending on maternal, fetal, and/or labor status. Emerging risk factors warrant closer surveillance. Women, or the unborn fetuses, who are at risk of infection need closer monitoring of maternal body temperature and pulse. Women with a labor epidural in place, those experiencing induction or augmentation of labor with oxytocin, or those who are hypertensive are more likely to have blood pressure fluctuations and need closer monitoring (Cunnigham et al., 2014; King et al., 2015).

Hourly or continuous blood pressure measurements have not been determined to serve a clinical purpose in the absence of pathology or interventions warranting closer evaluation, and are not consistent with the recommendations of some of the professional organizations involved in maternity care or expert opinions in the field (CABC, 2015; Cunningham et al., 2014; NICE, 2014). Excessive blood pressure readings are at least an annoyance and at most a tethering, detrimental intervention. This is especially true of the "double check" automated readings attached to short cables that restrict movement. These readings are frequently monitoring for nonexistent blood pressure problems (Holland & Lewis, 2014; Ogedegbe & Pickering, 2010). Increased freedom of movement enhances maternal autonomy and comfort, the progress of labor, and returns the decision to move to the woman.

### Monitoring Fetal Well-Being During Labor

Continuous electronic fetal monitoring (continuous EFM) is one of the most routine and tethering practices used in the United States with women at low risk for complications (Cahill & Spain, 2015). Recommendations for continuous EFM and for intermittent auscultation (IA) for monitoring fetal heart rate (FHR) vary across organizations (ACNM, 2015c; ACOG, 2009b; AWHONN, 2015; Ayres-de-Campos, Spong, & Chandraharan, 2015; Lewis & Downe, 2015). Outcomes with continuous EFM are not superior to IA (Ayres-de-Campos et al., 2015; Cahill & Spain, 2015).

ACOG, as part of its latest practice bulletin on FHR auscultation, released the findings of a meta-analysis of randomized controlled trials (RCTs), showing no benefit of continuous EFM over IA with low-risk women or any good evidence regarding recommended frequency and duration of IA (ACOG, 2009b). The recommendations of this ACOG practice bulletin were reaffirmed in 2015 (ACOG, 2016).

The most recent Cochrane meta-analysis on continuous EFM concluded that continuous EFM is associated with increased numbers of instrument-assisted births and more cesarean births without improvement in newborn outcomes (Alfirevic, Devane, & Gyte, 2013). Several subsequent studies have confirmed these findings (Jackson & Gregory, 2015; Jenniskens & Janssen, 2015; Rossignol, Chaillet, Boughrassa, & Moutquin, 2014)

The present ACOG guidelines do not take a position in favor of either continuous EFM or IA (ACOG, 2009b); but the AWHONN and International Federation of Gynecology and Obstetrics (FIGO) guidelines favor IA (AWHONN, 2015; Lewis & Downe, 2015). The ACNM (2015c) supports IA as the preferred method for women with low-risk pregnancies, stating, "IA is the preferred method for monitoring the FHR during labor for women at term who at the onset of labor are at low risk for developing fetal acidemia" (p. 631). IA minimally disrupts a woman in labor and does not tether her to the EFM machine. IA is a best practice supported by ACNM and unopposed by ACOG. IA promotes the woman's ability to choose to move during labor and provides comfort and progress of labor (ACNM, 2015c; AWHONN, 2015; Lewis & Downe, 2015). In addition, ambulation and being upright during labor are associated with a lower incidence of decelerations of FHR (King & Pinger, 2014).

Continuous or nearly continuous EFM has become the standard of care, and is favored or required in most hospital settings with limited accurate information available to the public for the purposes of informed consent (Torres, DeVries, & Low, 2014). One reason for this ubiquitous practice is the highly litigious environment in the United States (Eggemont, 2015; Maso et al., 2015). Another reason is the fallacious nature of the culture of safety, the perception that more technology predicts and protects birth outcomes (Brown, Johnstone, & Heazell, 2015; Conason & Pegalis, 2010). This perception needs to be addressed among maternity care clinicians.

## Pain Management in Labor

Much of the tethering observed in typical hospital labor management arises from the use of pharmacological intervention (Clark et al., 2015; Frey et al., 2015; Nicholson et al., 2015). In the United States, fear of pain is grounded in cultural beliefs around childbirth, which proliferate through the most popular consumer books on pregnancy and childbirth (Magee & Nakisbendi, 2012; McCarthy, 2014;

Murkoff & Mazel, 2008). Caregivers often assume that optimal or total pain relief is very important to most laboring women and that those women who avoid pharmacological pain-relief measures must be misinformed (Hawkins, 2015; Pugliese et al., 2013; Sng, Kwok, & Sia, 2015). Over the course of the past 15 years, a variety of studies in several countries have demonstrated that pain relief is not a major determinant of maternal satisfaction, unless expectations are not met (Bianchi & Adams, 2009; Cook & Loomis, 2012; Hodnett, 2002; Karlsdottir, Sveinsdottir, Olafsdottir, & Kristjansdottir, 2015; Leeman, Fontaine, King, Klein, & Ratcliffe, 2003; McLachlan et al., 2015; Van der Gucht & Lewis, 2015).

Pain relief and maternal satisfaction with pain relief are different issues altogether (Lindholm & Hildingsson, 2015; Madden, Turnbull, Cyna, Adelson, & Wilkinson, 2013). Feeling supported and comforted in labor appear to be primary drivers of maternal satisfaction, reducing rates of posttraumatic stress and decreasing the need for intervention in the physiologic birth process (Andersen, Melvaer, Videbech, Lamont, & Joergensen, 2012; Aune, Amundsen, & Skaget Ass, 2014; Garthus-Niegel, von Soest, Vollrath, & Eberhard-Gran, 2013; Goutaudier, Séjourné, Rousset, Lami, & Chabrol, 2012; Nikula, Laukkala, & Pölkki, 2015; Ross-Davie & Cheyne, 2014).

The authors of the only Cochrane Review to date on pain management in labor (Jones et al., 2012) found that the experience of pain in labor is variable and may be influenced by position, mobility, fear, anxiety, and/or confidence in one's ability to give birth. In addition, the majority of studies of pain relief in labor examine drug intervention (Capogna & Stirparo, 2013; Chen et al., 2014; Dualé et al., 2015; Heesen et al., 2015; Patel et al., 2014; Pugliese et al., 2013; Sng et al., 2015; Wassen et al., 2015), far fewer examine nondrug interventions (Bonapace, Chaillet, Gaumond, Paul-Savorie, & Marchand, 2013; Chen & Wang, 2014; Shirvani & Ganji, 2014), and comparisons across studies are difficult because of variability regarding how pain intensity is measured, including the woman's sense of control in labor (Jones et al., 2012).

### The Role of Pain in Labor

Anthropologists and evolutionary ecologists have suggested that the purpose of pain in labor is to alert the woman that birth is imminent, direct her to seek shelter, and to elicit caring behaviors among her support system (Lefebvre, 2012; Lowe, 2002). Others state that the character and purpose of pain in labor are poorly understood (Maul, 2007; Wong, 2010). Unmitigated pain and anxiety in protracted dysfunctional labors result in excessive catecholamine secretion, unbalancing the relationship between oxytocin and catecholamines in normal labor (Aral, Köken, Bozkurt, Sahin, & Demirel, 2014). Several studies' conclusions have also suggested that unmitigated, severe labor pain may contribute to postpartum depression and posttraumatic stress disorder (PTSD; Beck, Gable, Sakala, & Declercq, 2011; Garthus-Niegel, Knoph, von Soest, Nielsen, & Eberhard-Gran, 2014; James, 2015). Overarching themes in the birth stories among women with harrowing birth experiences are loss of sense of control, and poor communication around interventions and outcomes (e.g., episiotomy, instrumental vaginal birth, emergent cesarean birth, or a damaged neonate). Only a small portion of women who suffer from depressive disorders postpartum or PTSD report that they experienced severe, unmitigated labor pain (Beck et al., 2011; Garthus-Niegel et al., 2013).

## Pharmacological Pain Management in Normal Labor

### Epidural Analgesia

In comparison to all other available pharmacological analgesics deemed safe to use during labor, the evidence is convincing that epidural analgesia provides higher scores for maternal pain relief as well as satisfaction with pain relief (Attanasio, Kozhimannil, Jou, McPherson, & Camann, 2015; Gizzo, Noventa, et al., 2014; Grant, Tao, Craig, McIntire, & Leveno, 2015; Sng et al., 2014). The debate continues on the transient positive or adverse effects of epidurals on mother, fetus, and/or labor (Ismail, 2013; Miller, Cypher, Nielsen, & Flogia, 2013; Wassen et al., 2014); or the potential long-term adverse effects on mother, infant, and mother–infant dyad (Bannister-Tyrrell, Ford, Morris, & Roberts, 2014; Dozier et al., 2013; Goer, 2015; Lind, Perrine, & Li, 2014; Ranganathan et al., 2015). Complicating the debate is the fact that most of the epidural anesthesia research is reported by anesthesiologists.

Epidural analgesia for labor alters the physiology of labor and increases the risk for hypotension, increased temperature, difficulty with or inability to void, itching, nausea, longer pushing stage, and immobility (Goer & Romano, 2012; Sakala & Corry, 2008). It has been suggested that epidural analgesia interferes with the secretion of oxytocin and catecholamine peaks toward the end of labor, diminishing uterine contractility and the ejection reflex (Buckley, 2015). These physiologic alterations may contribute to the cascade of interventions by increasing the need for exogenous oxytocin and increasing the length of the second stage (Leveno, Nelson, & McIntire, 2015; Sindik et al., 2012).

Epidural analgesia limits mobility during labor because of the tethering effect of multiple lines, the necessity to continuous EFM, and frequent maternal blood pressure readings (Goer & Romano, 2012; Simkin & Archeta, 2011). Not only is ambulation compromised or unmanageable leading to bed confinement, but maternal position changes often require assistance. Other barriers to mobility also include inadequate leg strength and physical stamina (Goer & Romano, 2012).

Anim-Somouah, Smyth, and Jones (2011), in the latest Cochrane Review contrasting epidural use in labor versus no epidural use, concluded that epidural and combined spinal–epidural effectively manage labor pain but may contribute to adverse events, including cesarean birth for fetal distress, need for augmentation of labor with exogenous oxytocin, prolonged second stage, urinary retention, hypotension, fever, and continued motor blockade for a time after birth. As a result of the effects of pharmacological pain management, the woman is less capable of making decisions about her activity and movement in labor (Goer & Romano, 2012). Lack of decision-making capacity may adversely affect a women's perception of comfort and safety during labor.

*Parental Opioids in Labor*

Parental opioids have fallen into relative disuse as the use of labor epidurals has increased. Although hundreds of studies on labor epidural use are published every year, in the past 10 to 15 years, publication of studies on the effects of parental opioids on laboring women has been minimal. Therefore, the efficacy and safety of parenteral opioid administration to control labor pain has not been well demonstrated in the most current literature (Anderson, 2011).

Morphine (administered intramuscularly) is used primarily for sedation, that is, "therapeutic sleep" in the latent phase of labor (Anderson, 2011). Fentanyl (Sublimaze, administered most often intravenously) has been recently documented as having deleterious effects on breastfeeding initiation during the first postpartum hour (Brimdyr et al., 2015). However, other authors (Fleet, Jones, & Belan, 2014) reported subcutaneously administered fentanyl, not widely used in the United States, as having a significantly positive effect on maternal pain scores 30 minutes postadministration with comparable neonatal outcomes (i.e., Apgar scores, length of hospital stay, and breastfeeding on discharge) to the control group. In addition, the mothers remained alert and no antiemetic use was required.

Serious neonatal respiratory depression occurring after large dosages of intramuscular or intravenous opioid administration to laboring women has been well documented (Anderson, 2011). Jones et al. (2012) reviewed more than 100 studies of parenteral opioid administration for pain relief in labor and concluded that there is insufficient evidence on parental opioids being more effective than placebos but found evidence that opioids administered in labor cause nausea, vomiting, and FHR abnormalities. Although the administration of narcotics may theoretically not interfere with the ability of a laboring woman to ambulate, the potential side effects of nausea, vomiting, dizziness, and sedation make it less likely that the woman would choose mobility or that it would be safe for her to be out of bed. In addition, many institutions restrict ambulation of the woman under the influence of parental opioids as a safety measure to prevent falls (Anderson, 2011).

The authors of the latest Cochrane Review of parenteral opioids for management of labor pain (Ullman, Smith, Burns, Mori, & Dowswell, 2010) concluded that up to two thirds of women who receive opioids report moderate to severe pain within 1 to 2 hours after administration. Common side effects include maternal drowsiness, nausea, and vomiting. No clear evidence of adverse effects to the newborn was found. Given the limited utility of intravenous or intramuscular opioids for managing labor pain and their side effects, most notably the effect on maternal mobility, their widespread use during labor should not be promoted.

## Nonpharmacological Pain Management

In view of the numerous challenges to maternal mobility in labor with the use pharmacological pain management and the ensuing cascade of interventions, a strong case can be made for nonpharmacological management as the best practice to support physiologic birth. There are safe, cost-effective, and potentially satisfying methods of nonpharmacological pain management. Most nonpharmacological pain-control measures used in labor either facilitate or require freedom of movement. Freedom of movement alone is an effective intervention for relief of pain in labor, facilitating optimum fetal positioning, and shortening the length of labor (Chaillet et al., 2014; Ondeck, 2014). Jones et al. (2012) concluded that there is some evidence suggesting that immersion in water, relaxation, acupuncture, and massage may decrease labor pain with few adverse effects.

In 2002, Simkin and O'Hara published a groundbreaking review of studies with sufficient rigor to assess the efficacy of nonpharmacological pain relief. Five effective strategies were extrapolated from the literature:

- Continuous labor support
- Upright position
- Change of position
- Immersion in water
- Temporary pain-reduction measures

These five strategies have been further developed over the past two decades (Amran et al., 2014; Ruhl et al., 2006; Shilling, Difranco, & Simkin, 2004; Simkin, 2003; Simkin & Bolding, 2004; Simkin & Hull, 2011) and advanced for consumer dissemination through three editions of *The Labor Progress Handbook* (Simkin & Archeta, 2011). The first three strategies have been incorporated into the Lamaze Healthy Birth Practices (Green & Hotelling, 2014; Ondeck, 2014).

### Continuous Labor Support

Continuous support provided by partners or other relatives may be problematic as a result of lack of objectivity and experience. Labor support provided by a nurse or a midwife may be unpredictable because of inadequate staffing and the need to attend to other women. Continuous labor support by a trained layperson (such as a doula) has been identified as an effective pain-relieving strategy, especially for women laboring without strong family support (Green & Hotelling, 2014). A 2013 Cochrane Review corroborated these findings (Hodnett, Gates, Hofmeyr, & Sakala, 2013). This review combined the results from 21 RCTs involving more than 15,000 women. Continuous labor support provided by persons outside of the woman's social network, such as doulas, was the most effective (Hodnett et al., 2013).

Women who received continuous labor support were more likely to have a spontaneous vaginal birth and less likely to have interventions, including regional analgesia, cesarean birth, or instrumental vaginal birth (Hodnett et al., 2013). Labors were shortened by a mean of 58 minutes and there were few low 5-minute Apgar scores. The women with continuous labor support were less likely to report dissatisfaction with their labor experience and satisfaction with the birth was noted to be greater (Hodnett et al., 2013). Continuous labor support has meaningful benefits for women and infants and causes no known harm. Unfortunately, continuous labor support is the exception rather than the norm in U.S. obstetrical settings.

*Upright Position*

Maintenance of upright positioning in labor has demonstrated benefits for facilitating fetal descent, increasing uterine contractility, and shortening the length of labor (Kumud & Chopra, 2013). In their review, Simkin and O'Hara (2002) examined the research conducted by Caldeyro-Barcia and associates in the 1950s and 1960s (Diaz, Schwarcz, Fescina, & Caldeyro-Barcia, 1980), which concluded that upright positioning during labor caused more frequent and stronger uterine contractions, and facilitated cervical dilation. Maternal pain perception in relation to position was not evaluated (Diaz et al., 1980). Simkin and O'Hara (2002) also evaluated five studies that addressed maternal pain perception in relation to position. The women were their own controls. The women rated labor pain in various positions: sitting versus side-lying and standing versus supine. None of the participants found supine positioning as comfortable as any of the alternatives. The authors of a recent Cochrane Review (Lawrence, Lewis, Hofmeyr, & Styles, 2013) found that various upright positions, commonly employed by laboring women in other countries, reduced the length of the first stage of labor as well as the need for epidural analgesia.

*Change of Position*

Cultural influences and maternal expectations inform a woman about birth position (e.g., kneeling, squatting, sitting, lying, or standing). The lithotomy position and flat dorsal positions for birth were American inventions, dating back to the first half of the 1800s, and are not evidence based (Gupta & Nikoderm, 2000). Although it is now less common for women to birth flat on their backs, variations of the lithotomy position are still the most common positions for birth (Priddis, Dahlen, & Schmied, 2012).

Historically, two observational studies in U.S. hospitals in the mid-1980s noted that, without specific nursing instruction, many laboring women moved around in bed, yet few assumed upright positions or ambulated during labor (Carlson et al., 1986; Rossi & Lindell, 1986). Carlson et al. (1986) noted that the most common position assumed during the first stage of labor was lying on the left side, usually twice as often as lying on the right side. Although the study was intended to observe labor position without coaching, it is likely that cultural influences (e.g., prior labor experience, shared stories, prenatal education classes, coaching by labor room personnel, and depictions of labor in popular culture) influenced maternal position more than spontaneous inclination (Carlson et al., 1986). Now, 30 years later, some of these cultural norms are beginning to change with women opting for a greater variety of labor and birth positions (Gizzo, Di Gangi, et al., 2014). Fostering a culture of normal physiologic birth can influence women to listen to their bodies and make their own decisions about optimal position during labor and birth.

Epidural analgesia limits birth positions. For women without epidurals, side-lying and upright positions were found in a Cochrane Review to be associated with decreased severity of pain, fewer heart rate abnormalities for the fetus, shorter pushing phase (though not statistically significant), less use of episiotomies, and less use of interventions, such as forceps and vacuum extraction for birth, but an increase in blood loss greater than 500 mL was reported (Gupta, Hofmeyr, & Shehmar, 2012). The authors of this Cochrane Review suggest several benefits to upright positioning in labor and support women in making their own choices about positioning in second-stage labor (Gupta et al., 2012).

In another Cochrane Review, Kemp, Kingswood, Kibuka, and Thornton (2013) examined women utilizing recumbent or upright positions in second-stage labor with or without epidural analgesia. The authors found no difference in the rate of instrumental vaginal birth, cesarean section, or length of second-stage labor. Although the data at this juncture are insufficient, the authors concluded that women should assume whatever position they find most comfortable for the second stage (Kemp et al., 2013).

### Hydrotherapy, Including Water Immersion

The use of water as therapy in labor has become increasingly popular in the United States (Brickhouse, Isaacs, Batten, & Price, 2015; Lee, Liu, Lu, & Gau, 2013; Weaver, 2014). Although intrapartum hydrotherapy most often brings water birth to mind, there is also the use of warm showers, and water immersion during the first and second stages of labor to increase maternal comfort during subsequent land birth (Lee et al., 2013; Liu et al., 2014; Stark, 2013). Initial concerns over bathing with ruptured membranes have not been confirmed as harmful (Harper, 2014).

In the latest Cochrane Review (Cluett & Burns, 2009 [last assessed as up to date, 2011]), the authors reported there is no increased risk of maternal or neonatal infection from immersion in water during labor. This review of 11 RCTs ($n = 3,000$ women) demonstrated a significant reduction in analgesia/anesthesia of all types when women used water immersion as a method of pain relief in labor, and a decrease in the length of the first stage of labor. There was no difference between water birth versus land birth in perineal trauma, maternal/neonatal infection, score of 5-minute Apgar less than 7, or neonatal intensive care unit (NICU) admission (Cluett & Burns, 2009).

To address neonatal safety concerns, Davies, Pearce, and Wong (2015) engaged in a systemic review and meta-analysis of 12 studies. In the evaluation of neonatal morbidity and mortality, the differences in outcome between the water-birth and land-birth groups were too small to reach statistical significance.

More than a decade ago, Simkin and O'Hara (2002) reviewed and reported the physiological changes that may contribute to the efficacy of water immersion during labor. Warmth and buoyancy release muscle tension and may create a sense of well-being that decreases catecholamine production, facilitating labor progress, especially in anxious women. Buoyancy promotes the freedom of movement and maternal positioning known to facilitate optimal fetal positioning. Hydrostatic pressure on peripheral tissues helps the fetus achieve and maintain a flexed position in direct proportion to the amount of surface area immersed. Fluid moves from peripheral tissues to the intravascular space, and blood is redistributed to the thorax. The expanded blood volume triggers the release of atrial natriuretic factor suppressing the production of vasopressin in the posterior pituitary gland. Because oxytocin is also produced by the posterior pituitary, it is possible that oxytocin is suppressed along with vasopressin. This phenomenon may account for the gradual slowing of labor noted when water immersion lasts longer than 90 minutes. This theory may also explain why immersion in early labor might slow labor progress.

The essential directives for safe water birth have not significantly changed over the past 15 years. It is recommended that water temperature should be at body temperature to avoid a rise in maternal core body temperature. The woman should immerse herself to cover her abdomen but leave the shoulders and upper chest exposed to facilitate heat dissipation while maintaining buoyancy and warmth. Bathing episodes should be limited to 90 minutes to prevent oxytocin suppression (Nutter, Shaw-Battista, & Marowitz, 2014; Simkin & O'Hara, 2002). ACNM (2014) supports water immersion as a safe and drug-free measure that reduces labor pain and enhances movement (see Chapter 22).

### Temporary Pain-Reduction Measures

Interest in temporary, nonpharmacological pain-reduction measures is as old as childbirth (Dick-Read, 2013). There was an initial 2006 Cochrane Review on non-pharmacological measures (Smith, Collins, Cyna, & Crowther, 2006). At that time, Smith and colleagues (2006) reported insufficient evidence on the efficacy of the use of mind–body techniques, relaxation, white noise, music, massage, reflexology, acupressure, acupuncture, aromatherapy, and homeopathy. The authors concluded that hypnosis decreases the need for labor augmentation, increases the incidence of spontaneous vaginal birth, and has a high rate of maternal satisfaction. Acupuncture may decrease the need for oxytocin augmentation and analgesia, including epidural analgesia, but differences in needling techniques decreased the strength of these conclusions. The authors proposed that using more than one of these techniques sequentially or simultaneously may provide greater pain relief and enhance maternal satisfaction (C. A. Smith et al., 2006).

Subsequent Cochrane Reviews evaluating relaxation techniques (Smith, Levett, Collins, & Crowther, 2011); acupuncture and acupressure (Smith, Collins, Crowther, & Levett, 2011); aromatherapy (Smith, Collins, & Crowther, 2011); hypnosis (Madden, Middleton, Cyna, Matthewson, & Jones, 2012); and massage, reflexology, and other manual methods for pain management in labor (Smith, Levett, Collins, & Jones, 2012) concluded with recommendations for further research because of insufficient evidence secondary to the prevalent lack of RCTs or quasi-RCT data. The authors determined that hypnosis use in labor shows promise (Madden et al., 2012); massage, acupressure, and acupuncture may have a role in decreasing pain as well as improving the laboring woman's emotional outlook, including satisfaction with pain management and the experience of labor (Smith, Collins, et al., 2011; Smith, Levett, et al., 2011); and acupressure and acupuncture may lead to a decrease in the need for pharmacological management (Smith, Collins, et al., 2011). Yet another Cochrane Review by Jones et al. (2012) concluded there was insufficient evidence to determine whether hypnosis, biofeedback, sterile water papules, aromatherapy, or transcutaneous electrical nerve stimulation (TENS) is more effective than placebo in ameliorating labor pain.

The lack of side effects of all these modalities is significant in promoting freedom of movement and physiologic birth. All nonpharmacological interventions reviewed have demonstrated safety, efficacy, and high rates of maternal satisfaction. These interventions are cost-effective and represent best practices in implementing the recommendation from the BirthTOOLS toolkit (ACNM, 2015d).

## BEST PRACTICES TO FOSTER PHYSIOLOGIC BIRTH

In 2011, a joint position statement was endorsed by ACNM, ACOG, AWHONN, the American College of Osteopathic Obstetricians and Gynecologists, the Society for Maternal–Fetal Medicine, the American Academy of Family Physicians, and the American Academy of Pediatrics. The position statement supported birth as a physiologic process, stating most women should be able to labor and birth with minimal to no intervention (Lawrence et al., 2012).

ACNM, the National Association of Certified Professional Midwives (NACPM), and the Midwives Alliance of North America (MANA) recently formulated a description of characteristics of physiologic birth (Kennedy et al., 2015). This description was the impetus for the creation of BirthTOOLS, a toolkit for clinicians that promotes safe and physiologic birth (ACNM, 2015d). In this toolkit, areas specifically identified as disruptive to physiologic birth are lack of support persons, nutritional deprivation, use of opiates, regional analgesia, general anesthesia, and situations leading the woman to feel unsupported or threatened (ACNM, 2015d). Examples of such situations could include limiting positions or restricting change of positions, and inflexible guidelines on the use of hydrotherapy, touch, or massage. The BirthTOOLS toolkit contains evidence-based guidance organized into the following sections:

- Promoting progress in the first stage of labor
- Assessment of fetal well-being
- Comfort and coping in labor
- Nutrition and hydration during labor (ACNM, 2015d)

King and Pinger (2014) identified best practices that promote physiologic birth in the *Pearls of Midwifery*. Some specific *pearls* or concepts related to untethering are:

- Oral nutrition in labor is safe, optimizing outcomes
- Ambulation and freedom of movement in labor are safe, satisfying for women, and facilitate labor
- Hydrotherapy is safe and effective in decreasing pain during active labor
- Continuous labor support should be standard care
- IA should be standard care for low-risk women (King & Pinger, 2014)

Clinicians have access to a variety of evidence-based resources to learn, adopt, and integrate best practices for untethering. Women and families have access to information enabling them to make informed choices. The evidence-based information on best practices for untethered labor and birth is being disseminated. There is positive change underway in the direction of promoting untethering and physiologic birth.

---

**USING THE EVIDENCE FOR BEST PRACTICE**

**Case Study 18.1    Untethered in Labor: Birth Outcome and Maternal Satisfaction**

Samantha Jo (S.J.) is a 25-year-old gravida 2 para 1 woman at 39 weeks, 3 days gestation. S.J. arrives at the hospital in active first-stage labor. S.J. denies spontaneous rupture of membranes or vaginal bleeding and reports good fetal movement. S.J. is accompanied by her husband and her doula. The midwife determines S.J. is 6-cm dilated, 90% effaced, and—1 station with bulging bag of waters. S.J.'s contractions are moderate to strong by palpation, and she rates her pain as 8 of 10. S.J. is admitted for labor care and is assigned a nurse who is currently caring for a woman who gave birth about 2 hours ago. S.J.'s husband reports he is relieved that she is being admitted because he wanted to come to the hospital hours ago, but Ginny, their doula, explained that S.J. should have to stop and breathe with each contraction while ambulating at home before coming to the hospital.

S.J. is given a choice of either wearing her own clothes or the hospital's gown. The nurse listens to fetal heart tones per intermittent monitoring protocol and takes S.J.'s vital signs, explaining to S.J. that her blood pressure should be assessed again in 4 hours and fetal heart tones should be assessed again in 15 minutes. S.J.'s nurse brings her a water pitcher and offers light food and juice from the unit kitchen. The nurse orients S.J., her husband, and the doula to the room and encourages her to sit on a birth ball, stand, ambulate, bathe, or walk in the hallways as S.J. pleases. S.J.'s midwife remains close at hand, assesses S.J.'s comfort, offers reassurance, and answers questions. The midwife encourages S.J. to use a variety of positions and bathing to facilitate labor and increase comfort while assisting S.J. to position herself on a birthing ball. After 4 hours of active laboring while alternating bathing, walking, and resting, S.J. gives birth to an 8-pound male infant with an Apgar score of 9/9.

**Exemplar of Best Practice**

S.J. benefited from continuous labor support by a family member and a trained doula of her choice. S.J. was admitted when clearly in active labor. S.J.'s nurse and midwife joined S.J. and her support persons in establishing her plan of care and assessed her sense of well-being as well as her physical needs for comfort and sustenance. Evidence-based practices were used to manage S.J.'s discomfort, including frequent position changes, a variety of nonpharmacological pain-mitigating measures, oral intake, and appropriate monitoring of maternal and fetal vital signs.

---

# REFERENCES

Alfirevic, Z., Devane, D., & Gyte, G. M. (2013). Continuous cardiotocography (CTG) as a form of electronic fetal monitoring (EFM) for fetal assessment during labour. *Cochrane Database of Systematic Reviews, 2013*(5). doi:10.1002/14651858.CD006066.pub2

American College of Nurse-Midwives (ACNM). (2014). Hydrotherapy during labor and birth [Position statement]. Retrieved from http://www.midwife.org/ACNM/files/ACNMLibrary Data/UPLOADFILENAME/000000000286/Hydrotherapy-During-Labor-and-Birth-April -2014.pdf

American College of Nurse-Midwives (ACNM). (2015a). A focus on physiologic birth: What is physiologic birth? Retrieved from http://www.birthtools.org/What-Is-Physiologic-Birth

American College of Nurse-Midwives (ACNM). (2015b). A menu of change: Nutrition and hydration during labor. Retrieved from http://birthtools.org/MOC-Nutrition-Hydration-During -Labor.

American College of Nurse-Midwives (ACNM). (2015c). Intermittent auscultation for intrapartum fetal heart rate surveillance. *Journal of Midwifery & Women's Health, 60*(5), 626–632. doi:10.1111/jmwh.12372

American College of Nurse-Midwives (ACNM). (2015d). BirthTOOLS.org: Tools for optimizing the outcomes of labor safely. Retrieved from http://birthtools.org

American College of Obstetricians and Gynecologists (ACOG). (n.d.). *ACOG Committee Opinion No. 441: Oral intake during labor* (Reaffirmed 2013). Retrieved from http://www .acog.org/Resources-And-Publications/Committee-Opinions/Committee-on-Obstetric -Practice/Oral-Intake-During-Labor

American College of Obstetricians and Gynecologists (ACOG). (2009a). ACOG Committee Opinion No. 441: Oral intake during labor. Obstetrics & Gynecology, *114*(3), 703–715. doi:10.1097/AOG.0b013e3181ba0649

American College of Obstetricians and Gynecologists (ACOG). (2009b). Intrapartum fetal heart rate monitoring: Nomenclature, interpretation, and general management principles (Practice Bulletin No. 106). *Obstetrics & Gynecology, 114*(1), 192–209. doi:10.1097/ AOG.0b013e3181aef106

American College of Obstetricians and Gynecologists (ACOG). (2016). Practice bulletin— Clinical management guidelines for obstetricians-gynecologists. Retrieved from https:// www.acog.org/-/media/List-of-Titles/PBListOfTitles.pdf

Amran, N. L., Klein, M. C., Mok, H., Simkin, P., Lindstrom, K., & Grant, J. (2014). How birth doulas help clients adapt to changes in circumstances, clinical care, and client preferences during labor. *Journal of Perinatal Education, 23*(2), 96–103. doi:10.1891/1058 -1243.23.2.96

Andersen, L., Melvaer, L., Videbech, P., Lamont, R., & Joergensen, J. (2012). Risk factors for developing post-traumatic stress disorder following childbirth: A systematic review. *Acta Obstetricia et Gynecologica Scandinavica, 91*(11), 1261–1272. doi:10.1111/j.1600-0412 .2012.01476x

Anderson, D. (2011). A review of systemic opioids commonly used for labor pain relief. *Journal of Midwifery and Women's Health, 56*(4), 222–239. doi:10.1111/j.1542-2011.2011.00061.x

Anim-Somouah, M., Smyth, R. M., & Jones, L. (2011). Epidural versus non-epidural or no analgesia in labor. *Cochrane Database of Systematic Reviews, 2011*(12). doi:10.1002/14651858 .CD000333.pub.3

Aral, I., Köken, G., Bozkurt, M., Sahin, F. K., & Demirel, R. (2014). Evaluation of the effects of maternal anxiety on the duration of vaginal labour delivery. *Clinical and Experimental Obstetrics and Gynecology, 41*(1), 32–36.

Attanasio, L., Kozhimannil, K. B., Jou, J., McPherson, M. E., & Camann, W. (2015). Women's experiences with neuraxial labor analgesia in the Listening to Mothers II Survey: A content analysis of open-ended responses. *Anesthesia and Analgesia, 121*(4), 974–980. doi:10.1213/ANE.0000000000000546

Aune, I., Amundsen, H. H., & Skaget Ass, L. C. (2014). Is a midwife's continuous presence during childbirth a matter of course? Midwives experiences and thoughts about factors that may influence their continuous support of women during labour. *Midwifery, 30*(1), 89–95. doi:10.1016/j.midw.2013.02.001

Ayres-de-Campos, D., Spong, C. Y., & Chandraharan, E. (2015). FIGO consensus guidelines on intrapartum fetal monitoring: Cardiotocography. *International Journal of Gynaecology and Obstetrics, 131*(1), 13–24. doi:10.1016/j.ijgo.2015.06.020

Bannister-Tyrrell, M., Ford, J. B., Morris, J. M., & Roberts, C. L. (2014). Epidural analgesia in labour and the risk of caesarean delivery. *Paediatric and Perinatal Epidemiology, 28*(5), 400–411. doi:10.1111/ppe.12139

Beck, C. T., Gable, R. K., Sakala, C., & Declercq, E. (2011). Posttraumatic stress disorder in new mothers: Results from a two-stage U.S. national survey. *Birth, 38*(3), 216–227. doi:10.1111/j.1523-536X.2011.00475.x

Bianchi, A. L., & Adams, E. D. (2009). Labor support during the second stage of labor for women with epidurals: Birth in this era is technology driven. *Nursing for Women's Health, 13*(1), 38–47. doi:10.1111/j.1751-486X.2009.01372.x

Bonapace, J., Chaillet, N., Gaumond, I., Paul-Savoie, E., & Marchand, S. (2013). Evaluation of the Bonapace Method: A specific educational intervention to reduce pain during childbirth. *Journal of Pain Research, 6*, 653–661. doi:10.2147/JPR.S46693

Brickhouse, B., Isaacs, C., Batten, M., & Price, A. (2015). Strategies for providing low-cost water immersion therapy with limited resources. *Nursing for Women's Health, 19*(6), 526–532. doi:10.1111/1751-486X.12247

Brimdyr, K., Cadwell, K., Widström, A. M., Svensson, K., Neumann, M., Hart, E. A., . . . Phillips, R. (2015). The association between common labor drugs and suckling when skin-to-skin during the first hour after birth. *Birth, 42*(4), 319–328. doi:10.1111/birt.12186

Brody, H., & Sakala, C. (2013). Revisiting "The maximin strategy in modern obstetrics." *Journal of Clinical Ethics, 24*(3), 198–206.

Brown, R., Johnstone, E. D., & Heazell, A. E. (2015). Professionals' views of fetal monitoring support the development of devices to provide objective longer term assessment of fetal wellbeing. *Journal of Maternal–Fetal and Neonatal Medicine.* Advance online publication. doi:10.3109/14767058.2015.1059808

Buckley, S. (2015). *Hormonal physiology of childbearing: Evidence and implications for women, babies, and maternity care.* New York, NY: Childbirth Connection.

Cahill, A. G., & Spain, J. (2015). Intrapartum fetal monitoring. *Clinical Obstetrics and Gynecology, 58*(2), 263–268. doi:10.1097/GRF.0000000000000109

Capogna, G., & Stirparo, S. (2013). Techniques for the maintenance of epidural anesthesia. *Current Opinion in Anaesthesiology, 26*(3), 261–267. doi:10.1097/ACO.0b013e328360b069

Carlson, J. M., Diehl, J. A., Sachtleben-Murray, M., McRae, M., Fenwick, L., & Friedman, E. A. (1986). Maternal position during parturition in normal labor. *Obstetrics and Gynecology, 68*(4), 443–447.

Centers for Disease Control and Prevention (CDC). (2015). Births: Preliminary data for 2014. *National Vital Statistics Report, 64*(6), 1–19. Retrieved from http://www.cdc.gov/nchs/data/nvsr/nvsr64/nvsr64_06.pdf

Chaillet, N., Belaid, C., Crochetière, C., Roy, L., Gagné, G. B., Moutquin, J. M., . . . Bonapace, J. (2014). Nonpharmacologic approaches for pain management during labor compared with usual care: A meta-analysis. *Birth, 41*(2), 122–137. doi:10.1111/birt.12103

Chen, S., Lin, P., Yang, Y., Yang, Y., Lee, C., Fan, S., & Chen, L. (2014). The effects of different epidural analgesia formulas on labor and mode of delivery in nulliparous women. *Taiwanese Journal of Obstetrics and Gynecology, 53*(1), 8–11. doi:10.1016/j.tjog.2012.01.039

Cheng, E. R., Declercq, E. R., Belanoff, C., Stotland, N. E., & Iverson, R. E. (2015). Labor and delivery experiences of mothers with suspected large babies. *Maternal and Child Health Journal, 19*(12), 2578–2586. doi:10.1007/s10995-015-1776-0

Childbirth Connection. (2010). 90 Years baby! Retrieved from http://www.childbirthconnection.org/pdfs/90-year-timeline.pdf

Childbirth Connection. (2016). History. Retrieved from http://www.childbirthconnection.org/article.asp?ck=10076

Clark, S. L., Meyers, J. A., Frye, D. K., Garthwaite, T., Lee, A. J., & Perlin, J. B. (2015). Recognition and response to electronic fetal heart rate patterns: Impact on newborn outcomes and primary cesarean delivery rate in women undergoing induction of labor. *American Journal of Obstetrics and Gynecology, 212*(1), 191.e1–191.e6. doi:10.1016/j.ajog.2014.11.019

Cluett, E. R., & Burns, E. (2009). Immersion in water in labour and birth. *Cochrane Database of Systematic Reviews, 2009*(7). doi:10.1002/14651858.CD000111.pub3

Commission for the Accreditation of Birth Centers (CABC). (2015). *Indicators of compliance with standards for birth centers.* Retrieved from https://www.birthcenteraccreditation.org/go/get-cabc-indicators

Conason, R. L., & Pegalis, S. E. (2010). Neurologic birth injury: Protecting the legal rights of the child. *Journal of Legal Medicine, 31*(3), 249–286. doi:10.1080/01947648.2010.505816

Cook, K., & Loomis, C. (2012). Impact of choice and control on women's childbirth experiences. *Journal of Perinatal Education, 21*(3), 158–168. doi:10.1891/1058-1243.21.3.158

Cunningham, F. G., Leveno, K. J., Bloom, S. L., Spong, C. Y., Dashe, J. S., Hoffman, B. L., . . . Sheffield, J. S. (2014). *Williams obstetrics* (24th ed.). New York, NY: McGraw-Hill.

Davies, D., Pearce, M., & Wong, N. (2015). The effect of waterbirth on neonatal mortality and morbidity: A systematic review and meta-analysis. *JBI Database of Systematic Reviews and Implementation Reports, 13*(10), 180–231. doi:10.11124/jbisrir-2015-2105

Davies, L., & Deery, R. (Eds.). (2014). *Nutrition in pregnancy and childbirth: Food for thought.* New York, NY: Routledge

Declercq, E. R., Sakala, C., Corry, M. P., & Applebaum, S. (2007). Listening to Mothers II: Report of the Second National U.S. Survey of Women's Childbearing Experiences. *Journal of Perinatal Education, 16*(4), 9–14. doi:10.1624%2F105812407X244769

Declercq, E. R., Sakala, C., Corry, M. P., Applebaum, S., & Herrlich, A. (2014). Listening to Mothers III: Pregnancy and birth: Report of the Third National U.S. Survey of Women's Childbearing Experiences. *Journal of Perinatal Education, 23*(1), 9–16. doi:10.1891/1058-1243.23.1.9

Diaz, A. G., Schwarcz, R., Fescina, R., & Caldeyro-Barcia, R. (1980). Vertical position during the first stage of the course of labor, and neonatal outcome. *European Journal of Obstetrics & Gynecology and Reproductive Biology, 11*(1), 1–7. doi:10.1016/0028-2243(80)90046-5

Dick-Read, G. (2013). *Childbirth without fear: The principles and practice of natural childbirth.* London, UK: Printer & Martin.

Dozier, A., Howard, C., Brownell, E., Wissler, R., Glantz, J., Ternullo, S., . . . Lawrence, R. (2013). Labor epidural anesthesia, obstetric factors, and breastfeeding cessation. *Maternal and Child Health Journal, 17*(4), 689–698. doi:10.1007/s10995-012-1045-4

Dualé, C., Nicolas-Courbon, A., Gerbaud, L., Lemery, D., Bonnin, M., & Pereira, B. (2015). Maternal satisfaction as an outcome criterion in research on labor analgesia: Data analysis from the recent literature. *Clinical Journal of Pain, 31*(3), 235–246. doi:10.1097/AJP.0000000000000106

Eggermont, M. (2015). Intrapartum care and substandard care: Judicial recommendations to reduce risk of liability. *Archives of Gynecology and Obstetrics, 292*(1), 87–95. doi:10.1007/s00404-014-3612-y

Fleet, J., Jones, M., & Belan, I. (2014). Subcutaneous administration of fentanyl in childbirth: An observational study on the clinical effectiveness of fentanyl for mother and neonate. *Midwifery, 30*(1), 36–42. doi:10.1016/j.midw.2013.01.014

Frey, H. A., Tuuli, M. G., England, S. K., Roehl, K. A., Odibo, A. O., Macones, G. A., & Cahill, A. G. (2015). Factors associated with higher oxytocin requirements in labor. *Journal of Maternal–Fetal and Neonatal Medicine, 28*(13), 1614–1619. doi:10.3109/14767058.2014.963046

Garthus-Niegel, S., Knoph, C., von Soest, T., Nielsen, C. S., & Eberhard-Gran, M. (2014). The role of labor pain and overall birth experience in the development of posttraumatic stress symptoms: A longitudinal cohort study. *Birth, 41*(1), 108–115. doi:10.1111/birt.12093

Garthus-Niegel, S., von Soest, T., Vollrath, M. E., & Eberhard-Gran, M. (2013). The impact of subjective birth experiences on post-traumatic stress symptoms: A longitudinal study. *Archives of Women's Mental Health, 16*(1), 1–10. doi:10.1007/s00737-012-0301-3

Gizzo, S., Di Gangi, S., Noventa, M., Bacile, V., Zambon, A., & Nardelli, G. B. (2014). Women's choice of position during labour: Return to the past or a modern way to give birth? A cohort study in Italy. *BioMed Research International, 2014*, 1–7. doi:10/1155/2014/638093

Gizzo, S., Noventa, M., Fagherazzi, S., Lamparelli, L., Ancona, E., Di Gangi, S., . . . Nardelli, G. B. (2014). Update on best available options in obstetrics anaesthesia: Perinatal outcomes, side effects and maternal satisfaction. Fifteen years systematic literature review. *Archives of Gynecology and Obstetrics, 290*(1), 21–34. doi:10.1007/s00404-014-3212-x

Goer, H. (2015). Epidurals: Do they or don't they increase cesareans? *Journal of Perinatal Education, 24*(4), 209–212. doi:10.1891/1058-1243.24.4.209

Goer, H., & Romano, A. (2012). *Optimal care in childbirth: The case for a physiological approach.* Seattle, WA: Classic Day.

Goutaudier, N., Séjourné, N., Rousset, C., Lami, C., & Chabrol, H. (2012). Negative emotions, childbirth pain, perinatal dissociation and self-efficacy as predictors of postpartum post-traumatic stress symptoms. *Journal of Reproductive and Infant Psychology, 30*(4), 352–362. doi:10.1080/02646838.2012.738415

Grant, E. N., Tao, W., Craig, M., McIntire, D., & Leveno, K. (2015). Neuraxial analgesia effects on labor progression: Facts, fallacies, uncertainties and the future. *British Journal of Obstetrics and Gynaecology, 122*(3), 288–293. doi:10.1111/1471-0528.12966

Green, J., & Hotelling, B. A. (2014). Healthy birth practice #3: Bring a loved one, friend, or doula for continuous labor support. *Journal of Perinatal Education, 23*(4), 194–197. doi:10.1891/1058-1243.23.4.194

Gupta, J. K., Hofmeyr, G. J., & Shehmar, M. (2012). Position in the second stage of labour for women without epidural anesthesia. *Cochrane Database of Systematic Reviews, 2012*(5). doi:10.1002/14651858.CD002006.pub3

Gupta, J. K., & Nikoderm, C. (2000). Maternal posture in labor. *European Journal of Obstetrics, Gynecology, and Reproductive Biology, 92*(2), 273–277. doi:10.1016/S0301 -2115(99)00272-9

Harper, B. (2014). Birth, bath, and beyond: The science and safety of water immersion during labor and birth. *Journal of Perinatal Education, 23*(3), 124–134. doi:10.1891/1058-1243 .23.3.124

Hawkins, J. L. (2015). 150 years in pursuit of optimal pain relief during labour. *International Journal of Obstetrics and Gynaecology, 122*(7), 993. doi:10.1111/1471-0528.13401

Heesen, M., Böhmer, J., Klör, S., Hoffman, T., Rosssaint, R., & Straube, S. (2015). The effect of adding a background infusion to patient-controlled epidural labor analgesia on labor, maternal, and neonatal outcomes: A systematic review and meta-analysis. *Anesthesia and Analgesia, 121*(1), 149–158. doi:10.1213/ANE.0000000000000743

Hodnett, E. (2002). Pain and women's satisfaction with the experience of childbirth: A systematic review. *American Journal of Obstetrics and Gynecology, 186*(5), S160–S172. doi: 10.1016/S0002-9378(02)70189-0

Hodnett, E. D., Gates, S., Hofmeyr, G. J., & Sakala, C. (2013). Continuous support for women during childbirth. *Cochrane Database of Systematic Reviews, 2013*(7). doi:10.1002/14651858 .CD003766.pub5

Holland, M., & Lewis, P. S. (2014). An audit and suggested guidelines for in-patient blood pressure measurement. *Journal of Hypertension, 32*(11), 2166–2170. doi:10.1097/HJH .0000000000000306

Ismail, S. (2013). Labor analgesia: An update on the effect of epidural anesthesia on labor outcome. *Journal of Obstetric Anesthesia and Critical Care, 3*(2), 70–73. doi:10.4103/2249 -4472.123297

Jackson, S., & Gregory, K. D. (2015). Management of the first stage of labor: Potential strategies to lower the cesarean delivery rate. *Clinical Obstetrics and Gynecology, 58*(2), 217–226. doi:10.1097/GRF.0000000000000102

James, S. (2015). Women's experiences of symptoms of posttraumatic stress disorder (PTSD) after traumatic childbirth: A review and critical appraisal. *Archives of Women's Health, 18*(6), 761–771. doi:10.1007/s00737-015-0560-x

Jenniskens, K., & Janssen, P. A. (2015). Newborn outcomes in British Columbia after cesarean section: Potential strategies to lower the cesarean delivery rate. *Journal of Obstetrics and Gynaecology Canada, 37*(3), 207–213.

Jones, L., Othman, M., Dowswell, T., Alfirevic, A. Gates, S., Newburn, M., . . . Neilson, J. P. (2012). Pain management for women in labor: An overview of systematic reviews. *Cochrane Database of Systematic Reviews, 2014*(3). doi:1002/14651858.CD009234.pub.2

Kachalia, A., & Bates, D. W. (2014). Disclosing medical errors: The view from the USA. *Surgeon, 12*(2), 64–67. doi:10.1016/j.surge.2013.12.002

Karlsdottir, S. I., Sveindottir, H., Olafsdottir, O. A., & Kristjansdottir, H. (2015). Pregnant women's expectations about pain intensity during childbirth and their attitudes towards pain management: Findings from an Icelandic national study. *Sexual and Reproductive Healthcare, 6*(4), 211–218. doi:10.1016/j.srhc.2015.05.006

Kemp, E., Kingswood, C. J., Kibuka, M., & Thornton, J. G. (2013). Position in the second stage of labor for women with epidural anaesthesia. *Cochrane Database of Systematic Reviews, 2013*(1). doi:10.1002/14651858.CD008070.pub2

Kennedy, H. P., Cheyney, M., Lawlor, M., Myers, S., Schuiling, K., & Tanner, T. (2015). The development of a consensus statement of normal physiologic birth: A modified Delphi study. *Journal of Midwifery & Women's Health, 60*(2), 140–145. doi:10.1111/jmwh.12254

King, T. L., Brucker, M. C., Kriebs, J. M., Fahey, J. O., Gegor, C. L., & Varney, H. (2015). *Varney's midwifery* (5th ed.). Burlington, MA: Jones & Bartlett.

King, T. L., & Pinger, W. (2014). Evidence based practice for intrapartum care: The pearls of midwifery. *Journal of Midwifery & Women's Health, 59*(6), 572–585. doi:10.1111/jmwh.12261

Kozhimannil, K. B., Law, M. R., & Virning, B. A. (2013). Cesarean delivery rates vary tenfold among US hospitals; reducing variation may address quality and cost issues. *Health Affairs, 32*(3), 527–535. doi:10.1377/hlthaff.2012.1030

Kumud, R. A., & Chopra, S. (2013). Effect of the upright positions on the duration of labor. *Nursing and Midwifery Research Journal, 9*(1), 10–20.

Lawrence, A., Lewis, L., Hofmeyr, G. J., & Styles, C. (2013). Maternal positions and mobility during first stage labour. *Cochrane Database of Systematic Reviews, 2013*(10). doi:10.1002/14651858.CD003934.pub4.

Lawrence, H. C., III, Copel, J. A., O'Keeffe, D. F., Bradford, W. C., Scarrow, P. K., Kennedy, H. P., . . . Olden, C. R. (2012). Quality patient care in labor and delivery: A call to action. *American Journal of Obstetrics and Gynecology, 207*(3), 147–148. doi:10.1016/j.ajog.2012.07.018

Lee, S. L., Liu, C. Y., Lu, Y. Y., & Gau, M. L. (2013). Efficacy of warm showers on labor pain and birth experience during the first labor stage. *Journal of Obstetric, Gynecologic, and Neonatal Nursing, 42*(1), 19–28. doi:10.1111/j.1552-6909.2012.01424.x

Leeman, L., Fontaine, P., King, V., Klein, M. C., & Ratcliffe, S. (2003). The nature and management of labor pain: Part 1. Nonpharmacologic pain relief. *American Family Physician, 68*(6), 1109–1112.

Lefebvre, L. (2012). An adaptive framework for parturition and predatory pain. *Contemporary Hypnosis and Integrative Therapy, 29*(1), 30–36.

Leveno, K. J., Nelson, D. B., & McIntire, D. D. (2015). Second stage of labor: How long is too long? *American Journal of Obstetrics and Gynecology.* Advance online publication. doi:10.1016/j.ajog.2015.10.926

Lewis, D., & Downe, S. (2015). FIGO consensus guidelines on intrapartum fetal monitoring: Intermittent auscultation. *International Journal of Gynaecology and Obstetrics, 131*(1), 9–12. doi:10.1016/j.ijgo.2015.06.019

Lind, J. N., Perrine, C. G., & Li, R. (2014). Relationship between use of labor pain medications and delayed onset of lactation. *Journal of Human Lactation, 30*(2), 167–173. doi:10.1177/0890334413521189

Lindholm, A., & Hildingsson, I. (2015). Women's preferences and received pain relief in childbirth—A prospective longitudinal study in a northern region of Sweden. *Sexual and Reproductive Healthcare, 6*(2), 74–81. doi:10.1016/j.srhc.2014.10.001

Liu, Y., Liu, Y., Huang, X., Du, C. Peng, J., Huang, P., & Zhang, J. (2014). A comparison of maternal and neonatal outcomes between water immersion during labor and conventional labor and delivery. *BMC Pregnancy and Birth, 14*, 160. doi:10.1186/1471-2393-14-160

Madden, K., Middleton, P. Cyna, A. M., Matthewson, M., & Jones, L. (2012). Hypnosis for pain management during labour and birth. *Cochrane Database of Systematic Reviews, 2012*(11). doi:10.1002/14651858.CD009356.pub2

Madden, K. L., Turnbull, D., Cyna, A. M., Adelson, P., & Wilkinson, C. (2013). Pain relief for childbirth: The preferences of pregnant women, midwives and obstetricians. *Women and Birth, 26*(1), 33–40. doi:10.1016./j.wombi.2011.12.002

Magee, S., & Nakisbendi, M. D. (2012). *The pregnancy countdown book: Nine months of practical tips, useful advice, and uncensored truths.* Philadelphia, PA: Quirk Books.

Makvandi, S., Latifnejad Roudsari, R., Sadeghi, R., & Karimi, L. (2015). Effect of birth ball on labor pain relief: A systematic review and meta-analysis. *Journal of Obstetrics and Gynaecology Research, 41*(11), 1679–1686. doi:10.1111/jog.12802

Maso, G., Piccoli, M., De Seta, F., Parolin, S. Banco, R., Camacho Mattos, L., . . . Alberico, S. (2015). Intrapartum fetal heart rate monitoring interpretation of labor: A critical appraisal. *Minerva Ginecologica, 67*(1), 65–79.

Maul, A. (2007). An evolutionary interpretation of the significance of physical pain experienced by human females: Defloration and childbirth pains. *Medical Hypotheses, 69*(2), 403–409. doi:10.1016/j.mehy.2007.01.005

McCarthy, J. (2014). *Belly laugh: The naked truth about pregnancy and childbirth* (10th ed.). Philadelphia, PA: Da Capo Press.

McLachlan, H. L., Forster, D. A., Davey, M., Farrell, T., Flood, M., Shafiei, T., & Waldenström, U. (2015). The effect of primary midwife-led care on women's experience of childbirth: Results from the COSMOS randomised control trial. *British Journal of Obstetrics and Gyneacology.* Advance online publication. doi:10.1111/1471-0528.13713

Miller, N. R., Cypher, R. L., Nielsen, P. E., & Flogia, L. M. (2013). Maternal pulse pressure at admission is a risk factor for fetal heart rate changes after initial dosing of a labor epidural: A retrospective cohort study. *American Journal of Obstetrics and Gynecology, 209*(4), 382.e1–382.e8. doi:10.1016/ajog.2013.05.049

Moore, J., & Low, L. K. (2012). Factors that influence the practice of elective induction of labor: What does the evidence tell us? *Journal of Perinatal and Neonatal Nursing, 26*(3), 242–250. doi:10.1097/JPN.0b013e31826288a9

Murkoff, H., & Mazel, S. (2008). *What to expect when you are expecting* (4th ed.). New York, NY: Workman.

National Institute for Health and Care Excellence (NICE). (2014). Intrapartum care for healthy women and babies. Retrieved from https://www.nice.org.uk/guidance/CG190/chapter/About-this-guideline#copyright

Nicholson, J. M., Kellar, L. C., Henning, G. F., Waheed, A., Colon-Gonzalez, M., & Ural, S. (2015). The association between the regular use of preventive labour induction and improved birth outcomes: Findings of a systematic review and meta-analysis. *Journal of Obstetrics and Gynaecology, 112*(6), 773–784. doi:10.1111/1471-0528.13301

Nikula, P., Laukkala, H., & Pölkki, T. (2015). Mothers' perceptions of labor support. *American Journal of Maternal/Child Nursing, 40*(6), 373–380. doi:10.1097/NMC.0000000000000190

Ogedegbe, M. D., & Pickering, M. D. (2010). Principles and techniques of blood pressure measurement. *Cardiology Clinics, 28*(4), 571–586. doi:10.1016/j.ccl.2010.07.006

Ondeck, M. (2014). Healthy birth practice #2: Walk, move around, and change positions throughout labor. *Journal of Perinatal Education, 23*(4), 188–193. doi:10.1891/1058-1243 .23.4.188

Patel, N. P., El-Wahab, N., Fernando, R., Wilson, S., Robson, S. C., Columb, M. O., & Lyons, G. R. (2014). Fetal effects of combined spinal-epidural vs epidural labor analgesia: A prospective randomized double-blind study. *Anaesthesia, 69*(5), 458–467. doi:10.1111/anae.12602

Priddis, H., Dahlen, H., & Schmied, V. (2012). What are the facilitators, inhibitors, and implications of birth positioning? A review of the literature. *Women and Birth, 25*(3), 100–106. doi:10.1016/j.wombi.2011.05.001

Pugliese, P. L., Cinnella, G., Raimondo, P., De Capraris, A., Salatto, P., Sforza, D., . . . Dambrosio, M. (2013). Implementation of epidural analgesia for labor: Is the standard of effective analgesia reachable for all women? An audit of two years. *European Review for Medical and Pharmacological Sciences, 17*(9), 1262–1268.

Ranganathan, P., Golfeiz, D., Phelps, A. L., Singh, S., Shnol, H., Paul, N., . . . Vallejo, M. C. (2015). Chronic headache and backache are long-term sequelae of unintentional dura puncture in the obstetric population. *Journal of Clinical Anesthesia, 27*(3), 201–206. doi:10.1016/j.jclinane.2014.07.008

Rooks, J. P. (2012). Labor pain management other than neuraxial: What do we know and where do we go next? *Birth, 39*(4), 318–322. doi:10.1111/birt.12009

Ross-Davie, M., & Cheyne, H. (2014). Intrapartum support: What do women want? A literature review. *Evidence Based Midwifery, 12*(2), 52–58.

Rossi, M. A., & Lindell, S. G. (1986). Maternal positions and pushing techniques in a nonprescriptive environment. *Journal of Obstetric, Gynecologic, and Neonatal Nursing, 15*(3), 203–208. doi:10.1111/j.1552-6909.1986.tb01387.x

Rossignol, M., Chaillet, N., Boughrassa, F., & Moutquin, J. (2014). Interrelations between four antepartum obstetric interventions and cesarean delivery of women at low risk: A systematic review and modeling of the cascade of interventions. *Birth, 41*(1), 70–78. doi:10.1111/ birt.12088

Ruhl, C., Adams, E. D., Besuner, P., Bianchi, A., Lowe, N. K., Ravin, C. R., . . . Simkin, P. (2006). Labor support: Exploring its role in modern and high-tech birthing practices. *AWHONN Lifelines, 10*(1), 58–65. doi:10.1111/j.1552-6356.2006.00003.x

Sakala, C., & Corry, M. P. (2008). Evidence based maternity care: What is it and what it can achieve. Retrieved from http://www.milbank.org/uploads/documents/0809MaternityCare/ 0809MaternityCare.pdf

Sakala, C., Yang, Y. T., & Corry, M. P. (2013). Maternity care and liability: Pressing problems, substantive solutions. *Women's Health Issues, 23*(1), e7–e13. doi:10.1016/j.whi.2012.11.001

Sanders, R. (2015). Midwifery facilitation: Exploring the functionality of labor discomfort. *Birth, 42*(3), 202–205. doi:10.1111/bir.12183

Sharts-Hopko, N. C. (2010). Oral intake during labor: A review of the evidence. *Journal of Maternal/Child Nursing, 35*(4), 197–203. doi:10.1097/NMC.0b013e3181db48f5

Shilling, T., Difranco, J, & Simkin, P. (2004). #2: Freedom of movement throughout labor. *Journal of Perinatal Education, 13*(2), 11–15. doi:10.1624%2F105812404X109483

Shirvani, M. A., & Ganji, Z. (2014). The influence of cold pack on labour pain relief and birth outcomes: A randomised controlled trial. *Journal of Clinical Nursing, 23*(17–18), 2473–2480. doi:10.1111/jocn.12413

Simkin, P. (1986). Stress, pain, and catecholamines in labor: Part 2. Stress associated with childbirth events: A pilot survey of new mothers. *Birth, 13*(4), 234–240.

Simkin, P. (2003). Maternal positions and pelves revisited. *Birth, 30*(2), 130–132. doi:10.1046/j.1523-536X.2003.00232.x

Simkin, P. (2010). The fetal occiput posterior position: State of the science and new perspective. *Birth, 37*(1), 61–71. doi:10.1111/j.1523-536X.2009.00380.x

Simkin, P., & Arecheta, R. (2011). *The labor progress handbook: Early interventions to prevent and treat dystocia* (3rd ed.). Oxford, UK: Wiley-Blackwell.

Simkin, P., & Bolding, A. (2004). Update on nonpharmacologic approaches to relieve labor pain and prevent suffering. *Journal of Midwifery and Women's Health, 49*(6), 189 501. doi:10.1016/j.jmwh.2004.07.007

Simkin, P., & Hull, K. (2011). Pain, suffering, and trauma in labor and prevention of subsequent posttraumatic stress disorder. *Journal of Perinatal Education, 20*(3), 166–176. doi:10.1891/1058-1243.20.3.166

Simkin, P. P., & O'Hara, M. (2002). Nonpharmacologic relief of pain during labor: Systematic reviews of five methods. *American Journal of Obstetrics and Gynecology, 186*(Suppl. 5), S131–S159. doi:10.1016/S0002-9378(02)70188-9

Simpson, K. R., & Creehan, P. A. (2014). *Perinatal nursing* (4th ed.). Philadelphia, PA: Lippincott Williams & Wilkins.

Sindik, N., Petrović, O., Manestar, M., Franciscović, V., Klavić, M., & Marić, M. (2012). Vaginal delivery and continuous epidural analgesia: Should we change our clinical approach? *Collegium Antropologicum, 36*(2), 499–504.

Singata, M., Tranmer, J., & Gyte, G. M. (2013). Restricting oral fluid and food intake during labour. *Cochrane Database of Systematic Reviews, 2013*(8). doi:10.1002/14651858.CD003930.pub3

Smith, C. A., Collins, C. T., & Crowther, C. A. (2011). Aromatherapy for pain management in labour. *Cochrane Database of Systematic Reviews, 2011*(7). doi:10.1002/14651858.CD009215

Smith, C. A., Collins, C. T., Crowther, C. A., & Levett, K. M. (2011). Acupuncture or acupressure for pain management in labour. *Cochrane Database of Systematic Reviews, 2011*(7). doi:10.1002/14651858.CD009232

Smith, C. A., Collins, C. T., Cyna, A. M., & Crowther, C. A. (2006). Complementary and alternatives therapies for pain management in labour. *Cochrane Database of Systematic Reviews, 2006*(4). doi:10.1002/14651858.CD003521.pub2

Smith, C. A., Levett, K. M., Collins, C. T., & Crowther, C. A. (2011). Relaxation techniques for pain management in labour. *Cochrane Database of Systematic Reviews, 2011*(12). doi:10.1002/14651858.CD009514

Smith, C. A., Levett, K. M, Collins, C. T., & Jones, L. (2012). Massage, reflexology and other manual methods for pain management in labour. *Cochrane Database of Systematic Reviews, 2012*(2). doi:10.1002/14651858.CD009290.pub2

Smith, V., Begley, C. M., Clarke, M., & Devane, D. (2012). Professionals' views of fetal monitoring during labour: A systematic review and thematic analysis. *BMC Pregnancy and Childbirth, 12*(1), 166–183. doi:10.1186/1471-2393-12-166

Sng, B. L., Kwok, S. C., & Sia, A. H. (2015). Modern neuraxial labour analgesia. *Current Opinion in Anesthesiology, 28*(3), 285–289. doi:10.1097/ACO.0000000000000183

Sng, B. L., Leong, W. L., Zeng, Y., Siddiqui, F. J., Assam, P. N., Lim, Y., . . . Sia, A. T. (2014). Early versus late initiation of epidural analgesia for labour. *Cochrane Database of Systematic Reviews, 2014*(10). doi:10.1002/14651858.CD007238.pub2

Stark, M. A. (2013). Therapeutic showering in labor. *Clinical Nursing Research, 22*(3), 359–374. doi:10.1177/1054773812471972

Thompson, S., Kohli, R., Jones, C., Lovejoy, N., McGraves-Lloyd, K., & Finison, K. (2015). Evaluating health care delivery reform initiatives in the face of 'cost of disease.' *Population Health Management, 18*(1), 6–14. doi:10.1089/pop.2014.0019

Torres, J., DeVries, R., & Low, L. K. (2014). Consumer information on fetal heart rate monitoring during labor: A content analysis. *Journal of Perinatal and Neonatal Nursing, 28*(2), 135–143. doi:10.1097/JPN.0000000000000035

Ullman, R., Smith, L. A., Burns, E., Mori, R., & Dowswell, T. (2010). Parenteral opioids for maternal pain relief in labour. *Cochrane Database of Systematic Reviews, 2010*(9). doi:10.1002/14651858.CD007396.pub2

Vallejo, M. C., Cobb, B. T., Steen, T. L., Singh, S., & Phelps, A. L. (2013). Maternal outcomes in women supplemented with a high-protein drink in labour. *Australian and New Zealand Journal of Obstetrics and Gynaecology, 53*(4), 369–374. doi:10.1111/ajo.12079

Van der Gucht, N., & Lewis, K. (2015). Women's experiences of coping with pain during childbirth: A critical review of qualitative research. *Midwifery, 31*(3), 349–358. doi:10.1016./j.midw.2014.12.005

Van Teijlingen, E. R., Lowis, G. W., McCaffery, P., & Porter, M. (Eds.). (2011). Midwifery and the medicalization of childbirth: Comparative perspectives. Hauppague, NY: Nova Science.

Wassen, M., Smits, L., Scheepers, H., Marcus, M., Van Neer, J., & Roumen, F. (2015). Routine labor epidural analgesia versus labour analgesia on request: A randomized non-inferiority trial. *British Journal of Obstetrics and Gynaecology, 122*(3), 344–350. doi:10.1111/1471-0528.12854

Wassen, M. H., Winkens, B., Dorssers, E. I., Marcus, M. A., Moonen, R. J., & Roumen, F. E. (2014). Neonatal sepsis is mediated by maternal fever in labour epidural analgesia. *Journal of Obstetrics and Gynaecology, 34*(8), 679–683. doi:10.3109/01443615.2014.925858

Weaver, M. H. (2014). Waterbirth in the hospital setting. *Nursing for Women's Health, 18*(5), 365–369. doi:10.1111/1751-486X.12144

Wolk, S. W., Sine, D. M., & Paull, D. E. (2014). Institutional disclosure: Promise and problems. *Journal of Healthcare Risk Management, 33*(3), 24–32. doi:10.1002/jhrm.21132

Wong, C. A. (2010). Advances in labor analgesia. *International Journal of Women's Health, 1*, 139–154. doi:10.2147/IJWH.S4553

Zwecker, P., Azoulay, L., & Abenhaim, H. A. (2011). Effect of fear of litigation on obstetric care: A nationwide analysis of obstetrical practice. *Journal of Perinatology, 28*(4), 277–284. doi:10.1055/s-0030-1271213

# CHAPTER NINETEEN

# VAGINAL BIRTH AFTER CESAREAN: EMOTION AND REASON

Mayri Sagady Leslie

## THE DILEMMA OF VAGINAL BIRTH AFTER CESAREAN

Few issues in maternal–infant health have garnered the spectrum of emotional response generated by vaginal birth after cesarean (VBAC). Issues include equitable access to care, the reproductive right of women to have the option of VBAC, plus complex, and, at times, heterogeneous evidence on VBAC outcomes. The American College of Nurse-Midwives (ACNM) states that "all women who have experienced Cesarean birth have the right to safe and accessible options when giving birth in subsequent pregnancies" (ACNM, 2011a, p. 1). In addition, women have the right to evidence-based information, informed consent, and qualified maternity care providers, "regardless of geographic location, socio-economic status or type of medical coverage" (ACNM, 2011a, p. 1).

Midwives face many issues when caring for mothers eligible for VBAC. Central to these issues is the need for ongoing support of the mother's personal journey as she makes her choice between VBAC and elective repeat cesarean delivery (ERCD). Also included in the framework is providing informed, passionate, and empathetic care based on current evidence. Both mother and midwife are influenced by their own personal values and preferences. These values and preferences should be a recognized and significant component of care. Other important factors include the woman's current health and health history, her socioeconomic and cultural environment, evolving evidence and professional guidelines, institutional policies affecting VBAC availability, and the overarching political–cultural environment in maternity and midwifery care concerning this topic.

This chapter explores the scientific evidence for VBAC practice in the United States, discusses best practices for midwives caring for women planning a VBAC, and make recommendations for expanding VBAC accessibility and availability.

## Measuring VBAC

Being familiar with the terminology and methodology of measuring VBAC and cesarean birth is critical to understanding the research, and for effective communication with colleagues and families. Table 19.1 provides a comprehensive list of cesarean and VBAC terms and how they are calculated. The outdated term *trial of labor* (TOL; also called *trial of labor after cesarean* [TOLAC]) suggests that a VBAC labor is only a "trial." Any woman in labor has the potential of having a cesarean; hence, the term "trial" could be applied to all labors. These emotionally charged terms have been avoided in this text. However, many research studies and professional documents use them. In this chapter, the contemporary term labor after cesarean (LAC) is used except in quoted material.

Estimating the number of VBACs in the United States has been challenging. Changes in the U.S. birth certificate resulted in a period of noncomparable data between 2005 and 2014 (Childbirth Connection, 2015a; Figure 19.1). In 2014, states representing 90% of U.S. births reported a VBAC rate of 10.6%, the highest rate since 2005 when the VBAC rate was 10.1% (Hamilton, Martin, Osterman, & Curtin, 2015). This most currently reported rate is still in stark contrast to the 1989 rate of 28.6%. The website cesareanrates.com (Arnold, 2015a) provides current VBAC rates by state based on public data where available. In addition, a sister site, VBACFinder.com, provides hospital VBAC rates based on the same data (Arnold, 2015b).

**TABLE 19.1   Vaginal Birth After Cesarean (VBAC) and Cesarean Terms and Measures**

| Measure | |
|---|---|
| Total cesarean rate: | $\dfrac{\text{Total births by cesarean}}{\text{Total number of births}}$ |
| Primary cesarean rate: | $\dfrac{\text{Number of cesarean births with no previous cesarean birth}}{\text{Number of primary cesarean births plus number of vaginal births (not VBACs)}}$ |
| Repeat cesarean rate: | $\dfrac{\text{Number of cesarean births with a previous cesarean birth}}{\text{Number of VBACs plus number of repeat cesarean births}}$ |
| VBAC rate: | $\dfrac{\text{Number of vaginal births with a previous cesarean birth}}{\text{Number of VBACs plus number of repeat cesarean births}}$ |
| VBAC success rate: | $\dfrac{\text{Number of vaginal births with a previous cesarean birth planning VBAC at time of labor}}{\text{Number of all births with a previous cesarean planning a VBAC at time of labor}}$ |
| ERCD rate: | $\dfrac{\text{Number of repeat cesareans eligible for VBAC at time of labor}}{\text{Number of VBACs plus number of repeat cesarean births eligible for VBAC at time of labor}}$ |

Adapted from MacDorman et al. (2011).

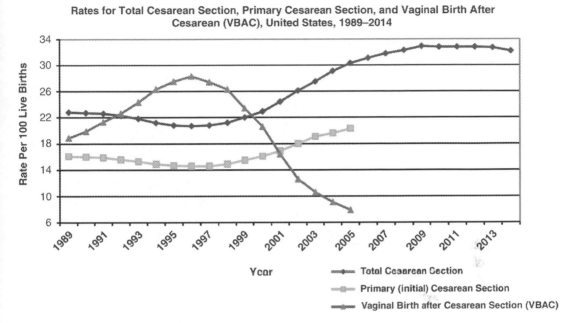

**Figure 19.1**   Vaginal birth after cesarean (VBAC) and cesarean birth rates from U.S. birth certificate data 1989 to 2014.
Used with permission from Childbirth Connection (2015).

Based on 2013 birth certificate data, Curtin, Gregory, Korst, and Uddin (2015) reported a VBAC success rate of approximately 70% for all women after one previous cesarean birth, not solely low-risk women; and 51% for all women having two or more previous cesarean births. The percentage of successful vaginal births for low-risk women having their first baby (no prior cesarean) was 89% (Curtin et al., 2015). In a systematic review of 203 studies, VBAC success rates ranged from 49% to 87% (Guise et al., 2010). These findings suggest that a woman planning a VBAC and one planning a vaginal birth for her first baby have a relatively equal likelihood of succeeding at having a vaginal birth.

## VBAC in Hospitals, Birth Centers, and at Home

In 2007, the U.S. VBAC rate was 3.6% for home births compared with 1.6% in birth centers and 1.0% in hospitals (MacDorman, Declercq, & Menacker, 2011). The availability of VBACs in hospitals has diminished significantly over the course of the past 20 years. Professional guidelines, restriction of practice, institutional policy changes, and providers' refusal to offer the option to mothers created what is called the "VBAC ban." With 30 years of advocacy and support for VBAC, the International Cesarean Awareness Network (ICAN), a consumer-based organization, gathered important data which showed that the VBAC ban was in effect in approximately 30% of all U.S. hospitals in 2011. This database is in the process of being updated and can be found at the ICAN website (ICAN, 2016a). As an example, 22 counties in New Mexico dropped from 100% VBAC availability in 1998 to 32% by 2008 (Leeman, Beagle, Espey, Ogburn, & Skipper, 2013).

VBAC availability in hospitals has been noted to be associated with the type of hospital and its birth volume with fewer options for VBAC in rural as compared to urban and university hospitals (Eden et al., 2012). In 2014, the authors of a study of 7 million hospital births found that VBAC rates were 5% in the rural setting and 10% in urban births (Kozhimannil, Hung, Prasad, Casey, & Moscovice, 2014). Researchers in New Mexico found that a hospital that did not offer the VBAC option was, on average, 121 miles from the nearest hospital that did (Leeman et al., 2013). In addition, the findings of a 2007 study of 17 hospitals revealed that although more women chose VBAC in the university versus community hospital, the VBAC success rate was about 75% for both (DeFranco et al., 2007). However, VBAC success rates vary greatly between hospitals (Kozhimannil et al., 2014).

A large 2004 study on the outcomes of VBAC in birth centers compared birth center outcomes to the outcomes of comparable (or even higher risk) populations in U.S. hospitals (Lieberman, Ernst, Rooks, Stapleton, & Flamm, 2004). The perinatal death rate in the birth center population evaluated at the time of the study exceeded hospital rates in all comparable studies. The authors recommended that VBAC should take place within the hospital setting rather than birth centers (Lieberman et al., 2004). This recommendation resulted in a shift away from VBAC availability in U.S. birth centers.

In 2013, an outcome study of 14,437 U.S. birth center births from 2007 to 2010 included few VBAC labors (0.3%) because "few birth centers were allowing TOLACs during the study period" (Stapleton, Osborne, & Illuzi, 2013, p. 4). Seventy percent of the VBACs at the birth centers were successful. Overall, the neonatal mortality rate for the birth center births was 0.4/1,000 births compared to the 2007 U.S. rate of 0.75/1,000 for infants of more than 2,500 g (Stapleton et al., 2013). Today, the Commission for the Accreditation of Birth Centers (CABC) states that "CABC accredited birth centers may choose to offer Trial of Labor after Cesarean" (2014, para. 1). The mother must have a history of not more than one prior cesarean birth with a low transverse incision. In addition, CABC (2014) details further specific requirements that had been defined to safeguard maternal and fetal safety.

Women may choose to have a VBAC at home because of a strong preference for home birth, for circumstantial reasons (e.g. VBAC bans), or both. A large study of data from the Midwives' Alliance of North America examined planned VBAC at home between 2004 and 2009 (Cox, Bovbjerg, Cheyney, & Leeman, 2015). Birth outcomes of women with a prior cesarean birth ($n = 1,052$) were compared to those of births of women with no prior cesarean ($n = 12,092$). The overall VBAC success rate was 87%. The rate was higher when the mother also had a prior vaginal birth (90.2%) or a previous VBAC (95.6%). Transfer rates to the hospital were significantly higher for these VBAC mothers (18% vs. 7% for all others).

Failure to progress was the main reason for transfer of care. Uterine ruptures for women with previous cesarean birth were 1.90/1,000 births compared with 0.08 for the control group (Cox et al., 2015).

An earlier study by Latendresse, Murphy, and Fullerton (2005) reported on birth after cesarean at home (*n* = 57). The overall VBAC success rate was 94.7%, with 87.7% of the VBACs occurring in the home. There was no incidence of uterine rupture or scar dehiscence. One infant was stillborn—a postdate infant with meconium present during labor. The study size was not sufficient to make statistical inferences about maternal or neonatal mortality. An important fact when considering these results is that more than half of the women with prior cesarean births in this study also had a previous VBAC (56.1%)—a known factor to increase VBAC success (Latendresse et al., 2005).

## Influence of the Clinician on VBAC

The midwife can have a significant influence on the option for a VBAC and the management pathways used during labor. A qualitative study of the perspectives of midwives and physicians on barriers to VBAC found the following concerns: fear of liability, minimizing risk, the convenience of a cesarean, the marginalization of midwives, and the availability of a surgical team as needed (Cox, 2011). The VBAC guidelines from the American College of Obstetricians and Gynecologists (ACOG, 1999) demonstrate these themes.

Why women choose a VBAC versus an ERCD after they have had one or more cesarean birth is multifactorial. One study's authors (Metz et al., 2013) determined that the strongest effect on this decision was the type of health care provider available to the women. This finding bears further evaluation. An analysis of birth certificate data from 22 states in 2007 found VBAC rates of 1.4% for nurse-midwives compared with 2.5% of births attended by other midwives and 1.0% of births attended by physicians (MacDorman et al., 2011).

Midwifery care for VBACs has been sparsely studied. It is important to note that the previous discussion of VBAC in birth centers and at home almost entirely reflects midwifery care in those settings. Avery, Carr, and Burkhardt (2004) reported the results of 649 VBACs in eight nurse-midwifery practices. The overall VBAC success rate was 72%. Sixteen percent of mothers in this study had experienced a prior VBAC. An earlier study in 1997 looked at midwifery care in a hospital-based birth center. The VBAC success rate was 98.3%. The number of mothers who had had a previously successful VBAC was much higher than the more recent study (84% vs. 16%), thus limiting the comparability of the findings (Harrington, Miller, McClain, & Paul, 1997).

A 2005 survey of ACOG members found that among 73% of the respondents, less than half of obstetricians' patients with previous cesarean births had VBAC labors. Male providers were more likely to perform repeat cesareans than their female counterparts (*p* = .005). Among the survey participants, 58% self-reported a VBAC success rate of 50% to 80% (Coleman, Erickson, Schulkin, Zinberg, & Sachs, 2005).

A systematic review by Catling-Paull, Johnston, Ryan, Fourer, and Homer (2011) examined nonclinical factors that increased provider uptake of VBAC and affected their VBAC success. Findings that were significantly associated with increasing VBACs included a conservative approach to cesareans, use of opinion leaders, and providing individual feedback data to providers. The lack of impact, and, at times, the negative impact of professional guidelines on the VBAC rate has also been reviewed (Catling-Paull et al., 2011; Roberts, Deutchman, King, Fryer, & Miyoshi, 2007; Zweifler et al., 2006). For example, charge nurses were surveyed at 243 hospitals in California after the recommendations from the National Institutes of Health (NIH; 2010) and ACOG (2010) encouraged increased use of VBAC (Barger, Dunn, Bearman, DeLain, & Gates, 2013). The research findings revealed that 44% of hospitals did not allow VBAC, and the only changes that had occurred since 2010 were that five hospitals had added a VBAC option, whereas four others stopped making it available. The authors (Barger et al., 2013) concluded that NIH and ACOG recommendations had had a minor impact in affecting the availability of VBAC. Catling-Paull et al. (2011) determined that in contrast to national directives, the greatest positive difference in increasing VBAC occurs when local policies or guidelines are enacted.

## THE EVIDENCE ON OUTCOMES OF VBAC AND ERCD

Considering the evidence on the clinical outcomes of VBAC requires an informed, multiview perspective. Frequently, the evidence is reported based on the overall outcomes between VBAC and ERCD. Although this reporting method encompasses the majority of previous research, this approach does not provide evidence of outcomes classified by type of birth, which is an important distinction for providers and consumers alike. The types of birth include VBAC labors that end in a vaginal birth, those that result in a cesarean birth after VBAC labor, and planned ERCDs without labor. Using these categories, a review of the 2013 U.S. birth certificate data compared outcomes on four maternal morbidities: maternal transfusion, ruptured uterus, unplanned hysterectomy, and admission to the intensive care unit (ICU; Curtin et al., 2015). For all categories, a successful VBAC was the safest type of birth. Cesarean birth after a VBAC labor held the highest risk for maternal transfusion, ruptured uterus, and ICU admission (Curtin et al., 2015). The VBAC success rate should be kept in mind when considering the outcomes of these categories. Although cesarean birth after a VBAC labor holds higher risks, theoretically, in a practice where the VBAC success rate is 75%, one in four women will experience a cesarean after a VBAC labor.

Another important distinction is to understand what birth experiences preceded the VBAC. These prior birth experiences could include single or multiple cesarean births, previous spontaneous vaginal births, as well as previous successful VBACs. Mercer et al. (2008) reviewed the outcomes of the VBACs of 13,532 women across 19 U.S. centers. In a progressive fashion, the more successful VBACs a mother had, the lower the risk for adverse maternal and neonatal outcomes. In addition, as the number of VBACs a woman had increased, the VBAC success rate also increased from 68.3% for the first VBAC, and 87.6% and 90.9% for the second and third VBACs, respectively (Mercer et al., 2008).

The evidence base for VBAC is sparse in areas and occasionally requires considering evidence from more than 10-year-old studies. The majority of the discussion that follows is based on the 2010 review of 203 studies on VBAC. Additional research is presented when available.

## Maternal Outcomes

Maternal outcomes from the systematic review by Guise et al. (2010) and the birth certificate review by Curtin et al. (2015) are indicated in Table 19.2. The most significant outcomes are discussed next. When available, data for term pregnancies have been displayed. Because the majority of midwifery clients have

**TABLE 19.2  Outcomes of Vaginal Birth After Cesarean (VBAC) Compared With Elective Repeat Cesarean Delivery (ERCD)**

| Outcomes | Guise et al. (2010; per 100,000 births) | | Curtin et al. (2015; per 100,000 births) | | |
|---|---|---|---|---|---|
| | VBAC TOL | ERCD | VBAC TOL With Vaginal Birth | VBAC TOL With Cesarean | ERCD |
| Hysterectomy<br>  All gestational ages<br>  Term | 170<br>140 | 280<br>160 | 51.1 | 158.7 | 143.9 |
| Transfusion | | | 366.8 | 731.4 | 458 |
| Uterine rupture | 325 | 26 | 43.8 | 495.4 | 65.6 |
| Uterine rupture and IOL<br>  IOL any gestational age<br>  IOL term<br>  IOL > 40 weeks | 1,000<br>1,500<br>3,200 | | | | |
| ICU admission | | | 131.4 | 356 | 265.3 |
| Maternal mortality<br>  All gestational ages<br>  Term births only | 3.8<br>1.9 | 13.4<br>9.6 | | | |
| Perinatal mortality | 130 | 50 | | | |
| Neonatal mortality | 110 | 50 | | | |

IOL, induction of labor; TOL, trial of labor.

Neonatal mortality, birth up to 28 days of life; perinatal mortality, 20 weeks gestation up to 28 days of life.

Adapted from Guise et al. (2010) and Curtin et al. (2015).

term pregnancies; these outcomes may be more relevant to the midwife reader's clinical practice than the overall statistics often provided. Data are provided as percentage per 100,000 births.

In the United States, maternal mortality represents a growing concern. From 1990 to 2013, the maternal mortality rate rose from 12 per 100,000 births to 28 (World Health Organization, 2013). Maternal death is a rare event for both VBAC and ERCD. However, there is a substantial difference in risk between the two groups (1.9/100,000 for VBAC vs. 9.6/100,000 for ERCD at term). For all gestational ages, there will be nine fewer deaths per 100,000 women when VBAC is chosen. Guise et al. (2010) rated the strength of the evidence on maternal mortality as high.

Uterine rupture is the most significant adverse event associated with VBAC and drives much of the debate and decision making on the issue. To be included in the review on uterine rupture (Guise et al., 2010), all studies had to define the event as a "complete separation through the entire thickness of the uterine wall (including serosa)" (p. 51). Hence, no scar dehiscence is included in these data. It is important to note that none of the studies in this review collected data on induction of labor (IOL), a factor known to increase the risk of uterine rupture. The strength of the evidence on uterine rupture was rated as moderate (Guise et al., 2010).

Women who experience rupture have an increased risk for hysterectomy (14%–33%; Landon et al., 2004). In the Guise at al. (2010) review, perinatal mortality from uterine rupture ranged from 2.8% to 6%. No evidence has been found to support maternal age, gestational age, preterm cesarean birth, or type of scar as influential factors in uterine rupture (Landon et al., 2004; Lydon-Rochelle, Cahill, & Spong, 2010).

Specific methods of induction and augmentation related to uterine rupture were also discussed by Guise et al. (2010). This subset of studies did not use a strictly anatomical definition of *rupture* and in some cases included dehiscence. IOL substantially increases the risk of uterine rupture in a woman who has chosen a VBAC and the risk increases with gestational age (Guise et al., 2010). Augmentation of labor was reviewed and was not found to be a significant factor for uterine rupture. The strength of the evidence on induction methods and uterine rupture was considered low. Palatnik and Grobman (2015) found that although IOL at 39 to 41 weeks was associated with an increased VBAC success rate (odds ratio [OR] = 1.31; 95% confidence interval [CI; 1.03–1.67]), a relationship was also demonstrated with a higher uterine rupture rate (OR = 2.73; 95% CI [1.22–6.12]).

The risk of uterine rupture associated with VBAC is the primary reason for ACOG's recommendation that an immediately available physician, anesthesia, and other staff ready to respond to an emergency be present in hospitals when VABCs are offered (ACOG, 1999). This recommendation was a key factor in the initiation of VBAC bans, as many hospitals could not meet these standards. Minkoff and Fridman (2010) reported that no evidence to date had demonstrated improved outcomes in hospitals where this standard had been applied. The authors posit that if the standard requiring an in-house physician for VBAC is valid because of the risk of uterine rupture, then it should be equally valid for all

**TABLE 19.3   Incidence of Adverse Labor Events**

| Event | Incidence/Births | Source |
|---|---|---|
| Uterine rupture w/VBAC TOL | 8/1,000 | Guise et al. (2010) |
| Placental abruption | 11–13/1,000 | Ananth and Wilcox (2001) |
| Cord prolapse | 14–62/1,000 | Murphy and Mackenzie (1995) |
| Shoulder dystocia | 6–14/1,000 | MacKenzie et al. (2007) |

TOL, trial of labor (for all gestational ages); VBAC, vaginal birth after cesarean.

mothers at risk for events, such as placental abruption, cord prolapse, and shoulder dystocia, which happen approximately as frequently with other types of births (Minkoff & Fridman, 2010; Table 19.3).

The risk for hysterectomy at term is not different between VBAC and ERCD. When considering all gestational ages, there is a slightly higher risk with ERCD (Guise et al., 2010). Overall, maternal transfusion risk has not been found to be significantly different between VBAC and ERCD. However, study findings are inconsistent (Guise et al., 2010). One study found that more than one VBAC is associated with fewer transfusions (Mercer et al., 2008).

Increased basal metabolic rate has been linked to decreased VBAC success rates. Women who enter labor in an obese or morbidly obese state are at highest risk for adverse outcomes such as uterine rupture or dehiscence, wound infection, and increased hospital stays. The babies of this subset of women are at risk for greater birth weight (> 4,000 g) and injury during the birthing process (Guise et al., 2010).

Women with one prior cesarean birth and a history of a subsequent ERCD or a cesarean birth after an unsuccessful VBAC may again have the option to choose between VBAC and ERCD: "Women with two previous low transverse Cesarean deliveries may be considered candidates for TOLAC" (ACOG, 2010, p. 458). If the women have a third or subsequent cesarean birth, the health risks significantly increase. This is an important component of informed choice as 50% of all pregnancies in the United States are unplanned (Centers for Disease Control and Prevention, 2010). The primary adverse outcomes with multiple cesareans are hysterectomy, placenta previa, and placenta accreta (Guise et al., 2010; Silver, 2010).

## Infant Outcomes

The *perinatal mortality rate* (PMR) is defined by the National Center for Vital Statistics to include the deaths of infants less than 28 days of age and fetal deaths of 20 weeks or more gestation (MacDorman & Kirmeyer, 2009). The rate includes antepartum stillbirth, intrapartum demise, and neonatal deaths to 28 days. The overall PMR for VBAC in the review by Guise at al. (2010) was 130/100,000 births.

For ERCD and women who had a cesarean birth after a VBAC, the rate was 50/100,000 births. The PMR associated with uterine rupture resulted in an overall risk of 20/100,000 VBACs. The strength of the evidence on PMR was low to moderate (Guise et al., 2010).

Of the studies reviewed by Guise et al. (2010), six found no significant differences on neonatal intensive care unit (NICU) admissions between VBAC and ERCD. One study found an increase in NICU admissions in babies whose mothers had an ERCD without labor versus a successful VBAC. The strength of evidence on NICU admissions is low. In the same analysis, Apgar scores, birth trauma, and sepsis were not significantly different when comparing VBAC to ERCD. For each of these findings, the strength of the evidence was low. Studies that reviewed neonatal respiratory events had conflicting findings and a lack of consensus. The strength of evidence was low (Guise et al., 2010). Other authors report that infants born after an ERCD have an increased risk of transient tachypnea of the newborn, persistent pulmonary hypertension, respiratory morbidity, and respiratory distress syndrome (O'Shea, Klebanoff, & Signore, 2010; Patel & Jain, 2010).

## BEST PRACTICES

## Education and Counseling

Education of potential VBAC clients has been shown to increase the rates of women choosing VBAC (Calvello et al., 2015). ACNM provides an excellent client education resource: "Birth Options After Having a Cesarean" (ACNM, 2015). Another invaluable resource is "Counseling Women With a Previous Cesarean Birth: Toward a Decision-Making Partnership" (Cox, 2014). In addition, Childbirth Connection (2015b), a Project of the National Partnership for Women and Families, offers excellent resources for mothers considering VBAC. These sources are also recommended to all readers by the author as a model for educating women about VBAC, and the cross-cutting issues that impact making an informed choice.

In the nationwide study Listening to Mothers III, women with a history of a previous cesarean birth were asked whether they felt pressured to have a cesarean for their second birth. Over a fourth (28%) of the mothers who had a VBAC for their second birth said they had experienced pressure to have a cesarean and 23% of those who had an ERCD felt pressured as well (Declercq, Sakala, Corry, Applebaum, & Herrlich, 2014). In keeping with respect for autonomy and beneficent clinical practice, providers should carefully consider how they discuss options.

### Screening Tools in Counseling VBAC-Eligible Women

A number of tools have been developed to screen pregnant women for VBAC eligibility. Eden et al. (2010) evaluated 16 prediction models and found that all models demonstrated reasonable ability to identify mothers who would have a VBAC, but that none were effective at consistently identifying who would have an ERCD. In the same analysis, one study reviewed tools that had been successful at predicting who would have a VBAC, yet failed to predict that 50% of the mothers who were scored with unfavorable risk factors went on to have successful vaginal births (Dinsmoor & Brock, 2004). The VBAC calculator is a readily available consumer-oriented online tool (Maternal–Fetal Medicine Units Network, n.d.). Although tools such as this one may be useful, the impact of provider management decisions and the birth environment contribute significantly to the woman's ability to decide her mode of birth.

### Decision Aids for VBAC Eligible Women

In a randomized controlled trial, Shorten, Shorten, Keogh, West, and Morris (2005) studied the effects of using a decision aid. At 12 to 18 weeks gestation, eligible women were given a booklet reviewing the benefits and risks of VBAC. Knowledge, decisional conflict, and birth preference were subsequently measured twice during the pregnancy. Mode of birth was collected, and satisfaction was measured postpartum at 6 to 8 weeks. Although there was no significant change in planned mode of birth, the booklet was effective in improving knowledge and reducing decisional conflict. An excellent example of a VBAC decision aid comes from the Best Birth Clinic in Vancouver: a patient information book that discusses planned repeat cesarean and VBAC options. The graphics in this document are especially consumer friendly (BC Women's Cesarean Task Force & Best Birth Clinic, 2010).

## Supporting Informed Choice

Among women deciding about VBAC, 48% will make their decision before they are pregnant again. Among those who remain undecided, 34% to 39% will choose VBAC midway through their pregnancies (Guise et al., 2010).

Four domains of influence on a mother's decision regarding VBAC or ERCD are described in a study by Konheim-Kalkstein, Barry, and Galoth (2014): perception of risk, memory of the first cesarean birth, locus of control (internal vs. external), and sources of information used in decision making. In the review by Guise et al. (2010), women's self-efficacy, involvement in decision making, and access to counseling and educational programs were all associated with an increased choice for VBAC. Childbirth education earlier in prenatal care was also associated with more women choosing VBAC. Women who did not receive counseling or education from providers were more likely to choose ERCD (Guise et al., 2010).

Metz et al. (2014) investigated decisions made by 3,120 women eligible for VBAC in 14 regional centers and reported that 29.7% chose LAC. Those with a prior vaginal birth or who are currently in the care of a midwife were more likely to opt for LAC. Level of knowledge about VBAC in contrast to ERCS is another factor in decision making for VBAC. Scaffidi, Posmontier, Bloch, and Wittman-Price (2014) reported that mothers with a higher level of VBAC and ERCD knowledge were 3.9 times more likely to choose a VBAC than those with a lower level of knowledge.

Eden, Hashima, Osterweil, Nygren, and Guise (2004) reviewed 11 studies examining factors affecting women's preferences for modes of birth. Ease of recovery and a desire to return home quickly to care for other children were the most commonly cited reasons for choosing VBAC. Four of the studies reported that safety of the mother and baby was an important factor, but not usually the prime factor (Eden et al., 2004). In a different qualitative study of mothers' perceptions on VBAC, "maternal instincts about what is best for the baby" emerged as one of the three key themes among women who either previously had a VBAC or had attempted VBAC (Phillips, McGrath, & Vaughan, 2009, p. 80). The authors describe the mothers as having "a single-minded belief in the significance of a natural birth for the newborn" (Phillips et al., 2009, p. 80). In a different study, Konheim-Kalkstein, Whyte, Miron-Shatz, and Stellmack (2015) analyzed content on a VBAC discussion board and found that those women planning a VBAC strongly relied on online information and peer communities in their planning.

Planning VBAC or ERCD needs to be a shared decision between the midwife and the woman, using unbiased, best evidence, the woman's preference, and the realities of the environment. Counseling should occur in a milieu of trust, values clarification, and risk–benefit exploration. The midwife listens to the preferences of the mother and is aware of her own preferences, values, and potential biases. As part of this shared decision-making process, decision aids may be used (Kaimal & Kuppermann, 2010).

### Informed Consent

Informed consent should be grounded in the ethical principles of respect for autonomy and beneficence. Chervenak and McCullough (2011) proposed a series of eight steps to include when working with patients considering their options for birth after a previous cesarean (Table 19.4).

Best practice for informed consent dictates that the midwife should be able to answer questions in a balanced manner, comparing outcomes from planned VBAC versus planned ERCD with consideration as to the mother's unique circumstances and history. Jordan and Murphy (2009) address the concept of informed compliance versus informed consent, influenced by how one discusses risk. Informed compliance refers to biased communication regarding medical risk such that it influences decision making (Bassett, Iyer, & Kazanjian, 2000). How risk is communicated makes a considerable difference on how women perceive their options. For example, counseling a mother about her risk of uterine rupture using the data derived from Guise et al. (2010) can be presented in multiple ways:

- The risk of uterine rupture in this pregnancy is 0.3% (absolute risk)
- The risk of uterine rupture in this pregnancy is 11.5 times higher than a woman who had no previous cesarean birth (relative risk; 0.3/0.026)
- VBAC creates five additional uterine ruptures for every 1,000 cesarean births (attributable risk)

**TABLE 19.4   Steps for Discussing the Option of VBAC With Women**

| Discussion Points |
| --- |
| ● Recognize the capacity of each pregnant patient to deal with medical information and not underestimate that capacity. |
| ● Recognize the validity of the values and beliefs of patients. |
| ● Offer all medically reasonable alternatives for managing a patient's pregnancy (i.e., technically possible alternatives supported by evidence-based and beneficence-based clinical judgment about maternal and fetal outcomes). |
| ● Provide information about the clinical benefits and risks of each medically reasonable alternative. |
| ● Recommend a medically reasonable alternative when in evidence-based clinical judgment, it is clearly superior. |
| ● Recommend against technically possible alternatives that are not supported in evidence-based and beneficence-based clinical judgment. |
| ● Ensure that a patient's decision-making process is voluntary. |
| ● Elicit a patient's value-based preference. |

VBAC, vaginal birth after cesarean.

Adapted with permission from Share with Women Column (ACNM, 2015).

Original source adapted with permission from *Journal of Midwifery and Women's Health* (Chervenak et al., 2011).

Each of these statements is based on the same statistical findings but could elicit a different response in a woman considering VBAC versus ERCD. Polit and Beck (2012) recommend that relative and attributable risks in comparison to absolute risks should be the framework of all risk discussions.

## Providing Midwifery Care

Essential components of midwifery care for a woman who has chosen VBAC includes decision support, emotional support, and midwifery clinical care. These practices overlap in function and embrace the midwifery model of care. Decision support involves providing information, respecting, nurturing, and promoting the mother's autonomy while recognizing one's own preferences and biases. Decision support may be an evolving process during pregnancy as the mother considers her options. Emotional support is the second critical function the midwife provides. Many women with previous cesarean births have emotional issues lingering into their next pregnancy. At the heart of this support is empowerment and trust: in birth, in her body, in her own power, and in the midwife. Midwifery clinical care embraces normalcy in pregnancy, labor, birth, and postpartum. Best practice for the midwife involves using the best evidence around these three critical functions to inform practice (Kennedy & Shannon, 2004).

ACNM (2011b) provides a clinical bulletin: "Care for Women Desiring Vaginal Birth After Cesarean." The bulletin provides 10 detailed practice implications recommended for midwifery care of VBAC clients. These recommendations include formal counseling and discussion of risk, reviewing the probability of

**TABLE 19.5　Factors Associated With Increased Likelihood of a Successful Vaginal Birth After Cesarean**

| Modifiable Factors | Nonmodifiable Factors |
|---|---|
| • No induction or augmentation<br>• Greater dilatation on admission<br>• Greater dilatation at rupture of membranes<br>• Effacement reaches 75%–90%<br>• Delivering at public and urban hospitals<br>• BMI < 30 | • Previous vaginal birth<br>• Previous vaginal birth after cesarean<br>• Spontaneous labor<br>• Gestational age ≤ 40 weeks<br>• Greater maternal height<br>• Infant weight < 4,000 g |

BMI, body mass index.

Adapted from Guise et al. (2010).

VBAC success, and the use of a specific informed consent document. The antepartum care of a woman with a previous cesarean is very similar to the care of all women. Decision and emotional support during the prenatal period are critical and are discussed next. When available, after reading the original operative note, documentation of the scar from previous cesarean(s) should be included in the chart, and the operative note should also be included as part of the current chart. Ongoing evaluation of modifiable and nonmodifiable risk factors that can impact VBAC success is critical (Guise et al., 2010; NIH, 2010). Equally important is working with women to make changes to improve modifiable factors (Table 19.5).

Intrapartum clinical care recommendations from ACNM (2011b) include fetal heart rate assessment in labor by either continuous electronic monitoring or intermittent monitoring following the guideline for high-risk patients. In addition, every effort should be made to support a spontaneous labor. IOL is reserved for circumstances when the benefit outweighs the risk and should occur in a hospital in consultation with a physician who would be able to perform a cesarean, should one be needed. The use of prostaglandin for cervical ripening is discouraged and misoprostol is contraindicated (ACNM, 2011b).

For midwives facing VBAC bans or restricted practice of VBACs, utilizing levels of risk assessment for VBAC women (low, medium, or high) can decrease the need for the immediately available physician standard, making VBAC more accessible to women. See the Northern New England Perinatal Quality Improvement Network (n.d.) for additional strategy details.

## Changing Clinical Practice

### Promoting the Normalcy of Birth

In a qualitative study of exemplary midwives, Kennedy and Shannon (2004) identified the core processes of midwifery care. "Support of normalcy," the primary process, included belief in the normalcy of birth, tolerance for wide variations of normal, belief and trust in women's strength, presence—the physical act of being *with woman*, and teaching students to believe and trust in normal birth (Kennedy & Shannon, 2004). The first four processes are especially critical in the care of women who have chosen VBAC as they often face resistance and doubt in themselves and from others.

The option for mothers to choose VBAC is more than an issue of safety and clinical outcomes. In an era in which both professionals and consumer advocates point to the right of mothers to have patient-choice cesareans, the right to choose VBAC or vaginal birth has significantly decreased. Leeman and Plante (2006) raise this issue as they point to the importance of retaining patient-choice vaginal birth. In many communities today, as previously discussed, VBAC bans by providers and hospitals have taken away the woman's right to choose. In such an environment, a woman may be coerced into choosing elective cesarean birth using an overestimation of VBAC risk, an approach that violates the principle of informed consent. Other options for a woman facing a ban include seeking VBAC from providers or institutions away from her local environment, which may or may not be covered by her insurance, resulting in a decision that can have financial and social implications and/or make the option nonviable, further contributing to health disparity for women with low resources. Finally, the woman could obtain VBAC care with a skilled provider in an out-of-hospital setting (birth center or home), or choose to be without a skilled attendant at home.

Lack of access to all options denies the woman her full reproductive rights, which should include the choice of a VBAC in the hospital in her own community attended by a midwife or physician of her choosing. Although some women may prefer to give birth in a birth center or at home, such choices should not be the only option. Not all women seeking VBAC are good candidates for such settings. Midwives can serve as advocates for their client's reproductive rights by working to prevent new VBAC bans, helping to displace existing ones, and ensuring full options are available to those women the midwives serve.

Another aspect of supporting VBAC as a choice entails understanding its cost-effectiveness. Childbirth is the number one reason for both hospitalization and medical office visits in the United States. Although cesarean births represent one third of all births, they account for nearly half of the childbirth-related expenses of hospitalization, $7.8 billion annually. Repeat cesarean birth is the number one indicator for cesareans and accounts for one third of all procedures (Agency for Healthcare Research and Quality, 2010). VBAC is a cost-effective alternative to escalating cesarean rates and escalating health care costs. Increasing the number of VBACs would reduce the number of ERCDs. Wymer, Shi, and Plunkett (2014) determined that, from a cost perspective, an initial VBAC is nearly as cost-effective as an ERCD for a second birth. However, with each subsequent birth, VBAC becomes less costly and more effective. Another pertinent factor to consider is the lifetime cost-effectiveness of VBAC versus ERCD and the impact on quality of life. In a setting in which the probability of a successful VBAC is at least 47.2% or more, using a VBAC strategy versus ERCD results in savings of $164.2 million and an additional 500 quality-adjusted life-years (Gilbert et al., 2013).

### Promoting Vaginal Birth

Frequently missing in the discussion on the choice between VBAC and ERCD are the benefits of vaginal birth. Although the dialogue focuses on comparative risk, the discussion often does not take into consideration the benefits of vaginal birth to both mother and baby. As a best practice, midwives need to include discussion of the emotional as well as physiological benefits to the mother and family.

Gut colonization of the newborn is another key point that can be overlooked. Within 3 days of birth, babies born by vaginal birth, as compared to those born by cesarean, have better gut colonization with bacteria important for immune system development (Biasucci et al., 2010). Lack of early colonization with *Lactobacillus* as well as Bifidobacteria has been associated with the subsequent development of allergies (Biasucci et al., 2010). Vaginal birth also optimizes early breastfeeding without the disturbances of cesarean birth.

### Reducing Primary Cesareans

Reduction of primary cesareans is a critical strategy that eliminates the need to choose between VBAC and ERCD in the next pregnancy. The primary cesarean rate was 22.8% in 2013 for 90% of the total U.S. births (Childbirth Connection, 2015a). Primary cesareans account for approximately 60% of all cesareans and the probability of a subsequent cesarean for these mothers is 90% (Osterman & Martin, 2014).

In addition, the relationship between primary cesarean birth and VBACs in hospitals is important. In a study of 234 California hospitals in 2009, an inverse relationship was determined. The higher the VBAC rate of the hospital, the lower the primary cesarean rate (Rosenstein et al., 2013). In 2014, ACOG and the Society for Maternal–Fetal Medicine (SMFM) published their consensus for strategies on the safe prevention of primary cesareans (ACOG & SMFM, 2014).

### Encouraging Consumer Advocacy

Consumers have considerable impact on health care policy decisions (Romano, Gerber, & Andrews, 2010). For instance, the ICAN has a volunteer workforce and a public website with extensive resources on VBAC (ICAN, 2016b). "The Birth Survey" is a joint project of the Grassroots Advocates Committee and the Coalition for Improving Maternity Services (n.d.). On the site, mothers share their experiences of providers and birth setting. In addition to their own advocacy efforts, a best practice for the midwife is empowering women and their supporters in consumer-driven advocacy that can change practice. Linking current patients to consumer advocacy groups can also provide a culture of normalcy for a mother considering or planning a VBAC.

## CONCLUSION

Encouraging open discussion and speaking to key talking points in VBAC advocacy help to shape the discourse. The midwife, as an expert in birth, has a respected voice and can contribute toward effecting change. A summary of strategic ideas and talking points for changing the VBAC environment include the following:

- The more women who choose VBAC, the more successful VBACs become (when VBAC rates fall, it is the number of women electing to try VBAC that declines, not the success rate).
- The more successful primary VBACs, the more repeat VBACs.
- The more repeat VBACs, the higher the success rate, improved outcomes, and increased cost-effectiveness.

As evidence-based providers who are experts in normal birth, midwives are ideally suited to provide care for mothers desiring VBAC. In addition, as experienced collaborative care providers, midwives can effect change for the reproductive rights of women by offering them the chance for truly informed consent and choice, hallmarks of the midwifery model of care.

---

### USING THE EVIDENCE FOR BEST PRACTICE

**Case Study 19.1   VBAC: Navigating Between Emotion and Reason**

Clara, a 25-year-old, gravida 4 para 2012, enters midwifery care at 12 weeks gestation in good health with no significant medical issues. Her obstetrical history includes a previous uncomplicated vaginal birth followed by a cesarean birth for breech. After offering Clara the option for a VBAC or ERCD, the midwife discusses the risk and benefits of each birth mode, providing Clara with written educational materials and website link information.

At her next visit at 16 weeks, Clara informs her midwife that she has decided to have ERCD as she is afraid of uterine rupture and of losing her baby. Clara recalls hearing somewhere that many babies could die from ruptures. After confirming that Clara wishes to discuss the statistics, the midwife provides the correct information about absolute, attributable, and relative risks.

At the end of this conversation, Clara states that the prospects of a VBAC are not as frightening as she had thought. The midwife discusses community support groups and classes available for women considering VBAC. Clara tells the midwife that her friend Sarah has just had a VBAC and that maybe Sarah can be a source for further discussion. The midwife reassures Clara that she can plan either VBAC or ERCD, and can change her mind again if she wishes.

Clara continues to discuss the possibility of VBAC with the midwife during subsequent prenatal visits. At her 32-week visit, Clara informs the midwife that she is sure she wants to attempt a VBAC and has arranged to work with a doula. Oral and written informed consent are obtained per institution policy. Clara, her partner, and the nurse-midwife make a general birth plan that includes avoiding induction and augmentation during labor and staying home in early labor.

At 40 5/7 weeks, Clara goes into spontaneous labor. In early labor, the doula stays with Clara and her partner at home as a support person. When labor progresses,

*(continued)*

> **USING THE EVIDENCE FOR BEST PRACTICE (continued)**
>
> Clara, her partner, and the doula leave for the hospital, where the midwife determines that Clara is 7- to 8-cm dilated, 100% effaced, and −1 station. Labor progresses well with the membranes rupturing spontaneously right before the birth. Clara gives birth to a robust baby girl with Apgar scores of 8 and 9. She breastfeeds her new daughter immediately.
>
> **Exemplar of Best Practice**
>
> The midwife used the scientific evidence to present the options of VBAC and ERCD in an unbiased manner, allowing Clara time to process information and to change her mind. This approach assisted Clara in making an informed decision about her mode of birth. The midwife also provided appropriate educational materials and assisted in developing a birth plan employing best practices for a VBAC.

# REFERENCES

Agency for Healthcare Research and Quality. (2010). Healthcare cost and utilization project (HCUP). Retrieved from http://hcupnet.ahrq.gov

American College of Nurse-Midwives (ACNM). (2011a). Vaginal birth after cesarean delivery [Position statement]. Retrieved from http://www.midwife.org/ACNM/files/ACNM LibraryData/UPLOADFILENAME/000000000090/VBAC%20Dec%202011.pdf

American College of Nurse-Midwives (ACNM). (2011b). Care for women desiring vaginal birth after cesarean [Clinical Bulletin]. *Journal of Midwifery and Women's Health, 56*(5), 517–525. doi:10.1111/j.1542-2011.2011.00112.x

American College of Nurse-Midwives (ACNM). (2015). Birth options after having a cesarean. *Journal of Midwifery and Women's Health, 60*(4), 475–476. doi:10.1111/jmwh.12354

American College of Obstetricians and Gynecologists (ACOG). (1999). ACOG Practice Bulletin No. 5: Vaginal birth after previous cesarean delivery. *International Journal of Gynaecology and Obstetrics, 66*(2), 197–204. doi:10.1016/S0020-7292(99)80021-6

American College of Obstetricians and Gynecologists (ACOG). (2010). ACOG Practice Bulletin No. 115: Vaginal birth after previous cesarean delivery. *Obstetrics & Gynecology, 116*(2, Pt. 1), 450–463. doi:10.1097/AOG.0b013e3181eeb251

American College of Obstetricians and Gynecologists (ACOG), & Society for Maternal–Fetal Medicine (SMFM). (2014). Safe prevention of primary cesarean delivery (Obstetric Care Consensus No. 1). *Obstetrics & Gynecology, 123*(3), 693–711. doi:10.1097/01.AOG.0000 444441.0411.1d

Ananth, C. V., & Wilcox, A. J. (2001). Placental abruption and perinatal mortality in the United States. *American Journal of Epidemiology, 153*(4), 332–337.

Arnold, J. (2015a). Hospital cesarean rates by state. Retrieved from http://www.Cesareanrates.com

Arnold, J. (2015b). VBACFinder. Retrieved from http://www.vbacfinder.com

Avery, M. D., Carr, C. A., & Burkhardt, P. (2004). Vaginal birth after cesarean section: A pilot study of outcomes in women receiving midwifery care. *Journal of Midwifery and Women's Health, 49*(2), 113–117. doi:10.1016/j.jmwh.2003.12.014

Barger, M. K., Dunn, J. T., Bearman, S., DeLain, M., & Gates, E. (2013). A survey of access to trial of labor in California hospitals in 2012. *BMC Pregnancy and Childbirth, 13*(1), 1–10. doi:10.1186/1471-2393-13-83

Bassett, K. L., Iyer, N., & Kazanjian, A. (2000). Defensive medicine during hospital obstetrical care: A byproduct of the technological age. *Social Science & Medicine, 51*(4), 523–537. doi:10.1016/S0277-9536(99)00494-3

BC Women's Cesarean Task Force, & Best Birth Clinic. (2010). Vaginal birth after cesarean and planned repeat cesarean birth. Retrieved from http://www.powertopush.ca/wp-content/uploads/2010/05/Best-Birth-Clinic-VBAC-Patient-Info-Booklet-with-BC-Data_web.pdf

Biasucci, G., Rubini, M., Riboni, S., Morelli, L., Bessi, E., & Retetangos, C. (2010). Mode of delivery affects the bacterial community in the newborn gut. *Early Human Development, 86*(Suppl. 1), 13–15. doi:10.1016/j.earlhumdev.2010.01.004

Calvello, S., Shaikh, M., Malek, S., Mboge, B., Kaplan, & Knapp, K. (2015, October). *Impact of education on trial of labor after cesarean section.* Poster session presented at meeting of the American Public Health Association, Chicago, IL.

Catling-Paull, C., Johnston, R., Ryan, C., Foureur, M. J., & Homer, C. S. (2011). Non-clinical interventions that increase the uptake and success of vaginal birth after cesarean section. *Journal of Advanced Nursing, 67*(8), 1662–1676. doi:10.1111/j.1365-2648.2011.05662.x

Centers for Disease Control and Prevention. (2010). Unintended pregnancy prevention. Retrieved from http://www.cdc.gov/reproductivehealth/UnintendedPregnancy

Chervenak, F. A., & McCullough, L. B. (2011). An ethical framework for the informed consent process for trial of labor after cesarean delivery. *Clinics in Perinatology, 38*(2), 227–231. doi:10.1016/j.clp.2011.03.002

Childbirth Connection. (2015a). Cesarean section: Cesarean section trends in the United States 1989–2014. Retrieved from http://www.childbirthconnection.org/article.asp?ck=10554

Childbirth Connection. (2015b). VBAC or repeat C-section: What you need to know. Retrieved from http://www.childbirthconnection.org/article.asp?ck=10212

Coleman, V. H., Erickson, K., Schulkin, J., Zinberg, S., & Sachs, B. P. (2005). Vaginal birth after cesarean delivery: Practice patterns of obstetrician-gynecologists. *Journal of Reproductive Medicine, 50*(4), 261–266. doi:10.1097/01.ogx.0000180847.45288.49

Commission for the Accreditation of Birth Centers (CABC). (2014). Common questions: Can an accredited birth center do TOLAC/VBACs? Retrieved from https://www.birthcenteraccreditation.org

Cox, K. J. (2011). Providers' perspectives on the vaginal birth after cesarean guidelines in Florida, United States: A qualitative study. *BMC Pregnancy Childbirth, 11*(1), 1–9. doi:10.1186/1471-2393-11-72

Cox, K. J. (2014). Counseling women with a previous cesarean birth: Toward a shared decision-making partnership. *Journal of Midwifery and Women's Health, 59*(3), 237–245. doi:10.1111/jmwh.12177

Cox, K. J., Bovbjerg, M. L., Cheyney, M., & Leeman, L. M. (2015). Planned home VBAC in the United States 2004–2009: Outcomes, maternity care practices, and implications for shared decision making. *Birth.* Advance online publication. doi:10.1111/birt.12188

Curtin, S. C., Gregory, K. D., Korst, L. M., & Uddin, S. F. (2015). Maternal morbidity for vaginal and cesarean deliveries, according to previous cesarean history: New data from the birth certificate, 2013. *National Vital Statistics Reports, 64*(4), 1–13. Retrieved from http://www.cdc.gov/nchs/data/nvsr/nvsr64/nvsr64_04.pdf

Declercq, E. R., Sakala, C., Corry, M. P., Applebaum, S., & Herrlich, A. (2014). Major survey findings of Listening to Mothers (SM) III: Pregnancy and birth: Report of the Third National US Survey of Women's Childbearing Experiences. *Journal of Perinatal Education, 23*(1), 9–16. doi:10.1891/1058-1243.23.1.9

DeFranco, E. A., Rampersad, R., Atkins, K. L., Odibo, A. O., Stevens, E. J., Peipert, J. F., . . . Macones, G. A. (2007). Do vaginal birth after cesarean outcomes differ based on hospital setting? *American Journal of Obstetrics and Gynecology, 197*(4), 400.e1–400.e6. doi:10.1016/j.ajog.2007.06.014

Dinsmoor, M. J., & Brock, E. L. (2004). Predicting failed trial of labor after primary cesarean delivery. *Obstetrics & Gynecology, 103*(2), 282–286. doi:10.1097/01.AOG.0000110544.42128.7a

Eden, K. B., Denman, M. A., Emeis, C. L., McDonagh, M. S., Fu, R., Janik, R. K., . . . Guise, J. M. (2012). Trial of labor and vaginal delivery rates in women with a prior cesarean. *Journal of Obstetric, Gynecologic, and Neonatal Nursing, 41*(5), 583–598. doi:10.1111/j.1552-6909.2012.01388.x

Eden, K. B., Hashima, J. N., Osterweil, P., Nygren, P., & Guise, J. M. (2004). Childbirth preferences after cesarean birth: A review of the evidence. *Birth, 31*(1), 49–60. doi:10.1111/j.0730-7659.2004.0274.x

Eden, K. B., McDonagh, M., Denman, M. A., Marshall, N., Emeis, C., Fu, R., . . . Guise, J. M. (2010). New insights on vaginal birth after cesarean: Can it be predicted? *Obstetrics & Gynecology, 116*(4), 967–981. doi:10.1097/aog.0b013e3181f2de49

Gilbert, S. A., Grobman, W. A., Landon, M. B., Varner, M. W., Wapner, R. J., Sorokin, Y., . . . Mercer, B. M. (2013). Lifetime cost-effectiveness of trial of labor after cesarean in the United States. *Value in Health, 16*(6), 953–964. doi:10.1016/j.jval.2013.06.014

Grassroots Advocates Committee, & Coalition for Improving Maternity Services. (n.d.). Homepage. Retrieved from http://thebirthsurvey.com/index.html

Guise, J. M., Eden, K., Emeis, C., Denman, M. A., Marshall, N., Fu, R., . . . McDonagh, M. (2010a). *Vaginal birth after cesarean: New insights* (Evidence Report/Technology Assessment No. 191. Prepared by the Oregon Health & Science University Evidence Based Practice Center under Contract No. 290-2007-10057-1. AHRQ Publication No. 10-E003). Rockville, MD: Agency for Healthcare Research and Quality. Retrieved from http://www.ahrq.gov/sites/default/files/wysiwyg/research/findings/evidencebased-reports/vbacup-evidence-report.pdf

Hamilton, B. E., Martin, J. A., Osterman, M. J, & Curtin, S. C. (2015). Births: Preliminary data for 2014. *National Vital Statistics Reports, 54*(6), 1–19. Retrieved from http://www.cdc.gov/nchs/data/nvsr/nvsr64/nvsr64_06.pdf

Harrington, L. C., Miller, D. A., McClain, C. J., & Paul, R. H. (1997). Vaginal birth after cesarean in a hospital-based birth center staffed by certified nurse-midwives. *Journal of Nurse-Midwifery, 42*(4), 304–307. doi:10.1016/S0091-2182(97)00019-0

International Cesarean Awareness Network (ICAN). (2016a). VBAC policy database. Retrieved from http://www.ican-online.org/hospital-vbac-policy-database

International Cesarean Awareness Network (ICAN). (2016b). Homepage. Retrieved from http://www.ican-online.org

Jordan, R. G., & Murphy, P. A. (2009). Risk assessment and risk distortion: Finding the balance. *Journal of Midwifery and Women's Health, 54*(3), 191–200. doi:10.1016/j.jmwh.2009.02.001

Kaimal, A. J., & Kuppermann, M. (2010). Understanding risk, patient and provider preferences, and obstetrical decision making: Approach to delivery after cesarean. *Seminars in Perinatology, 34*(5), 331–336. doi:10.1053/j.semperi.2010.05.006

Kennedy, H. P., & Shannon, M. T. (2004). Keeping birth normal: Research findings on midwifery care during childbirth. *Journal of Obstetric, Gynecologic, and Neonatal Nursing, 33*(5), 554–560. doi:10.1177/0884217504268971

Konheim-Kalkstein, Y. L., Barry, M. M., & Galoth, K. (2014). Examining influences on women's decision to try labour after previous cesarean section. *Journal of Reproductive and Infant Psychology, 32*(2), 137–147. doi:10.1080/02646838.2013.875133

Konheim-Kalkstein, Y. L., Whyte, R., Miron Shatz, T., & Stellmack, M. A. (2015). What are VBAC women seeking and sharing? A content analysis of online discussion boards. *Birth, 42*(3), 277–282. doi:10.1111/birt.12167

Kozhimannil, K. B., Hung, P., Prasad, S., Casey, M., & Mascovice, I. (2014). Rural–urban differences in obstetric care, 2002–2010, and implications for the future. *Medical Care, 52*(1), 4–9. doi:10.1097/MLR.0000000000000016

Landon, M. B., Hauth, J. C., Leveno, K. J., Spong, C. Y., Leindecker, S., Varner, M. W., & Gabbe, S. G. (2004). Maternal and perinatal outcomes associated with a trial of labor after prior cesarean delivery. *New England Journal of Medicine, 351*(25), 2581–2589. doi:10.1056/NEJMoa040405

Latendresse, G., Murphy, P. A., & Fullerton, J. T. (2005). A description of the management and outcomes of vaginal birth after cesarean birth in the homebirth setting. *Journal of Midwifery and Women's Health, 50*(5), 386–391. doi:10.1016/j.jmwh.2005.02.012

Leeman, L. M., Beagle, M., Espey., E., Ogburn, T., & Skipper, B. (2013). Diminishing availability of trial of labor after cesarean delivery in New Mexico hospitals. *Obstetrics & Gynecology, 122*(2, Pt. 1), 242–247. doi:10.1097/AOG.0b013e31829bd0a0

Leeman, L. M., & Plante, L. A. (2006). Patient-choice vaginal delivery? *Annals of Family Medicine, 4*(3), 265–268. doi:10.1370/afm.537

Lieberman, E., Ernst, E. K., Rooks, J. P., Stapleton, S., & Flamm, B. (2004). Results of the national study of vaginal birth after esarean in birth centers. *Obstetrics & Gynecology, 104*(5, Pt. 1), 933–942. doi:10.1097/01.AOG.0000143257.29471.82

Lydon-Rochelle, M. T., Cahill, A. G., & Spong, C. Y. (2010). Birth after previous cesarean delivery: Short-term maternal outcomes. *Seminars in Perinatology, 34*(4), 249–257. doi:10.1053/j.semperi.2010.03.004

MacDorman, M. F., Declercq, E., & Menacker, F. (2011). Recent trends and patterns in cesarean birth and vaginal birth after cesarean (VBAC) deliveries in the United States. *Clinics in Perinatology, 38*(2), 179–192. doi:10.1016/j.clp.2011.03.007

MacDorman, M. F., & Kirmeyer, S. (2009). Fetal and perinatal mortality, United States, 2005. *National Vital Statistics Reports, 57*(8), 1–19. Retrieved from http://www.cdc.gov/nchs/data/nvsr/nvsr57/nvsr57_08.pdf

MacKenzie, I. Z., Shah, M., Lean, K., Dutton, S., Newdick, H., & Tucker, D. E. (2007). Management of shoulder dystocia: Trends in incidence and maternal and neonatal morbidity. *Obstetrics and Gynecology, 110*(5), 1059–1068.

Maternal–Fetal Medicine Units Network. (n.d.). VBAC calculator. Retrieved from https://mfmunetwork.bsc.gwu.edu/PublicBSC/MFMU/VGBirthCalc/vagbirth.html

Mercer, B. M., Gilbert, S., Landon, M. B., Spong, C. Y., Leveno, K. J., Rouse, D. J., . . . Ramin, S. M. (2008). Labor outcomes with increasing number of prior vaginal births after cesarean delivery. *Obstetrics & Gynecology, 111*(2, Pt. 1), 285–291. doi:10.1097/AOG.0b013e31816102b9

Metz, T. D, Stoddard, G. J., Henry, E., Jackson, M., Holmgren, C., & Esplin, S. (2013). How do good candidates for trial of labor after cesarean (TOLAC) who undergo elective repeat cesarean differ from those who choose TOLAC? *American Journal of Obstetrics and Gynecology, 208*(6), 458.e1–458.e6. doi:10.1016/j.ajog.2013.02.011

Minkoff, H., & Fridman, D. (2010). The immediately available physician standard. *Seminars in Perinatology, 34*(5), 325–330. doi:10.1053/j.semperi.2010.05.005

Murphy, D. J., & MacKenzie, I. Z. (1995). The mortality and morbidity associated with umbilical cord prolapse. *British Journal of Obstetrics and Gynaecology, 102*(10), 826–830.

National Institutes of Health (NIH). (2010). National Institutes of Health consensus development conference statement: Vaginal birth after cesarean: New insights. Retrieved from http://consensus.nih.gov/2010/images/vbac/vbac_statement.pdf

Northern New England Perinatal Quality Improvement Network. (n.d.). VBAC overview. Retrieved from http://www.nnepqin.org/VBAC.asp

O'Shea, T. M., Klebanoff, M. A., & Signore, C. (2010). Delivery after previous cesarean: Long-term outcomes in the child. *Seminars in Perinatology, 34*(4), 281–292.

Osterman, M. J., & Martin, J. A. (2014). Trends in low-risk cesarean delivery in the United States, 1990–2013. *National Vital Statistics Reports, 62*(6), 1–16.

Palatnik, A., & Grobman, W. A. (2015). Induction of labor versus expectant management for women with a prior cesarean delivery. *American Journal of Obstetrics and Gynecology, 112*(3), 358.e1–358.e6. doi:10.1016/j.ajog.2015.01.026

Patel, R. M., & Jain, L. (2010). Delivery after previous cesarean: Short-term perinatal outcomes. *Seminars in Perinatology, 34*(4), 272–280. doi:10.1053/j.semperi.2010.03.007

Phillips, E., McGrath, P., & Vaughan, G. (2009). "I wanted desperately to have a natural birth": Mothers' insights on vaginal birth after caesarean (VBAC). *Contemporary Nurse, 34*(1), 77–84. doi:10.5172/conu.2009.34.1.077

Polit, D. F., & Beck, C. T. (2012). *Nursing research* (9th ed.). Philadelphia, PA: Lippincott Williams & Wilkins.

Roberts, R. G., Deutchman, M., King, V. J., Fryer, G. E., & Miyoshi, T. J. (2007). Changing policies on vaginal birth after cesarean: Impact on access. *Birth, 34*(4), 316–322. doi:10.1111/j.1523-536X.2007.00190.x

Romano, A. M., Gerber, H., & Andrews, D. (2010). Social media, power, and the future of VBAC. *Journal of Perinatal Education, 19*(3), 43–52. doi:10.1624%2F105812410X514431

Rosenstein, M. G., Kuppermann, M., Gregorich, S. E., Cottrell, E. K., Caughey, A. B., & Cheng, Y. W. (2013). Association between vaginal birth after cesarean delivery and primary cesarean delivery rates. *Obstetrics & Gynecology, 122*(5), 1010–1017. doi:10.1097/AOG.0b013 e3182a91e0f

Scaffidi, R. M., Posmontier, B., Bloch, J. R., & Wittman-Price, R. (2014). Relationship between personal knowledge and decision self-efficacy in choosing trial of labor after cesarean. *Journal of Midwifery and Woman's Health, 59*(3), 246–253. doi:10.1111/jmwh.12173

Shorten, A., Shorten, B., Keogh, J., West, S., & Morris, J. (2005). Making choices for childbirth: A randomized controlled trial of a decision-aid for informed birth after cesarean. *Birth, 32*(4), 252–261. doi:10.1111/j.0730-7659.2005.00383.x

Silver, R. M. (2010). Delivery after previous cesarean: Long-term maternal outcomes. *Seminars in Perinatology, 34*(4), 258–266. doi:10.1053/j.semperi.2010.03.006

Stapleton, S. R., Osborne, C., & Illuzzi, J. (2013). Outcomes of care in birth centers: Demonstration of a durable model. *Journal of Midwifery and Women's Health, 58*(1), 3–14. doi:10.1111/jmwh.12003

World Health Organization. (2013). Trends in maternal mortality: 1990 to 2013. Estimates by WHO, UNICEF, UNFPA, The World Bank and the United Nations Population Division. Retrieved from http://www.who.int/reproductivehealth/publications/monitoring/maternal -mortality-2013/en

Wymer, K. M., Shi, Y. C., & Plunkett, B. A. (2014). The cost-effectiveness of a trial of labor accrues with multiple subsequent vaginal deliveries. *American Journal of Obstetrics and Gynecology, 211*(1), 56.e1–56.e12. doi:10.1016/j.ajog.2014.01.033

Zweifler, J., Garza, A., Hughes, S., Stanich, M. A., Hierholzer, A., & Lau, M. (2006). Vaginal birth after cesarean in California: Before and after a change in guidelines. *Annals of Family Medicine, 4*(3), 228–234. doi:10.1370/afm.544

CHAPTER TWENTY

# THE LIMITS OF CHOICE: ELECTIVE INDUCTION AND CESAREAN DELIVERY ON MATERNAL REQUEST

Kerri D. Schuiling and Joan K. Slager

## CONTROVERSIAL ISSUES AND CHOICE

The midwifery model of care frames childbirth as a normally occurring event in women's lives. Within the context of normal childbearing, midwives hold fast to the belief that less intervention is better for both mother and baby. Unfortunately, in our society, birth is often viewed as risky, and technology as reliable and progressive. Today, childbirth in the United States is occurring within a technocratic context in which interventions, such as induction of labor and cesarean delivery on maternal request (CDMR), are almost normalized. This chapter presents the discourse and current research around elective induction of labor (EIOL) and CDMR. Current evidence for best practices is provided as a foundation for decision making about clinical practice. The ethics of choice and the meaning of risk are explored.

## The Issues

The various reasons a woman may request a cesarean birth include belief that it is safer for the baby, fear of a traumatic vaginal delivery resulting in long-term incontinence, and fear of labor pain (Romero, Coulson, & Galvin, 2012). The number of cesarean births rose by 60% from 1996 to 2009 (Martin, Hamilton, & Osterman, 2013) and increased by more than 70% in six states from 1996 to 2007 (Menacker & Hamilton, 2010). However, from 2009 to 2012 a slight decline (less than 1%) in the number of cesarean births was observed. Unfortunately, the rate of cesarean births in the United States still remains above 32% (Martin et al., 2013).

Accompanying the rise in cesarean births is the fact that induction of labor is commonplace. EIOL is labor that is induced in the absence of standard medical indications (Caughey et al., 2009a; Lydon-Rochelle et al., 2007). The widespread acceptance of scheduling *social induction* has fallen under the scrutiny of many quality organizations because of its relation to cesarean birth and birth of a premature infant (Beebe, Beaty, & Rayburn, 2007; Vardo, Thornburg, & Glantz, 2011). Complications caused by prematurity result in significant perinatal morbidity and mortality as well as emotional and physical costs to parents and society.

Induction of labor frequently results in increased health care costs, longer labor, and an increased potential for morbidity for both mother and baby, contributing to longer hospital stays. Such inductions are typically done for provider and/or patient convenience and are viewed by many clinicians as contrary to a culture of patient safety (Simpson, 2010).

## Methods of Induction

Methods used to induce labor are considered either mechanical or pharmacologic. One mechanical method is the use of balloon catheters that place pressure on the cervix, thereby causing mechanical dilation and prompting the release of endogenous prostaglandin. Another method is sweeping of membranes, which stimulates the release of prostaglandins in the hope of ripening the cervix and stimulating the onset of labor. Dinoprostone, a retrievable insert, is a pharmacological method used to soften and ripen the cervix in preparation for induction of labor. Oxytocin and misoprostol are examples of pharmacological methods used to initiate labor. Oxytocin is one of the more common and oldest drugs used to induce labor. However, reports warn about the hazards associated with oxytocin, the drug most commonly associated with preventable adverse outcomes.

The Institute for Safe Motherhood and the Institute for Safe Medication Practices designated intravenous oxytocin as a *high-alert medication* and has added it to a list of pharmacological agents with risk that may necessitate increased safety measures (Clark, Simpson, Knox, & Garite, 2009; Simpson & Knox, 2009). The American College of Obstetricians and Gynecologists (ACOG, 2009 [reaffirmed 2015]) recommends that oxytocin be used only by clinicians who are educated about its use and familiar with its effects. The maximum safe dose of oxytocin has not been established, and clinicians are encouraged to use the least amount of drug to effect labor stimulation. Furthermore, ACOG encourages hospitals to develop guidelines for its preparation and administration (ACOG, 2009 [reaffirmed 2015]).

## ELECTIVE INDUCTION OF LABOR

## Reasons for EIOL

EIOL occurs for a variety of nonmedical reasons (such as potential for rapid labor, distance from hospital, and psychosocial indications; ACOG, 2009 [reaffirmed 2015]). Women may also wish to end their pregnancies because of physical discomfort, arriving at the hospital too late for epidural placement, scheduling issues, and timing of available family support.

## Rates of EIOL

The rate of induction of labor for singleton births began to rise in 1996 and continued to rise steadily until 2010 when it reached a high of 23.8%. A slight decline in the induction rate began to be observed in 2011 (23.7%) and again in 2012 (23.3%; Osterman & Martin, 2014). However, the number of women who have their labors induced may be overestimated. The rates of induction without medical indication are typically derived from birth certificate data. Bailit and the Ohio Perinatal Quality Collaborative (2010), in a study representing 20 hospitals, found that birth certificates overestimated rates of elective induction by about 10%. Nonetheless, a significant number of childbearing women experience induced labor.

Elective induction rates vary by gestational age. However, the overall rates for induction have fallen slightly since 2010 with the largest decrease observed in pregnancies that are 38 weeks gestation. The decrease in induction of labor, particularly at 35 to 38 weeks, is most likely the result of a change in obstetrical practice because research findings suggests that there is a greater risk of fetal morbidity and mortality at this time (Osterman & Martin, 2014).

## Decision Making on EIOL

Decision making about whether to induce labor electively should include weighing the risks against the benefits. When the benefits of a facilitated birth outweigh the risks of continuing the pregnancy, it is reasonable to consider elective induction (Caughey et al., 2009a). Regardless of the reason for EIOL, ACOG recommends confirmation that the fetus is at term or that the fetal lungs are mature prior to EIOL. Further, EIOL should not occur prior to 39 completed weeks of gestation, regardless of the outcome of fetal lung maturity testing (ACOG, 2009/2015).

Although there are a variety of ways to date a pregnancy, validating whether a pregnancy is at term (37–42 weeks gestation) is still not an exact science. Recent evidence suggests that this 5-week window allows for much discrepancy in newborn outcomes. Thus, ACOG (2013a) convened a work group in 2012 to address the disparity in newborn morbidity that resulted in the refinement of the definition of *term pregnancy*. Deliveries occurring at or beyond 37 completed weeks were defined as *early term* (37 0/7–38 6/7 weeks), *full term* (39 0/7–41 6/7 weeks), and *post term* (42 0/7 weeks gestation and beyond; ACOG, 2013a).

EIOL at term for nulliparous women is associated with increased risk for cesarean birth, postpartum hemorrhage, neonatal resuscitation, increased hospital costs, and longer lengths of stay without improvement of neonatal outcomes (Ehrenthal, Jiang, & Strobino, 2010; Kaimal et al., 2011; Vardo et al., 2011).

Other studies' findings do not demonstrate the same increase in risks. For example, the authors of a retrospective cross-sectional study of 131,243 low-risk deliveries of which 13,242 were electively induced concluded that EIOL at term, regardless of parity or cervical status, was associated with decreased risks of cesarean delivery and other maternal and neonatal morbidities when compared with expectant management (Gibson, Waters, & Bailit, 2014). Current researchers suggest the comparison must be EIOL with expectant management and not spontaneous onset of labor because the latter cannot be a choice. It just occurs naturally.

Infants between the gestational ages of 37 to 39 completed weeks gestation are often erroneously considered term by the general public, thus meeting the fetal requisites for EIOL or planned cesarean birth. The evidence suggests otherwise. A study of 12,821 infants born by elective cesarean birth at 37 completed weeks gestation revealed that these infants had a two- to fourfold increase in neonatal complications compared to 39 completed weeks gestation (Tita et al., 2009). Complications included respiratory distress requiring admission to the neonatal intensive care unit (NICU), sepsis, and hypoglycemia. Even those infants born at 38 and 4/7 weeks experienced statistically significant higher morbidity than infants who had completed 39 weeks gestation (Tita et al., 2009).

The American College of Nurse-Midwives (ACNM) takes the position that induction of labor should be offered to women only for medical indications that are supported by scientific evidence and if the benefit of birth outweighs the risk of prematurity (ACNM, 2005). Furthermore, the ACNM identifies that spontaneous labor offers substantial benefits to the mother and her newborn and that disruption of the normal process without a medical indication actually represents a risk for potential harm (ACNM, 2010).

Women will continue to request EIOL. It is the clinician's responsibility to provide education that is informative, accurate, and evidence based. Simpson, Newman, and Chirino (2010a) surveyed 1,349 women about their attendance at prepared childbirth classes and their experience with labor and birth. The purpose of the study was to explore nulliparous women's reasons for requesting EIOL. It is interesting to note that 63% of the women who attended childbirth education classes and who did not request EIOL stated that their childbirth educators provided helpful information to assist them in their decision making. Women also identified their physicians as a powerful influence on their decision making about requesting EIOL. Women were more likely to have EIOL if their physician suggested it (Simpson et al., 2010a).

Another study compared women who attended childbirth education and viewed a video about the risks and benefits of EIOL to women who did not attend the classes and did not view the video. Reported findings revealed that elective induction rates differed significantly based on class attendance (Simpson, Newman, & Chirino, 2010b). Childbirth education can help women to make decisions about EIOL.

## The Evidence on EIOL

An early retrospective study of EIOL using record review of 1,135 women with singleton pregnancies at low risk for complications (vertex presentation between 38 and 41 weeks gestation and eligible for vaginal birth) revealed that the majority of the women ($n = 872$) had spontaneous labor. Among those women who had their labors induced ($n = 263$), there was a significantly increased risk for cesarean birth. In addition, those women who had labor induced followed by vaginal birth still incurred higher hospital costs ($273 and higher) and longer stays in the hospital than noninduced vaginal births (Maslow & Sweeny, 2000).

A larger (n = 7,804) retrospective chart review of nulliparous women at term with a singleton fetus in the vertex position revealed that labor induction was significantly associated with cesarean birth (Ehrenthal et al., 2010). When a nulliparous woman with an unfavorable cervix (Bishop score ≤ 6) undergoes induction of labor, her risk of cesarean birth doubles (ACOG, 2009/2015). A retrospective chart review of nulliparous women (n = 485) with singleton pregnancies at term revealed a 33.6% cesarean birth rate and found that EIOL was significantly related to increased length of stay, epidural use, postpartum hemorrhage, and neonatal oxygen requirement (Vardo et al., 2011).

The Agency for Healthcare Research and Quality (AHRQ) sponsors evidence-based, peer-reviewed reports through its evidence-based-practice centers (EPCs). A large systematic review was undertaken to answer four key questions around EIOL:

- What evidence describes the maternal risks of elective induction versus expectant management?
- What evidence describes the fetal/neonatal risks of elective induction versus expectant management?
- What is the evidence that certain physical conditions/patient characteristics are predictive of a successful induction of labor?
- How is a failed induction defined? (Caughey et al., 2009b)

The initial literature search identified 3,722 potentially relevant articles of which 76 met inclusion criteria. Nine were randomized controlled trials (RCTs) comparing expectant management with EIOL. This study stands out from others because EIOL is compared with expectant management, not spontaneous labor. The researchers (Caughey et al., 2009b) explain that comparing EIOL with spontaneous labor is problematic:

> Expectant management of the pregnancy involves nonintervention at any particular point in time and allowing the pregnancy to progress to a future gestational age. Thus, women undergoing expectant management may go into spontaneous labor or may require indicated induction of labor at a future gestational age. (p. v)

These researchers (Caughey et al., 2009b) posit that comparing EIOL with spontaneous labor is a fundamental flaw and can result in misleading conclusions. Two systematic reviews by these authors (Caughey et al., 2009a, 2009b) concluded that expectant management of pregnancy was associated with 22% higher odds of cesarean birth than EIOL and a 50% higher risk of meconium-stained amniotic fluid. The majority of studies that were included in the meta-analysis focused on women who were pregnant at 41 weeks gestation or beyond. In addition, women whose pregnancies and labor were expectantly managed were more likely to have meconium-stained amniotic fluid than their EIOL comparisons. However, the observational studies that were included showed a consistently lower risk of cesarean birth for women who had EIOL (Caughey et al., 2009a, 2009b). Thus, the primary finding of the second systematic review suggests that EIOL at 41 weeks gestation may be associated with a decrease in the risk of cesarean birth and meconium-stained amniotic fluid (Caughey et al., 2009b).

Keirse (2010) questions the definition of EIOL by Caughey et al. (2009b, p. 1) in their second systematic review. Caughey et al. (2009b) define *EIOL* as "induction of labor without a medical indication," but Keirse points out that the authors advise that EIOL may be done for "ending the ongoing risk for complications in the pregnancy" and to "limit their patients' physical risks" (Caughey et al., 2009b, p. 1). Keirse begs the question as to whether medical inductions occur only for patient comfort, pointing out that ACOG has defined the weeks of gestation as a medical indication for induction (Keirse, 2010).

Berghella, Blackwell, Ramin, Sibai, and Saade (2011) conducted a search of the MEDLINE database using the terms *elective* and *obstetrics*. Berghella et al. (2011) found more than 2,200 publications that included both terms, revealing that elective was used most often in relation to surgical intervention as opposed to medical procedures. These authors posit that the term *elective* lacks scientific specificity. Berghella et al. (2011) suggest that the term elective be deleted and that clinicians carefully document the specific indication for induction. If the terms elective and *medically indicated* are used, then there must be agreement on scientific definitions (Berghella et al., 2011).

King, Pilliod, and Little (2010) conducted a systematic review on EIOL that included meta-analyses of RCTs and other study designs since 1999. King et al. (2010) compared expectant management (awaiting spontaneous labor between 37 and 41 weeks) until labor occurred with EIOL. There were several limitations identified, including the small number of studies that focus on EIOL among women at low risk for complications and whose pregnancies are between 37 and 41 weeks gestation (King et al., 2010). These studies are older and did not include parity or cervical status. Four key questions were addressed in this review:

- What are the benefits and harms of EIOL at term (37–41 weeks gestation) compared with expectant management?
- Do the benefits and harms of EIOL at term vary by gestational age or other maternal or fetal characteristics?
- What are the appropriate medical indications for induction of labor?
- What are potential ways to reduce elective inductions of labor? (King et al., 2010, p. 1)

The findings of this review suggest that the commonly identified reasons for EIOL are not strongly supported by evidence except for gestational age beyond 41 weeks and prelabor rupture of the membranes at term (King et al., 2010). The evidence was moderately strong for EIOL increasing the risk of NICU admission for an infant less than 39 weeks; the evidence level was low for a significant increase in risk of cesarean birth and increased risk of operative vaginal delivery and very low for increased hospitalization stay (King et al., 2010). However, observational studies' findings suggested an increased cesarean rate among nulliparous preterm women with low Bishop scores. The authors state that there is a moderate level of evidence that quality-improvement programs focusing on avoiding inappropriate EIOL is an effective strategy in decreasing cesarean births, especially for nulliparous women with low Bishop scores (King et al., 2010).

## CESAREAN DELIVERY ON MATERNAL REQUEST

In low-resource regions of the world, a low cesarean birth rate often reflects poor access to health care. However, in a high-resource country, such as the United States, the escalating rate of cesarean sections is reason for concern. The Centers for Disease Control and Prevention (CDC) provides annual data on the number of births and trends in mode of birth. In 2013, the most recent year for which definitive birth data are available, there were a total of 3.93 million births in the United States. Of this total, 32.7% were cesarean births, representing a slight decline from the rates identified in 2011 and 2012, which held stable at 32.8% (Martin, Hamilton, Osterman, Curtin, & Matthews, 2015). In the United States, one mother in three will have a cesarean birth. Although some of the increase in cesarean births may be the result of an increase in both EIOL and CDMR, the percentage of CDMRs that contribute to this rate is probably less than 3% (Ecker, 2013). ACOG (2013b/2015) defines CDMR as a primary prelabor cesarean delivery upon maternal request in the absence of any fetal or maternal indications.

ACNM takes the position that the practice of CDMR is not supported by scientific evidence, and that without an evidence base to endorse CDMR, there is potential for harm. Therefore, ACNM (2005) endorses vaginal birth as the optimal mode of birth for women who do not have a medical indication for a cesarean birth. Conversely, ACOG (2013b/2015) takes the position that there is insufficient evidence to compare the benefits and risks of CDMR with planned vaginal birth, that most studies on CDMR have proxy outcomes that do not adjust adequately for confounding variables, and finally the results must be interpreted with caution.

ACOG (2013b [reaffirmed 2015]) makes the following recommendations:

- In the absence of maternal or fetal indications for cesarean delivery, a plan for a vaginal birth is safe and appropriate and should be recommended.
- In cases for which CDMR is planned, CDMR should not be performed prior to 39 completed weeks gestation.
- CDMR should not be motivated by the unavailability of effective pain management.
- CDMR is particularly not recommended for women desiring several children given that the risks of placenta previa, accreta, and gravid hysterectomy increase with each cesarean birth.

## The Evidence

There are few studies on CDMR or on maternal–fetal outcomes after CDMR. Recognizing the need for more knowledge about CDMR and the health outcomes of mothers and babies, the National Institutes of Health (NIH) convened a state-of-the-science conference on CDMR in 2006. A panel of 18 individuals (non-aligned with the Department of Health and Human Services and representing medicine, nursing, midwifery, reproductive physiology, public health sciences, and other disciplines) conducted and presented systematic reviews (NIH, 2006). The following are the conclusions of this groundbreaking conference:

- The incidence of cesarean birth without a medical indication is increasing in the United States, in part because of CDMR.
- The evidence is insufficient to fully evaluate the benefits and risks of CDMR.
- Until there is quality evidence available, decisions around CDMR should be individualized and consistent with ethical principles.
- CDMR is not recommended for women who desire several children because of the associated risks of cesarean birth (e.g., placenta previa, placenta accreta).
- Because of the significant neonatal risks of respiratory complications prior to 39 completed weeks gestation, CDMR should not be performed prior to 39 weeks.
- CDMR should not be motivated by unavailability of effective pain relief.
- The NIH or another federal agency should establish and maintain a website that provides up-to-date information on the benefits and risks related to mode of birth (NIH, 2006).

Risser and King (2010) conducted a systematic review of studies on elective cesarean birth and CDMR. The goal was to provide answers to three key questions:

- What are the benefits and harms of elective cesarean birth compared with spontaneous labor or elective induction?
- Do the benefits and harms of elective cesarean birth at term vary by gestational age or other maternal or fetal characteristics?
- What are the appropriate medical indications for planned cesarean birth? (Risser & King, 2010).

In many of the reviewed studies, proxies were used for elective cesarean birth and CDMR because the intended birth route was not identified or was too difficult to determine (Risser & King, 2010). This study-design feature is important when applying the results of a given study because of the inherent methodological issues in using proxies. Therefore, recommendations must be weighed against the limitations of the systematic review. The primary findings suggest that neonatal morbidity and potential neonatal mortality are associated with elective cesarean birth as compared to vaginal birth (Risser & King, 2010). The evidence, as reported by Risser and King (2010), further indicates that, in order to reduce neonatal mortality, elective cesarean birth should not be performed prior to 39 completed weeks gestation. Women desirous of large families should not undergo CDMR because of the related risks with succeeding pregnancies. Overall, the authors found that elective cesarean does not appear to confer medical benefits (Risser & King, 2010). (See Risser and King [2010] for detailed discussion of elective cesarean section outcomes.)

### Maternal Benefits and Risks

There are few studies that compare the risks and benefits of CDMR with planned vaginal birth. Because of lack of data, researchers use proxy descriptors, such as scheduled, elective cesarean birth with no indicated risk, to compare outcomes of CDMR with vaginal birth (Miesnik & Reale, 2007). Findings from studies using proxies must be used with caution because of the diverse meanings and perceptions around the descriptors.

ACOG identified potential maternal benefits of CDMR: decreased risk of postpartum hemorrhage and transfusion, fewer surgical complications, and a decrease in urinary incontinence the first year after birth (ACOG, 2010). CDMR may decrease the incidence of pelvic organ prolapse (POP). However, study outcomes indicate that parity, not mode of birth, provides the greater risk for the development of POP (Richter, 2006).

The risks of fever, infection, pneumonia, and thromboembolic events are increased with a cesarean birth. Although there are surgical risks of potential damage to the bladder, ureters, and other abdominal structures related to cesarean birth, these risks are reduced when compared to vaginal birth, although the evidence for this finding is weak. There is increased risk of placenta previa or accreta in subsequent pregnancies among women who undergo cesarean birth. If there is scarring from a cesarean birth and it results in abnormal placentation in a succeeding pregnancy, future reproductive capability may be compromised (Miesnik & Reale, 2007).

### Neonatal Benefits and Risks

Planned cesarean birth can have some benefits for neonates; for example, a lower mortality rate, lower infection rate, and reduced risks of intracranial hemorrhage, neonatal asphyxia, and encephalopathy. Fewer birth injuries occur to the neonate born via cesarean birth. Further, neonatal mortality may be reduced with CDMR at 40 weeks gestation because a vaginal birth between 40 and 42 weeks gestation can increase the risk of stillbirth (ACOG, 2013c [reaffirmed 2015]).

Respiratory distress syndrome (RDS) is a significant risk for preterm infants. A study ($n = 1,284$ cesarean births) focused on neonatal outcomes in elective cesarean births following uncomplicated pregnancies over a 3-year period

(Zanardo et al., 2014). This study concluded that RDS could be significantly reduced if elective cesarean births occurred at least at 39 weeks gestation. The incidence of RDS after elective cesarean term birth was 22/1,000 births as compared to vaginal births (9/1,000 births). There was, however, a significant reduction in the incidence of RDS from week 37 +0/7 to 37 +6/7 weeks gestation and thereafter falling to 5.9/1,000 births for infants born at or after 40 +0/7 weeks (Zanardo et al., 2004).

A retrospective cohort study of mode of delivery conducted in Shanghai, China, described the risks and benefits of CDMR in a Chinese population of 66, 226 women. A total of 16,333 women (24.7%) underwent CDMR and the frequency of neonatal RDS was higher in the CDMR group (Liu, Landon, Cheng, & Chen, 2015).

Although the establishment of fetal lung maturity may be valuable in decision making related to elective birth, the late preterm infant (despite documentation of mature lecithin/sphingomyelin ratios or the presence of phosphatidyl glycerol indicating mature fetal lung status) may still develop RDS, interventricular hemorrhage, or necrotizing enterocolitis. ACOG (2013c [reaffirmed 2015]) takes the position that if birth is medically indicated, amniocentesis for fetal lung maturity in well-dated pregnancies should not be used to time the delivery. The rationale for this is straightforward. If there is a compelling indication for delivery because of either maternal or newborn benefit, the delivery would need to proceed regardless of maturity testing. However, if delivery could be safely delayed, then there is no indication for delivery (ACOG, 2013c [reaffirmed 2015]).

A study comparing adverse outcomes of infants born preterm (32–33 6/7 weeks gestation), late preterm (34–36 6/7 weeks), and term (37 weeks or later) revealed that late preterm infants had significantly increased risk of poor outcomes when compared to term infants. Perinatal and morbidity rates increased for every week less than 39 weeks gestation (Bastek et al., 2008). These findings support ACOG's recommendation that elective induction/cesarean birth should not occur prior to 39 completed weeks gestation (ACOG, 2009 [reaffirmed 2015]).

A large retrospective study comparing the outcomes of neonates born following documentation of fetal lung maturity prior to 39 completed weeks gestation ($n = 459$) with those born at 39 or 40 weeks gestation ($n = 13,339$) demonstrated that neonates born between 36 and 38 weeks, even after documented fetal lung maturity, are at a higher risk of adverse outcomes, including RDS (Bates et al., 2010). There is a significant risk of morbidity and mortality for neonates born prior to 39 completed weeks gestation. CDMR should not occur prior to 39 completed weeks gestation, regardless of fetal lung maturity. Efforts need to be directed at decreasing the rate of late preterm birth (Fuchs & Wapner, 2006).

Cesarean birth can negatively impact breastfeeding and bonding in the postpartum because of the recovery time and pain associated with the surgery. Breastfeeding and bonding may be negatively impacted if the infant is in the NICU. Women requesting CDMR need to be counseled that the surgery itself, even if the outcome is good, may impact immediate mother–infant bonding and feeding. There is a potential for newborns born by cesarean to spend more time separated from their mothers (Miesnik & Reale, 2007).

## THE PUBLIC HEALTH IMPACT OF EIOL AND CDMR

Many women believe that cesarean birth is safer than a vaginal birth (Weaver, Statham, & Richards, 2007). However, the request for cesarean birth remains low and there is little to no distinction made between elective cesarean birth and CDMR. The former is often recommended or suggested by the physician and may be for reasons unrelated to medical indications, such as provider convenience. CDMR is requested by the pregnant woman. (Wilson, 2007).

### Population-Based Effects

There are public health population-based impacts with increased cesarean birth. Plante (2006) identifies that for every 5% increase in elective cesarean birth, the United States can expect to see the following changes in larger population-based outcomes:

- Increase in maternal deaths (14–32), surgical complications (5,000–24,000), infections (4,000–6,000), venous thrombosis (200–300)
- Increase in postpartum readmission (2,200), hospital days (930,000), increased medical error, longer wait time for elective operations
- Increase in NICU admissions (33,000) and RDS (8,000)
- $750 million to $1.7 billion in expenditures (Plante, 2006)

"What makes sense on an individual patient level may be ill-advised on a population basis and patient request is a poor substitute for policy" (Plante, 2006, p. 813).

### Financial Impact

It is well documented that increasing the number of EIOL and CDMR increases costs to society. A recent study comparing three approaches to reduce the number of elective cesarean births found that a hard-stop approach (a hospital-developed policy that would prohibit purely elective cesarean births prior to 39 weeks gestation) had the potential to lower the late preterm birth rate to 1.7% (Clark et al., 2010). This finding means that one-half million NICU-days could be avoided, saving close to $1 billion annually (Clark et al., 2010).

Zupancic (2008) examined the economic implications of an increase in elective cesarean births. He emphasizes that the most important economic issue with CDMR is whether there is health benefit to mother, baby, or society that offsets the cost. There are few well-constructed studies that present evidence of cost–benefit determination. As EIOL and CDMR increase, one cost is expansion of nurse staffing to meet safe staffing guidelines (Simpson, 2010).

### Impact on Health Outcomes

Once intervention occurs, a cascade of events follows, such as insertion of intravenous lines, continuous electronic fetal monitoring, confinement to bed, use of high-alert medication such as oxytocin, and potential for increased pain and iatrogenic infections (Simpson, 2010). Some posit that elective cesarean birth is a socially constructed technological process. The transformation of cesarean birth from emergent to elective impacts health outcomes, essentially reconstructing the way women view birth. It gives credence to birth as fraught with risk, a disease to be cured.

The conversation around cesarean birth has shifted from safety to one of women's choice, particularly interesting when considering the biomedical context in which women have very few choices but now are given choices about labor induction and surgical birth. Because obstetricians usually are the health care providers who perform cesarean births, they hold the power that can marginalize the voices of the women as well as the midwives and nurses who care for them during labor (Hewer, Boschma, & Hall, 2009). CDMR may, in fact, increase a woman's fears about birth and create more anxiety: the woman is now burdened with refusing versus choosing. Pregnant women as well as midwives and nurses need to be well informed and active in the debates about health outcomes of EIOL and CDMR (Hewer et al., 2009).

## EVIDENCE-BASED BEST PRACTICES

Even though the research is sparse and the findings sometimes controversial, there are evidence-based best practices that can inform the practice of midwifery around these issues. The following best practices are recommended:

- EIOL and/or CDMR should not occur prior to 39 completed weeks gestation.
- Women need to be fully informed about the risks and benefits of EIOL and CDMR and the weak to moderate strength of the evidence. The risks of using a high-alert medication, such as oxytocin, to induce labor should be included in counseling.
- Confirmation of fetal lung maturity is not to be used as an indication for EIOL or CDMR.
- EIOL and CDMR carry the risk of longer hospitalization time and may impede breastfeeding and bonding as a result of maternal–infant separation following surgery or from neonatal complications.
- Women desirous of having several children should not undergo CDMR.
- Practices and care facilities should develop policies around EIOL and CDMR that are based on the best evidence, safety, and cost.
- Pregnant women should be encouraged to take childbirth education classes in which the benefits and risks of EIOL and CDMR are fully explained and there is time for discussion and reflection.
- Birth certificates need to identify whether labor was electively induced and whether cesarean birth was elective or requested by the mother without medical indications.

### USING THE EVIDENCE FOR BEST PRACTICE

**Case Study 20.1   Prenatal Education About the Risks of Intervention**

Emily is a 25-year-old gravida 1 para 0. She began prenatal care during the first trimester of her pregnancy and her prenatal course was uneventful. In her last month of pregnancy, she began requesting induction of labor as a result of common discomforts of pregnancy and because her husband was a truck driver with only 2 vacation days left for the year.

Cervical exams at 38 and 39 weeks gestation revealed a closed, unripe cervix. The patient was counseled about the risks of induction of labor with an unripe cervix and the increased likelihood of cesarean birth. At 40 weeks, her provider agreed to electively induce labor and Emily was admitted to labor and delivery at 40 2/7 weeks. Cervical exam revealed that the cervix was dilated 1 to 2 cm, 50% effaced, soft, and posterior. The vertex presentation was noted to be at −2 station. Bishop's score was 4. Pitocin induction of labor was initiated and continued for 9 hours. The patient achieved contractions every 2 minutes, but there was no cervical change. She was discharged home that evening with a diagnosis of "failed induction of labor."

Emily returned the following day in prodromal labor and was dilated 2 cm, 100% effaced, and −2 station. The Bishop's score was now 6. Artificial rupture of membranes was performed, after which she received epidural anesthesia, Pitocin augmentation, and progressed to 7 cm before developing uterine tachysystole. Discontinuation of the Pitocin resulted in spacing of the contractions. Attempts to restart the Pitocin resulted in uterine hyperstimulation. During one episode of tachysystole, the fetal heart rate decelerated to 80 bpm. Emily then underwent an urgent primary cesarean birth for nonreassuring fetal heart rate and failure to progress. Her baby boy weighed 6 pounds, 13 ounces, with Apgar scores of 8 and 9.

**Exemplar of Best Practice**

This case study exemplifies the cascade of events that can occur with technological intervention. Using evidence-based information in counseling, this woman's health care provider potentially could have helped Emily to avoid the risks of EIOL, primary cesarean birth, and potential complications in future pregnancies. As an exemplar of best practice, the midwife needs to ensure that the client and her family have the opportunity to discuss and reflect on the evidence for best practice and be aware of the risks associated with intervention in a normal process. Ongoing education during the pregnancy and encouraging participation in childbirth classes are two exemplars of best practices available to midwives that may prevent EIOL, primary cesarean birth, or maternal–infant complications in current or subsequent pregnancies.

## REFERENCES

American College of Nurse-Midwives (ACNM). (2005). Elective primary cesarean section [Position statement]. Retrieved from http://www.midwife.org/ACNM/files/ACNM LibraryData/UPLOADFILENAME/000000000062/Elective%20Primary%20CS%20 Mar%2006.pdf

American College of Nurse-Midwives (ACNM). (2010). Induction of labor [Position statement]. Retrieved from http://www.midwife.org/ACNM/files/ACNMLibraryData/UPLOADFILE NAME/000000000235/Induction%20of%20Labor%2010.10.pdf

American College of Obstetricians and Gynecologists (ACOG). (2009 [reaffirmed 2015]). ACOG Practice Bulletin No. 107: Induction of labor. *Obstetrics & Gynecology, 114* (2, Pt. 1), 386–397. doi:10.1097/AOG.0b013e3181b48ef5

American College of Obstetricians and Gynecologists. (2010). *Cesarean delivery on maternal request*. Retrieved from http://www.acog.org/Resources_And_Publications/Committee_Opinions/Committee_on_Obstetric_Practice/Cesarean_Delivery_on_Maternal_Request.aspx

American College of Obstetricians and Gynecologists (ACOG). (2013a). ACOG Committee Opinion No. 579: Definition of term pregnancy. *Obstetrics & Gynecology, 122*(5), 1139–1140. doi:10.1097/01.AOG.0000437385.88715.4a

American College of Obstetricians and Gynecologists (ACOG). (2013b [reaffirmed 2015]). ACOG Committee Opinion No. 559: Cesarean delivery on maternal request. *Obstetrics & Gynecology, 121*(4), 904–907. doi:10.1097/01.AOG.0000428647.67925.d3

American College of Obstetricians and Gynecologists (ACOG). (2013c [reaffirmed 2015]). ACOG Committee Opinion, No. 560: Medically indicated late-preterm and early-term deliveries. *Obstetrics & Gynecology, 121*(4), 908–910. doi:10.1097/01.AOG.0000428648.75548.00

Bailit, J. L., & Ohio Perinatal Quality Collaborative. (2010). Rates of labor induction without medical indication are overestimated when derived from birth certificate data. *American Journal of Obstetrics & Gynecology, 203*(3), 269.e1–269.e3. doi:10.1016/j.ajog.2010.07.004

Bastek, J. A., Sammel, M. D., Paré, E., Srinivas, S. K., Posencheg, M. A., & Elovitz, M. A. (2008). Adverse neonatal outcomes: Examining the risks between preterm, late preterm, and term infants. *American Journal of Obstetrics & Gynecology, 199*(4), 367.e1–367.e8. doi:10.1016/j.ajog.2008.08.002

Bates, E., Rouse, D. J., Mann, M. L., Chapman, V., Carlo, W. A., & Tita, A. T. (2010). Neonatal outcomes after demonstrated fetal lung maturity before 39 weeks gestation. *Obstetrics & Gynecology, 116*(6), 1288–1295. doi:10.1097/AOG.0b013e3181fb7ece

Beebe, L., Beaty, C., & Rayburn, W. (2007). Immediate neonatal outcomes after elective induction of labor. *Journal of Reproductive Medicine, 52*(3), 173–175.

Berghella, V., Blackwell, S. C., Ramin, S. M., Sibai, B. M., & Saade, G. R. (2011). Use and misuse of the term "elective" in obstetrics. *Obstetrics & Gynecology, 117*(2, Pt. 1), 372–376. doi:10.1097/AOG.0b013e31820780ff

Caughey, A. B., Sundaram, V., Kaimal, A. J., Cheng, Y. W., Gienger, A., Little, S. E., . . . Bravata, D. M. (2009a). *Maternal and neonatal outcomes of elective induction of labor*. Evidence Report/Technology Assessment No. 176. (Prepared by the Stanford University-UCSF Evidence based Practice Center. AHRQ Publication No. 09-E005). Rockville, MD: Agency for Healthcare Research and Quality. Retrieved from http://www.ncbi.nlm.nih.gov/books/NBK38683

Caughey, A. B., Sundaram, V., Kaimal, A. J., Gienger, A., Cheng, Y. W., McDonald, K. M., . . . Bravata, D. M. (2009b). Systematic review: Elective induction of labor versus expectant management of pregnancy. *Annals of Internal Medicine, 151*(4), 252–263. doi:10.7326/0003-4819-151-4-200908180-00007

Clark, S. L., Frye, D. R., Meyers, J. A., Belfort, M. A., Dildy, G. A., Kofford, S., & Perlin, J. A. (2010). Reduction in elective delivery at < 39 weeks of gestation: Comparative change and the impact on neonatal intensive care admission and stillbirth. *American Journal of Obstetrics & Gynecology, 203*(5), 449.e1–449.e6. doi:10.1016/j.ajog.2010.05.036

Clark, S. L., Simpson, K. R., Knox, G. E., & Garite, T. J. (2009). Oxytocin: New perspectives on an old drug. *American Journal of Obstetrics & Gynecology, 200*(1), 35.e1–35.e6. doi:10.1016/j.ajog.2008.06.010

Ecker, J. (2013). Elective cesarean delivery on maternal request. *Journal of the American Medical Association, 309*(18), 1930–1936. doi:10.1001/jama.2013.3982

Ehrenthal, D. B., Jiang, X., & Strobino, D. M. (2010). Labor induction and the risk of cesarean delivery among nulliparous women at term. *Obstetrics & Gynecology, 116*(1), 35–42. doi:10.1097/AOG.0b013e3181e10c5c

Fuchs, K., & Wapner, R. (2006). Elective cesarean section and induction and their impact on late preterm births. *Clinics in Perinatology, 33*(4), 793–801. doi:10.1016/j.clp.2006.09.010

Gibson, K. S., Waters, T. P., & Bailit, J. L. (2014). Maternal and neonatal outcomes in electively induced low-risk term pregnancies. *American Journal of Obstetrics & Gynecology, 211*(3), 249.e1–249.e16. doi:10.1016/j.ajog.2014.03.016

Hewer, N., Boschma, G., & Hall, W. A. (2009). Elective caesarean section as a transformative technological process: Players, power and context. *Journal of Advanced Nursing, 65*(8), 1762–1771. doi:10.1111/j.1365-2648.2009.05021.x

Kaimal, A. J., Little, S. E., Odibo, A. O., Stamilio, D. M., Grobman, W. A., Long, E. F., . . . Caughey, A. B. (2011). Cost-effectiveness of elective induction of labor at 41 weeks in nulliparous women. *American Journal of Obstetrics & Gynecology, 204*(2), 137.e1–137.e9. doi:10.1016/j.ajog.2010.08.012

Keirse, M. J. (2010). Elective induction, selective deduction, and cesarean section. *Birth, 37*(3), 252–256. doi:10.1111/j.1523-536X.2010.00413.x

King, V. J., Pilliod, B. S., & Little, A. (2010). Rapid review: Elective induction of labor Medicaid Evidence based Decisions Project. Portland, OR: Oregon Health & Science University, 1–62. Retrieved from https://www.ohsu.edu/xd/research/centers-institutes/evidencebased-policy-center/evidence/med/upload/Elective-Induction-of-Labor_PUBLIC_RR_Final_12_10.pdf

Liu, X., Landon, M. B., Cheng, W., & Chen, Y. (2015). Cesarean delivery on maternal request in China: What are the risks and benefits? *American Journal of Obstetrics & Gynecology, 212*(6), 817.e1–817.e9. doi:10.1016/j.ajog.2015.01.043

Lydon-Rochelle, M. T., Cárdenas, V., Nelson, J. C., Holt, V. L., Gardella, C., & Easterling, T. R. (2007). Induction of labor in the absence of standard medical indications: Incidence and correlates. *Medical Care, 45*(6), 505–512. doi:10.1097/MLR.0b013e3180330e26

Martin, J. A., Hamilton, B. E., & Osterman, M. J. (2013). Births in the United States, 2013 (NCHS Data Brief, No. 175). Retrieved from http://www.cdc.gov/nchs/data/databriefs/db175.pdf

Martin, J. A., Hamilton, B. E., Osterman, M. J., Curtin, S. C., & Matthews, T. J. (2015). Births: Final data for 2013. *National Vital Statistics Reports, 64*(1), 1–68. Retrieved from http://www.cdc.gov/nchs/data/nvsr/nvsr64/nvsr64_01.pdf

Maslow, A. S., & Sweeny, A. L. (2000). Elective induction of labor as a risk factor for cesarean delivery among low-risk women at term. *Obstetrics & Gynecology, 95*(6, Pt. 1), 917–922. doi:10.1016/S0029-7844(00)00794-8

Menacker, F., & Hamilton, B. E. (2010). Recent trends in cesarean delivery in the United States (NCHS Data Brief No. 35). Retrieved from http://www.cdc.gov/nchs/data/databriefs/db35.htm

Miesnik, S. R., & Reale, B. J. (2007). A review of the issues surrounding medically elective cesarean delivery. *Journal of Obstetric and Neonatal Nursing, 36*(6), 605–615. doi:10.1111/j.1552-6909.2007.00196.x

National Institute of Health (NIH). (2006). NIH state-of-the-science conference statement on cesarean delivery on maternal request. *NIH Consensus and State-of-the-Science Statements, 23*(1), 1–29.

Osterman, M. J., & Martin, J. A. (2014). Recent declines in induction of labor by gestational age (NCHS Data Brief No. 155, pp. 1–8). Retrieved from http://www.cdc.gov/nchs/data/databriefs/db155.pdf

Plante, L. A. (2006). Public health implications of cesarean on demand. *Obstetrical & Gynecological Survey, 61*(12), 807–815. doi:10.1097/01.ogx.0000248826.44123.73

Richter, H. E. (2006). Cesarean delivery on maternal request versus planned vaginal delivery: Impact on development of pelvic organ prolapse. *Seminars in Perinatology, 30*(5), 272–275. doi:10.1053/j.semperi.2006.07.008

Risser, A., & King, V. (2010). Rapid review: Elective cesarean section: Medicaid Evidence based Decisions Project. Portland, OR: Oregon Health & Science University, 1–62. Retrieved from https://www.ohsu.edu/xd/research/centers-institutes/evidencebased-policy-center/evidence/med/upload/Elective-Delivery-Elective-Cesarean_PUBLIC_Rapid-Review_Final_12_1_10.pdf

Romero, S. T., Coulson, C. C., & Galvin, S. L. (2012). Cesarean delivery on maternal request: A western North Carolina perspective. *Maternal and Child Health Journal, 16*(3), 725–734. doi:10.1007/s10995-011-0769-x

Simpson, K. R. (2010). Reconsideration of the costs of convenience: Quality, operational, and fiscal strategies to minimize elective labor induction. *Journal of Perinatal & Neonatal Nursing, 24*(1), 43–52. doi:10.1097/JPN.0b013e3181c6abe3

Simpson, K. R., & Knox, G. E. (2009). Oxytocin as a high-alert medication: Implications for perinatal safety. *American Journal of Maternal/Child Nursing, 34*(1), 8–15. doi:10.1097/01.NMC.0000343859.62828.ee

Simpson, K. R., Newman, G., & Chirino, O. R. (2010a). Patient education to reduce elective labor inductions. *American Journal of Maternal/Child Nursing, 35*(4), 189–194. doi:10.1097/NMC.0b013e3181d9c6d6

Simpson, K. R., Newman, G., & Chirino, O. R. (2010b). Patients' perspectives on the role of prepared childbirth education in decision making regarding elective labor induction. *Journal of Perinatal Education, 19*(3), 21–32. doi:10.1642/10581240X514396

Tita, A. T., Landon, M. B., Spong, C. Y., Lai, Y., Leveno, K. J., Varner, M. W., . . . Mercer, B. M. (2009). Timing of elective repeat cesarean delivery at term and neonatal outcomes. *New England Journal of Medicine, 360*(2), 111–120. doi:10.1056/NEJMoa0803267

Vardo, J. H., Thornburg, L. L., & Glantz, J. C. (2011). Maternal and neonatal morbidity among nulliparous women undergoing elective induction of labor. *Journal of Reproductive Medicine, 56*(1–2), 25–30.

Weaver, J. J., Statham, H., & Richards, M. (2007). Are there "unnecessary" cesarean sections? Perceptions of women and obstetricians about cesarean sections for nonclinical indications. *Birth, 34*(1), 32–41. doi:10.1111/j.1523-536X.2006.00144.x

Wilson, B. L. (2007). Assessing the effects of age, gestation, socioeconomic status, and ethnicity on labor inductions. *Journal of Nursing Scholarship, 39*(3), 208–213. doi:10.1111/j.1547-5069.2007.00170.x

Zanardo, V., Simbi, A. K., Franzoi, M., Soldà, G., Salvadori, A., & Trevisanuto, D. (2004). Neonatal respiratory morbidity risk and mode of delivery at term: Influence of timing of elective caesarean delivery. *Acta Paediatrica, 93*(5), 643–647. doi:10.1111/j.1651-2227.2004.tb02990.x

Zupancic, J. A. (2008). The economics of elective cesarean section. *Clinics in Perinatology, 35*(3), 591–599. doi:10.1016/j.clp.2008.07.001

# CHAPTER TWENTY-ONE

# EVIDENCE-BASED MANAGEMENT OF PRELABOR RUPTURE OF THE MEMBRANES AT TERM

Amy Marowitz

## PREMATURE RUPTURE OF MEMBRANES AT TERM: RISK FOR MATERNAL AND INFANT INFECTION

*Prelabor rupture of the membranes* (PROM) at term is defined as spontaneous rupture of the amniotic membranes prior to the onset of labor in a term gestation. This situation is encountered regularly by midwives because PROM occurs in about 8% to 10% of term pregnancies (Gunn, Mishell, & Morton, 1970; Hannah et al., 1996; Zamzami, 2006). PROM is a well-established risk factor for maternal and neonatal infection (Chang, Lee, Baqui, Tan, & Black, 2013; Seaward et al., 1997, 1998; Soper, Mayhall, & Froggatt, 1996).

Interventions to hasten birth are often employed when PROM occurs in an effort to lessen the risk of infection (American College of Obstetricians and Gynecologists [ACOG], 2013). However, the duration of rupture is not the only risk factor, and multiple variables may interact in a synergistic fashion to result in infection (Chang et al., 2013).

One of the primary management decisions to be made with term PROM is choosing between expectant management (waiting for spontaneous onset of labor) and induction of labor. Although approximately 60% of women with term PROM will begin labor spontaneously within 24 hours of rupture (de Graça Krupa, Cecatti, de Castro Surita, Milanez, & Parpinelli, 2005; Gunn et al., 1970; Walker, 2003), expectant management of term PROM is an uncommon management approach today (Radoff, 2014; Tran, Cheng, Kaimal, & Caughey, 2008). However, it is a reasonable option that should be presented to the woman along with the option of labor induction.

### The Evidence on Management of Term PROM

Early research from the 1950s and 1960s showed a significantly higher perinatal mortality when the membranes rupture before the onset of labor and increasing mortality with length of time ruptured (Burchell, 1964; Calkins, 1952; Lanier, Scarbrough, Fillingim, & Baker, 1965). Some studies showed a much higher perinatal mortality when the membranes were ruptured more than 24 hours before birth (Calkins, 1952; Lanier et al., 1965; Taylor, Morgan, Bruns, & Drose, 1961). These findings prompted concern about duration of rupture as the greatest risk for infection, resulting in recommendations for aggressive management to hasten birth by inducing labor shortly after rupture of membranes. A number of authors writing at this time recommended ensuring birth by 24-hours postrupture, even if a cesarean birth was required (Lanier et al., 1965; Webster, 1969).

The following excerpt from the classic article by Shubeck et al. (1966) summarizes the prevailing view from this era:

> With rupture of membranes, the clock of infection starts to tick; from this point on isolation and protection of the fetus from external microorganisms virtually ceases. . . . Fetal mortality, largely due to infection, increases with the time from rupture of membranes to the onset of labor. (p. 22)

In the years since these studies were conducted, many methodological flaws have been identified in the early research. The studies were retrospective in nature and based on chart reviews or, in the case of Shubeck et al. (1966), analysis of one large data bank, the Collaborative Project. Information about management aspects of labor that could impact infection risk, such as repeated vaginal exams, was not addressed. Antibiotic therapy for anaerobic organisms, the pathogens commonly responsible for intrapartum infection, was not used at the time. Thus, maternal and neonatal outcomes in the presence of infection were significantly poorer as compared to today. In one of these early studies, the perinatal mortality rate following infection was reported at 50% (Lanier et al., 1965).

Another problem with the early studies was that the outcomes of preterm PROM and term PROM were not considered separately. The risks of fetal and neonatal infection and associated mortality markedly increase with preterm birth following PROM (ACOG, 2013). Despite problems with these early studies, the recommendation for aggressive intervention following PROM was readily accepted by many providers and continues to today.

In the 1970s and 1980s, concern mounted regarding the high rate of cesarean birth that resulted from aggressive management (Conway, Prendiville, Morris, Speller, & Stirrat, 1984; Duff, Huff, & Gibbs, 1984; Kappy et al., 1982). Research on PROM management focused on comparing induction with expectant management. Several of these studies showed similar perinatal mortality and maternal and neonatal complications with both options, but a higher cesarean birth rate with routine induction (Conway et al., 1984; Duff et al., 1984; Kappy et al., 1982).

## The TERMPROM Study

Identifying evidence-based best practice was limited by the methodology of these earlier studies. Most of the studies were not randomized and had relatively small numbers. There was limited homogeneity among the studies in the definition of *expectant management*, how induction was operationalized, and the criteria used to diagnose infection. These methodological issues prompted the standardization of definitions as well as the implementation of a large randomized trial to compare induction and expectant management of term PROM.

The Term Prelabor Rupture of the Membranes (TERMPROM) study was a multicenter, multinational trial in which 5,041 women with term PROM were randomly assigned to one of four groups:

- Immediate induction with oxytocin
- Immediate induction with prostaglandin $E_2$ ($PGE_2$)
- Expectant management up to 4 days followed by induction with oxytocin if labor did not begin spontaneously during this time frame
- Expectant management up to 4 days followed by $PGE_2$ if labor did not begin spontaneously during this time frame (Hannah et al., 1996)

The 4-day limit for expectant management was determined arbitrarily, based on the investigators' assumption that few women would be willing to wait longer than 4 days for the spontaneous onset of labor (Hannah et al., 1996).

The primary outcomes examined were rates of maternal and neonatal infection and cesarean birth rates. There was no difference in rates of neonatal infection or cesarean birth between the expectant management and the induction groups, with a lower rate of maternal infection in the induction-with-oxytocin group (4% as compared to 8% in the expectant management group). The rate of maternal infection for the induction-with-$PGE_2$ group was slightly higher than for the induction-with-oxytocin group (6.2%; Hannah et al., 1996).

The Cochrane Collaboration completed a systematic review of term PROM management (Dare, Middleton, Crowther, Flenady, & Varatharaju, 2006). The findings of this review closely mirror those of the TERMPROM study, which is not surprising considering that the TERMPROM study was the largest of 12 trials reviewed accounting for 5,041 of almost 7,000 total participants. The other 11 studies had between 59 and 566 participants. The majority of the studies in the Cochrane Review allowed for only 24 hours of expectant management. Thus, the TERMPROM study is of considerable importance because of its large size, randomized design, and longer expectant management time frame.

## Limitations of the TERMPROM Study

The importance of this study within the current body of literature on term PROM management has resulted in close scrutiny, revealing several limitations and questions about the finding of increased risk of maternal infection with expectant management. Limitations include potential overdiagnosis of chorioamnionitis, vaginal exams as an independent risk factor for infection, and the vaginal presence of group B streptococcus (GBS).

### Potential Overdiagnosis of Chorioamnionitis

Accurate diagnosis of chorioamnionitis can be difficult because there are no definitive diagnostic criteria. The signs and symptoms, such as fever, foul-smelling fluid, and abdominal tenderness, are either nonspecific or subjective. Fever can result from a multitude of processes such as other infections or the use of epidural analgesia. Foul-smelling fluid is a subjective assessment, and it may be difficult to distinguish between abdominal tenderness from infection and normal sensations from labor contractions. The accuracy of diagnosis of chorioamnionitis is increased if it is based on two or more clinical criteria, generally fever plus at least one other clinical sign such as abdominal tenderness, foul-smelling fluid, elevated white blood cell (WBC) count, or maternal or fetal tachycardia (Tita & Andrews, 2010).

In the TERMPROM study, the diagnosis of chorioamnionitis was based on the presence of any one of the following criteria:

- Fever before or during labor, defined as a temperature of more than 37.5°C (99.5°F) on two occasions greater than or equal to 1 hour apart, or one temperature of 38°C (100.4°F)
- WBC count of more than 20,000
- Foul-smelling amniotic fluid (Hannah et al., 1996)

Fever was defined atypically in the TERMRPOM study. A more typical definition of fever as a diagnostic criterion for chorioamnionitis is a temperature of more than 38°C/100.4°F on two occasions greater than or equal to 1 hour apart, or one temperature of 38.3°C/101°F (Tita & Andrews, 2010). This lower temperature threshold for fever, in combination with the use of one criterion instead of the more typical and accurate number of two or more, may have resulted in an overdiagnosis of chorioamnionitis in the TERMPROM study.

### Vaginal Exams: An Independent Risk Factor for Infection

In the TERMPROM study, women in the expectant management groups had significantly more vaginal exams than women in the induction groups (Hannah et al., 1996). This variable is important because the number of vaginal exams performed during labor is an independent risk factor for maternal infection. Regardless of the duration of ruptured membranes or duration of labor, the greater the number of vaginal exams, the higher the risk of infection (Tita & Andrews, 2010). This finding is well supported by epidemiological studies examining risk factors for chorioamnionitis (Hastings-Tolsma et al., 2013; Newton, Prihoda, & Gibbs, 1989; Soper et al., 1996; Soper, Mayhall, & Dalton, 1989). In one study, Soper et al. (1989) noted that the risk of chorioamnionitis with ruptured membranes was 3% with two vaginal exams and 63% after eight vaginal exams.

Secondary analysis of data from the TERMPROM study on the predictors of chorioamnionitis supports this finding (Seaward et al., 1997). The authors examined a number of factors, including duration of rupture of membranes, duration of labor, time from membrane rupture to active labor, and GBS colonization status. They found that the number of vaginal exams was the most important factor in predicting both chorioamnionitis and postpartum endometritis. In this study, the risk of chorioamnionitis was 2% with fewer than three vaginal exams and 20% after eight or more vaginal exams. The risk gradually increased as the number of exams rose from three to eight (Seaward et al., 1997). In addition to the number of vaginal exams, elapsed time between the first exam and birth is also significant in terms of infection risk (Schutte, Treffers, Kloosterman, & Soepatmi, 1983).

In the TERMPROM study, most women had a vaginal exam upon admission to the study (Hannah et al., 1996). This clinical practice is likely to have had a greater impact on subsequent infection among the expectant management groups because these women had a longer interval between admission and birth than those in the induction groups. In the secondary analysis of the TERMPROM data, Seaward et al. (1997) found that the duration of the latency period (time from rupture of membranes to onset of labor) had little effect on the development of infection when few vaginal exams were done.

### Group B Streptococcus

Maternal GBS colonization is a known risk factor for both maternal and neonatal infection (Centers for Disease Control and Prevention [CDC], 2010). The TERMPROM study was completed prior to the current CDC guidelines for universal screening for GBS during pregnancy and intrapartum prophylaxis with antibiotics for GBS-positive women. However, in the TERMPROM study, all women had a GBS culture upon entry to the study, allowing for analysis of this factor on outcome. Most culture results were not available before birth, and most GBS-positive women did not receive intrapartum antibiotic prophylaxis (Hannah et al., 1997). Although this factor potentially affected women who were induced or managed expectantly, GBS colonization may have had a greater impact on the expectant management groups because of a longer duration of rupture and a greater number of vaginal exams.

In a secondary analysis of the TERMPROM study data, the influence of maternal GBS status on infection risk was examined (Hannah et al., 1997; Seaward et al., 1997, 1998). In this analysis, the authors found maternal GBS colonization to be a risk factor for chorioamnionitis, postpartum endometritis, and neonatal infection (Seaward et al., 1997, 1998).

## Additional Research

A 2014 observational cohort study provides additional information about expectant management with term PROM (Pintucci, Meregalli, Colombo, & Florilli, 2014). In this study, 1,439 low-risk women who experienced term PROM were expectantly managed for 48 hours unless there was an indication for induction such as maternal fever, fetal heart rate abnormalities, or postterm pregnancy. Those with positive GBS cultures received prophylactic antibiotics. One digital vaginal exam was done upon admission; repeat exams were deferred until active labor. Diagnostic criteria for chorioamnionitis and neonatal infection in this study were similar to those used in the TERMPROM study (Hannah et al., 1996).

The incidence of chorioamnionitis was 1.2% (Pintucci et al., 2014) as compared to 4% for the induction-with-oxytocin group, 6.2% for the induction-with-PGE$_2$ group, and 8% for the expectant management group in the TERMPROM study. The neonatal infection was comparable to that seen in the TERMPROM study (Hannah et al., 1996).

A statistically significant increase in the rate of neonatal infection was seen with chorioamnionitis (odds ratio [OR] = 12.48; 95% confidence interval [CI; 5.58–27.9]; $p < .01$), greater than eight digital vaginal exams in labor (OR = 3.32; 95% CI [1.54–7.15]; $p < .0039$) and positive maternal GBS status (OR = 2.73; 95% CI [1.34–5.55]; $p < .0085$). These findings support those of the TERMPROM study, secondary analysis of that study (Hannah et al., 1996), and other studies (Newton et al., 1989; Schutte et al., 1983). Increasing the duration of ruptured membranes was not associated with increased rates of neonatal infections.

Caution must be used when comparing the results Pintucci and colleagues (2014) and the TERMPROM study. The study design and some of the management protocols were different. However, the study by Pintucci and colleagues adds to the body of evidence supporting expectant management as a safe option for selected women with term PROM.

## Expert Statements on the Management of Term PROM

Many clinicians use recommendations from professional organizations to help guide management decisions. Organizations providing recommendations for intrapartum care include the ACOG; the American College of Nurse-Midwives (ACNM); and, in Canada, the Association of Ontario Midwives (AOM). An examination of the discrepancies in the recommendations from these organizations is instructive in understanding some of the controversies related to the management of term PROM.

ACOG has published three practice bulletins on management of term PROM since the TERMPROM study was published. Each bulletin briefly addresses the issue of term PROM and then evaluates induction versus expectant management. The recommendations in these bulletins differ, though the TERMPROM study was used as the primary supporting data for all three. In the ACOG Practice Bulletin Number 1 (1998), the authors state:

> Risk of Cesarean delivery and risk of neonatal infectious complications do not appear to depend on the mode of management . . . although the risks of maternal infection may increase with expectant management . . . labor may be induced at the time of presentation or patients may be observed for up to 24 to 72 hours. (p. 81)

In contrast, in the 2007 ACOG Practice Bulletin Number 80, the authors state, "For women with PROM at term, labor should be induced at the time of presentation, generally with oxytocin infusion, to reduce the risk of chorioamnionitis" (p. 1014).

The 2007 ACOG Practice Bulletin did not include a rationale for the change in management recommendations. Fahey (2008) proposed that this change was based on newer evidence demonstrating the association between chorioamnionitis and increased risk of cerebral palsy. In addition, there has been an increase in the rates of elective induction and, presumably, greater acceptance of labor induction in the intervening years (Fahey, 2008).

The recommendations changed slightly in the 2013 ACOG Practice Bulletin Number 139. The authors recommend the following in regard to management of term PROM:

[I]f spontaneous labor does not occur near the time of presentation, labor should be induced . . . expectant management may be acceptable for a patient who declines induction of labor (if) clinical and fetal conditions are reassuring and she is adequately counseled regarding the risks. (ACOG, 2013, p. 921)

In 2008, ACNM published a position statement on the management of PROM at term, which was last revised in 2012. The authors stated, "The researchers found a higher incidence of uterine infection in the expectant management arm of this trial [the TERMPROM]. However . . . the study had several important limitations that affected the incidence of maternal infection" (ACNM, 2012, p. 1).

ACNM recommended that women be informed of the risks and benefits of management options and supported to choose between expectant management and induction if certain conditions are met. The conditions for expectant management include:

- A term, uncomplicated, singleton, vertex pregnancy with clear amniotic fluid
- Absence of identified infection, including GBS, hepatitis B and C, HIV
- Absence of fever and no evidence of significant risk for fetal acidemia in the fetal heart rate and fetal heart rate pattern (ACNM, 2012, p. 1)

AOM's clinical practice guideline on management of term PROM was published in 2010. The authors recommend that midwives "offer clients with PROM > 37 weeks' gestation the option of induction or expectant management. In the absence of abnormal findings . . . expectant management is as appropriate as induction of labor" (AOM, 2010, p. 10).

These organizations have used the same literature to arrive at different conclusions regarding the management of term PROM. It is noteworthy that the authors of the TERMPROM study state, "Induction of labor . . . and expectant management are reasonable options for women and their babies if membranes rupture before the start of labor at term" (Hannah et al., 1996, p. 1010).

## BEST PRACTICES

### Expectant Management

When the option of expectant management is chosen, a number of additional management decisions must occur. There is little current literature addressing best practices for expectant management of term PROM.

#### Where to Await Labor

A woman awaits labor at home or at the hospital. Evidence on which to base this decision is sparse. Women in the expectant management groups of the TERMPROM study were not randomized to home or hospital for this time period, though data on location for expectant management in the TERMPROM study were available and examined during secondary analysis (Hannah et al., 2000). In this analysis, expectant management at home was associated with higher rates of maternal and neonatal infection and cesarean section. However, the lack of randomization and control for variables that increase infection risk (such as vaginal exams and GBS status) detract from the validity of the data. No rigorous follow-up studies have been done on this issue.

The AOM practice bulletin on PROM addresses the locale issue, recommending that women be at home for the latency period as a result of the weakness of the evidence for women to be in the hospital during this time (AOM, 2010). Whether or not this recommendation would be readily accepted in settings in the United States is unclear. However, in some sites it may be impractical or impossible for women to await the onset of labor in the hospital during longer latency periods, especially in busy units with space and staffing limitations. Given the lack of strong evidence on the safest location for expectant management prior to the onset of labor and the absence of a physiologic explanation for an increased risk of infection with this approach, awaiting labor at home may be a reasonable option for women choosing expectant management.

#### Monitoring Maternal and Fetal Well-Being

In studies on expectant management, type and frequency of monitoring during the latency period varied considerably, with monitoring frequencies of every 4 hours to once a day (Duff et al., 1984; Hannah et al., 1996; Kappy et al., 1982). Outcome studies with different guidelines for monitoring have not been undertaken; therefore, decisions should be based on clinical judgment and conventional practices. A thorough evaluation comprises maternal vital signs; fetal heart tones per intermittent or continuous auscultation; complete blood count (CBC); assessment of color and odor of amniotic fluid; and maternal coping, including hydration and nutritional status, degree of fatigue, emotional status, and adequacy of family support. In their clinical practice guideline on management of term PROM, AOM (2010) recommends a complete, daily assessment. Location of expectant management may influence monitoring frequency, as hospital policies may require a specific interval.

### Expectant Management With GBS-Positive Women

In the secondary analysis of the TERMPROM study data, the influence of maternal GBS status on infection risk was examined in several publications (Hannah et al., 1997; Seaward et al., 1997, 1998). In these analyses, the authors found maternal GBS colonization a risk factor for chorioamnionitis, postpartum endometritis (Seaward et al., 1997), and neonatal infection (Seaward et al., 1998). In addition, the authors found that induction mediated this risk presumably because of its impact on other risk factors for infection, specifically, the number of vaginal exams, duration of rupture, and duration of labor (Hannah et al., 1996).

As mentioned previously, this study took place prior to the current policy of routine antepartum GBS cultures and intrapartum antibiotic prophylaxis for GBS-positive women. Most GBS-positive women in the TERMPROM study did not receive antibiotics (Hannah et al., 1997). It is not known how the administration of prophylactic antibiotics to GBS-positive women with ruptured membranes as per CDC (2010) recommendation would have impacted these outcomes.

Based on the evidence described earlier, ACNM (2012) recommends against offering GBS-positive women expectant management. AOM takes a different stance, citing lack of evidence on which to base management given current policies related to GBS screening and prophylaxis for colonized women. AOM (2010) recommends offering induction or expectant management for 18 hours. This time frame is based on research results indicating a sharp increase in risk of early-onset GBS infection of the newborn when membranes have been ruptured for 18 hours or more (Benitz, Gould, & Druzin, 1999). However, the current relevance of these findings is unknown, as the study included rupture before and after the onset of labor, and also occurred before the era of routine GBS culture and treatment.

Current evidence indicates that GBS colonization without intrapartum antibiotic prophylaxis is one of several known risk factors for maternal and neonatal infection in the presence of term PROM. In addition, CDC (2010) makes a clear recommendation to begin antibiotic prophylaxis with the rupture of membranes. Therefore, regardless of the plan for induction or expectant management, women with term PROM with a positive GBS status should be advised of this recommendation.

### Frequency of Vaginal Exams

Strong and consistent evidence shows that digital vaginal exams are a risk for infection (Hastings-Tolma et al., 2013; Seaward et al., 1997; Soper et al., 1996). In the TERMPROM secondary analysis, the number of vaginal exams was the risk factor most strongly predictive of infection, and the risk increases in a linear fashion with the number of exams (Seaward et al., 1997). The elapsed time between the first vaginal exam and birth may be a factor as well (Schutte, Treffers, Klossterman, & Soepatmi, 1983).

ACOG, ACNM, and AOM are all in agreement on the issue of digital exams in the presence of ruptured membranes. ACOG (2007) recommends that "digital cervical examinations should be avoided in patients with PROM unless they are in active labor or imminent delivery is anticipated" (p. 9). ACNM (2012) indicates "Expectant management requires minimization of digital vaginal exams, including avoidance of a baseline vaginal exam" (p. 1). AOM (2010) provides explicit guidance regarding the use of vaginal exams, advising "in order to reduce the risk of maternal and neonatal infection, avoid digital vaginal exams for women with PROM whenever possible, until active labour or upon induction of labour" (p. 10).

Avoidance of vaginal exams prior to labor is important but, in order to minimize infection risk as much as possible, these exams must be used judiciously once labor has begun. The midwife's approach to labor management in respect to expectations for labor progress is an important consideration. Allowance for a normal latent phase of labor is critical. The gradual, physiologic changes of latent labor are a necessary prelude for active labor. There is no evidence that latent or active labor progress should be assessed or managed differently in the presence of PROM (Pintucci et al., 2014).

Unless there are signs of infection, all women should be allowed adequate time to progress in labor regardless of membrane status. In fact, overconcern about labor progress with PROM can lead to more vaginal exams than necessary, inadvertently increasing risk of infection (Hastings-Tolma et al., 2013).

### Out-of-Hospital Birth

Expectant management of term PROM when an out-of-hospital birth is planned requires unique considerations. Women seeking out-of-hospital birth may be particularly interested in expectant management of term PROM. For these women, choosing induction of labor usually means changing the intended place of birth.

Many midwives attending births in the home or birth center follow guidelines requiring transfer to hospital care if active labor has not begun with 24 hours of rupture. Under these circumstances, women may feel pressured to stimulate labor with methods such as castor oil ingestion or nipple stimulation in an attempt to avoid going to the hospital. Midwives, in turn, may feel pressured to be overly vigilant regarding labor progress, doing more vaginal exams than usual, resulting in an increased risk of infection.

Expectant management for up to 96 hours in the absence of signs of infection or other complications is a potentially reasonable option for women in the out-of-hospital setting. Most women will begin labor in this time period (de Graça Krupa et al., 2005; Gunn et al., 1970; Walker, 2003). For those who do not, transfer to the hospital for induction with oxytocin would parallel the guidelines in the TERMPROM study (Hannah et al., 1996).

There are some small studies supporting the efficacy of castor oil (Davis, 1984) and nipple stimulation (Curtis, Resnick, Evens, & Thompson, 1999) in inducing labor with term PROM. The advantage of these approaches is that they do not necessarily require hospital transfer. However, there is no evidence to guide decisions on whether or not these methods should be used as a substitute for oxytocin after 96 hours of rupture, or used earlier to reduce the need for oxytocin. In addition, it is not known whether the risk of infection is impacted by the use of either intervention in addition to, or as a substitute for oxytocin induction.

Management of prelabor rupture of membranes at term in the out-of-hospital setting requires detailed discussions with the woman and her family about potential risks and benefits of all options. Also, it is important to anticipate the repercussions of different decisions in terms of number of vaginal exams and maternal status. Clearly, if transfer to the hospital for oxytocin induction is required at 96 hours postrupture or earlier, it is optimal for the woman to be well rested, hydrated, and nourished, and to have minimal or no digital vaginal exams prior to the time of hospital admission.

## Induction of Labor

Prelabor rupture of membranes is a legitimate indication for induction of labor. Many women will choose this option for a variety of reasons. After the decision for induction is made, there are other management issues to consider.

### Induction and Vaginal Exams

Minimizing vaginal exams reduces the risk of infection with PROM even when induction is undertaken, and this approach should be a priority (ACOG, 2013; AOM, 2010). As with expectant management, issues related to expectations for labor progress are linked to frequency of vaginal exams. The midwife must allow for the normal latent phase, and use reasonable and judicious parameters in evaluating active labor progress (ACOG, 2013). Vaginal exams should be performed only if the information gleaned would change the management of the labor (AOM, 2010).

### Induction and Cervical Ripening

Another issue related to induction for PROM is the use of cervical ripening with prostaglandins ($PGE_2$ or $PGE_1$) or mechanical methods for the woman with an unripe cervix. In the TERMPROM study, women randomized to the induction-with-$PGE_2$ group had a slightly higher rate of chorioamnionitis than those in the induction-with-oxytocin group. There was no difference in the cesarean birth rate (Hannah et al., 1996). However, use of $PGE_2$ was not based on cervical ripeness. Therefore, this study does not address the benefits of using $PGE_2$ for the woman with PROM who also has an unripe cervix.

Misoprostol (Cytotec) is a $PGE_1$ prostaglandin preparation introduced after the TERMPROM study was completed. In a 2005 meta-analysis, misoprostol was found to be comparable to oxytocin in terms of rates of maternal and neonatal complications as an induction agent for term PROM (Lin, Nuthalapaty, Carver, Case, & Ramsey, 2005). In a 2011 randomized comparative trial, immediate induction with $PGE_2$ and misoprostol was found to be equally safe and efficacious in cervical ripening for term PROM (Chaudhuri, Mitra, Banerjee, Biswas, & Bhattacharyya, 2011).

Mechanical methods used to promote cervical ripening, such as *Laminaria japonica* (an osmotic dilator) and Foley bulb dilators, have also been introduced since the publication of the TERMPROM study. Though not widely studied as a means of cervical ripening with term PROM, there is evidence that these mechanical methods, *Laminaria japonica* (Kurasawa et al., 2014) and Foley catheter bulbs (Mackeen, Walker, Ruhstaller, Schuster, & Sciscione, 2014), are safe and effective for this use.

## Planning for Expectant Management

Incorporating a guideline for the option of expectant management with term PROM into a midwifery practice may be challenging. Successful implementation requires advanced planning, beginning with dialogue with medical and nursing colleagues. This dialogue should include a discussion of current evidence and recommendations of professional midwifery organizations. Also, it may be helpful to explain in detail how education on and informed consent about different options will occur, and the central role of shared decision making in the midwifery approach to care.

It may be necessary to discuss with nursing administration the feasibility of awaiting labor in the hospital. Nursing staff must be made aware of the critical importance of minimizing vaginal exams, including avoiding a baseline exam on arrival when a woman has PROM and is not in active labor.

Consultation with pediatrics is also important. Some pediatric departments or specific providers routinely perform partial or full septic work-ups on neonates based on the duration of rupture. If a discussion of the evidence does not result in a change of this practice, an explanation of the policy should be included in the discussion with the woman, as it may influence her decision related to induction versus expectant management, or duration of expectant management.

A brief discussion with women during prenatal care about options associated with PROM may be beneficial (AOM, 2010). This discussion can easily be incorporated into the usual teaching on rupture of membranes.

## CONCLUSION

The optimal management of term PROM is not clear. Research from the 1950s and 1960s showed a sharp increase in complications once the membranes have been ruptured for 24 hours. Concerns about an elevated risk after 24 hours of rupture persist despite the fact that contemporary research findings have demonstrated otherwise. Scientific understanding of the relationship between ruptured membranes and infection risk has evolved since the 1960s. The amniotic membranes are no longer seen as an impenetrable barrier; in fact, pre-existing infection is thought to be the cause of some prelabor ruptures (ACOG, 2007). Also, factors other than duration of ruptured membranes are known to increase the risk of infection (Seaward et al., 1997, 1998; Soper et al., 1996).

The TERMPROM study has contributed to our knowledge regarding management of prelabor rupture of membranes at term. However, women in the expectant management arm of this study were exposed to practices that increased their risk of infection and it is likely that chorioamnionitis was overdiagnosed. Therefore, the finding of increased maternal infection with expectant management is questionable and this study should not be used to rule out the option of expectant management. A randomized trial utilizing more widely accepted criteria for the diagnosis of chorioamnionitis restricted the use of digital vaginal exams, and contemporary guidelines for screening of and prophylaxis for GBS would fill some significant gaps in the evidence.

The differences in the recommendations for term PROM in current practice bulletins suggest philosophical differences among professions. ACNM (2012) addresses this directly in its bulletin, stating:

> [W]omen have a right to self determination in their care . . . women should receive counseling and informed consent about the risks and benefits of management options of PROM at term . . . [and] be allowed to select expectant management as a safe alternative to induction labor. (p. 1)

No one management approach is right for all women and in all situations. The goal of midwifery management with term PROM should be minimizing infection risk within the framework of the midwifery model of care and the woman's preferred care options.

## USING THE EVIDENCE FOR BEST PRACTICE

### Case Study 21.1  Management of PROM at Term

Rachel, a 31-year-old gravida 1 para 0, started care in a midwifery practice in the first trimester. Her pregnancy was normal with a negative GBS culture at 37 weeks. At 39 weeks and 5 days, Rachel called the midwife at 9:30 a.m., stating she had just experienced a large gush of fluid and was leaking a moderate amount of clear fluid. She arrived at the hospital birthing unit at 11 a.m. Maternal vital signs were normal, the fetal heart rate tracing was category 1, the fetus was cephalic by external examination, and a speculum exam revealed nitrazine-positive, clear fluid coming from the cervical os, and a relatively closed cervix. Microscopy showed positive ferning. Rachel was not having contractions.

Rachel had been educated briefly about term PROM during prenatal care. The midwife now discussed potential risks and benefits of expectant management and induction based on current evidence. Rachel decided on expectant management. The midwife offered the options of staying at home or in the antepartum unit. Rachel chose to go home. A complete blood count was done and the midwife did discharge teaching, including nothing per vagina, rest, hydration, nourishment, and taking her temperature every 4 hours while awake. Rachel was instructed to contact the midwife

(continued)

## USING THE EVIDENCE FOR BEST PRACTICE (continued)

if she had a temperature of more than 99.5°F, meconium in the amniotic fluid, decreased fetal movement, bleeding more than spotting, or the onset of regular, strong contractions. She was instructed to return the next morning and that she could request an induction at any time.

The next morning, Rachel returned to the hospital at 9 a.m. She slept most of the night and awakened at 6 a.m. with mild contractions every 8 to 10 minutes. She was drinking, eating, voiding without difficulty, and coping well with contractions. She continued to leak small amounts of clear fluid. Vital signs and WBC count were normal, and the fetal heart rate tracing was category 1. Vaginal exam was deferred. The midwife reviewed coping with the latent phase and encouraged delaying admission until active labor. Rachel agreed with this plan.

She returned to the hospital at 6 p.m. with moderate to strong contractions every 3 to 4 minutes. All parameters were normal. A vaginal exam revealed she was 4 cm dilated, 100% effaced, at 0 station, leaking clear fluid, and had cephalic presentation. The contractions became progressively closer and stronger over the next several hours, and all parameters remained normal. The midwife deferred vaginal exams, observing contraction pattern and maternal discomfort as signs of progressive labor. At midnight, Rachel experienced increasing vaginal and rectal pressure. Vaginal exam revealed Rachel was 9-cm dilated, 100% effaced, and +1 station. Rachel began pushing at 1:30 a.m. and at 3:00 a.m. gave birth to a 7 lb, 2 oz girl with Apgar scores of 8 and 9.

### Exemplar of Best Practice

This case study exemplifies evidence-based best practice for term PROM. Rachel was screened for GBS during pregnancy, educated briefly on term PROM during prenatal care, given options, and allowed to choose between induction and expectant management when term PROM occurred. Infection risk was reduced by deferring vaginal exam until active labor as well as minimizing vaginal exams during active labor.

# REFERENCES

American College of Nurse-Midwives (ACNM). (2012). Premature rupture of membranes (PROM) at term [Position statement]. Retrieved from http://www.midwife.org/ACNM/files/ACNMLibraryData/UPLOADFILENAME/000000000233/PROM%20Mar%202012.pdf

American College of Obstetricians and Gynecologists (ACOG). (1998). Premature rupture of membranes. Clinical management guidelines for obstetrician-gynecologists (ACOG Practice Bulletin No. 1). *International Journal of Gynaecology and Obstetrics, 63*(1), 75–84.

American College of Obstetricians and Gynecologists (ACOG). (2007). Premature rupture of membranes. Clinical management guidelines for obstetrician-gynecologists (ACOG Practice Bulletin No. 80). *Obstetrics and Gynecology, 109*(4), 1007–1019. doi:10.1097/01.AOG.0000263888.69178.1f

American College of Obstetricians and Gynecologists (ACOG). (2013). Premature rupture of membranes. Clinical management guidelines for obstetrician-gynecologists (ACOG Practice Bulletin No. 139). *Obstetrics and Gynecology, 122*(4), 918–930. doi:10.1097/01.AOG.0000435415.21944.8f

Association of Ontario Midwives (AOM). (2010). Management of prelabour rupture of membranes at term (AOM Clinical Practice Guideline No. 13). Retrieved from http://www.ontario midwives.ca/images/uploads/guidelines/No13CPG_PROM_final.pdf

Benitz, W. E., Gould, J. B., & Druzin, M. L. (1999). Risk factors for early-onset group B streptococcal sepsis: Estimation of odds ratios by critical literature review. *Pediatrics, 103*(6), e77. doi:10.1542/peds.103.6.e77

Burchell, R. C. (1964). Premature spontaneous rupture of the membranes. *American Journal of Obstetrics and Gynecology, 88*(2), 251–255.

Calkins, L. A. (1952). Premature spontaneous rupture of the membranes. *American Journal of Obstetrics and Gynecology, 64*(4), 871–877.

Centers for Disease Control and Prevention (CDC). (2010). *Prevention of perinatal group B streptococcal disease.* [Revised guideline]. *Morbidity & Mortality Weekly Report, 59*(RR-10), 1–36. Retrieved from http://www.cdc.gov/mmwr/pdf/rr/rr5910.pdf

Chang, G. J., Lee, A. C., Baqui, A. H., Tan, J., & Black, R. E. (2013). Risk of early-onset neonatal infection with maternal infection or colonization: A global systematic review and meta-analysis. *PLoS Medicine, 10*(8), e1001502. doi:10.1371/journal.pmed.1001502

Chaudhuri, S., Mitra, S. N., Banerjee, P. K., Biswas, P. K. & Bhattacharyya, S. (2011). Comparison of vaginal misoprostol tablets and prostaglandin $E_2$ for the induction of labor in premature rupture membranes at term: A randomized comparative trial. *Journal of Obstetrics and Gynaecology Research, 37*(11), 1564–1571. doi:10.1111/j.1447-0756.2011 .01575.x

Conway, D. I., Prendiville, W. J., Morris, A., Speller, D. C., & Stirrat, G. M. (1984). Management of spontaneous rupture of the membranes in the absence of labor in primigravida women at term. *American Journal of Obstetrics and Gynecology, 150*(8), 947–951. doi:10.1016/0002 -9378(84)90388-0

Curtis, P., Resnick, J. C., Evens, S., & Thompson, C. J. (1999). A comparison of breast stimulation and intravenous oxytocin for the augmentation of labor. *Birth, 26*(2), 115–122. doi:10.1046/j.1523-536x.1999.00115.x

Dare, M. R., Middleton, P., Crowther, C. A., Flenady, V. J., & Varatharaju, B. (2006). Planned early birth versus expectant management (waiting) for prelabour rupture of membranes at term (37 weeks or more). *Cochrane Database of Systematic Reviews, 2006*(1). doi:10.1002/ 14651858.CD005302.pub2

Davis, L. (1984). The use of castor oil to stimulate labor in patients with premature rupture of membranes. *Journal of Midwifery, 29*(6), 366–370. doi:10.1016/0091-2182(84)90166-6

de Graça Krupa, F., Cecatti, J. G., de Castro Surita, F. G., Milanez, H. P., & Parpinelli, M. A. (2005). Misoprostol versus expectant management in premature rupture of membranes at term. *British Journal of Obstetrics and Gynaecology, 112*(9), 1285–1290. doi:10.1111/j.1471 -0528.2005.00700.x

Duff, P., Huff, R. W., & Gibbs, R. S. (1984). Management of premature rupture of membranes and unfavorable cervix in term pregnancy. *Obstetrics and Gynecology, 63*(5), 697–702.

Fahey, J. O. (2008). Clinical management of intra-amniotic infection and chorioamnionitis: A review of the literature. *Journal of Midwifery and Women's Health, 53*(3), 227–235. doi:10.1016/j.jmwh.2008.01.001

Gunn, G. C., Mishell, D. R., Jr., & Morton, D. G. (1970). Premature rupture of the fetal membranes: A review. *American Journal of Obstetrics and Gynecology, 106*(3), 469–483.

Hannah, M. E., Hodnett, R. D., Willan, A., Foster, G. A., Di Cecco, R., & Helewa, M. (2000). Prelabor rupture of the membranes at term: Expectant management at home or in the hospital? *Obstetrics and Gynecology, 96*(4), 533–538. doi:10.1016/S0029-7844(00)00971-6

Hannah, M. E., Ohlsson, A., Farine, D., Hewson, S. A., Hodnett, E. D., Myhr, T. L., . . . Willan, A. R. (1996). Induction of labor compared with expectant management for prelabor rupture of the membranes at term. TERMPROM study group. *New England Journal of Medicine, 334*(16), 1005–1010. doi:10.1056/NEJM199604183341601

Hannah, M. E., Ohlsson, A., Wang, E. E., Matlow, A., Foster, G. A., Willan, A. R., . . . Seaward, P. G. (1997). Maternal colonization with group B streptococcus and prelabor rupture of membranes at term: The role of induction of labor. TERMPROM study group. *American Journal of Obstetrics and Gynecology, 177*(4), 780–785. doi:10.1016/S0002-9378(97)70268-0

Hastings-Tolsma, M., Bernard, R., Brody, M. G., Hensley, T., Koschorek, K., & Patterson, E. (2013). Chorioamnionitis: Prevention and management. *American Journal of Maternal/Child Nursing, 38*(4), 206–212. doi:10.1097/NMC.0b013e3182836bb7

Kappy, K. A., Cetrulo, C. L., Knuppel, R. A., Ingardia, C. J., Sbarra, A. J., Scerbo, J. C., & Mitchell, G. W. (1982). Premature rupture of the membranes at term. A comparison of induced and spontaneous labors. *Journal of Reproductive Medicine, 27*(1), 29–33.

Kurasawa, K., Yasmamoto, M., Usami, Y., Mochimaru, A., Mochizuki, A., Aoki, S., . . . Hirhara, F. (2014). Significance of cervical ripening in pre-induction treatment for premature rupture of membranes at term. *Journal of Obstetrics and Gynaecology Research, 40*(1), 32–39. doi:10.1111/jog.12116

Lanier, L. R., Jr., Scarbrough, R. W., Jr., Fillingim, D. W., & Baker, R. E., Jr. (1965). Incidence of maternal and fetal complications associated with rupture of the membranes before onset of labor. *American Journal of Obstetrics and Gynecology, 93*(3), 398–404.

Lin, M. G., Nuthalapaty, F. S., Carver, A. R., Case, A. S., & Ramsey, P. S. (2005). Misoprostol for labor induction in women with term premature rupture of membranes: A meta-analysis. *Obstetrics and Gynecology, 160*(3), 593–601. doi:10.1097/01.AOG.0000172425.56840.57

Mackeen, A. D., Walker, L., Ruhstaller, K., Schuster, M., & Sciscione, A. (2014). Foley catheter vs. prostaglandin as ripening agent in pregnant women with premature rupture of membranes. *Journal of the American Osteopathic Association, 114*(9), 686–692. doi:10.7556/jaoa.2014.137

Newton, E. D., Prihoda, T. J., & Gibbs, R. S. (1989). Logistic regression analysis of risk factors for intra-amniotic infection. *Obstetrics and Gynecology, 73*(4), 571–575.

Pintucci, A., Meregalli, V., Colombo, P., & Florilli, A. (2014). Premature rupture of membranes at term in low risk women: How long should we wait in the "latent phase?" *Journal of Perinatal Medicine, 42*(2), 189–196. doi:10.1515/jpm-2013-0017

Radoff, K. A. (2014). Orally administered misoprostol for induction of labor with prelabor rupture of membranes at term. *Journal of Midwifery & Women's Health, 59*(3), 254–263. doi:10.1111/jmwh.12195

Schutte, M. F., Treffers, P. E., Kloosterman, G. J., & Soepatmi, S. (1983). Management of premature rupture of membranes: The risk of vaginal examination to the infant. *American Journal of Obstetrics and Gynecology, 146*(4), 395–400.

Seaward, P. G., Hannah, M. E., Myhr, T. L., Farine, D., Ohlsson, A., Wang, E. E., . . . Hodnett, E. D. (1997). International Multicentre Term Prelabor Rupture of Membranes Study: Evaluation of predictors of chorioamnionitis and postpartum fever in patients with prelabor rupture of membranes at term. *American Journal of Obstetrics and Gynecology, 177*(5), 1024–1029. doi:10.1016/S0002-9378(97)70007-3

Seaward, P. G., Hannah, M. E., Myhr, T. L., Farine, D., Ohlsson, A., Wang, E. E., . . . Ohel, G. (1998). International multicentre term PROM study: Evaluation of predictors of neonatal infection in infants born to patients with premature rupture of membranes at term. Premature rupture of the membranes. *American Journal of Obstetrics and Gynecology, 179*(3, Pt. 1), 635–639. doi:10.1016/S0002-9378(98)70056-0

Shubeck, F., Benson, R. C., Clark, W. W., Jr., Berendes, H., Weiss, W., & Deutschberger, J. (1966). Fetal hazard after rupture of the membranes. A report from the collaborative project. *Obstetrics and Gynecology, 28*(1), 22–31.

Soper, D. E., Mayhall, C. G., & Dalton, H. P. (1989). Risk factors for intraamniotic infection: A prospective epidemiologic study. *American Journal of Obstetrics and Gynecology, 161*(3), 562–568. doi:10.1016/0002-9378(89)90356-6

Soper, D. E., Mayhall, C. G., & Froggatt, J. W. (1996). Characterization and control of intra-amniotic infection in an urban teaching hospital. *American Journal of Obstetrics and Gynecology, 175*(2), 304–310. doi:10.1016/S0002-9378(96)70139-4

Taylor, E. S., Morgan, R. L., Bruns, P. D., & Drose, V. E. (1961). Spontaneous premature rupture of the membranes. *American Journal of Obstetrics and Gynecology, 82*, 1341–1348.

Tita, A. T., & Andrews, W. W. (2010). Diagnosis and management of clinical chorioamnionitis. *Clinics in Perinatology, 37*(2), 339–354. doi:10.1016/j.clp.2010.02.003

Tran, S. H., Cheng, Y. W., Kaimal, A. J., & Caughey, A. B. (2008). Length of rupture of membranes in the setting of premature rupture of membranes at term an infectious maternal morbidity. *American Journal of Obstetrics and Gynecology, 198*(6), 700.e1–700.e5. doi:10.1016/j.ajog.2008.03.031

Walker, J. (2003). Pre labour rupture of membranes at term. *Midwifery Matters, 97*, 6–8.

Webster, A. (1969). Management of premature rupture of the fetal membranes. *Obstetrical and Gynecological Survey, 24*(6), 485–496.

Zamzami, T. Y. (2006). Prelabor rupture of membranes at term in low-risk women: Induce or wait? *Archives of Gynecology and Obstetrics, 273*(5), 278–282. doi:10.1007/s00404-005-0072-4

# THE MIDWIFE AS CATALYST: PROMOTING INSTITUTIONAL CHANGE WITH INTRAPARTUM IMMERSION HYDROTHERAPY

Elizabeth Nutter and Jenna Shaw-Battista

Routine intrapartum care practices in the United States frequently obstruct physiologic childbirth, even among healthy women who desire to birth naturally. Only 64% of women in the United States in 2013 experienced spontaneous vaginal birth (Martin, Hamilton, Osterman, Curtin, & Matthews, 2015). Most women who give birth in the United States receive numerous obstetrical interventions, including some form of pharmacological pain relief, for example, epidural analgesia and anesthesia despite potential negative impacts on maternal and fetal circulation, labor progress, and the normal birth rate (Declercq, Sakala, Corry, & Applebaum, 2006).

## PHYSIOLOGIC CHILDBIRTH AND INTRAPARTUM HYDROTHERAPY

Physiologic childbirth, sometimes called normal birth, is defined as the spontaneous onset and progression of labor culminating in a vaginal birth of a term neonate and placenta, with minimal maternal blood loss (American College of Nurse-Midwives [ACNM], Midwives Alliance of North America [MANA], & National Association of Certified Professional Midwives [NACPM], 2012). Physiologic childbirth is often defined as not using pharmacological pain-relief methods that alter maternal and neonatal physiology during parturition. Almost all North American maternity care provider organizations preclude general or spinal anesthesia from published definitions of normal physiologic childbirth, and some include epidural analgesia and anesthesia, nitrous oxide, and/or sedatives and narcotics as part of physiologic childbirth (ACNM, MANA, & NACPM, 2012; Maternity Care Working Party, 2007; Society of Obstetricians and Gynaecologists of Canada, Association of Women's Health, Obstetric and Neonatal Nurses of Canada, Canadian Association of Midwives, College of Family Physicians of Canada, & The Society of Rural Physicians of Canada, 2008).

The consensus statement by the ACNM, MANA, and NACPM outlines the many positive health effects of physiologic labor and birth for women and infants (ACNM et al., 2012). Physiologic birth promotes optimal neuroendocrine function with increased release of endogenous oxytocin, endorphins, and beneficial catecholamines in response to healthful levels of biophysical stress during labor (eustress), thereby reducing the need for labor augmentation with accompanying risk of fetal compromise and need for operative intervention. Facilitation of optimal physiological processes during labor and birth further supports normal newborn cardiopulmonary transition and thermoregulation after birth, along with successful lactation and enhanced maternal–infant bonding (ACNM et al., 2012).

Intrapartum hydrotherapy is the therapeutic use of water for labor pain relief and relaxation. Hydrotherapy can be provided to childbearing women in a shower, bathtub, pool, or other available body of clean water. The term *intrapartum immersion* is only used to signify hydrotherapy via submersion and is differentiated by the timing of use during labor or birth. *Water labor* is defined as the use of immersion during some portion of labor followed by conventional birth in the air. *Water birth* is defined as the emergence of the neonate underwater, regardless of immersion hydrotherapy earlier in labor or the location of placental delivery. Delineation of these terms is essential as the effects of immersion hydrotherapy are distinct from use of the shower, and the quality of research evidence differs for water labor and water birth (Nutter, Meyer, Shaw-Battista, & Marowitz, 2014a).

Research demonstrates that intrapartum hydrotherapy may facilitate physiologic birth and decrease routine obstetric interventions that characterized maternity care in the United States (Declercq et al., 2006; Martin et al., 2015). This is achieved through the reduced use of analgesia and anesthesia among women who employ hydrotherapy as intrapartum immersion can resolve labor dystocia and reduce the need for labor augmentation with oxytocin (Burns, Boulton, Cluett, Cornelius, & Smith, 2012; Cluett & Burns, 2009; Cluett, Pickering, & Brooking, 2001; Cluett, Pickering, Getliffe, & St. George-Saunders, 2004).

The frequency of intrapartum immersion hydrotherapy in the United States is unknown and is not collected as part of national vital statistics data or routine institutional quality-assessment activities. In a nationally representative survey sample of women who gave birth in the United States in 2005, just 6% of respondents reported using a shower or tub in labor (Declercq et al., 2006). The pain-relieving effect of hydrotherapy is underutilized, despite being favorably compared to other nonpharmacological comfort measures and equivalent to pain relief offered by narcotic and sedative administration (Chaillet et al., 2014; Declercq et al., 2006; Simkin & Bolding, 2004). Research also demonstrates higher rates of hydrotherapy utilization among women in midwife-led and interprofessional collaborative maternity care practices in the United States (Albers, 1998; Shaw-Battista, 2009; Stark & Miller, 2009).

In contrast, intrapartum immersion hydrotherapy has been well integrated into interprofessional maternity care in the United Kingdom since the 1980s, and is widely used to support laboring women and physiologic childbirth (Burns et al., 2012; National Institute for Health and Care Excellence [NICE],

2014). The United Kingdom monitors maternal and neonatal morbidity and mortality without observing negative outcomes related to intrapartum immersion (Houston, 2010).

International organizations uniformly endorse the use of immersion hydrotherapy during labor but offer a wide range of positions on the state of the science about potential risks and benefits of water birth. The American Congress of Obstetricians and Gynecologists (ACOG) and the American Academy of Pediatrics (AAP) endorse immersion only during the first stage of labor (ACOG, 2014) and only support water birth if it occurs in a clinical trial. ACNM supports immersion hydrotherapy during labor and birth with trained attendants who follow evidence-based guidelines based on the best available data (ACNM, 2014). The Royal College of Obstetricians and Gynaecologists (RCOG) and Royal College of Midwives (RCM) support immersion in water during labor and concluded in 2006 that the state of the science did not support endorsing or prohibiting water birth. In addition, the Royal Colleges' joint statement suggested that organizations provide intrapartum immersion services for women who make an informed choice and stated that women have the right to this pain-relief method under the care of high-quality care by providers (Alfirevic & Gould, 2006).

Maternal–child health professional organizations cite literature to justify taking a position on the provision of intrapartum immersion practice. Skeptics question the safety of water birth and report that no fetal or neonatal benefits have been demonstrated (ACOG, 2014). Research suggests that physiologic labor and birth have positive short- and long-term health implications for both mother and infant (ACNM et al., 2012) despite interprofessional disagreements about the quality and findings of water birth research.

## INTRAPARTUM IMMERSION HYDROTHERAPY: THE EVIDENCE

### Positive Effects

A recent integrative review of water birth research revealed that women who labor and give birth in the water are unlikely to experience medical interventions that can disrupt physiologic birth (Nutter et al., 2014a). Research demonstrates a significant reduction in the use of paracervical and/or neuraxial analgesia by women who try intrapartum immersion during labor, with no increase in infection or other adverse effects on the fetus, newborn, or mother (Cluett & Burns, 2009; Nutter et al., 2014a; Young & Kraske, 2013). Intrapartum immersion reduces anxiety, vasopressin, oxytocin, and cortisol while increasing maternal relaxation and reducing pain perception (Benfield et al., 2010; Eberhard, Stein, & Geissbuehler, 2005). Buoyancy, ease of movement, and an increased number of maternal positions in labor have also been reported as benefits of hydrotherapy (Ohlsson et al., 2001; Stark, Rudell, & Haus, 2008). Lastly, women utilizing intrapartum immersion report an increased sense of control and high levels of satisfaction with their birth experience (Cluett & Burns, 2012; Geissbühler & Eberhard, 2000; Hall & Holloway, 1998).

Intrapartum immersion literature also demonstrates healthful outcomes and suggests benefits associated with hydrotherapy during childbirth. Along with the reduced use of pharmacological pain-relief methods, labor augmentation with synthetic oxytocin and episiotomy are less commonly associated with water birth compared to conventional birth (Geissbuehler & Eberhard, 2000; Shaw-Battista, 2009; Zanetti-Dällenbach et al., 2007; Zanetti-Dällenbach, Lapaire, Maertens, Holzgreve, & Hösli, 2006). Women who utilize immersion hydrotherapy are more likely to experience intermittent auscultation compared to continuous electronic fetal monitoring (CEFM) in risk-adjusted analyses despite the availability of waterproof monitors (Shaw-Battista, 2009).

To date, only one study has rigorously evaluated the risk of perinatal mortality and morbidity among babies born in water (Gilbert & Tookey, 1999). This surveillance study ($n = 4{,}032$ water births) analyzed standard perinatal outcomes data in the U.K. National Health Service, surveying every pediatric provider in the British Isles on a monthly basis about newborns who may have had complications of intrapartum immersion hydrotherapy. No perinatal deaths were directly attributed to water birth. The study concluded that perinatal outcomes among low-risk women after water birth showed no increased risk (perinatal mortality relative risk [RR] of 0.9/1,000, confidence interval [CI] 99%) compared to women who gave birth conventionally (RR of 1.2/1,000 live births, CI 95%; Gilbert & Tookey, 1999).

## Controversy

Although intrapartum immersion during the first stage of labor has been demonstrated to be safe for the mother and neonate when evidence-based clinical protocols are followed, controversy remains about the strength of research in support of water birth safety and its demonstrable benefits (ACOG, 2014). Isolated cases of neonatal complications have been reported in the literature attributed to water birth (ACOG, 2014; Byard & Zuccollo, 2010; Pinette, Wax, & Wilson, 2004). Descriptions of cases vary widely among reports and frequently fail to describe key details such as water birth procedures, long-term outcomes, whether the water birth was planned, and the type of attendant, if present at the time of birth. Case reports should not be considered generalizable information although they guide researchers and may help health care providers to learn from others' experiences and reflect on their own practices (Melnyk & Fineout-Overholt, 2014).

One possible complication of water birth, occurring in approximately 2.4 per 1,000 water births, is a partially torn or snapped umbilical cord (cord avulsion; Nutter et al., 2014a). There is insufficient research demonstrating the rate of neonatal morbidity following cord avulsion with intrapartum immersion, although the risk of neonatal hemorrhage is likely to be related to delayed recognition and management (Schafer, 2014).

There is an absence of well-designed randomized controlled trials of water birth, and limited patient and provider knowledge on intrapartum immersion. Rare case reports of adverse sequelae undermine routine support of intrapartum immersion in the United States. Nonetheless, the number of patients seeking intrapartum immersion and water birth is expected to continue as consumer demand and availability of birth pools in hospitals increase (Burns et al., 2012).

## Barriers in Implementing Evidence-Based Practice

Clinical practices are often influenced by factors unrelated to research and optimal practices and outcomes. Medical interventions have frequently been incorporated into routine obstetrics without sufficient evidence to support change or demonstrate maternal and/or fetal–neonatal safety or benefit. For example, research clearly demonstrates that use of CEFM increases the rate of operative delivery without decreasing the likelihood of cerebral palsy, infant mortality, or other measures of neonatal well-being (Alfirevic, Devane, & Gyte, 2013). Despite level-one evidence of maternal and neonatal risk, continuous fetal heart rate (FHR) monitoring remains the most frequently performed obstetrical intervention in obstetrics in the United States (Ananth, Chauhan, Chen, D'Alton, & Vintzileos, 2013). To date, there is currently no joint call by pediatric and obstetric organizations to cease CEFM outside of a research protocol because of risk avoidance. Unlike CEFM, intrapartum hydrotherapy is a practice with international consensus on safety and benefit in labor (NICE, 2014), and is significantly underused in the United States (Declercq et al., 2006).

Barriers to hydrotherapy are not limited to those impacting the physiologic birth rate, interprofessional disagreements on the state of the science, or lack of provider knowledge about evidence-based intrapartum immersion guidelines. Cultural factors, systems issues, and the practice styles of individual health care providers all impact women's choices for pain-relief methods, including labor and birth in water (Kennedy & Lyndon, 2008; Stark & Miller, 2009).

### *Provider Concerns*

ACOG and AAP (2014) suggest that the safety and efficacy of water birth for the newborn has not been established and that water birth should be considered experimental and should only be performed in clinical trials. This opinion did not address the challenges to water birth research, which is costly and complicated for numerous practical, statistical, and ethical reasons. The experience of childbirth is uniquely personal, significant, and poorly suited to reductive descriptions with simple statistics. This raises ethical questions about randomized controlled trials, particularly when women are prevented from using an evidence-based labor pain treatment option unless they enroll in an intrapartum immersion trial and are randomized to the water birth intervention (Shaw-Battista, 2015; Walsh, 2011). Although observational studies cannot establish causality, they do help to address a key question: What are outcomes of healthy women and their neonates who self-select immersion hydrotherapy in a controlled environment with an experienced attendant at birth?

Existing data indicate nurses and midwives have knowledge and concerns about intrapartum hydrotherapy. For example, Stark and Miller (2009) evaluated nurses' perceived barriers to the use of warm-water immersion during labor and found that participants had knowledge about the safety and effectiveness of intrapartum immersion along with concerns about personal safety, the effort required for hydrotherapy provision, and the health care environment as a limiting factor. Nurses employed in facilities with certified nurse-midwives (CNM) reported fewer perceived barriers related to the work environment than nurses who primarily care for women attended by physicians during labor and birth (Stark & Miller, 2009).

Meyer, Weible, and Weober (2010) reported on the water birth perceptions, exposure, and experience of CNMs in Georgia. Findings included CNMs' perception of water birth benefits and concerns raised about maintaining water temperature and the physical demands placed on the provider. Young and Kraske's (2013) literature review identified commonly cited reasons for concern about water birth: water aspiration, neonatal and maternal infection, maternal and fetal thermoregulation, workforce skills and education, and emergency procedures in case of maternal collapse. They concluded that preventing a woman from accessing water immersion during birth based on concerns of water aspiration, infection, and thermoregulation was not evidence based. Practice issues related to workforce competencies and emergency procedures can be mitigated with appropriate policy, guidelines, continuing education, simulations, and/or clinical practice with mentorship by experienced water birth providers (Young & Kraske, 2013).

### Shared Decision Making

Water birth is an example of ethical care in shared decision making. Walsh states, "practitioners have a responsibility to make the best clinical judgment we can in partnership with women, even if this means going against normative practice" (Walsh, 2011, p. 4). Although science can help to advance our understanding of the impacts of obstetrical intervention and address gray areas in clinical decision making, evidence is not a neutral concept because studies require support from funders with specific priorities, research findings are not always definitive, and various interest groups stand to gain or lose from the adaption of their particular interpretation of the literature. To compound these issues, research often fails to include the critical perspective of childbearing women whose preferences, values, and informed consent should be paramount when formulating a plan of care.

### Timely Implementation

Another barrier to hydrotherapy is the general failure to translate research into clinical practice and policy in a timely manner, if at all. This limitation to evidence-based practice is one of the most consistent findings reported in clinical and health services research (Grimshaw, Eccles, Lavis, Hill, & Squires 2012). Water birth is an example of a clinical practice that began at the request of childbearing families without the evidence of proven safety or benefits, rather than introduction by researchers or maternity care providers (Rosser, 1994). At this point, intrapartum hydrotherapy is an example of failure to implement high-quality, experimental data about the safety and benefit of immersion during labor as an alternative to pharmacological pain-relief methods.

### Institutional Change

Incorporating research evidence into clinical practice is vital and complex, requiring a multifaceted strategy to promote organizational change (Chaillet et al., 2014). Studies of organizational strategies to incorporate evidence into practice and change provider behavior are instructive to new initiatives despite the limited success and failure rates of 60% to 70% (Burns & Jackson, 2011; Leslie, Erickson-Owens, & Cseh, 2015).

Emerging research may help to improve the success rate of organizational and individual initiatives to improve the quality of care through integration of best practices identified in health sciences research. For example, Leslie et al. (2015) performed qualitative research that examined how individual midwives and physicians increased use of evidence based practices. They identified five key themes that are essential to success:

- Trusting colleagues
- Believing the evidence
- Honoring mothers and families
- Knowing personal certainty
- Protecting the integrity of the mother and the baby (Leslie et al., 2015)

Collectively, these themes supported providers successfully moving from a decision to actualization of change (Leslie et al., 2015).

In a systematic review of the literature, Chaillet and colleagues (2006) found that key factors in implementation of evidence-based guidelines in obstetrics may differ from other medical specialties as a result of unique variables that influence professional behaviors among maternal–child health care providers. They suggested that obstetric nurses might be receptive to educational programs, clinical audits, and feedback to promote evidence-based clinical practice change. They also reported that a multipronged approach with an opinion leader as the change agent might facilitate acceptance of a given intervention. These findings were consistent with other limited evidence on effective strategies used to promote change in midwifery and maternity care (Nutter, Shaw-Battista, & Marowitz 2014b; Walsh, 2011).

The least effective strategies include dissemination of informational resources and continuing-education classes. Activities with moderate success include performance feedback, identification of peer-nominated leaders, and interprofessional collaboration to develop clinical consensus and strengthen teamwork. According to the literature on general practice change, the most effective strategies for incorporating and maintaining new water birth services are likely to be outreach visits by experts to meet with providers in their practice settings, ongoing mentoring for providers as they begin to incorporate the practice, involvement by local leaders and influential providers, and ongoing assessment of care processes and outcomes to address concerns, quality, and safety (Chaillet et al., 2006; Nutter, et al, 2014b; Walsh, 2011).

## BEST PRACTICES FOR MIDWIVES

Although the evidence on water birth is largely observational research, the potential benefits, including maternal comfort, autonomy, and choice, seem to outweigh any rare risk of harm in low-risk women and their healthy newborns. Morbidity and mortality are rare in both conventional and water births among women with straightforward term pregnancies and singleton vertex infants who constitute most of the U.S. childbearing population, including hydrotherapy research participants (Nutter et al., 2014a). Alfirevic and Gould (2006) state that "one could argue that the anecdotal evidence is reassuring, given thousands of women have given birth under water in the last few decades" (p. 2).

### Shared Decision Making in Midwifery Care

The midwifery model of care informs a therapeutic relationship that facilitates shared decision making and respect for women's autonomy. Through this lens, the choice of intrapartum immersion, including water birth, can be supported among women who understand the limited state of water birth science and choose hydrotherapy for pain control in labor.

Available literature on immersion hydrotherapy provides a considerable amount of information about how to limit risk of harm and incorporate the best available data. Research demonstrates that trained professionals can utilize evidence-based clinical guidelines, practice infection control, adhere to eligibility criteria, and comply with water birth delivery procedures. These measures can achieve excellent outcomes among healthy women and newborns for whom adverse outcomes are rare (Alfirevic & Gould, 2006). For these reasons, the benefits and potential risks of labor and birth in water must be discussed with women along with other labor pain relief methods, and their associated risks and benefits, in order to facilitate informed choice.

Maternity care organizations with neutral or supportive position statements on water birth stress the importance of respecting maternal autonomy in the decision to use immersion hydrotherapy during labor or birth following informed consent discussions with knowledgeable care providers. For example, the U.K.'s Royal Colleges of Obstetricians-Gynaecologists and Midwives supports giving women the opportunity to labor and birth in water as desired, and recommends prenatal education about the option for all women at low risk for perinatal complications (Alfirevic & Gould, 2006).

### Utilizing Inclusion and Exclusion Criteria

Water birth research protocols and hydrotherapy procedures can inform and improve clinical practices related to intrapartum immersion.

### Inclusion Criteria

Inclusion criteria based on the best available evidence are:

- A singleton pregnancy at term (at least 37 0/7 weeks gestation) with a cephalic presentation
- Stable maternal vital signs and category I or category II FHR pattern
- Women with GBS are eligible for intrapartum immersion with routine management and antibiotic prophylaxis (Nutter et al., 2014b)

### Exclusion Criteria

Water birth research has not typically included women with a high-risk pregnancy or health condition. Exclusion criteria for intrapartum immersion commonly include:

- Any condition requiring continuous FHR
- Abnormal vaginal bleeding
- Maternal fever greater than 100.4°F
- Recent administration of sedating medication (e.g., opioid administration within 1–2 hours)
- Other conditions that could compromise maternal airway self-protection
- General or regional anesthesia
- Untreated skin infection or active herpes simplex virus lesion
- Blood-borne pathogens (HIV, hepatitis B or C)
- Musculoskeletal compromised mobility or other condition that could compromise a woman's ability to leave the tub quickly in an emergency
- Category III FHR pattern
- History of a postpartum hemorrhage (> 1,000 mL)
- Anticipated shoulder dystocia or neonatal resuscitation (Nutter et al., 2014b)

## Managing the Labor and Birth

### Labor in Water

The woman's entire abdomen should be submersed in water to facilitate movement and to maximize benefits and comfort. The water temperature should never exceed 100°F as fetal hyperthermia may ensue, potentially causing dilated cerebral vasculature and increased oxygen consumption resulting in fetal hypoxia (Nutter et al., 2014b). Warm water may be cooled as per women's preferences during the first stage of labor but should be regulated to 97° to 99.9°F during the second stage of labor and water birth. This will minimize the risk of newborn bath water inhalation, which could result from an abrupt decrease in the ambient temperature at the time of birth into cooler water. During hydrotherapy, the water temperature should be assessed and documented hourly in the medical record (Nutter et al., 2014b).

Women may be advised that they can enter the tub at any time. Intrapartum hydrotherapy can be used to aid in prodromal labor, serving as a form of therapeutic rest for the laboring mother. In a mother strongly desiring an unmedicated birth, it may be best to delay immersion hydrotherapy until active labor as it is probably the most effective nonpharmacological method to reduce labor pain (Simkin & Bolding, 2004). Immersion hydrotherapy may also be considered with labor dystocia as an alternative to other forms of augmentation, based upon the randomized trials demonstrating efficacy on par with synthetic oxytocin augmentation (Cluett & Burns, 2009; Cluett et al. 2001, 2004).

Maternal and fetal well-being are monitored during intrapartum hydrotherapy as in conventional childbirth. Fetal monitoring can be accomplished with a fetoscope, waterproof Doppler, or with waterproof electronic fetal monitoring equipment, if continuous observation is indicated. The FHR pattern and contraction pattern must be documented every 30 minutes during the first stage of labor and every 5 to 15 minutes during the second stage depending on risk status (AAP & ACOG, 2007).

If the FHR pattern changes, the midwife should evaluate the mother's vital signs and fetal intrauterine resuscitation measures can be undertaken according to standard practice, for example, the woman may be advised to change position in the tub, and an oral or intravenous fluid bolus may be considered. If the FHR is normal upon reassessment following treatment, the woman may remain in the water with close observation. If the worrisome FHR changes do not promptly resolve with position changes or other interventions, the woman should be assisted out of the tub for CEFM. If the FHR tracing is subsequently reassuring, it may become appropriate for the woman to re-enter the bath for labor and/or birth depending on her preferences and overall health status. If a category III FHR tracing is observed, the midwife should assist the woman in exiting the tub and promptly initiate CEFM and other interventions as needed.

### Water-Birth Procedures

During water birth, the best approach is "hands off" to perineal management in the second stage. The midwife should encourage the mother's pushing efforts with quiet verbal encouragement and guidance. If the baby emerges spontaneously, it is not necessary to feel for the presence of a nuchal cord. Time of birth is noted when the baby's entire body is outside of the mother, and any delay between the birth of the head and body should be noted per standard practice.

The baby must be born completely underwater, without exposure to air until the newborn's face is brought gently to the surface immediately after birth. If a woman raises herself out of the water during the birth and exposes the fetal head to air, she must be advised to remain standing or exit the tub with assistance to ensure the birth is completed in the air to avoid the potential risk of water inhalation by the newborn. In the event that a newborn's head is delivered into water but the body is born outside of the tub, the birth should be documented as a water birth with a narrative description of any event of complication, for example, the woman spontaneously got up during the birth and was asked to remain standing, or the woman was asked to exit the tub when the Gaskin maneuver failed to resolve a shoulder dystocia.

After birth into water, the infant should be brought directly but gently to the surface within 5 to 10 seconds while taking care to prevent tension on cord, minimizing avulsion. Cord entanglement can be quickly resolved underwater before bringing the newborn to the water surface for the first breath. Women should be asked to stand above the water or exit the tub in the event that a short umbilical cord prevents bringing the newborn's face to the surface. The newborn's face and head should not be re-submerged in water under any circumstance after being brought to the water's surface whether or not respiration has been initiated (Nutter et al., 2014b).

If a cord avulsion occurs, careful cord management during water birth and immediate evaluation of the newborn umbilicus is required (Nutter et al., 2014b). Cord clamps should be readily available and used immediately in case of cord avulsion or blood in the tub for which a source cannot be immediately identified. Delayed cord clamping can occur following an uncomplicated water birth, after pulsations have ceased or the placenta delivers. Once the umbilical cord is clamped and cut, a cord blood sample may be obtained and the placenta may be delivered via maternal pushing efforts per routine procedure (Nutter, 2013).

### Newborn Care

After water birth, maintain the warmth of the bath water to support newborn thermoregulation. Vigorous newborns may be held skin to skin by their mothers with their lower extremities, abdomen, and chest underwater. Dry the baby's exposed neck and head to reduce heat loss. Standard newborn Apgar scores should be obtained at 1 and 5 minutes after birth, not delayed until the newborn is removed from the tub. If respirations are not initiated within 30 seconds of water birth, the cord should be clamped and cut to enable removal of the newborn from the tub for immediate treatment, regardless of heart rate and tone, or any early resuscitation measures, for example, drying and stimulation (Nutter, 2013).

### Management of the Third Stage of Labor

As for conventional birth, the goal of third-stage management following water birth is to achieve placental delivery and minimize the blood loss, while facilitating skin-to-skin contact and bonding between mother and child. The placenta can be delivered in or out of the water at the discretion of the midwife and the mother's preference. If the placenta has not been delivered within 15 to 30 minutes, or blood loss is noted to be excessive or otherwise abnormal, the mother should be assisted out of the tub to complete the third stage of labor and receive treatment to prevent or treat hemorrhage. Prophylactic synthetic oxytocin can be given intramuscularly or intravenously during immersion hydrotherapy as per the standard guidelines and the woman's informed consent for active management of the third stage of labor. An estimation of blood loss and postnatal observations of the woman and newborn should be conducted and documented in the usual fashion. If the placenta is delivered in the tub, the woman may be assisted into a bed afterward to facilitate identification and repair of any genital lacerations.

### Water Birth Equipment

In addition to standard instruments and other delivery equipment, water birth midwives should consider obtaining several additional items for hydrotherapy provision (Nutter, 2013). A waterproof thermometer and Doppler or electronic fetal monitoring equipment are essential. Standard precautions can be achieved with exam gloves of sufficient length to cover the forearm when submerged during exams or fetal monitoring, with a waterproof gown, and eye protection. A scoop or net can be helpful to remove any fecal debris. Large warm towels or blankets are needed when the woman and newborn exit the water. Optional equipment includes a waterproof flashlight or mirror to aid visualization underwater and a low stool, exercise ball, and/or kneeling pads for the midwife, other providers, and birth companions.

## Establishing a Water Birth and Immersion Hydrotherapy Service

The first step in establishing a water birth and immersion hydrotherapy service is to conduct a thorough needs assessment among key stakeholders and determine the level of support available to initiate this service. The steps of innovation and change, as described previously, should be used. Once there is institutional buy-in for the service, there are a number of key steps in implementation.

### Development of Clinical Guidelines

The clinical guidelines, policies, and procedures for water birth management and the use and cleaning of the tub need to have clear delineations of staff roles and responsibilities. Clear guidelines facilitate participation of hospital and practice administrators, infection control, and facilities maintenance staff, to improve teamwork, communication, and standard hygiene practices, and to monitor quality of care and perinatal outcomes. A written consent form should be required following discussion of risks and benefits and alternative pain-relief options.

### Quality Improvement

Within the first 6 months that water birth is available or on a random, ongoing basis, chart audits of clinical outcomes and adherence to policies and procedures should be conducted to assess for best practices. Some examples of items to flag include offering all healthy childbearing women the intrapartum immersion hydrotherapy in the first stage of labor, and written consent for every water birth. Formal research should be conducted whenever feasible.

A key area of quality improvement is obtaining feedback from childbearing families. A range of strategies should be used. Some examples include open-ended interviews by the midwife at hospital discharge, postpartum satisfaction surveys, and comparisons of overall maternal postpartum satisfaction with care for the maternity unit before and after the option of water birth.

### Staff Competencies

Initial and ongoing competency of all the staff is essential. Some methods of assessing competence include regularly scheduled obstetrical emergency simulations with hydrotherapy, continuing-education activities, and perhaps most effective, mentoring and supervision of the water births attended by new or inexperienced midwives and staff.

### Childbirth Education

Including intrapartum immersion in childbirth education classes for families can be done in a face-to-face class or, for families who lack transportation or schedule flexibility, alternative methods could be language-appropriate written materials or the development of a remote asynchronous or live class via online video or an interactive learning activity.

## CONCLUSION

The midwife is in a key position to act as a catalyst for institutional change in promoting a safe alternative or adjunct to analgesia and anesthesia in childbirth. Midwives are encouraged to assume this leadership role in implementing change.

---

### USING THE EVIDENCE FOR BEST PRACTICE

**Case Study 22.1   Developing and Implementing a Water Birth Practice**

A midwife has accepted a position in a hospital where immersion hydrotherapy is rarely utilized, and when used is only implemented during labor, not birth. The midwife listens to a number of childbearing women who express interest in water birth, saying they have read about it online or talked with friends about their birth experiences. These clients also requested warm-water immersion to cope with pain in labor and reduce the likelihood of pain medications and anesthesia. Water birth did not seem to be their primary goal, but rather a safe and natural childbirth experience. The midwife spoke with her nursing and physician colleagues, learning that they were interested in exploring the possibility of intrapartum immersion as a nonpharmacological pain-relief option.

Then the midwife developed a survey to assess the knowledge and attitudes of hospital staff and affiliated health care providers. The survey results revealed concerns about maintaining water temperature and the provider's physical safety. The survey allowed the midwife to identify key supportive stakeholders and convene an interprofessional working group to identify best practices and draft clinical guidelines. The midwife also conducted focus groups to assess community interest in

*(continued)*

USING THE EVIDENCE FOR BEST PRACTICE (continued)

water birth. An unanticipated benefit of this community engagement were donated funds to purchase a tub and hydrotherapy equipment.

After the service was approved, in order to allay provider concerns, the midwife personally supervised the purchase of a tub with an automatic heater and temperature-regulation device, kneeling pads, and raised platforms to support good body mechanics. One year later, the midwife attended the first water birth. After this first birth, many healthy women in the practice chose intrapartum immersion hydrotherapy during some or all of their labors and births.

**Exemplar of Best Practice**

This case study exemplifies the role of the midwife as a catalyst for institutional change and in promoting physiologic birth through hydrotherapy. Among the many exemplary actions taken by the midwife-as-change-agent were conducting a needs assessment among key stakeholders, using the evidence in developing clinical guidelines, and establishing a childbirth education class about intrapartum immersion. These actions were all key to program implementation and sustainability.

# REFERENCES

Albers, L. (1998). Midwifery management of pain in labor: The CNM Data Group, 1996. *Journal of Nurse-Midwifery, 43*(2), 77–82. doi:10.1016/S0091-2182(97)00150-X

Alfirevic, Z., Devane, D., & Gyte, G. M. L. (2013). Continuous cardiotocography (CTG) as a form of electronic fetal monitoring (EFM) for fetal assessment during labour. *Cochrane Database of Systematic Reviews, 2013*(5). doi:10.1002/14651858.CD006066.pub2

Alfirevic, Z., & Gould, D. (2006). Royal College of Obstetricians and Gynecologists/Royal College of Midwives joint statement No. 1: Immersion in water in labour and birth. Retrieved from http://www.waterbirth.org/assets/documents/rcog_rcm_birth_in_water.pdf

American Academy of Pediatrics (AAP), & American College of Obstetricians and Gynecologists (ACOG). (2007). *Guidelines for perinatal care* (6th ed.). Elk Grove Village, IL: Authors.

American College of Nurse-Midwives (ACNM]). (2014). Hydrotherapy during labor and birth [Position statement]. Retrieved from http://www.midwife.org/ACNM/files/ACNMLibrary Data/UPLOADFILENAME/000000000286/Hydrotherapy-During-Labor-and-Birth-April -2014.pdf

American College of Nurse-Midwives (ACNM), Midwives Alliance of North America (MANA), & National Association of Certified Professional Midwives (NACPM). (2012). *Supporting healthy and normal physiologic childbirth: A consensus statement by ACNM, MANA and NACPM.* Silver Spring, MD: ACNM. Retrieved from http://mana.org/pdfs/ Physiological-Birth-Consensus-Statement.pdf

American College of Obstetricians and Gynecologists (ACOG). (2014). ACOG Committee Opinion No. 594: Immersion in water during labor and delivery. *Obstetrics and Gynecology, 123*(4), 912–915. doi:10.1097/01.AOG.0000445585.52522.14

Ananth, C. V., Chauhan, S. P., Chen, H. Y., D'Alton, M. E., & Vintzileos, A. M. (2013). Electronic fetal monitoring in the United States: Temporal trends and adverse perinatal outcomes. *Obstetrics and Gynecology, 121*(5), 927–933. doi:10.1097/AOG.0b013e318289510d

Benfield, R. D., Hortobagyi, T., Tanner, C. J., Swanson, M., Heitkemper, M. M., & Newton, E. R. (2010). The effects of hydrotherapy on anxiety, pain, neuroendocrine responses, and contraction dynamics during labor. *Biological Research for Nursing, 12*(1), 28–36. doi: 10.1177/1099800410361535

Burns, B., & Jackson, P. (2011). Success and failure in organizational change: An exploration of the role of values. *Journal Change Management, 11*(2), 133–162. doi:10.1080/14697017.2 010.524655

Burns, E. E., Boulton, M. G., Cluett, E., Cornelius, V. R., & Smith, L. A. (2012). Characteristics, interventions, and outcomes of women who used a birthing pool: A prospective observational study. *Birth, 39*(3), 192–202. doi:10.1111/j.1523-536X.2012.00548.x

Byard, R. W., & Zuccollo, J. M. (2010). Forensic issues in cases of water birth fatalities. *American Journal of Forensic Medicine and Pathology, 31*(3), 258–260. doi:10.1097/PAF .0b013e3181e12eb8

Chaillet, N., Belaid, L., Crochetière, C., Roy, L., Gagné, G. P., Moutquin, J. M., & Rossignil, M. (2014). Nonpharmacologic approaches for pain management during labor compared with usual care: A meta-analysis. *Birth, 41*(2), 122–137. doi:10.1111/birt.12103

Cluett, E. R., & Burns, E. (2009). Immersion in water in labour and birth. *Cochrane Database of Systematic Reviews, 2009*(2). doi:10.1002/14651858.CD000111.pub3

Cluett, E. R., Pickering, R. M., & Brooking, J. I. (2001). An investigation into the feasibility of comparing three management options (augmentation, conservative and water) for nulliparae with dystocia in the first stage of labour. *Midwifery, 17*(1), 35–43. doi:http://dx.doi .org/10.1054/midw.2000.0233

Cluett, E. R., Pickering, R. M., Getliffe, K., & St. George-Saunders, N. J. (2004). Randomized controlled trial of labouring in water compared with standard of augmentation for management of dystocia in first stage of labour. *British Medical Journal, 328*, 314–319. doi:dx .doi.org/10.1136/bmj.37963.606412.EE

CNM Data Group. (1998). Midwifery management of pain in labor: The CNM Data Group, 1996. *Journal of Nurse-Midwifery, 43*(2), 77–82. doi:10.1016/S0091-2182(97)00150-X

Declercq, E. R., Sakala, C., Corry, M. P., & Applebaum, S. (2006). *Listening to Mothers II: Report of the Second National U.S. Survey of Women's Childbearing Experiences.* New York, NY: Childbirth Connection. Retrieved from http://www.childbirthconnection.org/pdfs/ LTMII_report.pdf

Eberhard, J., Stein, S., & Geissbuehler, V. (2005). Experience of pain and analgesia with water and land births. *Journal of Psychosomatic Obstetrics & Gynecology, 26*(2), 127–133. doi: 10.1080/01443610400023080

Geissbühler, V., & Eberhard, J. (2000). Waterbirths: A comparative study—A prospective study on more than 2,000 waterbirths. *Fetal Diagnosis and Therapy, 15*(5), 291–300.

Gilbert, R. E., & Tookey, P. A. (1999). Perinatal mortality and morbidity among babies delivered in water: Surveillance study and postal survey. *British Medical Journal, 319*, 483–487. doi:dx.doi.org/10.1136/bmj.319.7208.483

Grimshaw, J. M., Eccles, M. P., Lavis, J. N., Hill, S. J., & Squires, J. E. (2012). Knowledge translation of research findings. *Implementation Science, 7*(50), 1–17. doi:10.1186/1748-5908-7-50

Hall, S. M., & Holloway, I. M. (1998). Staying in control: Women's experiences of labour in water. *Midwifery, 14*(1), 30–36. doi:10.1016/S0266-6138(98)90112-7

Houston, J. (2010). Promoting a policy for use of water in labour and for birth in the United States. *MIDIRS Midwifery Digest, 20*(4), 471–475.

Kennedy, H. P., & Lyndon, A. (2008). Tensions and teamwork in nursing and midwifery relationships. *Journal of Obstetric, Gynecologic, & Neonatal Nursing, 37*(4), 426–435. doi:10.1111/j.1552-6909.2008.00256.x

Leslie, M. S., Erickson-Owens, D., & Cseh, M. (2015). The evolution of individual maternity care providers to delayed cord clamping: It is the evidence? *Journal of Midwifery & Women's Health, 60*(5), 561–569. doi:10.1111/jmwh.12333

Martin, J. A., Hamilton, B. E., Osterman, M. H., Curtin, S. C., & Matthews, M. S. (2015). Births: Final data for 2013. *National Vital Statistics Reports, 64*(1), 1–68. Hyattsville, MD: National Center for Health Statistics. Retrieved from http://www.cdc.gov/nchs/data/nvsr/nvsr64/nvsr64_01.pdf

Maternity Care Working Party. (2007). Making normal birth a reality: Consensus statement from the Maternity Care Working Party. Retrieved from https://www.nct.org.uk/sites/default/files/related_documents/Makingnormalbirthareality_NormalBirthConsensusStatement.pdf

Melnyk, B. M., & Fineout-Overholt, E. (2014). *Evidence based practice in nursing and healthcare: A guide to best practice* (3rd ed.). Philadelphia, PA: Lippincott Williams & Wilkins.

Meyer, S. L., Weible, C. M., & Woeber, K. (2010). Perceptions and practice of waterbirth: A survey of Georgia midwives. *Journal of Midwifery & Women's Health, 55*(1), 55–59. doi:10.1016/j.jmwh.2009.01.008

National Institute for Health and Care Excellence (NICE). (2014). Intrapartum care for healthy women and babies. (NICE guidelines [CG190]). Retrieved from https://www.nice.org.uk/guidance/CG190/chapter/About-this-guideline#copyright

Nutter, E. (2013). *Hydrotherapy and childbirth: An evidence based protocol to guide waterbirth in Army hospitals.* (Unpublished doctor of nursing practice capstone project). Frontier Nursing University, Hyden, KY.

Nutter, E., Meyer, S., Shaw-Battista, J., & Marowitz, A. (2014a). Waterbirth: An integrative analysis of peer-reviewed literature. *Journal of Midwifery and Women's Health, 59*(3), 286–319. doi:10.1111/jmwh.12194

Nutter, E., Shaw-Battista, J., & Marowitz, A. (2014b). Waterbirth fundamentals for clinicians. *Journal of Midwifery & Women's Health, 59*(3), 350–354. doi:10.1111/jmwh.12193

Ohlsson, G., Buchhave, P., Leandersson, U., Nordstrom, L., Rydhstrom, H., & Sjolin, I. (2001). Warm tub bathing during labor: Maternal and neonatal effects. *Acta Obstetricia et Gynecologica Scandinavica, 80*(4), 311–314. doi:10.1034/j.1600-0412.2001.080004311.x

Pinette, M. G., Wax, J., & Wilson, E. (2004). The risks of underwater birth. *American Journal of Obstetrics and Gynecology, 190*(5), 1211–1215. doi:10.1016/j.ajog.2003.12.007

Rosser, J. (1994). Is water birth safe? The evidence behind the controversy. *MIDIRS Midwifery Digest, 4*, 4–6.

Schafer, R. (2014). Umbilical cord avulsion in waterbirth. *Journal of Midwifery & Women's Health, 59*(1), 91–94. doi:10.1111/jmwh.12157

Shaw-Battista, J. C. (2009). *Optimal outcomes of labor and birth in water compared to standard maternity care.* San Francisco, CA: University of California.

Simkin, P., & Bolding, A. (2004). Update on nonpharmacologic approaches to relieve labor pain and prevent suffering. *Journal of Midwifery & Women's Health*, *49*(6), 489–504. doi:10.1016/j.jmwh.2004.07.007

Society of Obstetricians and Gynaecologists of Canada, Association of Women's Health, Obstetric and Neonatal Nurses of Canada, Canadian Association of Midwives, College of Family Physicians of Canada, & The Society of Rural Physicians of Canada. (2008). Joint policy statement on normal childbirth. *Journal of Obstetrics and Gynaecology Canada*, *30*(12), 1163–1165. Retrieved from http://www.jogc.com.proxy1.library.jhu.edu/abstracts/full/200812_SOGCClinicalPracticeGuidelines_3.pdf

Stark, M. A., & Miller, M. G. (2009). Barriers to the use of hydrotherapy in labor. *Journal of Obstetric, Gynecologic, and Neonatal Nursing*, *38*(6), 667–675. doi:10.1111/j.1552-6909 .2009.01065.x

Stark, M. A., Rudell, B., & Haus, G. (2008). Observing position and movements in hydrotherapy: A pilot study. *Journal of Obstetric, Gynecologic, & Neonatal Nursing*, *37*(1), 116–121. doi:10.1111/j.1552-6909.2007.00212.x

Young, K., & Kruske, S. (2013). How valid are the common concerns raised against water birth? A focused review of the literature. *Women and Birth*, *26*(2), 105–109. doi:10.1016/j .wombi.2012.10.006

Walsh, D. (2011). *Evidence and skills for normal labour and birth: A guide for midwives* (2nd ed.). New York, NY: Routledge.

Zanetti-Dällenbach, R., Lapaire, O., Maertens, A., Holzgreve, W., & Hösli, I. (2006). Water birth, more than a trendy alternative: A prospective, observational study. *Archives of Gynecology and Obstetrics*, *274*(6), 355–365. doi:10.1007/s00404-006-0208-1

Zanetti-Dällenbach, R. A., Tschudin, S., Zhong, X. Y., Holzgreve, W., Lapaire, O., & Hösli, I. (2007). Maternal and neonatal infections and obstetrical outcome in water birth. *European Journal of Obstetrics & Gynecology and Reproductive Biology*, *134*(1), 37–43. doi:10.1016/j .ejogrb.2006.09.012

# CHAPTER TWENTY-THREE

# NITROUS OXIDE'S PLACE IN LABOR AND BIRTH

Michelle R. Collins and Judith P. Rooks

Nitrous oxide ($N_2O$), or "laughing gas" as it is sometimes called, was used as a recreational drug before it was used as an analgesic for childbirth. For nearly a century, $N_2O$ has been used during labor and birth in countries such as the United Kingdom, Australia, New Zealand, Norway, and Finland. Use of $N_2O$ in large populations of childbearing women over as many years has created an extensive base of anecdotal evidence supporting its use during labor as safe for both the mother and the baby. Although it has not been widely available for use in the United States, there has been a recent resurgence in interest, both from birth professionals and pregnant women looking for expanded options for safe pain relief in childbirth. This chapter presents the historical context; existing evidence on the use of $N_2O$ during labor and birth; considerations for establishing an $N_2O$ analgesia service in a hospital; safety issues related to the mother, baby, and staff; and the logistics of using $N_2O$ in childbirth.

## HISTORY AND PRESENT USE

Use of $N_2O$ is often associated with industrial or dental use (Skiba et al., 2012). Industrial application of $N_2O$ includes use in rocket motors, racing engines, fertilizer production, and in the food industry for products requiring accelerants (e.g., canned whipped cream). Many Americans associate $N_2O$ with dentistry, where it is widely used, especially for children (Tobias, 2013). Emergency rooms and emergency transport systems also use $N_2O$, ideal for urgent situations in which the need for analgesia is often pressing. $N_2O$, like most analgesics, has potential for misuse and abuse. Those who abuse it as a recreational drug may experience sensory changes in their extremities, respiratory and cardiac changes, and altered mentation (Borok, Slowik, Ganesh, & Eljammal, 2014). Paradoxically, $N_2O$ is also used to treat addictions, particularly alcoholism (Amato, Minozzi, & Davoli, 2011).

$N_2O$ was used for analgesia during labor and childbirth in the United States between the 1930s and 1970s, with variable rates of use reported. "Twilight sleep," which was a combination of a narcotic, such as morphine and scopolamine, had become popular in the early 1900s and then fell from grace, leaving the door open for $N_2O$, which had already been used widely in Europe. In the early days of use by laboring women, $N_2O$ was sometimes combined with narcotics. Under the effect of both narcotics and inhalational agents, women were prone to loss of consciousness and vomiting with subsequent risk of aspiration (Zabriskie, 1943). In the 1940s, introduction of regional anesthesia during labor provided powerful pain relief and allowed women to be awake and aware during childbirth. Although regional anesthesia was (and still is) not available at all times in every American hospital with an obstetrics service, use of $N_2O$ diminished and eventually disappeared from the landscape of childbirth in America (Stewart & Collins, 2012).

There are important differences between use of $N_2O$ during dentistry and childbirth. In dentistry, $N_2O$ may be used at concentrations up to 70% at a continuous flow and is controlled by a member of the dental staff. In contrast, $N_2O$ for labor analgesia is provided at no higher than a 50% concentration of $N_2O$ with a 50% mixture of oxygen ($O_2$), is used intermittently, only during contractions, and is self-administered by the woman. Because of the way the delivery apparatus is constructed, there is no constant flow of $N_2O$ through the tubing to the patient, thus constituting what is defined as "intermittent" flow. The equipment used to provide $N_2O/O_2$ during labor is also different from that used to provide $N_2O$ during dentistry, which can be adjusted to vary the concentrations of the two gases. Because $N_2O$ delivery equipment is left in a room with the laboring woman and her support persons when midwives and other professionals are not in the room, it is crucial that the equipment delivers a fixed rate of 50% $N_2O$ and 50% $O_2$. As of 2015, only three devices had been approved to provide the $N_2O/O_2$ blend to a woman in labor. $N_2O$ used as a 50%/50% mixture with oxygen, or less, is classified as minimal sedation by the American Society of Anesthesiologists (ASA) Task Force on Sedation and Analgesia by Non-Anesthesiologists (2002).

The woman utilizing $N_2O$ during labor can choose either a face mask or a mouthpiece for delivery of the gas, depending on the equipment available at her birth site. If using the mask, she is instructed to make an airtight seal around her mouth and nose. If using the mouthpiece, she must use her lips to make an airtight seal around the mouthpiece. When the woman inhales, the negative pressure causes a demand valve in the equipment to open, allowing the $N_2O/O_2$ gas blend to flow into her lungs. When the woman exhales, the demand valve snaps shut, stopping the flow of $N_2O/O_2$, and the $N_2O$ in her blood begins to be eliminated in her exhalations, which are collected by an embedded scavenging device. The exhaled gas is then carried to a waste reservoir. The $N_2O$-contaminated gas is ultimately released into an inaccessible, external atmosphere and mixes with the outside air. Low concentrations of atmospheric $N_2O$ are not toxic. Most $N_2O$ in the Earth's atmosphere comes from natural processes, including denitrification of plant debris by bacteria in soils, and humans live with some environmental $N_2O$ (Ambus, Zechmeister-Boltenstern, & Butterbach-Bahl, 2006).

During labor, women directly control when and how often they inhale $N_2O$; having control contributes to satisfaction with $N_2O$ use (Rooks, 2011). Women find their own rhythm of inhaling and exhaling fairly quickly, although this rhythm may change as the frequency and intensity of contractions change. Initial patient teaching should instruct women to inhale through the mask or mouthpiece approximately 30 seconds before they anticipate their next contraction in order to best associate an adequate serum level of $N_2O$ with the peak of the contraction (Rooks, 2011).

## THE NEED FOR ACCESS TO $N_2O$ ANALGESIA DURING CHILDBIRTH

Narcotics and regional anesthesia have long been the main labor pain management modes widely available to laboring women in the United States (Osterman & Martin, 2011). Approximately 61% of American women who had singleton vaginal births in the 27 states surveyed in 2008 had received regional (epidural, spinal, or combined spinal and epidural) anesthesia (Osterman & Martin, 2011). State rates varied from a low of 22% in New Mexico to a high of 78% in Kentucky with 60% or more of the women in 20 of the 27 reporting states receiving regional anesthesia (Osterman & Martin, 2011). Some women, however, are not candidates for regional anesthesia and others do not desire regional anesthesia for childbirth. No one pharmacological form of pain relief is best for all women. The addition of $N_2O$ to the pharmacological options available to women birthing in the United States is necessary to give women expanded access to safe options (Rooks, 2011).

An epidural may cause a sudden drop in maternal blood pressure, necessitating frequent blood pressure measurement. Hypotensive episodes may necessitate intravenous fluid boluses as well as administration of oxygen if the fetal heart rate responds negatively to the hypotensive insult. Other epidural complications may include a severe headache (referred to as a "spinal headache") caused by leakage of spinal fluid after incidental puncture of the dura mater during epidural placement. Urinary retention and maternal fever are also associated complications with epidural use (Anim-Somuah, Smyth, & Jones, 2011). After epidural placement, the woman needs to maintain bedrest and requires assistance to alternate positions to facilitate optimal fetal positioning in the pelvis. Continuous fetal heart rate monitoring is also standard practice with epidural use. Labor may slow or stop, and the woman may experience shivering and difficulty in pushing. The laboring mother may need forceps or vacuum assistance for birth. Cesarean section for fetal distress is also a greater risk for women with epidural anesthesia (Anim-Somuah et al., 2011).

$N_2O$ is appropriate, even indicated, in specific clinical situations. $N_2O$ has significant anxiolytic effects in addition to analgesia (Collins, 2015). For a large number of women, anxiety about parturition is more intolerable than the actual pain associated with labor and birth. Fear and tension can inhibit the normal processes of labor (Smith, Levett, Collins, & Crowther, 2011). Decreasing a woman's fear and apprehension supports the physiology of labor. Even women who do not have significant anxiety about the birth process may be very apprehensive about procedures associated with labor and birth, such as insertion of an intravenous line or placement of regional anesthesia. Use of $N_2O$ during such procedures may facilitate a woman's tolerance and enhance comfort.

Because $N_2O$ can be initiated at any point during labor or the immediate postpartum period, it is especially attractive in many clinical situations. Some examples include use for the multiparous woman who requires no pain management in labor until late in the first stage, when placement of epidural anesthesia is not practical and concern over late narcotic use is reasonable. Another ideal situation for use of $N_2O$ is during the perineal inspection of a woman who has had an unmedicated labor and birth. As the adrenaline rush of birth dissipates, some women seem to have a heightened sensitivity to perineal touch, and are unable to tolerate even the slightest touch during perineal evaluation and/or repair of lacerations. The use of $N_2O$, in combination with local anesthesia if repair is necessary, can facilitate examination of the perineum, making the process much more tolerable. Many women do not initiate use of $N_2O$ until transition or the second stage. Inhaling $N_2O$ while pushing and through the birth has not been found to have adverse effects on newborns (Likis et al., 2012). Access to $N_2O$ in the labor suite is also ideal for postpartum bedside procedures such as manual removal of the placenta, repair of extensive lacerations, or dilation and curettage (D&C) done at the bedside.

Sometimes it is advisable or necessary to use adjunctive narcotic therapy with $N_2O$, especially for more invasive procedures such as a D&C. When narcotics are used adjunctively with $N_2O$, the combination may be considered conscious sedation. Additional monitoring and patient assessment may be necessary.

The American College of Nurse-Midwives (ACNM) supports the use of $N_2O$. Key components of the ACNM 2010 position statement "$N_2O$ for Labor Analgesia" are as follows:

- Women should have access to a variety of measures to assist them in coping with the challenges of labor, including $N_2O$.
- Research has supported the reasonable efficacy, safety, and unique and beneficial qualities of $N_2O$ as an analgesic for labor and its use as a widely accepted component of quality maternity care.
- Certified nurse-midwives and certified midwives should be trained to administer and oversee safe use of $N_2O$ analgesia during labor.
- Women should be educated about the use of $N_2O$ as an option for pain relief in labor.
- There is a need for ongoing research and evaluation of the use of analgesia during labor to facilitate inclusion of $N_2O$ as an option for women during labor throughout the United States (ACNM, 2010)

## EFFICACY AND SATISFACTION

Although $N_2O$ is clearly less effective than an epidural at reducing labor pain (Likis et al., 2012), the degree of maternal satisfaction with use of $N_2O$ versus regional anesthesia has not been well measured. This lack of evaluation of maternal satisfaction with $N_2O$ use is a factor to consider as the use of $N_2O$ is associated with greater mobility and fewer interventions than regional anesthesia. The Agency for Healthcare Research and Quality (AHRQ) review by Likis et al. (2012) of $N_2O$ labor analgesia included information from small studies that measured women's satisfaction with $N_2O$ for pain management as compared to epidural anesthesia (Baird, 1992; Bajoria, Ward, & Sooranna, 2001; Barker & Cotter, 2003). In a prospective cohort study of 20 women who used $N_2O$ (without pethidine), 60% of the women (12/20) were satisfied with the degree of pain relief (Bajoria et al., 2001). In another prospective cohort study of 200 women who used $N_2O$ without pethidine during labor, 33% (66/200) rated the pain relief from $N_2O$ as good (Baird, 1992). In a cross-sectional study of maternal satisfaction with pain relief provided by $N_2O$ without pethidine, 40 of 115 women who used $N_2O$ during labor (35%) were very satisfied with the pain relief provided (Barker & Cotter, 2003).

As pain relief with $N_2O$ is variable, it may be sufficient for some women's needs but it is not the solution for all women. Although $N_2O$ is not a potent analgesic at doses provided during labor, the anxiolytic effect, enhanced sense of control, and reduced perception of pain (even though the woman may still be aware that pain is present) make it a viable option for many women.

## SAFETY AND RISKS

Concerns include safety for women using $N_2O$, their fetuses, and the staff who provide care. Many of the noted effects fall into the category of unpleasant side effects, whereas a few could potentially harm the woman or her baby. Untoward effects in women that may cause discomfort but are not dangerous include dry mouth and/or nose (more common among women using masks instead of mouthpieces); nausea and/or vomiting; feeling dizzy or lightheaded; drowsiness; restlessness; parathesia (often described as tingling or pricking); dreams; amnesia or having a fogged memory of the labor and less often of the birth. Nausea is the most frequent side effect, reported in 17 of the 32 studies reporting "maternal harms" in the AHRQ review, with the percentages of women experiencing nausea varying from 0% to 13% (Likis et al., 2012). Vomiting was noted as a side effect in six of the 32 studies reviewed by AHRQ, with occurrence rates from 0% to 14%. Dizziness was reported in four studies in which $N_2O$ was utilized alone, with an occurrence range from 3% to 23%. Feeling drowsy with use of $N_2O$ as the sole agent ranged from 0% to 67%. Although sleepiness was reported in older studies in which $N_2O$ was used at greater than 50%, no studies included in the AHRQ review reported sleepiness as a side effect when not used in combination with sedatives or narcotics (Likis et al., 2012).

Maternal respiratory depression has been reported with $N_2O$ used at greater than 50% concentration or in combination with narcotics or sedatives. Respiratory depression is rarely, if ever, seen at 50%/50% concentration with intermittent flow, as opposed to continuous flow. When combined with the use of narcotics, sedatives, or other anesthetic gases, reported rates of unconsciousness varied from 0% to 1%, and usually occurred when someone other than the laboring women was holding the mask or mouthpiece to the woman's face. Respiratory depression is thought to be very unlikely when the patient is holding her own mask or mouthpiece (Likis et al., 2012). This step in the $N_2O$ use in labor design underscores why it is essential that the woman using $N_2O$ holds the mask or mouthpiece herself. When the level of $N_2O$ in the woman's blood approaches a level near that of affecting muscle control, the woman will have difficulty holding the mask or mouthpiece in a manner that creates an airtight seal and delivers additional $N_2O$. The resulting loss of negative pressure will cause the demand valve to snap closed and stop the supply of $N_2O$. Allowing someone else to hold it to her face bypasses this critical safety feature.

## Serious Complications From Long Exposure to High Concentrations of $N_2O$

### Deactivation of Vitamin $B_{12}$

$N_2O$ oxidizes a physiologically active form of vitamin $B_{12}$ (cobalamin), which leads to inactivation of the molecule. Vitamin $B_{12}$ is necessary to synthesize myelin, deoxyribonucleic acid (DNA), and ribonucleic acid (RNA; Sanders, Weimann, & Maze, 2008). Myelin is a mixture of proteins and lipids that form an insulating sheath around many nerve fibers, increasing the speed at which impulses are conducted. Except for the effects of $N_2O$ on consciousness, nausea and vomiting, and neuroapoptosis (discussed next), all known adverse effects of $N_2O$ are the result of inactivation of vitamin $B_{12}$. Extremely high doses of $N_2O$ and/or long-term exposure can reduce cobalamin function enough to cause adverse effects such as bone-marrow depression, megaloblastic anemia, and neuropsychiatric disorders. *Dose* is the concentration of $N_2O$ times the duration of the exposure. The effects reverse with time except when the dose is so high that it causes cells to die, which has occurred in rats exposed to very high concentrations of $N_2O$ (higher than those used during labor) for more than 6 hours. Any condition that reduces cobalamin function, such as Crohn's disease, celiac disease, gluten intolerance, pernicious anemia, long-term recreational abuse of $N_2O$, chronic malnutrition, or adherence to an extremely strict vegan diet without $B_{12}$ supplementation (animal products are the only food source of vitamin $B_{12}$), increases risks of complications from exposure to $N_2O$. Surgical patients who receive $N_2O$ anesthesia for greater than 6 hours are at increased risk (Sanders et al., 2008).

### Apoptosis

*Apoptosis* refers to cellular death in which a programmed sequence of events leads to the elimination of cells without releasing harmful substances into the surrounding tissue. By eliminating old, unnecessary, and unhealthy cells, apoptosis plays a critical role in maintaining health. The human body replaces up to a million cells per second. Too little or too much apoptosis plays a role in some disease processes. Cells that should be eliminated via apoptosis may persist, for example, in cancer. Conversely, too much apoptosis resulting in the death of too many cells, can cause grave tissue damage, as in Alzheimer's and Parkinson's diseases (Perier, Bové, & Vila, 2012; Rappaport, Mellon, Simone, & Woodcock, 2011).

Exposure to some anesthetic agents and gasses, especially ketamine, may cause the mistimed destruction of nerve cells. $N_2O$ alone has not been shown to result in apoptosis in rat fetuses with $N_2O$ concentrations of 75% or less (Sanders et al., 2008). Although $N_2O$ crosses the placenta, there are no significant differences in Apgar scores, umbilical cord blood-gas results, or the incidence of meconium-stained amniotic fluid (Rooks, 2011). In 2007, a Federal Drug Administration (FDA) task force studied the existing literature on $N_2O$ exposure and recommended no change in current practices regarding exposing children and fetuses to $N_2O$ (Creeley & Olney, 2010). Those recommendations remain unchanged.

## Contraindications

$N_2O$ should not be used by women who are physically unable to hold the mask or mouthpiece, whether because of impairment from any substance or a musculoskeletal condition. A true vitamin $B_{12}$ deficiency is another contraindication. Though exposing someone who is truly deficient in $B_{12}$ to an agent that could potentiate that deficiency could be harmful, women who are mildly deficient in $B_{12}$, for example, as a result of a dietary regimen (vegan or vegetarian), remain candidates for use of $N_2O$. Women who are truly deficient in $B_{12}$ usually have a chronic illness that caused the deficiency, such as celiac sprue, history of other malabsorption syndromes, or recent gastric bypass surgery. The $B_{12}$ status of these women would have been monitored during prenatal care as a direct result of the observation required by their health status. Routine serum evaluation of $B_{12}$ levels has not been routinely advocated for vegetarian or vegan women who did not require $B_{12}$ monitoring during pregnancy, especially with those receiving supplements.

Women at risk for the gas to become trapped (e.g., women who have had a collapsed lung or recent bariatric surgery), are not candidates for use of $N_2O$. Women who are not stable hemodynamically or who have conditions impairing their respiratory status (such as severe asthma, chronic obstructive pulmonary disease, or cystic fibrosis) may not be candidates for use of $N_2O$. Individualized clinical assessment is requisite for women with those conditions (Stewart & Collins, 2012).

## Occupational Risk for Midwives, Nurses, and Other Maternal Health Care Workers

Safety mechanisms specific to $N_2O$ limit the exposure of health care workers. In addition to limiting the concentration of $N_2O$ relative to oxygen used by laboring women, the intermittent use by most women, the adequate ventilation required in hospitals, use of a demand valve and scavenger system, and teaching laboring women to exhale into the mask or mouthpiece all limit the extent to which staff are exposed.

Health care workers' exposure to $N_2O$ can be measured via badges worn on their clothing that quantify the degree of exposure over a specified period of time. Hospitals/birth centers may choose to institute a policy of periodic badge usage and regular monitoring of exposure as part of quality review. The U.S. National Institute for Occupational Safety and Health (NIOSH) has set 25 parts per million (ppm) as the 8-hour time-weighted average ambient occupational exposure limit (OEL) for $N_2O$ (Rooks, 2011). Sweden, the United Kingdom, Norway, Italy, and Denmark have all set their OELs at 100 ppm. The American Conference of Governmental Industrial Hygienists (ACGIH), an organization open to all practitioners of industrial hygiene, occupational health, or environmental health or safety, recommends that the limit be set at 50 ppm (Rooks, 2011).

Several factors limit health care worker exposure to $N_2O$ used by laboring women as compared to use in dentistry. The continuous flow of $N_2O$ to the nasal mask that is used in dentistry, rather than flow initiated by the woman's inhalation, is a major factor. Intermittent flow decreases the amount of $N_2O$ in the ambient air. Dental patients may be given $N_2O$ at concentrations as high as 70%, whereas it is used only up to 50% concentrations during labor and birth. In addition, women exhale the gas through their mouths directly into the faces of dental personnel, as opposed to into a mask or mouthpiece during its use in labor and birth. Also, most U.S. hospitals maintain a specified number of complete ambient air turnovers per hour in hospital rooms; air changeovers are not required in dental offices (Rooks, 2011).

## BEST PRACTICES IN THE USE OF $N_2O$

### Patient Education

Patient counseling should include the side effects of nausea and vertigo as well as fatigue after prolonged periods of use (Collins, Starr, Bishop, & Baysinger, 2012). The woman should be taught how to form an appropriate seal with the mask over her mouth and nose or how to purse her lips around the mouthpiece. This technique will promote adequate inhalation sufficient to open the demand valve and adequate exhalation to make use of the scavenging system. The laboring woman needs to understand that, for best effect, it is optimal to begin inhaling approximately 30 seconds before she anticipates the beginning of the next contraction. Exhaling back into the mask or mouthpiece several times at the end of use helps to ensure low ambient contamination. The woman and any support persons at the bedside must understand that no one except the woman using $N_2O$ may hold and control the face mask or mouthpiece and that strict adherence to this rule is essential for the mother's safety. Although a woman may be mobile while using $N_2O$, a family or staff member should be in the room to ensure that she is steady on her feet.

## Safe Use for Labor Analgesia

Safe practice for $N_2O$ labor analgesia requires that:

- $N_2O$ is administered with oxygen ($O_2$) and $N_2O$ concentration does not exceed 50%
- $N_2O$ it is self-administered by the laboring women and she must hold the mask or mouthpiece without any assistance
- $N_2O$ delivery equipment is the approved equipment for this purpose and incorporates a demand valve to control the flow of gas and scavenging equipment to capture the woman's exhalations and aid in appropriate disposal

These measures help to prevent overdose or becoming hypoxic as well as protecting health care workers from contaminated ambient air (Rooks, 2011; Rosen, 2002; Sanders et al., 2008).

Use of $N_2O$ is appropriate in a variety of clinical situations. Identifying women who may benefit from using $N_2O$ requires a holistic view of the laboring woman. One woman may find great relief in the anxiolysis and wants to use it sooner than another woman who requires it for the discomfort of a rapid transition. For some women, $N_2O$ will provide adequate pain relief until they desire epidural placement. A fair percentage of women who begin using $N_2O$ convert to an epidural at some further point in their labor. If the use of $N_2O$ allows for a woman to maintain mobility for a longer period of time, delaying the bedrest inherent with regional anesthesia as well as other accompanying interventions (bladder catheter, intravenous line, pulse oximetry, continuous electronic fetal monitoring), it is a worthwhile venture. For many years, narcotics have been used during early labor with the expectation that the woman will have an epidural later during her labor. Using $N_2O$ early and converting to an epidural later is analogous to that situation, but avoids the complications associated with use of opioids.

Once the woman has initiated use, periodic evaluation by nurses or the obstetric provider (midwives or physicians) to assess usage, pain relief, and satisfaction is important (ACNM, 2010; Rooks, 2011). On occasion, women may position themselves on hands and knees, or leaning over their bed onto pillows, and situate the mask so that it is nestled into the pillows or bedding, eliminating the need to hold onto the breathing apparatus. Bedside providers need to be diligent in their observation that if the woman does this, she must be reminded that she still must hold onto her apparatus and manually bring it to her mouth. If the face mask or mouthpiece is supported by bedding, the safety mechanism of patient control is lost.

## Establishing a $N_2O$ Service

### Initial Steps

The important first step in establishing a nitrous service in a hospital is to assess the interest, resources, potential barriers, and culture of care, including the current epidural rate. This step is crucial because potentially formidable barriers can be anticipated and overcome with adequate forethought and planning. The second critical step is to construct a mission statement that documents the institution's commitment to offering $N_2O$ analgesia. This public commitment underscores the hospital's pledge to offer the option, while also sending a message to everyone in the institution. Third, and utterly critical to success in initiating a service, the key stakeholders involved in maternal–child care at the hospital must meet together to explore everyone's concerns, reservations, and ideas. This initial meeting of the minds serves to assess any barriers, real or anticipated, that may be present within the institution. This is crucial to success.

Many stakeholders are likely to have concerns; anesthesia personnel may be concerned about the use of an anesthetic gas outside of the operating room; nurses may be concerned about their role in patient use of the gas, how they will document the patient's usage, and risks to themselves from exposure to the gas. Validating, clarifying, and addressing all stakeholders' apprehensions is necessary at the beginning, as well as during implementation.

### Policy Development

Once all stakeholders agree to offer $N_2O$ to women in labor, the next step is to develop a policy and procedure. The authors suggest modeling the hospital's policy on what others have done. A certain amount of give and take from all sides is needed to construct a final policy that will be acceptable to all. While developing the policy, it is necessary to choose the nitrous delivery system that best fits the hospital's needs.

Currently, the three $N_2O$ delivery systems that have been approved for use in the United States all provide a blended mix of 50% oxygen with 50% $N_2O$. Two of them tap separate oxygen and $N_2O$ sources and carry the individual gases to the blender. The third device delivers the 50% $N_2O$/50% $O_2$ blend by use of proprietary premixed canisters. All three equipment options use the demand-valve system to initiate the flow of gas to the patient and incorporate a scavenging mechanism. Women who want to initiate $N_2O$ use must provide appropriate consent, whether written or verbal, whichever route is designated in the policy.

The policy makers need to keep in mind some established key facts. Because $N_2O$ has not been demonstrated to have any effect on the fetal heart rate or the contraction pattern, continuous electronic fetal monitoring is not required. If the woman's obstetrical condition warrants, the monitoring should be used, but not because she is using $N_2O$. Authors of various studies have found no greater rate of oxygen desaturation among women using $N_2O$ as compared with control groups, thus there is no requirement for pulse oximetry. In addition, because women may maintain full mobility while using $N_2O$, it is not necessary to incorporate bedrest into the institution's $N_2O$ policy.

No one but the laboring woman may inhale the $N_2O$ gas. Although this instance has not been identified as a problem in the literature, or reported anecdotally, if a person in the room with a laboring woman is discovered inhaling or is known to have inhaled it, either that person or the equipment must be removed from the room. Although not necessary for maternal or fetal safety, many hospitals require that a support person be at the bedside whenever the laboring woman is using N₂O. This person does not need to be a clinician.

## CONCLUSION

At present, there are limited safe, effective options for pharmacological pain relief during labor in the United States. N₂O has been widely used for nearly a century in many other countries, accruing an excellent safety record. The time has come for N₂O to become an option that is widely available to women giving birth in the United States.

## REFERENCES

Amato, L., Minozzi, S., & Davoli, M. (2011). Efficacy and safety of pharmacological interventions for the treatment of the alcohol withdrawal syndrome. *Cochrane Database of Systematic Reviews, 2011*(6). doi:10.1002/14651858.CD008537.pub2

Ambus, P., Zechmeister-Boltenstern, S., & Butterbach-Bahl, K. (2006). Sources of nitrous oxide emitted from European forest soils. *Biogeosciences, 3*(2), 135–145

American College of Nurse-Midwives (ACNM). (2010). Nitrous oxide for labor analgesia [Position statement]. *Journal of Midwifery & Women's Health, 55*(3), 292–296.

American Society of Anesthesiologists Task Force on Sedation and Analgesia by Non-Anesthesiologists. (2002). Practice guidelines for sedation and analgesia by non-anesthesiologists. *Anesthesiology, 96*(4), 1004–1017.

Anim-Somuah, M., Smyth, R. M., & Jones, L. (2011). Epidural versus non-epidural or no analgesia in labour. *Cochrane Database of Systematic Reviews, 2011*(12). doi:10.1002/14651858 .CD000331.pub3

Baird, P. A. (1992). Occupational exposure to nitrous oxide—Not a laughing matter. *New England Journal of Medicine, 327*(14), 1026–1027. doi:10.1056/NEJM199210013271411

Bajoria, R., Ward, S., & Sooranna, S. R. (2001). Atrial natriuretic peptide mediated polyuria: Pathogenesis of polyhydramnios in the recipient twin of twin-twin transfusion syndrome. *Placenta, 22*(8–9), 716–724. doi:10.1053/plac.2001.0715

Barker, T. A., & Cotter, L. (2003). Pregnancy following heart transplantation: A case report. *British Journal of Cardiology, 10*(1), 56–57.

Borok, Z., Slowik, N., Ganesh, S., & Eljammal, S. (2014). Acute respiratory distress syndrome associated with recreational abuse of nitrous oxide. *American Journal of Respiratory and Critical Care Medicine, 189*, A6491.

Collins, M. (2015). A case report on the anxiolytic properties of nitrous oxide during labor. *Journal of Obstetric, Gynecologic, and Neonatal Nursing, 44*(1), 87–92. doi:10.1111/1552 -6909.12522

Collins, M. R., Starr, S. A., Bishop, J. T., & Baysinger, C. L. (2012). Nitrous oxide for labor analgesia: Expanding analgesic options for women in the United States. *Reviews in Obstetrics & Gynecology, 5*(3–4), e126–e131.

Creeley, C. E., & Olney, J. W. (2010). The young: Neuroapoptosis induced by anesthetics and what to do about it. *Anesthesia & Analgesia, 110*(2), 442–448. doi:10.1213/ANE.0b013 e3181c6b9ca

Likis, F. E., Andrews, J. A. Collins, M. R., Lewis, R. M., Seroogy, J. J., Starr, S. A., . . . McPheeters, M. L. (2012). Nitrous oxide for the management of labor pain. *Comparative Effectiveness Reviews No. 67* (Prepared by the Vanderbilt Evidence-based Practice Center. AHRQ Publication No. 12-EHC071-EF). Rockville, MD: Agency for Healthcare Research and Quality. Retrieved from http://www.ncbi.nlm.nih.gov/books/NBK100802

Osterman, M. J., & Martin, J. A. (2011). Epidural and spinal anesthesia use during labor: 27-state reporting area, 2008. *National Vital Statistics Reports, 59*(5), 1–16. Retrieved from http://www.cdc.gov/nchs/data/nvsr/nvsr59/nvsr59_05.pdf

Perier, C., Bové, J., & Vila, M. (2012). Mitochondria and programmed cell death in Parkinson's disease: Apoptosis and beyond. *Antioxidants & Redox Signaling, 16*(9), 883–895. doi:10.1089/ars.2011.4074

Rappaport, B., Mellon, R. D., Simone, A., & Woodcock, J. (2011). Defining safe use of anesthesia in children. *New England Journal of Medicine, 364*(15), 1387–1390. doi:10.1056/NEJMp1102155

Rooks, J. P. (2011). Safety and risks of nitrous oxide labor analgesia: A review. *Journal of Midwifery & Women's Health, 56*(6), 557–565. doi:10.1111/j.1542-2011.2011.00122.x

Rosen, M. A. (2002). Nitrous oxide for relief of labor pain: A systematic review. *American Journal of Obstetrics and Gynecology, 186*(Suppl. 5), S110–S126. doi:10.1016/S0002-9378 (02)70186–5

Sanders, R. D., Weimann, J., & Maze, M. (2008). Biologic effects of nitrous oxide: A mechanistic and toxicologic review. *Anesthesiology, 109*(4), 707–722. doi:10.1097/ALN.0b013e318 1870a17

Skiba, U., Jones, S. K, Dragosits, U., Drewer, J., Fowler, D., Rees, R.M., . . . Manning, A. J. (2012). UK emissions of the greenhouse gas nitrous oxide. *Philosophical Transactions of the Royal Society B: Biological Sciences, 367*(1593), 1175–1185. doi:10.1098/rstb.2011.0356

Smith, C. A., Levett, K. M., Collins, C. T., & Crowther, C. A. (2011). Relaxation techniques for pain management in labour. *Cochrane Database of Systematic Reviews, 2011*(12). doi:10.1002/14651858.CD009514

Stewart, L. S., & Collins, M. (2012). Nitrous oxide as labor analgesia: Clinical implications for nurses. *Nursing for Women's Health, 16*(5), 398–409. doi:10.1111/j.1751-486X.2012.01763.x

Tobias, J. D. (2013). Applications of nitrous oxide for procedural sedation in the pediatric population. *Pediatric Emergency Care, 29*(2), 245–265. doi:10.1097/PEC.0b013e318280d824

Zabriskie, L. A. (1943). Anesthesia and analgesia in labor. In L. A. Zabriskie (Ed.), *Nurses handbook of obstetrics* (pp. 366–380). Philadelphia, PA: J. B. Lippincott.

# CHAPTER TWENTY-FOUR

# MANAGEMENT OF THE THIRD STAGE OF LABOR: IMPLEMENTING BEST PRACTICES

Mavis N. Schorn

With the excitement of a birth, the third stage of labor is often overlooked. However, postpartum hemorrhage (PPH) resulting from uterine atony is one of the highest causes for maternal mortality in the United States (Witcher & Sisson, 2015). Maternal death in the United States is a rare occurrence; however, the rate is increasing, with PPH one of its most common preventable causes (Knight et al., 2009; Witcher & Sisson, 2015). Kramer et al. (2013) analyzed 8.5 million births in a nationwide inpatient sample (from 1999 to 2008) and found that the incidence of severe PPH has tripled with other variables, providing minimal explanation for this increase. During the third stage, midwives facilitate maternal–infant bonding while being attentive to the health of the woman and her neonate. This chapter focuses on the contemporary evidence for supporting health and preventing complications in women during the third stage of labor.

## LENGTH OF THE THIRD STAGE OF LABOR: THE EVIDENCE

The current expectation for the length of the third stage of labor is based primarily on a study of more than 12,000 vaginal births that found the median length of the third stage was 6 minutes, with only 3.3% lasting more than 30 minutes (Combs & Laros, 1991). In another study of more than 45,000 vaginal births, Dombrowski, Bottoms, Saleh, Hurd, and Romero (1995) found that 50% of women who gave birth at term expelled their placentas within 5 minutes, with a mean third-stage duration of 7.5 minutes. Only 2.2% of women did not expel their placentas by 30 minutes. Magann et al. (2005) reviewed 6,588 vaginal births at a tertiary obstetric hospital with active management of the third stage of labor (AMTSL) as standard care and found that the median length of the third stage of labor was similar in women who had PPH and women who did not have a hemorrhage. However, after 30 minutes, the odds of having a PPH were six times higher than before 30 minutes. These studies continue to support the general guideline of 30 minutes or less as an expected length of the third stage of labor.

## Risk Factors for PPH

In addition to prolonged third-stage length, other factors contributing to an increased risk of PPH include hypertensive disorders, oxytocin induction or augmentation, placenta accreta, vacuum extraction, large-for-gestational-age neonates, and a history of retained placenta (Magann et al., 2013; Sheiner, Sarid, Levy, Seidman, & Hallak, 2005). Midwives need to be aware of the increased risk of PPH when the third stage is longer than 30 minutes as well as factors unrelated to the length of the third stage of labor but associated with PPH.

## AMTSL: THE EVIDENCE

AMTSL is a bundle of interventions implemented during the third stage of labor to decrease the incidence of PPH. Current international recommendations for AMTSL include administration of a uterotonic, controlled cord traction, and uterine massage. The 2004 joint statement of the International Confederation of Midwives (ICM) and the International Federation of Gynecology and Obstetrics (FIGO) and the 2014 recommendations of the World Health Organization (WHO) include AMTSL as optimal care to reduce blood loss and risk of PPH.

The Royal Australian and New Zealand College of Obstetricians and Gynaecologists, the Royal College of Obstetrician and Gynaecologists (RCOG), and the Society of Obstetricians and Gynaecologists of Canada (SOGC) have issued national guidelines recommending AMTSL for the prevention of PPH (Dahlke et al., 2015). RCOG and SOGC also recommend delayed cord clamping when possible (Dahlke et al., 2015). U.S. organizations have not supported AMTSL explicitly.

The Partnership for Maternal Safety, a workgroup within the Council on Patient Safety in Women's Health Care, developed an obstetric hemorrhage safety bundle (Main et al., 2015). The following organizations comprised this workgroup: American Association of Blood Banks, American Academy of Family Physicians, American College of Nurse-Midwives (ACNM), American College of Obstetricians and Gynecologists (ACOG), the Association of Women's Health, Obstetric and Neonatal Nurses (AWHONN), the Society for Maternal–Fetal Medicine (SMFM), and the Society for Obstetric Anesthesia and Perinatology (Main et al., 2015). The recommendations of this workgroup include informing women about the benefit of AMTSL in reducing the risk of PPH while also supporting selected women in forgoing prophylactic oxytocin. ACOG and AWHONN, however, recommend oxytocin administration after all births (ACOG, 2006; AWHONN, 2014, 2015).

The components of AMTSL have changed over time. The original components of AMTSL included prophylactic use of a uterotonic within 30 seconds of umbilical cord clamping and controlled cord traction. No reference to uterine massage was included (Prendiville, Elbourne, & McDonald, 2000; Prendiville, Harding, Elbourne, & Stirrat, 1988). The joint recommendation by ICM and FIGO (2004) included administration of uterotonic agents (preferably 10 units of oxytocin as an intramuscular injection), as well as controlled cord traction within 1 minute following birth of the neonate.

This recommendation also included uterine massage after placental expulsion but does not have any reference to cord clamping (ICM & FIGO, 2004). WHO (2014) added delayed cord clamping as a component of AMTSL along with administration of a uterotonic, controlled cord traction, and uterine massage. These recommendations included the use of oxytocin as the preferred uterotonic and highlighted oxytocin as the most important component of AMTSL (WHO, 2014). A systematic review comparing AMTSL and physiologic management revealed that the significant decrease in PPH with the use of AMTSL was found in a population of women with mixed risk of excessive bleeding; however, among women who were low risk for excessive bleeding, no significant difference in the rate of PPH was found between AMTSL and physiologic management of the third stage of labor (PMTSL; Begley, Gyte, Devane, McGuire, & Weeks, 2011). The changing components and the variation in the description of individual components included in AMTSL have not always been clearly described; they varied depending upon the source. The effectiveness of AMTSL cannot be assured when different combinations and timings of components of AMTSL are used in practice (Oladapo, 2010).

The changing components of the practice bundle that has been recommended since AMTSL was first tested and the varied descriptions by international and national guidelines have likely led to wide variation in adherence (Festin et al., 2003). At the same time, the components of physiologic management have been promoted without evaluation of the individual components or the synergistic effects of components as a cluster of best practice. The confusion surrounding the definition(s) of AMTSL and physiologic management compounds the difficulty of comparing the two practice bundles. An overview of the evidence on the individual components of AMTSL is presented next.

## Oxytocin as the Preferred Prophylactic Uterotonic

The most critical component of AMTSL for reducing the risk of PPH is the prophylactic use of a uterotonic. Among uterotonics studied, oxytocin has been the most effective and has been found to have the fewest side effects (Westhoff, Cotter, & Tolosa, 2013). In an effort to determine the effect of individual components of AMTSL, Sheldon, Durocher, Winikoff, Blum, and Trussell (2013) conducted a secondary data analysis of 39,202 hospital births in four countries and found that oxytocin was the only effective component for decreasing the risk of PPH when administered intravenously. Of the women who received prophylactic oxytocin only, without controlled cord traction or uterine massage, the rate of blood loss of 700 mL or greater was highest among women who received oxytocin by intramuscular administration (3.8%) and lowest among women who received oxytocin by intravenous administration (1.0%). When the other AMTSL interventions were combined with oxytocin, the route of oxytocin had no effect (Sheldon et al., 2013).

The timing of oxytocin administration, with the birth of the baby or following the placenta, has not been found to make a difference in reducing the risk of PPH. Studies have demonstrated equal efficacy without increased risk of a trapped placenta or other untoward outcomes (Soltani, Hutchon, & Poulose, 2010). No evidence has been found to suggest that administration of oxytocin with the birth of the neonate is harmful. However, for women who prefer to limit newborn exposure, administration can occur after the cord ceases pulsing or after placenta expulsion.

### Comparison to Ergot Alkaloid

Westhoff and colleagues (2013) conducted a systematic review of 20 randomized controlled trials (RCTs) to determine the effect of oxytocin administration on reduction in PPH risk, compared to both placebo and to ergot alkaloid (ergometrine, a drug commonly used in Europe in a manner similar to methergine use in the United States). They found that prophylactic oxytocin, *at any dose*, was found to decrease both PPH and the need for therapeutic uterotonics in comparison with placebo. The use of prophylactic oxytocin was associated with fewer side effects compared with the use of ergot alkaloids. There were no benefits found in combining oxytocin and ergometrine or providing ergometrine alone in preventing PPH (Westhoff et al., 2013).

### Comparison to Misoprostol

The prophylactic use of misoprostol, at various routes and doses, has been tested to determine effectiveness at reducing the rate of PPH. Villar, Gülmezoglu, Hofmeyr, and Forna (2002) conducted a systematic review of 16 RCTs that included 28,138 women to evaluate misoprostol as a prophylactic uterotonic in the third stage of labor. They found that misoprostol (administered orally or rectally at 400, 500, and 600 mcg doses) was less effective than injectable uterotonics (oxytocin or oxytocin-ergot preparations) in reducing severe blood loss. In addition, prostaglandin-related side effects increased as doses increased, including shivering, pyrexia, nausea, and diarrhea (Villar et al., 2002).

A systematic review of randomized trials involving 46 trials and more than 40,000 women compared misoprostol with either a placebo or another uterotonic in preventing or treating PPH (Hofmeyr et al., 2009). Another systematic review of randomized trials, examining 78 studies and more than 59,000 women, made similar comparisons (Hofmeyr, Gülmezoglu, Novikova, & Lawrie, 2013). Both reviews found that prophylactic misoprostol, at 400 and 600 mcg, resulted in fewer incidents of blood loss greater than 1,000 mL compared to a placebo. However, misoprostol at 600 to 800 mcg was less effective than other uterotonics and did not decrease blood loss any more effectively than at 400 mcg. Pyrexia was higher among women in all the misoprostol groups, increasing with dose. Misoprostol did not appear to increase or reduce severe maternal morbidity or mortality (Hofmeyr et al., 2013). In both reviews, 400 mcg of misoprostol was found to be just as effective as 600 mcg or higher doses for prevention of PPH, while causing less pyrexia (Hofmeyr et al., 2009, 2013). Misoprostol was not found to be more effective than oxytocin, either administered instead of or in addition to oxytocin. With the known side effects of misoprostol and no improved efficacy, oxytocin, as a single agent, continues to be the uterotonic of choice for PPH prophylaxis. The most current WHO recommendations focus on administration of a uterotonic as the most important AMTSL component and recommends that every woman be offered a uterotonic, preferably oxytocin, in the third stage of labor (Hofmeyr et al., 2013).

### Comparison to Herbal and Homeopathic Medications

The use of herbs or homeopathic medications as uterotonics has limited research, so their use is not evidence based. A Cochrane Review of five randomized studies involving 1,466 women was conducted to evaluate herbal and homeopathic medications in preventing PPH (Yaju, Kataoka, Eto, Horiuchi, & Mori, 2013). The evidence was insufficient to warrant future trials to assess these alternative remedies in the prevention of PPH.

## Continuous Cord Traction

Controlled cord traction is the process in which a birth attendant applies one hand on the maternal lower abdomen to secure the uterus and uses the other hand to apply continuous gentle tension on the umbilical cord to extract the placenta, increasing the tension with uterine contractions (Hofmeyr, Mshweshwe, & Gülmezoglu, 2015; ICM & FIGO, 2004). Controlled cord traction was included in the original AMTSL bundle without evaluation as a singular or synergistic benefit. Cord traction is a component of AMTSL that continues to be recommended if the birth is attended by a skilled birth attendant (Du, Ye, & Zheng, 2014; WHO, 2014). The potential risks of controlled cord traction include uterine inversion, avulsion of the umbilical cord, partial detachment of the placenta, and increased maternal discomfort. These risks necessitate a thorough evaluation as to whether controlled cord traction should continue to be incorporated as a component of the AMTSL, even if a skilled birth attendant is available (Du et al., 2014; WHO, 2014).

Two large RCTs designed to evaluate the effectiveness of controlled cord traction have found limited data to support its continued use. One trial included 16 hospitals and two primary health care centers in eight countries using AMTSL (Gülmezoglu et al., 2012). More than 12,000 women were randomly assigned to controlled cord traction or no cord traction, and blood loss was the primary outcome. Each woman, regardless of group assignment, received an injection of 10 units of oxytocin, via intramuscular route, within 1 minute of the birth. Blood lost during the third stage of labor was collected in a drape and weighed. The protocol required that uterine massage to express clots was performed after placenta expulsion. However, individual sites were allowed to vary the method of uterine massage so it was consistent with their existing practice. As only one case of uterine inversion occurred, cord traction was considered a safe intervention. However, investigators found that the omission of cord traction resulted in no significant improvement in the rate of PPH. They concluded that the administration of a uterotonic should be the focus of third-stage management.

Investigators from five university hospital settings in France conducted an RCT involving 4,058 women assigned to controlled cord traction (traction on the cord implemented with the first uterine contraction after birth) or to a control group in which the birth attendant waited for signs of placental separation and the mother's efforts to facilitate placental expulsion (Deneux-Tharaux et al., 2013). All women received oxytocin along with early cord clamping and cutting within 2 minutes of birth. Blood loss was measured in a calibrated collection bag. The women in the intervention group (who received controlled cord traction) had shorter third stages, fewer manual removals of placentas, and reported lower intensity of discomfort during the third stage. However, the number of women with blood loss greater than 500 mL, greater than 1,000 mL, and mean measured blood loss was not significantly different between the intervention and control groups.

Systematic reviews have concluded that continuous cord traction can be omitted from AMTSL without increasing the risk of severe PPH (Du et al., 2014; Hofmeyr et al., 2015). One systematic review and meta-analysis involving more than 30,000 participants found no significant difference between controlled cord traction and hands-off management in regard to the incidence of severe PPH, need for blood transfusion, or therapeutic uterotonics (Du et al., 2014). Hofmeyr and colleagues (2015) also conducted a systematic review of three trials with more than 27,000 women and found the provision of continuous cord traction in third-stage management did not reduce the risk of loss of 1,000 mL or more for women who received prophylactic uterotonics.

In evaluating the effectiveness of the individual components of AMTSL, Sheldon et al. (2013) found that controlled cord traction contributed to a reduction in PPH when oxytocin prophylaxis was either not administered or administered intramuscularly. When oxytocin was administered intravenously, continuous cord traction had no beneficial effect. More research is needed before concluding that controlled cord traction should be omitted in the absence of a uterotonic. However, based on current trials, if prophylactic oxytocin is administered, controlled cord traction can be omitted with no detrimental effect.

## Uterine Massage

Uterine massage following expulsion of the placenta is commonly conducted by midwives and physicians (Schorn, Minnick, & Donaghey, 2015). It is, however, not an original component of the AMTSL bundle of care (Prendiville et al., 1988). The ICM and FIGO recommendations included uterine massage as a component of AMTSL (ICM & FIGO, 2004). Uterine massage was recommended immediately and continuously after the expulsion of the placenta until the uterus contracted. In contrast, WHO recommends assessment of uterine tone to ensure a contracted uterus followed by assessment of uterine tone every 15 minutes for 2 hours, and, if there is uterine atony, provision of fundal massage (WHO, 2014),

There is very little data to support or refute the use of uterine massage. Abdel-Aleem, Hofmeyr, Shokry, and El-Sonoosy (2006) conducted a systematic review and found inconclusive benefit of uterine massage, compared to the use of oxytocin alone, in further reducing postpartum blood loss. They found only three studies evaluating uterine massage for the purpose of reducing the risk of PPH. In one trial, 200 women were randomized to AMTSL (oxytocin administration, controlled cord traction, and immediate cord clamping) or to AMTSL plus intermittent uterine massage that began after the birth and was administered every 10 minutes for 60 minutes (Abdel-Aleem et al., 2006). The mean blood loss and frequency of atonic PPH was reduced in the uterine massage group. However, the study did not have statistical significance (Abdel-Aleem et al., 2006).

Two studies using a similar protocol attempted to determine the effectiveness of sustained (continuous) uterine massage in reducing PPH (Abdel-Aleem et al., 2010; Chen et al., 2013). Abdel-Aleem et al. (2010) initiated uterine massage immediately after birth of the neonate ($n = 1,964$ women). Chen et al. (2013) did not initiate uterine massage until after the placenta was expelled ($n = 1,170$). Women in both studies were randomized into either routine management of oxytocin via intramuscular route or sustained uterine massage for 30 minutes, stimulating the whole surface of the uterus with steady repetitive movement, as firmly as tolerated by the mother. Abdel-Aleem et al. (2010) included a third group of women who received only sustained uterine massage with oxytocin administered following 30 minutes of uterine massage. All groups, in both studies, received continuous cord traction. The group that received the 30-minute uterine massage alone lost more blood compared to treatment with oxytocin with or without massage. In both studies, all women who received oxytocin did not have any significant difference in blood loss with the addition of uterine massage. A large secondary analysis of AMTSL interventions (Sheldon et al., 2013) revealed no evidence that uterine massage prevents PPH. The findings showed that uterine massage resulted in either an increased blood loss or no difference (Sheldon et al., 2013).

All three studies measured the blood lost during the third stage of labor through objective methods such as gravimetric and direct measurement in calibrated drapes. The level of discomfort by participants in the studies was not measured. Chen et al. (2013) reported that uterine massage had to be discontinued in 16 women because of the discomfort they were experiencing. Pain or discomfort was reported by more than 50% of the women receiving uterine massage at one study site but was not recorded at other study sites (Abdel-Aleem et al., 2010). These studies conclude that if oxytocin is used, uterine massage provided no additional benefit in decreasing the risk of PPH.

## Cord Clamping

Early cord clamping was in the original AMTSL bundle (Prendiville et al., 1988). This is the one intervention in the bundle that is no longer included by ICM/FIGO recommendations (Uwins & Hutchon, 2014). WHO (2012) specifically recommends delaying cord clamping for at least 1 to 3 minutes. The elimination of early cord clamping as a component of the AMTSL bundle is the result of finding neonatal benefit from delayed cord clamping rather than because it decreased risk of PPH. Nonetheless, a systematic review of 15 trials of 3,911 women found no significant difference between early and late cord clamping in regard to PPH or severe PPH (McDonald, Middleton, Dowswel, & Morris, 2013). Sheldon et al. (2013) also found no evidence that early cord clamping had any effect on the risk of PPH, providing evidence to eliminate early cord clamping as a component of AMTSL.

## PHYSIOLOGIC MANAGEMENT OF THE THIRD STAGE: THE EVIDENCE

The terms *physiologic management* and *expectant management* during the third stage of labor are often interchanged to describe a hands-off, conservative, or a wait-and-watch approach (Begley et al., 2011; Brucker, 2001; Kashanian, Fekrat, Masoomi, & Ansari, 2010; Maughan, Heim, & Galazka, 2006; Prendiville et al., 2000). Although AMTSL is clearly described in early studies, in the control group, expectant or physiologic management is often not as clear (Hastie & Fahy, 2009; Prendiville et al., 1988). Hastie and Fahy (2009) suggested that comparing expectant or physiologic management to AMTSL is actually a comparison of the use of uterotonics rather than active versus physiologic management. Components of physiologic management of the third stage of labor (PMTSL) that have been proposed include:

- No prophylactic uterotonic medication administered or uterotonic medications provided after placental expulsion, as needed, based on uterine tone
- No manipulation of the uterus before placental expulsion
- Upright maternal position
- Placenta separation without intervention
- Placenta expelled spontaneously by gravity or by maternal expulsion
- Environment maintained (quiet, private, warm)
- Umbilical cord not cut or clamped until cessation of pulsation
- Delayed cord clamping
- Immediate, uninterrupted skin-to-skin contact
- Early breastfeeding
- Mother and baby kept together (Begley, 1990; Burke, 2010; Fahy et al., 2010; Fry, 2007; Maughan et al., 2006)

Hastie and Fahy further developed principles of PMTSL in their Midwifery Guardianship model (2009). In addition to supporting PMTSL, they describe the midwife's role in maintaining expectation of a natural expulsion while promoting maternal–infant bonding. Hastie and Fahy suggested that this expectation may optimize birth physiology and hemostasis (2009).

A sentinel RCT of AMTSL versus PMTSL was conducted with 1,695 women, regardless of PPH risk (Prendiville et al., 1988). In this study, AMTSL components included administration of oxytocin-ergometrine, early cord clamping, and controlled cord traction. Physiologic management included no uterotonic administration, no cord cutting until the placenta was expelled, and no fundal manipulation or cord traction while women were encouraged to be in an upright position and to expel the placenta using their own effort. Of those allocated to AMTSL, 99% of the participants received all of the components. In the PMTSL group, 20% were administered a prophylactic oxytocic, 40% had cord traction, and approximately half of the participants had the cord clamped before the placenta was expelled. Only a small number of women allocated to the PMTSL group actually had physiologic management. The inclusion of women as participants regardless of their PPH risk status and the high-acuity settings in which the research was conducted biased AMTSL as standard practice, even prior to the initiation of the study (Hastie & Fahy, 2009).

Subsequent research also found PMTSL to be less effective in decreasing PPH than AMSTL. An RCT of AMTSL and PMTSL that included 1,429 low-risk women found a significant increase in frequency of PPH, defined as blood loss greater than 500 mL and postnatal anemia, in the women who receive physiologic management (Begley, 1990). Jangsten, Mattsson, Lyckestam, Hellström, and Berg (2011) conducted an RCT that included 1,802 low-risk women. Women received AMTSL or PMTSL. The PMTSL group had a significantly higher rate of PPH, defined as a blood loss greater than 1,000 mL. Blood loss of more than 1,000 mL occurred in 16.8% of the PMTSL women and 10% of the AMTSL women. Blood loss, both before and after placenta expulsion, was higher in the PMTSL group.

In contrast, a retrospective cohort review of 16,210 low-risk women who gave birth in New Zealand found that, after adjusting for known risk factors, women who experienced AMTSL had twice the risk of losing more than 1,000 mL blood compared with those women who expelled their placentas physiologically (Davis et al., 2012). A smaller retrospective cohort study also found a seven- to eightfold increase in PPH for 3,075 low-risk women who received AMTSL, compared to PMTSL (Fahy et al., 2010). It is possible that the retrospective design of these two studies created selection bias.

A systematic evaluation of the components of PMTSL is needed. Individual components should be tested as well combinations of components to examine synergistic effects. The population who might benefit from PMTSL is also unclear. Fry suggested that implementation of PMTSL should only be considered if the first and second stages of labor have been physiologic (2007).

## BLOOD LOSS MEASUREMENT: THE EVIDENCE

The normal amount of blood lost during the third stage of labor has been debated for centuries (Schorn, 2010). Determination of the amount of blood lost during the third stage of labor requires continuous attention. The contemporary focus on safety and best practice during the third stage of labor includes the importance of determining the amount of blood lost before it becomes excessive. Evaluation of any third-stage intervention used for the purpose of decreasing blood loss and preventing PPH must include objective blood loss measurement.

## Estimation

Studies have repeatedly determined that estimation of blood lost during the third stage of labor is inaccurate (Larsson, Saltveddt, Wilkund, Pahlen, & Andolf, 2006; Prasertcharoensuk, Swadpanich, & Lumbiganon, 2000; Schorn, 2010). A common critical error is underestimation of excessive blood loss (Lyndon, Lagrew, Shields, Main, & Cape, 2015; Prasertcharoensuk et al., 2000; Schorn, 2010). Blood loss simulations improve accuracy, but even following simulation, participant estimations remain significantly inaccurate (Maslovitz, Barkai, Lessing, Ziv, & Many, 2008).

Inaccurate recognition of excessive blood loss can lead to excessive loss and delay in treatment, both of which increase maternal morbidity and mortality. The California Maternal Quality Care Collaborative recommends that quantification of blood loss for all births is done during the third stage and continuously until bleeding slows (Lyndon et al., 2015). Other current quality-improvement groups advise quantitative measurement of blood loss rather than estimation to improve accuracy (Gabel & Weeber, 2012; Main et al., 2015). There have been multiple methods used to quantify blood loss (Schorn, 2010). However, direct and gravimetric measurement approaches are the most practical.

## Direct Measurement of Blood Loss

Direct measurement involves collection and measuring of blood in a calibrated container. It is necessary to begin the measurement after the birth of the neonate so that nonblood fluids or excretions are not included in the measurement. This requires coordination to remove fluids before the birth and to collect fluids after the birth. Direct measurement can be performed in a variety of ways, but collection in an underbuttocks drape with calibrated markings has been described and tested (Bamberg et al., 2015; Patel et al., 2006; Toledo, McCarthy, Hewlett, & Fitzgerald, 2007; Turpin, Osakunor, & Owiredu, 2015). Calibrated underbuttocks drapes, including markings on a collector bag for increasing quantity, assist the midwife in determining the amount of blood lost. Underbuttock drapes are simple, objective bedside tools used to identify the amount of blood lost. Turpin et al. (2015) and Toledo et al. (2007) found that PPH was underdiagnosed when visual estimation was compared to direct measurement. In an RCT of 106 vaginal births, Toledo et al. (2007) found the accuracy of the calibrated drape was within 15% of the actual volume, at all measured volumes, in contrast to an error rate of 16% to 41% with visual estimation, with error increasing proportionally with the volume lost.

Zhang et al. (2010) evaluated the use of a calibrated collector bag compared with visual estimation to assess postpartum blood loss and identify PPH. More than 25,000 women who gave birth in 78 maternity units in 13 European countries were enrolled. Although objective measurement with a calibrated bag has been shown to increase the accuracy of assessing blood loss compared to visual estimation, these researchers found no significant difference in the rates of PPH. It is possible that the use of a collector bag increased attention to early identification of PPH and thus reduced the rate (Zhang et al., 2010).

## Gravimetric Measurement of Blood Loss

Alternatively, a gravimetric measurement of blood loss can be used, which involves weighting blood-soaked items and clots. Each milliliter of fluid volume weighs 1 gram. If the weight of the dry items included is subtracted from the total weight, an indirect measure of blood can be obtained. This gravimetric method has been shown to be as much as 30% more accurate than visual estimation (Al Kadri, Al Anazi, & Tamim, 2011; Jones, 2015).

It is unclear which method of measuring blood loss is the best, direct (i.e., calibrated drapes) or indirect (i.e., gravimetric method). Although direct measurement with a calibrated drape has been found to be more accurate than gravimetric measurement (Ambardekar, Shochet, Bracken, Coyaji, & Winikoff, 2014), either quantitative method can be used (Bingham, Lyndon, Lagrew, & Main, 2011; Gabel & Weeber, 2012; Main et al., 2015). It may be advantageous to combine direct and indirect methods. Main et al. (2015) suggested collecting blood in a calibrated, underbuttocks drape immediately after the birth and also weighing blood-soaked items and clots not in the drape. The California Maternal Quality Care Collaborative Toolkit 2.0 recommends use of a calculator within an electronic medical record or a spreadsheet that includes standard dry weights for commonly used items (Lyndon et al., 2015).

## BEST PRACTICES: TRANSLATING THE EVIDENCE

There are several best practices midwives should consider in the management of the third stage of labor. A prenatal discussion with the woman about care during the third stage of labor enhances joint decision making and better understanding of the rationale behind practices. All women have some risk of excessive blood loss when they give birth. It is up to the midwife to determine whether the risk of blood loss is increased as a result of changing prenatal or intrapartum factors.

Once a woman enters the third stage of labor, midwives should expect placental expulsion within 30 minutes. Those women who do not complete the third stage within 30 minutes have an increased risk of PPH. Administration of a uterotonic, particularly oxytocin, is the most effective component of AMTSL for reduction of PPH. Administration of oxytocin may occur at the birth of the neonate or after placental expulsion; both options are equally effective and without increased risk. Prophylactic administration of misoprostol with oxytocin may increase maternal risk without any known benefit.

Early cord clamping is no longer a component of AMTSL and has not been demonstrated to decrease the risk of PPH. The use of controlled cord traction has an associated risk with little evidence to support its routine use as a component of AMTSL. Uterine massage, after the expulsion of the placenta, has not been found to be effective in preventing or reducing the risk of PPH. Sustained uterine massage may increase bleeding and should be avoided. The components of PMTSL are not clear. Uncertainty remains regarding optimal management of the third stage of labor.

## USING THE EVIDENCE FOR BEST PRACTICE

### Case Study 24.1    Supporting Normal Third Stage of Labor

Zoe is a 24-year-old healthy nulliparous woman in her third trimester who would like to discuss what to expect at her birth. She is planning on an unmedicated birth and would like only interventions necessary for safety. She asks about the third stage of labor and is interested in avoiding the routine practice of administering medication and pulling on the umbilical cord to hurry the expulsion of the placenta. Although agreeing with the desire to provide interventions only when necessary, the midwife explains that the administration of oxytocin reduces the risk of a hemorrhage during this critical time. The midwife explains that oxytocin can be deferred and administered only if Zoe has heavy bleeding but, if a hemorrhage occurs, she may need more than one medication to stop the bleeding and that once a hemorrhage occurs, the risk of complications related to the hemorrhage increases. The midwife also explains that cord pulling, or guiding the placenta out, would not be likely to occur. She explains that she encourages women to be upright and push out their own placentas. If Zoe cannot be upright, she can still bear down when she feels pressure from the placenta moving down the birth canal. If needed, the midwife may assist her by gently guiding the placenta out through controlled cord traction.

At 41 weeks gestation, Zoe gives birth to a 3,800-gram healthy girl in a semi-squatting position after an uncomplicated, unmedicated labor. She is at low risk for PPH, but the midwife exchanges the pads immediately under Zoe following the birth to collect blood loss. The midwife also suggests oxytocin (Pitocin) 10 international units administered intramuscularly for hemorrhage prevention as discussed prenatally. Zoe agrees to the oxytocin (Pitocin) and wants to stay upright to expel her placenta. She holds her baby closely; the baby is transitioning well with the cord still intact. Seven minutes after the birth, Zoe begins to feel contractions again and looks uncomfortable. The midwife notices an increase in blood trickling from her vagina. When asked whether she is feeling cramping or pressure, Zoe says she feels both. With encouragement, she bears down and expels the placenta. The cord is clamped and cut. Zoe is ready to sit and is guided to the bed while holding her baby. Assessing Zoe's fundus, the midwife finds it to be just below the umbilicus. The blood-soaked pad under Zoe during the third stage weighs 155 grams, thus the total blood loss is approximately 150 mL. The midwife is confident that Zoe's blood loss at this point is within the normal expected range. While Zoe enjoys and bonds with her new baby, the midwife inspects the placenta, finding it complete and normal. Once the baby is latched onto the breast, the midwife inspects the perineum and finds no lacerations.

### Exemplar of Best Practice

Prenatal discussion of third-stage management was an opportunity for shared decision making about Zoe's hemorrhage risk and treatment for prevention. After labor and birth proceeded in an uncomplicated manner, with no increased risk for hemorrhage, the midwife maintained physiologic management while implementing quantitative blood loss measurement and prophylactic oxytocin administration.

# REFERENCES

Abdel-Aleem, H., Hofmeyr, G. J., Shokry, M., & El-Sonoosy, E. (2006). Uterine massage and postpartum blood loss. *International Journal of Gynecology and Obstetrics, 93*(3), 238–239.

Abdel-Aleem, H., Singata, M., Abdel-Aleem, M., Mshweshwe, N., Williams, X., & Hofmeyr, G. J. (2010). Uterine massage to reduce postpartum hemorrhage after vaginal delivery. *International Journal of Gynecology and Obstetrics, 111*(1), 32–36.

Al Kadri, H. M., Al Anazi, B. K., & Tamim, H. M. (2011). Visual estimation versus gravimetric measurement of postpartum blood loss: A prospective cohort study. *Archives of Gynecology and Obstetrics, 283*(6), 1207–1213.

Ambardekar, S., Shochet, T., Bracken, H., Coyaji, K., & Winikoff, B. (2014). Calibrated delivery drape versus indirect gravimetric technique for the measurement of blood loss after delivery: A randomized trial. *BMC Pregnancy & Childbirth, 14*(276), 1–6.

American College of Obstetricians and Gynecologists (ACOG). (2006). ACOG Practice Bulletin: Clinical Management Guidelines for Obstetrician-Gynecologists Number 76, October 2006: Postpartum hemorrhage. *Obstetrics and Gynecology, 108*(4), 1039–1048.

Association of Women's Health, Obstetric and Neonatal Nurses (AWHONN). (2014). Oxytocin administration for management of third stage of labor (Practice Brief Number 2). Retrieved from http://www.pphproject.org/downloads/awhonn_oxytocin.pdf

Association of Women's Health, Obstetric and Neonatal Nurses (AWHONN). (2015). Guidelines for oxytocin administration after birth: AWHONN Practice Brief Number 2. *Journal of Obstetric, Gynecologic, and Neonatal Nursing, 44*, 161–163. doi:10.1111/1552-6909 .12528

Bamberg, C., Niepraschk-von Dollen, K., Mickley, L., Henkelmann, A., Hinkson, L., Kaufner, L., . . . Pauly, F. (2015). Evaluation of measured postpartum blood loss after vaginal delivery using a collector bag in relation to postpartum hemorrhage management strategies: A prospective observational study. *Journal of Perinatal Medicine, 44*(4), 443–449.

Begley, C. M. (1990). A comparison of "active" and "physiological" management of the third stage of labour. *Midwifery, 6*, 3–17.

Begley, C. M., Gyte, G. M., Devane, D., McGuire, W., & Weeks, A. (2011). Active versus expectant management for women in the third stage of labour. *Cochrane Database of Systematic Reviews* (11), CD007412.

Bingham, D., Lyndon, A., Lagrew, D., & Main, E. (2011). A state-wide obstetric hemorrhage quality improvement initiative. *American Journal of Maternal/Child Nursing, 36*, 297–302.

Brucker, M. (2001). Management of the third stage of labor: An evidence based approach. *Journal of Midwifery & Women's Health, 46*, 381–392.

Burke, C. (2010). Active versus expectant management of the third stage of labor and implementation of a protocol. *Journal of Perinatal & Neonatal Nursing, 24*, 215–228.

Chen, M., Chang, Q., Duan, T., He, J., Zhang, L., & Liu, X. (2013). Uterine massage to reduce blood loss after vaginal delivery. *Obstetrics & Gynecology, 122*, 290–295.

Combs, C. A., & Laros, R. K. (1991). Prolonged third stage of labor: Morbidity and risk factors. *Obstetrics & Gynecology, 77*, 863–867.

Dahlke, J. D., Mendez-Figueroa, H., Maggio, L., Hauspurg, A. K., Sperling, J. D., Chauhan, S. P., & Rouse, D. J. (2015). Prevention and management of postpartum hemorrhage: A comparison of 4 national guidelines. *American Journal of Obstetrics & Gynecology, 213,* 76.e1–76.e10.

Davis, D., Baddock, S., Pairman, S., Hunter, M., Benn, C., Anderson, J., . . . Herbison, P. (2012). Risk of severe postpartum hemorrhage in low-risk childbearing women in New Zealand: Exploring the effect of place of birth and comparing third stage management of labor. *Birth, 39*(2), 98–105. doi:10.1111/j.1523-536X.2012.00531.x

Deneux-Tharaux, C., Sentilhes, L., Maillard, F., Closset, E., Vardon, D., Lepercq, J., & Goffinet, F. (2013). Effect of routine controlled cord traction as part of the active management of the third stage of labour on postpartum haemorrhage: Multicentre randomised controlled trial (TRACOR). *British Medical Journal, 346.* doi:10.1136/bmj.f1541

Dombrowski, M. P., Bottoms, S. F., Saleh, A. A., Hurd, W. W., & Romero, R. (1995). Third stage of labor: Analysis of duration and clinical practice. *American Journal of Obstetrics & Gynecology, 172,* 1279–1284.

Du, Y., Ye, M., & Zheng, F. (2014). Active management of the third stage of labor with and without controlled cord traction: A systematic review and meta-analysis of randomized controlled trials. *Acta Obstetricia et Gynecologica, 93,* 626–633.

Fahy, K., Hastie, C., Bisits, A., Marsh, C., Smith, L., & Saxton, A. (2010). Holistic physiological care compared with active management of the third stage of labour for women at low risk of postpartum haemorrhage: A cohort study. *Women and Birth, 23,* 146–152.

Festin, M. R., Lumbiganon, P., Tolosa, J. E., Finney, K. A., Ba-Thike, K., Chipato, T., . . . Daly, S. (2003). International survey on variations in practice of the management of the third stage of labour. *Bulletin of the World Health Organization, 81*(4), 286–291.

Fry, J. (2007). Physiological third stage of labour: Support it or lose it. *British Journal of Midwifery, 15,* 693–695.

Gabel, K. T., & Weeber, T. A. (2012). Measuring and communicating blood loss during obstetric hemorrhage. *Journal of Obstetric, Gynecologic, and Neonatal Nursing, 41,* 551–558.

Gülmezoglu, A. M., Lumbiganon, P., Landoulsi, S., Widmer, M., Abdel-Aleem, H., Festin, M., . . . Elbourne, D. (2012). Active management of the third stage of labour with and without controlled cord traction: A randomized, controlled, non-inferiority trial. *Lancet, 379,* 1721–1727. doi:10.1016/S0140-6736(12)60206-2

Hastie, C., & Fahy, K. M. (2009). Optimising psychophysiology in third stage of labour: Theory applied to practice. *Women and Birth, 22,* 89–96.

Hofmeyr, G. J., Gülmezoglu, A. M., Novikova, N., & Lawrie, T. A. (2013). Postpartum misoprostol for preventing maternal and morbidity. *Cochrane Database of Systematic Reviews* (7). doi:10.1002/14651858.CD008982.pub2

Hofmeyr, G. J., Gülmezoglu, A. M., Novikova, N., Linder, V., Ferreira, S., & Piaggio, G. (2009). Misoprostol to prevent and treat postpartum haemorrhage: A systematic review and meta-analysis of maternal deaths and dose-related effects. *Bulletin of the World Health Organization, 87,* 666–677.

Hofmeyr, G. J., Mshweshwe, N. T., & Gülmezoglu, A. M. (2015). Controlled cord traction for the third stage of labour. *Cochrane Database of Systematic Reviews* (1). doi:10.1002/14651858.CD008020.pub2

International Confederation of Midwives (ICM), & International Federation of Gynaecologists and Obstetricians (FIGO). (2004). Joint statement: Management of the third stage of labour to prevent post-partum haemorrhage. *Journal of Midwifery & Women's Health, 49*(1), 76–77.

Jangsten, E., Mattson, L., Lyckestam, I., Hellström, A., & Berg, M. (2011). A comparison of active management and expectant management of the third stage of labour: A Swedish randomised controlled trial. *International Journal of Obstetrics & Gynaecology, 118,* 365–369.

Jones, R. (2015). Quantitative measurement of blood loss during delivery. *Journal of Obstetric, Gynecologic, & Neonatal Nursing, 44*(Suppl. 1), S41–S41.

Kashanian, M., Fekrat, M., Masoomi, Z., & Ansari, N. S. (2010). Comparison of active and expectant management on the duration of the third stage of labour and the amount of blood loss during the third and fourth stages of labour: A randomised controlled trial. *Midwifery, 26*(2), 241–245.

Knight, M., Callaghan, W. M., Berg, C., Alexander, S., Bouvier-Colle, M.-H., Ford, J. B., . . . Walker, J. (2009). Trends in postpartum hemorrhage in high resource countries: A review and recommendations from the International Postpartum Hemorrhage Collaborative Group. *BMC Pregnancy and Childbirth,* 1–9. doi:10.1186/1471-2393-9-55

Kramer, M. S., Berg, C., Abenhaim, H., Dahhou, M., Rouleau, J., Mehrabadi, A., & Joseph, K. S. (2013). Incidence, risk factors, and temporal trends in severe postpartum hemorrhage. *American Journal of Obstetrics & Gynecology, 209,* 449.e1–449.e7.

Larsson, C., Saltvedt, S., Wilkund, I., Pahlen, S., & Andolf, E. (2006). Estimation of blood loss after cesarean section and vaginal delivery has low validity with a tendency to exaggeration. *Acta Obstetricia et Gynecologica Scandinavica, 85,* 1448–1452.

Lyndon, A., Lagrew, D., Shields, L., Main, E., & Cape, V. (2015). *Improving health care response to obstetric hemorrhage.* (California Maternal Quality Care Collaborative Toolkit to Transform Maternity Care; Developed under contract #11-10006 with the California Department of Public Health). Sacramento, CA: Maternal, Child and Adolescent Health Division, California Department of Public Health.

Magann, E. F., Evans, S., Chauhan, S. P., Lanneau, G., Fisk, A. D., & Morrison, J. C. (2005). The length of the third stage of labor and the risk of postpartum hemorrhage. *Obstetrics & Gynecology, 105,* 290–293.

Magann, E. F., Lutgendorf, M. A., Keiser, S. D., Porter, S., Siegel, E. R., McKelvey, S. A., & Morrison, J. C. (2013). Risk factors for a prolonged third stage of labor and postpartum hemorrhage. *Southern Medical Journal, 106*(2), 131–135.

Main, E. K., Goffman, D., Scavone, B. M., Low, L. K., Bingham, D., Fontaine, P. L., . . . Levy, B. S. (2015). National partnership for maternal safety consensus bundle on obstetric hemorrhage. *Journal of Midwifery & Women's Health, 60*(4), 458–464.

Maslovitz, S., Barkai, G., Lessing, J. B., Ziv, A., & Many, A. (2008). Improved accuracy of postpartum blood loss estimation as assessed by simulation. *Acta Obstetricia et Gynecologica Scandinavica, 87*(9), 929–934.

Maughan, K. L., Heim, S. W., & Galazka, S. S. (2006). Preventing postpartum hemorrhage: Managing the third stage of labor. *American Family Physician, 73,* 1025–1028.

McDonald, S. J., Middleton, P., Dowswel, T., & Morris, P. S. (2013). Effect of timing of umbilical cord clamping of term infants on maternal and neonatal outcomes. *Cochrane Database of Systematic Reviews.* doi:10.1002/14651858.CD004074.pub3

Oladapo, O. (2010). What exactly is active management of third stage of labor? *Acta Obstetricia et Gynecologica Scandinavica, 89*(1), 4–6.

Patel, A., Goudar, S. S., Geller, S. E., Kodkany, B. S., Edlavitch, S. A., Wagh, K., . . . Derman, R. J. (2006). Drape estimation vs. visual assessment for estimating postpartum hemorrhage. *International Journal of Gynecology & Obstetrics, 93*(3), 220–224.

Prasertcharoensuk, W., Swadpanich, U., & Lumbiganon, P. (2000). Accuracy of the blood loss estimation in the third stage of labor. *BJOG: International Journal of Gynaecology & Obstetrics, 71,* 69–70.

Prendiville, W. J., Elbourne, D., & McDonald, S. (2007). Active versus expectant management in the third stage of labour. *Cochrane Database of Systematic Reviews* (4), 1–37. Retrieved from http://apps.who.int/rhl/reviews/langs/CD000007.pdf

Prendiville, W. J., Harding, J. E., Elbourne, D. R., & Stirrat, G. M. (1988). The Bristol third stage trial: Active versus physiological management of the third stage of labour. *British Medical Journal, 297,* 1295–1300.

Schorn, M. N. (2010). Measurement of blood loss: Review of the literature. *Journal of Midwifery & Women's Health, 55,* 20–27.

Schorn, M. N., Minnick, A., & Donaghey, B. (2015). An exploration of how midwives and physicians manage the third stage of labor in the United States. *Journal of Midwifery and Women's Health, 60*(2), 187–198

Sheiner, E., Sarid, L., Levy, A., Seidman, D. S., & Hallak, M. (2005). Obstetric risk factors and outcome of pregnancies complicated with early postpartum hemorrhage: A population-based study. *Journal of Maternal–Fetal and Neonatal Medicine, 18,* 149–154.

Sheldon, W. R., Durocher, J., Winikoff, B., Blum, J., & Trussell, J. (2013). How effective are the components of active management of the third stage of labor? *BMC Pregnancy and Childbirth, 13*(46), 1–8. doi:10.1186/1471-2393-13-46

Soltani, H., Hutchon, D. R., & Poulose, T. A. (2010). Timing of prophylactic uterotonics for the third stage of labour after vaginal birth. *Cochrane Database of Systematic Reviews* (8). doi:10.1002/14651858.CD006173.pub2

Toledo, P., McCarthy, R. J., Hewlett, B. J., & Fitzgerald, P. C. (2007). The accuracy of blood loss estimation after simulated vaginal delivery. *Obstetric Anesthesiology, 105,* 1736–1740.

Turpin, C. A., Osakunor, D. N. M., & Owiredu, W. K. B. A. (2015). Accuracy of blood loss determination after vaginal delivery: Visual estimation versus calibrated measurement. *British Journal of Medicine & Medical Research, 6,* 1121–1127.

Uwins, C., & Hutchon, D. (2014). Delayed umbilical cord clamping after childbirth: Potential benefits to baby's health. *Dove Medical Press Limited, 2014*(5), 161–171. Retrieved from https://www.dovepress.com/delayed-umbilical-cord-clamping-after-childbirth-potential-benefits-to-peer-reviewed-fulltext-article-PHMT

Villar, J., Gülmezoglu, A. M., Hofmeyr, J., & Forna, F. (2002). Systematic review of randomized controlled trials of misoprostol to prevent postpartum hemorrhage. *Obstetrics & Gynecology, 100,* 1301–1312.

Westhoff, G., Cotter, A. M., & Tolosa, J. E. (2013). Prophylactic oxytocin for the third stage of labour to prevent postpartum haemorrhage. *Cochrane Database of Systematic Reviews* (10). doi:10.1002/14651858.CD001808.pub2

Witcher, P. M., & Sisson, M. C. (2015). Maternal morbidity and mortality. *Journal of Perinatal and Neonatal Nursing, 29,* 202–212.

World Health Organization (WHO). (2012). WHO recommendations for the prevention and treatment of postpartum haemorrhage. Retrieved from http://apps.who.int/iris/bitstream/10665/75411/1/9789241548502_eng.pdf

World Health Organization (WHO). (2014). Active management of the third stage of labour: New WHO recommendations help to focus implementation. Retrieved from http://apps.who.int/iris/bitstream/10665/119831/1/WHO_RHR_14.18_eng.pdf

Yaju, Y., Kataoka, Y., Eto, H., Horiuchi, S., & Mori, R. (2013). Prophylactic interventions after delivery of placenta for reducing bleeding during the postnatal period. *Cochrane Database of Systematic Reviews* (11). doi:10.1002/14651858.CD009328.pub2

Zhang, W.-H., Deneux-Tharaux, C., Brocklehurst, P., Juszczak, E., Joslin, M., & Alexander, S. (2010). Effect of a collector bag for measurement of postpartum blood loss after vaginal delivery: Cluster randomised trial in 13 European countries. *British Medical Journal, 340,* C293. Retrieved from http://www.ncbi.nlm.nih.gov/pmc/articles/PMC2815270

# COLLABORATIVE PRACTICE: THE EVIDENCE FOR BEST PRACTICES

Barbara A. Anderson

*Midwifery is at a point of crisis: facing danger and opportunity. Across the globe, failure to provide an adequately educated and equitably distributed workforce poses a danger to the lives of mothers and infants. Yet, this crisis offers opportunities for leadership, innovation, and collaboration with our colleagues. Chapter 25 demonstrates how midwifery leadership can mobilize multidisciplinary systems to improve maternal and infant health. Chapters 26 and 27 describe a climate of learning and practice that breaks down silos, fosters communication, and acknowledges the value that each discipline brings to maternal and infant care. Section IV, "Collaborative Practice: The Evidence for Best Practices," examines the World Health Organization's mandate to create a culture of collaborative learning, preparing the workforce to deliver interprofessional care. This section also points to the call by the Institute of Medicine to forge multidisciplinary partnerships and collaborative practice.*

*Mary Breckinridge understood the need to collaborate across disciplines. On horseback, she visited the mountain women in rural Appalachian cabins, gathering evidence, identifying best practices, and delivering care. She then took that evidence and built collaborations for change. In that spirit, this section discusses building capacity for collaborative partnerships.*

# CHAPTER TWENTY-FIVE

# THE ROLE OF MIDWIFERY IN MOBILIZING COMMUNITIES TO IMPROVE MATERNAL AND NEWBORN HEALTH OUTCOMES

Jody R. Lori

## GLOBAL MATERNAL AND NEONATAL HEALTH

At the start of the millennium, the United Nations (UN) Millennium Development Goals (MDGs) targeted as these goals: a decrease in the maternal mortality ratio (MMR) by 75% and a reduction in under-5-year-old mortality by two thirds. In 2014, more than 71% of births across the world were assisted by a skilled provider, an increase from 59% in 1990. The MMR declined by 45%, and the global under-5-year-old mortality rate declined by more than 50% between 1990 and 2015 (UN, 2015a). Progress has been made. Looking toward the next global initiative, the UN Sustainable Development Goals (SDGs), the need for global community involvement to sustain this downward trend becomes self-evident (UN, 2015a).

The MDGs, adopted by the UN in 2000, target eight development goals for global focus. These are:

- To eradicate extreme poverty and hunger
- To achieve universal primary education
- To reduce child mortality
- To improve maternal health
- To combat HIV/AIDS, malaria, and other diseases
- To ensure environmental sustainability
- To develop a global partnership for development (UN, 2015a)

All 189 (now 193) UN member countries around the world have been part of this global initiative (UN, 2015a) and midwifery has been a key player. The MDGs energized the world to make substantial progress, but there is still far to go. The decline in neonatal mortality (infant deaths in the first 28 days of life) has been slower than in children aged 1 to 59 months, and now represents a larger share of the under-5-year-old mortality. Despite the reduction in maternal deaths, the MMR is 14 times higher in developing nations than in developed regions of the world. These inequities are targeted in the SDGs, which set goals that all countries should reduce the MMR by at least two thirds of their 2010 baseline level. The 2030 global target is to reduce fetal deaths to less than 70 deaths per 100,000 live births, and to reduce neonatal mortality to no more than 12 per 1,000 live births (UN, 2015b).

## Mobilizing Communities

One way to attain the SDGs globally is by mobilizing communities. The strategic framework for ending preventable maternal mortality (World Health Organization [WHO], 2015) calls for empowering women, girls, and communities and prioritizing country mobilization around these issues. Three major pillars have been identified to achieve improved maternal and newborn health and survival by the U.S. Agency for International Development (USAID). The first two pillars are advancing quality, respectful care and strengthening health systems and continuous learning (USAID, 2015). The third pillar is "enabling and mobilizing individuals and communities to improve healthy behaviors, expand use of appropriate services, and hold health systems accountable" (USAID, 2015, p. 17). USAID recognizes the community as an essential part of the health care system and recommends community mobilization to empower individuals and to assist communities in taking responsibility for their own care (USAID, 2015).

A broad range of community-based strategies use the term *community mobilization*, describing and operationalizing the concept in multiple ways. Many studies of community interventions have examined the effectiveness of an intervention targeted toward a passive audience. Mass campaigns for immunization programs are one example of mobilization strategies in which communities are passively involved (Rosato et al., 2008). Although mass campaigns can reach a wide audience through radio, billboards, or other media, these campaigns do not foster community ownership. Community mobilization activities are more than communities responding to direction from outsiders. These mobilization activities engage communities for action.

Community mobilization can have transformational power as a "capacity building process through which community members, groups or organizations plan, carry out, and evaluate activities on a participatory and sustained basis to improve their health and other conditions, either on their own initiative or stimulated by others" (Howard-Grabman & Snetro, 2003, p. 3). A number of key activities are involved in community mobilization, including:

- Developing an ongoing dialogue among community members
- Creating an environment in which individuals can empower themselves to address their health needs and those of the community in which they live
- Inclusion of those who are most affected by a health issue and also often the most marginalized
- Promoting partnerships through equity and diversity with community members in all phases of engagement to create locally appropriate responses to health issues

- Creating community organizations or strengthening existing ones to improve communities' health
- Linking communities with resources external to their environment to support their effort to improve health
- Committing the necessary time to work with communities to accomplish their goals (Howard-Grabman & Snetro, 2003)

Community mobilization can be used in situations in which the health problems of individuals, such as pregnant women and newborns, affect the health of the entire community.

## Empowerment Theory

Community mobilization draws on Freire's empowerment theory, described in *Pedagogy of the Oppressed* (Freire, 1996). One way to conceptualize community mobilization is as a behavior change model. There is a growing body of evidence that community mobilization strategies may change health behaviors and improve utilization of maternal health services for disadvantaged and marginalized groups in low-resource areas of the world (Babalola & Fatusi, 2009; Lawn et al., 2009; Mullany, Becker, & Hindin, 2007). Lee et al. (2009) describe community mobilization as a process of "enabling people to organize themselves, recognize opportunities, identify their collective potential, and utilize available resources to realize a shared goal through unified action" (p. S67). Community mobilization strategies to improve maternal and newborn health outcomes include multiple approaches to change individual behavior, increase collective knowledge, and promote broader community action (Lee et al., 2009). Unlike other models, community mobilization is not delivered in a linear form from implementers to communities. Rather, community mobilization allows communities to lead efforts for change by being the designers, implementers, and recipients of the change (Rath et al., 2010).

## Definition of Community

To begin, one must first identify and define the community. Communities exist in many different forms. A community can consist of individuals, groups, or organizations with a shared culture, language, geographical location, or set of common values (Mercy Corps, 2015). Communities can comprise groups of people interested in making social change within their specific group or working together to address a health care issue, such as maternal mortality, within a specific region. Specific groups within a community often have a common goal that will meet the interest of the entire community.

Community mobilization works through raising awareness, building community support, and empowering communities to take action on topics identified as important for the community. Community mobilization requires community-level decision making to prioritize topics. Community members then take the required actions agreed upon to effect change and evaluate the outcomes, making adjustments as needed. Community mobilization brings together diverse stakeholders to engage in a process in which individuals are accountable to one another and agree to work together for the good of the wider community. This community mobilization process can be used to empower members of the community to demand quality pregnancy-related services, and to improve maternal and newborn outcomes.

## Community Mobilization for Capacity Building

The need for strong community-based approaches has been identified as a sustainable and effective strategy for capacity building and scale-up of evidence-based practices. Some of the earliest work using community mobilization efforts to improve maternal and newborn health originated from the Warmi project, funded by the nongovernmental organization Save the Children and conducted in the early 1990s (O'Rourke, Howard-Grabman, & Seoane, 1998). The Warmi project focused on improving pregnancy outcomes for women living in remote, rural areas of Bolivia with limited access to skilled care. The project embraced strategies put forward at the 1978 landmark International Conference on Primary Health Care, held in Alma-Ata, Union of Soviet Socialist Republics (now Kazakhstan). The final document became known as the Alma-Alta Declaration (WHO, 1978). These strategies included:

- Enabling communities to become their own agents of change and allowing individuals and families to assume responsibility for their own health and the health of their communities
- Encouraging health providers to work with communities to acquire the capacity to appraise the situation, examine the options, and decide what their own contribution will be toward solving the problem (WHO, 1978)

Following the Alma-Ata Declaration, the importance of community participation was recognized as central to sustainable change. The four phases of community action (Figure 25.1) were developed from the Warmi project:

- Identifying and prioritizing problems
- Planning solutions as a group
- Acting together to implement solutions
- Evaluating results as a group (O'Rourke et al., 1998)

Using the community action cycle to mobilize communities for change, the Warmi project achieved a significant reduction in the perinatal mortality rate from 117 per 1,000 live births before the intervention to 43.8 per 1,000 live births after the intervention. In addition, there were significant changes in the proportion of women receiving prenatal care and those initiating breastfeeding on the first day postpartum (O'Rourke et al., 1998).

Community mobilization strategies work best when the community is acknowledged as the active agent of change.

By actively engaging communities, the broader determinants of maternal and newborn health can be addressed through collective action. Through sharing and

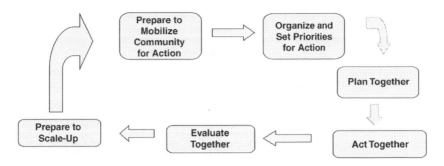

**Figure 25.1** Community action cycle: A dynamic framework to improve maternal and newborn outcomes.
Adapted from Howard-Grabman and Snetro (2003).

having their voices heard, community members' experiences are acknowledged and information is presented in a culturally appropriate way, and positively reinforced through peer support (O'Rourke et al., 1998).

## THE EVIDENCE FOR COMMUNITY MOBILIZATION

### Studies on Community Mobilization Intervention

Community mobilization strategies and interventions have been studied to address various public health issues, including gender-based violence (Ilika & Ilika, 2005), identification and treatment of malaria (Kindane & Morrow, 2000), and improvement of perinatal care and outcomes (More et al., 2012). Community mobilization empowers communities and promotes participation at every level—from problem identification to evaluating lessons learned from various interventions. Community mobilization builds capacity at the community level to take control of the specific community health issues (Lewycka et al., 2010).

In a 3-year randomized controlled trial (RCT) conducted in three contiguous districts in India, community mobilization and the community action cycles were used with women's groups. Pregnant women in the intervention groups met monthly to take part in participatory learning using the community action cycle. Meetings on clean delivery practices and care-seeking behaviors were facilitated by a trained, local community member through games, case study discussions, stories, and picture cards. Groups then devised their own strategies and culturally appropriate ways of implementation, including prevention of problems, home care support, consultation, and referral (Tripathy et al., 2010). These interventions resulted in a 32% decrease in the neonatal mortality rate in the intervention clusters after adjusting for clustering, stratification, and baseline differences (odds ratio = 0.68, 95% confidence interval, 0.59–0.78; Tripathy et al., 2010).

In a large RCT of nearly 30,000 women in Nepal utilizing community mobilization intervention with women's groups, neonatal mortality was reduced by 30% and maternal mortality was significantly lowered in women enrolled in the intervention groups (Manandhar et al., 2004). Similarly, building health-promotion capacities through community mobilization was positively associated with an increase in maternal health care–seeking behaviors among women from Guinea. Women in the intervention groups were more than twice as likely to attend four antenatal care visits, seek care for signs of complications, and give birth in a health facility (Brazier, Florentino, Barry, & Diallo, 2015).

A meta-analysis of community mobilization conducted by Lee et al. (2009) found a 71% increase in facility-based births and a 33% reduction in perinatal deaths. In addition, a twofold increase was noted when high-intensity mobilization strategies were employed within the study design. High-intensity strategies included active community engagement, presenting information within the cultural context of the setting, involving a wide range of community stakeholders, peer counseling, and home visitation programs. Although there was only moderate evidence from this meta-analysis, which included three RCTs, two quasi-experimental studies, and one before-and-after study, the authors concluded that the evidence is sufficient to generalize the findings in low- to middle-income countries (Lee et al., 2009). A second meta-analysis on community participation demonstrated largely positive impacts on newborn and maternal health when part of a package of interventions (Marston, Renedo, McGowan, & Portela, 2013).

In rural Zambia, a community mobilization intervention achieved significant improvements for pregnant women through increased knowledge of danger signs in pregnancy, use of emergency transport, and increased utilization (uptake) of antenatal care and skilled birth attendants (Ensor et al., 2014). Similarly, Rath et al. (2010) posit that their participatory learning and action cycle intervention with 244 women's groups was responsible for an increase in safe delivery practices leading to a substantial reduction in neonatal mortality.

In a study conducted in northern Nigeria, a three-pronged approach using community mobilization was used to promote the uptake of misoprostol to prevent postpartum hemorrhage following home birth. The three prongs included:

- Education for women and communities on birth preparedness and preventing postpartum hemorrhage through the use of misoprostol
- Training traditional birth attendants and community resource people to counsel pregnant women about bleeding after delivery
- Training community members in the storage and distribution of misoprostol (Prata, Ejembi, Fraser, Shittu, & Minkler, 2012)

In this study, 1,875 women were enrolled, with the majority (95%) giving birth at home. The authors found a significant impact on the successful distribution and uptake of misoprostol. The vast majority of women in the study (79%) took the misoprostol tablets prophylactically as instructed with only 2.1% experiencing a postpartum hemorrhage (Prata et al., 2012).

Although the evidence is mounting on the impact of community mobilization to improve maternal and newborn outcomes, there is a gap in the literature on how to measure community mobilization. Studies of community mobilization interventions most often report health outcomes or outputs of activities. Few of the studies measure the process of mobilization: what changes happen in relationships, perceptions, and beliefs at a community level. Altman, Kuhlmann, and Galavotti (2015) conducted a systematic review of community mobilization interventions targeting sexual, reproductive, and maternal health to better understand what specific programmatic components of community mobilization interventions produce change and influence health outcomes. The authors identified eight linking constructs from various community mobilization studies that help to measure the process of moving from simple participation in a group to mobilized, engaged communities (Kuhlman & Galavotti, 2015).

The following constructs have been explicitly used to measure the process of mobilization:

- Collective action, agency, efficacy, and collective identity
- Governance
- Perceived similarity, social acceptance/social cohesion
- Social networks/social support (Altman et al., 2015)

## Sustainability and Scale-Up

An essential element of community mobilization is participation. As participation from the community increases, community ownership and capacity also increase, which contributes to the likelihood of the project's sustainability over time (USAID, 2007). When taken to the highest level, community mobilization builds social networks, allows communities to set their own agendas, and shifts the power balance to community ownership (USAID, 2007). When communities remain active and empowered, sustained mobilization occurs and effective shared-governance ensues (Mercy Corps, 2015).

As with any intervention, the question of sustainability and scale-up is at the forefront for governments and funders. Is there evidence of sustainability among communities or groups that have been organized using community mobilization strategies? Following the trial in Nepal, in those areas where women's groups were mobilized, neonatal mortality rates remained lower for 3 to 6 years after the original studies were completed (Nair, Tripathy, Costello, & Prost, 2012). The community action cycle, as an understandable tool, can coalesce communities around self-identified problems and therefore encourages sustainability.

*Scale-up* refers to increasing the number or scope of activities. Yamey (2011) discusses successful scale-up and three broad areas of attributes needed for successful scale-up. The attributes identified included:

- *The tool or service*, for example, keeping the intervention simple and scientifically robust
- *The implementers*, for example, strong leadership and governance, engaging local stakeholders and implementers, a variety of implementers, and choosing the correct delivery strategy

● *The adopting community*, for example, an engaged and activated community, social and political will, and evidence as guide to the process (Yamey, 2011)

Community mobilization incorporates many of these attributes in its framework, but understanding the affordability of community mobilization is key to scale-up. Colbourn et al. (2015) examined the cost-effectiveness, and modeled the affordability of creating a community mobilization intervention designed to improve maternal and neonatal health in Malawi. The authors concluded that community mobilization through women's groups in Malawi is an affordable and cost-effective strategy to reduce neonatal and maternal mortality. Furthermore, it was determined that community mobilization could prevent a large proportion of disability-adjusted life-years (DALYs) from fetal, neonatal, and maternal deaths in the Malawi context (Colbourn et al., 2015).

Success does not mean reaching every community. Targeting areas with the highest maternal or newborn mortality to bring equitable, quality care to a larger group of people over a greater geographical area is a form of scale-up (USAID, 2007). Carefully choosing communities for scale-up can build momentum and provide the impetus for policy changes to support successful expansion.

## BEST PRACTICES FOR MIDWIFERY

There is an increasing body of literature describing successful community mobilization interventions to reduce maternal and newborn morbidity and mortality. This is especially true in communities with limited resources and poor access to care. Only when community mobilization is prioritized as a key intervention and integrated into national health plans to link women in impoverished urban or rural settings with skilled maternity care, will we begin to overcome the high rates of maternal and newborn mortality in some of the world's most marginalized communities. Midwifery practice is key to establishing these links and working with the community.

## Incorporating Community Mobilization Into the Midwifery Model of Care

The International Confederation of Midwives (ICM) lists the key midwifery concepts that define the role of midwives in promoting the health and well-being of women and childbearing families as:

● Partnership with women to promote self-care and health of mothers, infants, and families
● Respect for human dignity and full human rights
● Advocacy

- Cultural sensitivity, including working with women and health care providers to overcome harmful cultural practices
- Health promotion and disease prevention viewing pregnancy as a normal life event (ICM, 2010, p. 2)

The midwife is charged with health counseling and education, not only for the woman, but for the family and the community (ICM, 2010). Community mobilization is a tool that can be used by the practicing midwife to influence community behavior; increase awareness; and promote accessing skilled birth attendance, breastfeeding, family planning, and care-seeking for maternal and newborn problems (Lassi, Das, Salam, & Bhuta, 2014). Community mobilization can be used by midwives to reach the most vulnerable women who have very little voice in their reproductive choices and are the most marginalized. The midwifery model of care already treats women as full partners in their reproductive health care (ICM, 2010). Integrating community mobilization into existent programs provides an additional opportunity for midwives to empower women.

Community mobilization brings people together around a common concern and strengthens the capacity for leadership within a community. Although the core of community mobilization is a participatory process for decision making, ultimately the community is working toward improving equity within the setting.

## Steps for Successful Community Mobilization

The following steps are recommended for the midwife in promoting successful community mobilization:

- Know the community being served by understanding community members' interests, the local culture, and motivating factors for the community
- Work with existing leaders, both formal and informal, including government and key stakeholders as well as those without official positions
- Maintain regular and clear communication so that communities understand all elements of the community and the program
- Ask questions, listen, and be sure everyone is clear on the process
- Develop strong facilitation skills and obtain continuous feedback from the community
- Continually find ways to motivate and reenergize the community (Mercy Corps, 2015)

Case Study 25.1 offers an example of midwifery-led community mobilization. From 2010 to 2014, an operations research study funded by USAID was conducted using a community-based, participatory action model to examine the impact of maternity waiting homes (MWHs) in rural Liberia (Lori, Munro, et al., 2013). Key elements of the community action cycle were used to engage the community at each level of the research process. The phases of the project are described as well as the barriers, process, and outcomes (Figure 25.2).

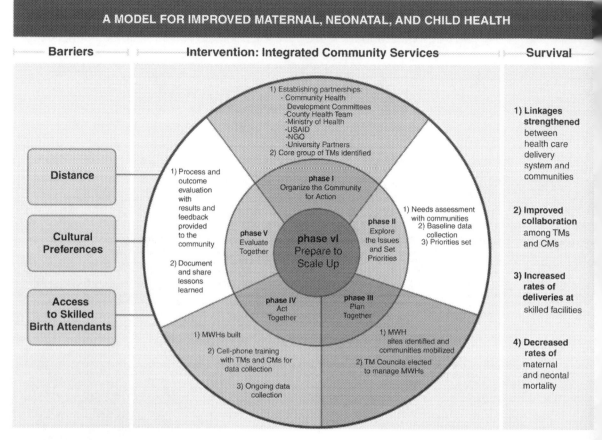

**Figure 25.2** The community action cycle used in the innovation, research, operations, and planned evaluation for mothers and children (I-ROPE) study.
CMs, certified midwives; MWH, maternal waiting home; NGO, nongovernmental organization; TMs, traditional midwives.
*Source:* Lori et al. (2013). Reprinted with permission from Elsevier.

Case Study 25.1 illustrates the use of community mobilization and the community action cycle in combatting high maternal and perinatal morbidity and mortality rates in Liberia, West Africa.

---

**USING THE EVIDENCE FOR BEST PRACTICE**

**Case Study 25.1    Community Mobilization to Improve Maternal Perinatal Health**

The Innovation, Research, Operations, and Planned Evaluation for Mothers and Children (I-ROPE) project introduced a MWH model to address Liberia's high maternal and perinatal morbidity and mortality rates by increasing facility-based birth.

The I-ROPE study adapted the general WHO concept of an MWH to the Liberian context by:

*(continued)*

**USING THE EVIDENCE FOR BEST PRACTICE (*continued*)**

- Establishing MWHs at primary health care facilities with basic emergency obstetric and newborn care capacity
- Organizing traditional midwives (TMs) and certified midwives (CMs) in collaborative teams

Using the community action cycle allowed for capacity building at the local level, enhancement of self-reliance, and long-term sustainability. Prior to construction of the MWHs during phase I, members of the research and implementation teams mobilized communities to identify the most pressing concerns and organized the community for action. Next, in phase II the issues were explored and priorities for action were set. During phase III, community members, the implementing agency, and researchers planned for action. Communities pledged the provision of raw materials and services (making bricks, hauling sand and gravel, cutting wood) and the donation of food and cooked meals for the construction teams. The communities agreed that each MWH would be run by a core group of TMs elected by the Community Health Development Committee and overseen by the CM at the respective health care facility. These groups were established by the Liberian Ministry of Health and Social Welfare (MOHSW), the chief administrative organization overseeing the health of the nation. MOHSW is charged with decision making in terms of health care facility management and provision of community health services under the National Strategy and Policy for Community Health Services (MOHSW, 2008). At each MWH, a TM council was elected and charged with responsibility for the day-to-day operation of the MWH. During phase IV, the community and partners acted together to begin both construction of the MWHs and the process of data collection. Finally, phase V concluded with an evaluation process, providing feedback to the communities at large and to the wider scientific community (Lori, Munro, et al., 2013; Lori, Wadsworth, Munro, & Rominski, 2013).

**Exemplar of Best Practice**

In addition to improvements in maternal mortality within communities served by MWHs, there was a significant increase in the number of team births attended by CMs and TMs together (Lori et al., 2013b). This finding reflects the strategy taken by the MOHSW in rebuilding the health system: to integrate and coordinate services with community involvement and participation. Mobilizing the community with midwifery leadership is exemplified in all phases of this project.

# REFERENCES

Altman, L., Kuhlmann, A. K., & Galavotti, C. (2015). Understanding the black box: A systematic review of the measurement of the community mobilization process in evaluations of interventions targeting sexual, reproductive, and maternal health. *Evaluation and Program Planning, 49*, 86–97. doi:10.1016/j.evalprogplan.2014.11.010

Babalola, S., & Fatusi, A. (2009). Determinants of use of maternal health services in Nigeria—Looking beyond individual and household factors. *BMC Pregnancy and Childbirth, 9*(43), 1–13. doi:10.1186/1471-2393-9-43. Retrieved from http://www.biomedcentral.com/content/pdf/1471-2393-9-43.pdf

Brazier, E., Florentino, R., Barry, M. S., & Diallo, M. (2015). The value of building health promotion capacities within communities: Evidence from a maternal health intervention in Guinea. *Health Policy and Planning, 30*(7), 885–894. doi:10.1093/heapol/czu089

Colbourn, T., Pulkki-Brännström, A. M., Nambiar, B., Kim, S., Bondo, A., Banda, L., . . . Skordis-Worrall, J. (2015). Cost-effectiveness and affordability of community mobilization through women's groups and quality improvement in health facilities (MaiKhanda trial) in Malawi. *Cost Effectiveness and Resource Allocation, 13*(1), 1–15. doi:10.1186/s21962-014-0028-2

Ensor, T., Green, C., Quigley, P., Badru, A. R., Kaluba, D., & Kureya, T. (2014). Mobilizing communities to improve maternal health: Results of an intervention in rural Zambia. *Bulletin of the World Health Organization, 92*(1), 51–59. doi:10.2471/BLT.13.122721

Freire, P. (1996). *Pedagogy of the oppressed* (2nd ed.). London, UK: Penguin.

Howard-Grabman, L., & Snetro, G. (2003). Toolkits: How to mobilize communities for health and social change. Retrieved from https://www.k4health.org/toolkits/pc-bcc/how-mobilize -communities-health-and-social-change

Ilika, A. M., & Ilika, U. R. (2005). Eliminating gender-based violence: Learning from the widowhood practices elimination initiative of a women organization in Ozublu, Anambra State of Nigeria. *African Journal of Reproductive Health, 9*(2), 65–75. doi:10.2307/3583463

International Confederation of Midwives (ICM). (2010). Essential competencies for basic midwifery practice. Retrieved from http://www.internationalmidwives.org/assets/uploads/ documents/CoreDocuments/ICM%20Essential%20Competencies%20for%20Basic%20 Midwifery%20Practice%202010,%20revised%202013.pdf

Kindane, G., & Morrow, R. H. (2000). Teaching mothers to provide home treatment of malaria in Tigra, Ethiopia: A randomized trial. *Lancet, 356*(9229), 550–555. doi:10.1016/S0140 -6736(00)02580-0

Lassi, Z. S., Das, J. K., Salam, R. A., & Bhuta, Z. A. (2014). Evidence from community level inputs to improve quality of care for maternal and newborn health: Interventions and findings. *Reproductive Health, 11*(Suppl. 2), 1–19. doi:10.1186/1742-4755-11-S2-S2. Retrieved from http://www.reproductive-health-journal.com/content/11/S2/S2

Lawn, J. E., Lee, A. C., Kinney, M., Sibley, L., Carlo, W. A., Paul, V. K., . . . Darmstadt, G. L. (2009). Two million intrapartum-related stillbirths and neonatal deaths: Where, why, and what can be done? *International Journal of Gynaecology and Obstetrics, 107*(Suppl. 1), S5–18, S19. doi:10.1016/j.ijgo.2009.07.016

Lee, A. C., Lawn, J. E., Cousens, S., Kumar, V., Osrin, D., Bhutta, Z. A., . . . Darmstadt, G. L. (2009). Linking families and facilities for care at birth: What works to avert intrapartum-related deaths? *International Journal of Gynaecology and Obstetrics, 107*(Suppl. 1), S65–S88. doi:10.1016/j.ijgo.2009.07.012

Lewycka, S., Mwansambo, C., Kazembe, P., Phiri, T., Mganga, A., Rosato, M., . . . Costello, A. (2010). A cluster randomised controlled trial of the community effectiveness of two interventions in rural Malawi to improve health care and to reduce maternal, newborn, and infant mortality. *Trials, 11*(88), 1–15. doi:10.1186/1745-6215-11-88. Retrieved from http:// www.trialsjournal.com/content/11/1/88

Lori, J. R., Munro, M. L., Rominski, S., Williams, G., Dahn, B. T., Boyd, C. J., . . . Gwenegale, W. (2013). Maternity waiting homes and traditional midwives in rural Liberia. *International Journal of Gynaecology and Obstetrics, 123*(2), 114–118. doi:10.1016/j.ijgo.2013.05.024

Lori, J. R., Wadsworth, A. C., Munro, M. L., & Rominski, S. (2013). Promoting access: The use of maternity waiting homes to achieve safe motherhood. *Midwifery, 29*(10), 1095–1102. doi:10.1016/j.midw.2013.07.020

Manandhar, D. S., Osrin, D., Shrestha, B. P., Mesko, N., Morrison, J., Tumbahangphe, K. M., . . . Costello, A. M. (2004). Effect of a participatory intervention with women's groups on birth outcomes in Nepal: Cluster-randomised controlled trial. *Lancet, 364*(9438), 970–979. doi:10.1016/S0140-6736(04)17021-9

Marston, C., Renedo, A., McGowan, C. R., & Portela, A. (2013). Effects of community participation on improving uptake of skilled care for maternal and newborn health: A systematic review. *PloS One, 8*(2), e55012. doi:10.1371/journal.pone.0055012

Mercy Corps. (2015). Guide to community mobilization programming. Retrieved from https://www.mercycorps.org/sites/default/files/CoMobProgrammingGd.pdf

Ministry of Health and Social Welfare (MOHSW). (2008). National strategy and policy for community health services. Republic of Liberia. Retrieved from http://www.basics.org/documents/National-Strategy-and-Policy-for-Community-Health-Services_Liberia.pdf

More, N. S., Bapat, U., Das, S., Alcock, G., Patil, S., Porel, M., . . . Osrin, D. (2012). Community mobilization in Mumbai slums to improve perinatal care and outcomes: A cluster randomized controlled trial. *PLoS Medicine, 9*(7), e1001257. doi:10.1371/journal.pmed.1001257

Mullany, B. C., Becker, S., & Hindin, M. J. (2007). The impact of including husbands in antenatal health education services on maternal health practices in urban Nepal: Results from a randomized controlled trial. *Health Education Research, 22*(2), 166–176. doi:10.1093/her/cyl060

Nair, N., Tripathy, P., Costello, A., & Prost, A. (2012). Mobilizing women's groups for improved maternal and newborn health: Evidence for impact, and challenges for sustainability and scale up. *International Journal of Gynaecology and Obstetrics, 119*(Suppl. 1), S22–S25. doi:10.1016/j.ijgo.2012.03.014

O'Rourke, K., Howard-Grabman, L., & Seoane, G. (1998). Impact of community organization of women on perinatal outcomes in rural Bolivia. *Revista Panamericana de Salud Pública, Pan American Journal of Public Health, 3*(1), 9–14. doi:10.1590/S1020-49891998000100002

Prata, N., Ejembi, C., Fraser, A., Shittu, O., & Minkler, M. (2012). Community mobilization to reduce postpartum hemorrhage in home births in Nigeria. *Social Science & Medicine, 74*(8), 1288–1296. doi:10.1016/j.socscimed.2011.11.035

Rath, S., Nair, N., Tripathy, P. K., Barnett, S., Rath, S., Mahhapatra, R., . . . Prost, A. (2010). Explaining the impact of a women's group led community mobilization intervention on maternal and newborn health outcomes: The Ekjut trial process evaluation. *BMC International Health and Human Rights, 10*(25), 1–13. doi:10.1186/1472-698X-10-25. Retrieved from http://www.healthynewbornnetwork.org/sites/default/files/resources/BMC_Rath.pdf

Rosato, M., Laverack, G., Grabman, L. H., Tripathy, P., Nair, N., Mwansambo, C., . . . Costello, A. (2008). Community participation: Lessons for maternal, newborn and child health. *Lancet, 372*(9642), 962–971. doi:10.1016/S0140-9736(08)61406-3

Tripathy, P., Nair, N., Barnett, S., Mahapatra, R., Borghi, J., Rath, S., . . . Costello, A. (2010). Effect of a participatory intervention with women's groups on birth outcomes and maternal depression in Jharkhand and Orissa, India: A cluster-randomised controlled trial. *Lancet, 375*(9721), 1182–1192. doi:10-1016/S0140-6736(09)62042-0

United States Agency for International Development (USAID). (2007). Demystifying community mobilization: An effective strategy to improve maternal and newborn health. Retrieved from http://pdf.usaid.gov/pdf_docs/pnadi338.pdf

United States Agency for International Development (USAID). (2015). Ending preventable maternal mortality: USAID maternal health vision for action evidence for strategic approaches. Retrieved from https://www.usaid.gov/sites/default/files/documents/1864/MH%20Strategy_web_red.pdf

United Nations (UN). (2015a). The Millennium Development Goals report. Retrieved from http://www.un.org/millenniumgoals/2015_MDG_Report/pdf/MDG%202015%20rev%20(July%201).pdf

United Nations (UN). (2015b). Transforming our world: The 2030 agenda for sustainable development. Retrieved from http://www.un.org/ga/search/view_doc.asp?symbol=A/70/L.1&Lang=E

World Health Organization (WHO). (1978, September). *Primary health care: Report of the International Conference on Primary Health Care.* Retrieved from http://www.searo.who.int/entity/primary_health_care/documents/hfa_s_1.pdf

World Health Organization (WHO). (2015). Strategies toward ending preventable maternal mortality (EPMM). Retrieved from http://apps.who.int/iris/bitstream/10665/153544/1/9789241508483_eng.pdf?ua=1

Yamey, G. (2011). Scaling up global health interventions: A proposed framework for success. *PLoS Medicine, 8*(6), e1001049. doi:10.1371/journal.pmed.1001049

# CHAPTER TWENTY-SIX

# THE EVIDENCE FOR INTERPROFESSIONAL EDUCATION IN MIDWIFERY

Denise Colter Smith and Mary Paul Backman

## INTERPROFESSIONAL EDUCATION

Health care delivery in the United States has changed dramatically over the past 40 years, and will continue to change with the implementation of the Affordable Care Act. Several challenges have been identified within the current health care system: a growing number of people seeking care, a lagging supply of health care providers, burgeoning costs, limited funding, and widening disparities (Armstrong, 2015; Himmelstein et al., 2014; Kozhimannil, Abraham, & Virnig, 2012; Lasser, Himmelstein, & Woolhandler, 2008). The question, still current, has been raised as to how midwives can improve the patient experience, the health of populations, and contain the costs of health care with these types of challenges (Berwick, Nolan, & Whittington, 2008).

Collaborative, or team-based, care is one strategy being implemented around the world and in the United States to fill these gaps in services and increase access to care (Reeves, Lewin, Espin, & Zwarenstein, 2010). In the document, "Framework for Action on Interprofessional Education and Collaborative Practice," the World Health Organization (WHO; 2010) identifies interprofessional education (IPE) as a strategy that will address the current workforce shortage issues and improve collaborative practice throughout the world, including the United States. This framework proposes that a health care workforce that has been trained to work together will be better prepared to deliver interprofessional care (WHO, 2010).

The primary objective of IPE is to prepare a workforce that can collaborate effectively, making the workforce *practice ready* as part of a team. IPE promotes collaboration through:

- Institutional support such as governance models and resource allocation
- Protocol development and implementation
- Workforce culture such as communication and conflict resolution
- An environment of care (WHO, 2010)

Because work environments have unique characteristics, IPE strategies differ from setting to setting. However, the WHO (2010) framework identifies the following competencies for all learners in the health professions:

- Teamwork
- Roles and responsibilities
- Communication skills
- Critical reflection in the workplace
- Effective relationships with patients
- Ethical practice

Health care educators, administrators, and policy makers should modify current education systems in ways that prepare professionals to work effectively in collaborative environments, escaping "silos" (WHO, 2010). Although it is important for individuals to learn professional identity and develop the knowledge and skills required to do their jobs proficiently, understanding one's role as part of the larger spectrum of health care services fosters the ability to provide safer and more effective care for patients. The workforce of today needs to be appropriately prepared to work alongside other professions, to communicate effectively, and to coordinate services to meet the needs of patients, their families, and the community (Interprofessional Education Collaborative Expert Panel [IECEP], 2011).

In this chapter, we present the principles and methods of IPE, discuss the relationship between IPE and interprofessional collaborative practice, review the evidence for IPE, and provide exemplars of IPE and interprofessional collaboration (IPC) in midwifery and medical education programs.

## Principles of IPE

IPE is defined as "when two or more professions learn with, from and about each other to improve collaboration and the quality of care" (Centre for Advancement of Interprofessional Education [CAIPE], 2015, para. 1). The majority of health professions, education programs offer little interactive learning, keeping instruction within their singular profession, that is, nurses train exclusively with nurses or medical students with physicians. This traditional approach to education does not equip individual clinicians for more complex environments. Implementing IPE is aimed at:

- Improving the quality of care
- Reducing errors
- Increasing patient satisfaction
- Improving clinical processes
- Improving patient outcomes (Reeves, Perrier, Goldman, Freeth, & Zwarenstein, 2013)

The WHO (2010) has outlined the goal of IPE programs as a coordinated effort to integrate essential content of all health professions curricula, develop

**TABLE 26.1   Methodologies for IPE**

| Method | Example |
| --- | --- |
| Exchange-based learning | Debates, case studies |
| Action-based learning | Problem-based learning, collaborative inquiry, continuous quality improvement |
| Observation-based learning | Joint visits to a patient by students from different professions; shadowing another profession |
| Simulation-based learning | Role-play, games, skills labs, experiential groups |
| Practice-based learning | Co-location across professions for placements; out-posting to another profession and interprofessional training wards |
| E-learning | Reusable learning objects relating to the preceding points |
| Blended learning | Combining e-learning with face-to-face learning |
| Received or didactic learning | Lectures |

*Source*: Barr et al. (2000).
Reprinted with open-access permission from http://caipe.org.uk/resources.

and use similar assessment strategies for evaluating effectiveness, establish a foundation for continuing interprofessional competency throughout the professional life span, promote scholarly development in the field, and develop a variety of learning approaches to facilitate this goal.

## Learning Strategies of IPE

Based upon the premise that IPE is a means of improving patient-centered care, then how, what, and when should it be learned? There are different approaches to learning, and no singular method has been identified as being the most important. Barr, Freeth, Hammick, Koppel, and Reeves (2000), on behalf of CAIPE, identify a number of educational strategies (Table 26.1). These methodologies can be used in both pre- and postlicensure environments, and multiple approaches can be combined to suit a particular situation or environment.

Several IPE working groups have presented frameworks for IPE program content to include principles, core competencies, and learning strategies. Together, these white papers and position statements present a composite picture of learning through IPE.

### IEPEC Core Competencies

In 2011, the Interprofessional Education Collaborative, a group of professional organizations of medical, nursing, pharmacy, and public health educators in the United States, convened an expert panel to develop core competencies for IPE, motivated by a vision that interprofessional collaborative practice should learn core competencies essential to providing safe, quality, team-based care. The core competencies within four respective domains are:

- Roles and responsibilities
- Values and ethics
- Communication
- Teams/teamwork (IEPEC, 2011)

Each of the four domains outlines specific competencies defining the domains, such as respecting the expertise of other professions, establishing clear roles and responsibilities, and building clear and effective methods of communication (IEPEC, 2011).

### Centre for Advancement of Interprofessional Education

Many of the global leaders in IPE come from countries with national health systems, such as the United Kingdom, Canada, and New Zealand. CAIPE, based in the United Kingdom, is an independent think tank for IPE that comprises individual and corporate members. CAIPE's work includes defining IPE, outlining principles of IPE, and reporting on IPE and collaborative practice under the auspices of the *Journal of Interprofessional Care*. The principles of IPE, based on review of the literature as well as the experiences of members who develop and implement IPE programs, are divided among three domains of values, process, and outcomes. These domains provide a framework for program development, implementation, and evaluation (Barr & Low, 2011). The CAIPE website provides resources on IPE.

### The Institute of Medicine

In 2003, the Institute of Medicine (IOM) published *Health Professions Education: A Bridge to Quality*, as part of a larger series of reports on improving health care quality. In the report, the committee identifies five competencies for health care education:

- Patient-centered care
- Evidenced-based practice
- Quality-improvement strategies
- Use of informatics
- Working in multidisciplinary teams (IOM, 2003)

The report's authors state that health care graduates should be able to "cooperate, collaborate, communicate, and integrate care in teams to ensure that care is continuous and reliable" (IOM, 2003, p. 4). Education, licensure, and certifying bodies should include interprofessional competencies as supplemental to basic competencies for their respective fields (IOM, 2003).

## INTERPROFESSIONAL COLLABORATIVE PRACTICE

As an emerging model, team-based, interprofessional collaborative practice is changing health care delivery. To be optimal and cost-effective, collaborative practice should utilize all members of the workforce to the full scope of practice, working together to develop shared goals. In the health care domain, those stakeholders include physicians, nurses, social workers, psychologists, pharmacists, and others. Mitchell and colleagues (2012) describe high-functioning team-based collaborative practice as being characterized by:

- Shared goals
- Clear roles
- Mutual trust
- Effective communication
- Measurable processes and outcomes

The IOM report *Core Principles & Values of Effective Team-Based Health Care* describes success in high-functioning collaborative practice as dependent upon the ability of individuals to integrate despite financial, structural, and cultural barriers. Personal values displayed by individuals who are effective members of high-functioning teams include honesty, discipline, creativity, humility, and curiosity (Mitchell et al., 2012).

In a historical review of IPC, Wood (1991) states, "Collaboration occurs when a group of autonomous stakeholders of a problem domain engage in an interactive process using shared rules, norms, and structures, to act or decide on issues related to that domain" (p. 146). D'Amour and Oandasan (2005) propose that IPC "conveys the idea of sharing and implies collective action oriented toward a common goal, in a spirit of harmony and trust, particularly in the context of health professionals" (p. 116). Smith (2015) defines *midwife–physician collaboration* as

a process in which midwives and physicians work together toward a common purpose: to provide safe, effective, patient-centered care for women and their families, guided by shared rules and structures, both formal and informal, which govern a mutually beneficial relationship, a relationship which seeks to optimize the context in which the collaboration is convened. (p. 137)

IPE is a primary mechanism for developing high-functioning, collaborative practice. Health care professionals need training preparing them with the knowledge, skills, and attitudes to deliver care in a collaborative environment (Reeves et al., 2013).

## IPE: THE EVIDENCE

A literature review by Brandt, Lutfiyya, King, and Chioreso (2014) attempted to identify whether IPE interventions had a measureable effect on the goals of the triple aim (care, health, and cost), and concluded that there were not enough studies to make any evaluation. A recent Cochrane Review (Reeves et al., 2013) identified 15 studies that analyzed the effectiveness of IPE interventions compared to no intervention. Seven of the 15 studies indicated positive outcomes in patient and provider satisfaction, positive team behaviors, reduction in errors, changes to working culture, and improved outcomes, such as with diabetes care. Four studies reported that there was no impact, and another four studies provided mixed results. Because of the small number of studies, the variety of interventions, and the various uses of outcome measures, conclusions were not generalizable. More robust work is needed to provide a solid base of evidence that IPE has a measurable effect on outcomes of care.

VanderWielen and colleagues (2014) conducted a survey of health care professions' students and asked the students to identify the benefits of IPE. Respondents spoke to the benefits of IPE, including enhanced knowledge and skills, being more aware of what other professions have to offer, and understanding that patients have many needs beyond the skills of a single practitioner. The respondents stated having gained improved communication skills, role clarity, and increased knowledge of the networks and resources to which they could refer patients.

In a literature review, Abu-Rish and colleagues (2012) evaluated the barriers to implementing IPE. The review included 83 studies, representing 20,000 students from multiple health professions. Barriers to implementing IPE were identified as scheduling (47%), leveling learner competencies (18.1%), preparation time (14.5%), and funding (12.0%). Administrative barriers were identified as primarily financial (38.6%) followed by lack of adequate personnel and staff support (14.5%; Abu-Rish et al., 2012).

## BEST PRACTICES FOR MIDWIVES IN IPC

IPC between midwives and physicians has grown substantially over the past 40 years, and case-study literature of successful collaborative practices has offered insight into how these collaborations come together, succeed, and sustain over time, as described in this chapter. Several collaborative practices were established primarily to meet a need within a community. Many were established to support medical education. In the following section, we describe the role of midwives in IPE, learning *from, about,* and *with* other professions.

### Learning From Other Professions

Midwives have had long-standing participation in the medical and resident education as described in the text that follows. In 2009, members of the American College of Nurse-Midwives (ACNM) formed the Medical Education Caucus to support members who teach medical students and residents. This body has expanded to include midwives working in nursing, midwifery, medical, and resident education (Radoff et al., 2015). In many education programs across the country, midwives teach physicians about midwifery care, professionalism, collaboration, and teamwork. The Medical Education caucus seeks to promote standards for education and evaluation of midwives in these roles.

A survey of six medical centers where midwives are involved in medical and resident education by Cooper (2009) described the background of the institutions, the role of midwives, the types of innovation in the program, obstacles to program development, and plans for future programs. The involvement cited most often was midwives' contribution to teaching patient-centered, interprofessional care. Midwives participated in curriculum instruction, incorporation of research into clinical practice, and evaluation of residents and students. Leadership and political and financial support are necessary for success. Over many years, respect for the role of midwives in these programs has been established.

McConaughey and Howard (2009) surveyed 74 midwifery practice directors, representing over 500 midwives, to describe the roles and responsibilities of midwives in medical education and graduate medical education (GME) programs. Eighty percent of the 74 practices teach obstetrics and gynecology residents, 60% teach family practice residents, 93% teach medical students, and 83% teach midwifery students. Unfortunately, many practices reported that they did not take any midwifery students because midwifery students interfere with the primary mission of teaching medical students and residents. Fifty-six percent of the midwives in those practices had faculty appointments and a few held tenured positions. Eighty percent of the respondents reported that they spent their time teaching in the clinical setting; 69% reported that they also taught in the classroom (McConaughey & Howard, 2009).

## Exemplars of Learning From Other Professions

### Women & Infants Hospital of Rhode Island and the Department of Obstetrics and Gynecology at the Alpert Medical School, Brown University

Angelini, O'Brien, Singer, and Coustan (2012) described a joint effort in building an academic, educational practice model with midwives as members of the teaching faculty for both medical students and residents. This collaborative practice has been in existence for over 40 years. A team of clinicians provide care for women in the low-risk unit on labor and delivery, including the chief resident, a first- or second-year resident, a staff obstetrician, a midwife, and three to four medical students. The midwife serves as the clinical instructor for low-risk patients while collaborating with attending obstetricians as needed for patients who require management of complications. Some key elements of the teaching and practice model include enhanced communication, exposure to midwifery services, focused didactic teaching by midwives on labor care, fetal assessment, and hand skills for birth, such as suturing (Angelini et al., 2012).

For over 11 years, midwives in this project have presented a leadership development workshop for residents, guiding them in developing their leadership and communication styles and promoting team building (Angelini et al., 2012). The program has been received well by the learners, and feedback from this program has been very positive (Steinhardt, 2015).

### Baystate Medical Center and Baystate Midwifery Education Program

At Baystate Medical Center in Springfield, Massachusetts, midwives and physicians support education programs for the Tufts University School of Medicine; the Baystate Midwifery Education Program; and 10 residency programs, including five obstetrics-gynecology residents per year (DeJoy et al., 2011). A team of obstetricians and midwives teach low-risk labor management: integrating teaching on patient safety, teamwork, evidenced-based care, professionalism, and communication while utilizing a curriculum that includes classroom teaching, clinical instruction, and formal evaluation. The program has been a successful exemplar of IPE for medical students, midwifery students, and residents in the same clinical setting (DeJoy et al., 2011).

### University of California, San Francisco

The midwifery practice at the University of California, San Francisco (UCSF) has provided midwifery care at San Francisco General Hospital since 1975. The site provides training to both midwifery and medical students, with faculty appointments in both the Department of Obstetrics and Gynecology and the School of Nursing. Described as "visionary," the program is committed to training midwives and physicians in a collaborative environment, emphasizing quality improvement, excellent outcomes, and a belief in the complementary nature of midwifery and medicine. UCSF also utilizes the CenteringPregnancy® model as part of collaborative learning (Hutchison et al., 2011).

### University of Maryland Medical Center

For more than 15 years, the collaborative practice at the University of Maryland Medical Center has demonstrated a sustainable practice model (Blanchard & Kreibs, 2012). IPE has enhanced the ability to provide midwifery care in a high-acuity, urban setting. Midwives at the University of Maryland teach medical students during preclinical rotations and clerkships, provide didactic education to residents and midwifery students, and supervise residents in obstetric triage and normal births. Midwives teach and coach in history taking and physical examination, hands-on clinical skills, and skills in communication and leadership (Blanchard & Kreibs, 2012). The Department of Obstetrics and Gynecology utilizes TeamSTEPPS® training, an evidence-based teamwork system to enhance safety, communication and teamwork with staff and students (Agency for Healthcare Research and Quality [AHRQ], 2015).

## Learning About Other Professions

There are similarities and differences in the accreditation of midwifery and medical education programs and in how these professions are certified and licensed. Licensing of physicians in the United States varies by state. At a minimum, each state requires that a physician graduating from a U.S. medical education program must pass all three steps in the United States Medical Licensing Examination® (USMLE) and complete at least 1 year of GME prior to licensing. Some states require up to 3 years of GME to obtain licensure. Graduates of international medical education programs also must pass the USMLE and meet additional GME requirements to obtain licensure.

For obstetricians-gynecologists, residency programs in the United States are accredited by the Accreditation Council for Graduate Medical Education (ACGME), which identifies six core competencies for graduates: patient care, medical knowledge, interpersonal and communication skills, professionalism, practice-based learning and improvement, and systems-based practice. This accreditation council establishes the minimal competency in procedures prior to graduation from residency programs (ACGME, 2013). The Council on Resident Education in Obstetrics and Gynecology (CREOG) writes and updates curricula that align with the six ACGME competencies (American College of Obstetricians and Gynecologists [ACOG], 2015). CREOG examinations are often used for assessing knowledge and, in some residency programs, as a means of predicting adequate preparation for board examination. However, these examinations are not mandatory for graduates of all residency programs.

The American Board of Obstetrics and Gynecology (ABOG) is a voluntary certification examination available to graduates of residency programs. The examination has both an oral and written component, in addition to a certificate maintenance component (ABOG, 2015). Board certification may be a requirement for credentialing and privileging in some organizations.

Midwifery education programs (certified nurse-midwives [CNMs] and certified midwives [CMs]) in the United States are accredited by the Accreditation Commission for Midwifery Education (ACME), based upon competencies from the American College of Nurse-Midwives Core Competencies for Basic Midwifery Practice. These competencies are:

- Hallmarks of midwifery
- Professional responsibilities
- Components of midwifery care, including the midwifery management process, fundamentals, midwifery care of women, and midwifery care of the newborn (ACNM, 2015a)

ACME establishes a minimum number of procedures as a graduation requirement (ACNM, 2015a). The American Midwifery Certification Board (AMCB) regulates midwifery certification. Initial certification is by examination and certificate maintenance is either by reexamination or extensive continuing education. Midwives who pass this examination are certified as a CNM or CM (ACNM, 2015b).

Licensing of midwives is a politically complex issue. The minimum requirements for midwifery licensure in all 50 states include graduation from an ACME-accredited program and certification by the AMCB. In most states, a valid license as a registered nurse (RN) is required before a midwifery license can be issued. In a few states, education or licensure as an RN is not required for midwifery licensure, hence the credential CM. Regulatory agencies for midwifery vary by state. Independent boards of midwifery exist in two states and in others boards of medicine or nursing oversee midwifery regulation. Licenses for midwifery in many states are considered advanced practice registered nursing (APRN) licensure. There are still a few states that require written collaborative agreements with a physician before the APRN is issued (ACNM, 2015b). Midwives and midwifery advocates have been working diligently to remove these barriers to practice.

## Learning *With*: IPE and Collaborative Practice

There are various methods for delivering IPE and times within the education cycle when IPE is optimal. Whether online, simulation-based learning, clinical-based learning, or didactics, there are numerous opportunities for IPE in pre- and postlicensure settings. Some examples could include:

- Team safety and communication training, that is, TeamSTEPPs
- Fetal heart monitoring, interpretation, and management
- Obstetrics emergency simulation-based training, that is, Advanced Life Support in Obstetrics (ALSO) or Emergencies in Clinical Obstetrics (ECO)
- Interprofessional journal club or evidenced-based practice reviews
- Coding, documentation, or business practice development
- Quality-improvement activities

### Exemplars of "Learning With"

#### Bronx Lebanon Medical Center

The collaborative practice at Bronx Lebanon Medical Center comprises 20 attending physicians, 17 residents, 17 midwives, and three physician assistants, attending more than 3,000 births, 9,000 triage visits, and 70,000 outpatient visits per year (Marshall et al., 2012). IPE is an important component of this practice, including interprofessional weekly grand rounds, team training, continuing education, emergency simulation drills, risk management training, and training in fetal heart rate monitoring and intrapartum management. In addition, midwives and physicians participate in medical student clerkships, which provide medical students with a glimpse of working collaboratively.

#### East Carolina University

In an adventurous project, educators in women's health at East Carolina University developed a standardized curriculum by mapping a set of core competencies from conception through menopause, used by six disciplines (family medicine, obstetrics and gynecology, nursing, midwifery, nurse-practitioner, and physician assistant; Taleff, Salstrom, & Newton, 2009). Faculty from the six disciplines identified health promotion, disease prevention, laboratory and diagnostic interpretation, physical examination, differential diagnosis, development of management plans, and anticipatory guidance as the basis of the core competencies. Additional areas identified were patient-centered care, cultural competence, effective communication, and collaborative practice.

The purposes of the project were to optimize the resources of the university and to provide a curriculum that could be used by other education programs. The authors of this work anticipate that this program is futuristic and will break through barriers to IPE. They state, "[The curriculum] distributes workload, invites experts to share resources and ideas, and decreases the duplication of resources across university departments or schools" (Taleff et al., 2009, p. 308).

*Madigan Army Medical Center*
This full-scope midwifery service is staffed by seven midwives at a medium- to large-sized medical center in the U.S. Department of Defense, attending approximately 2,000 births per year (combined midwifery, obstetric, and family medicine; Nielsen et al., 2012). The authors of this chapter describe their experience with this service. The goals of the service are to:

- Provide prenatal and well-woman care and attend the births for families who desire the midwifery model of care
- Participate as fully recognized faculty in the obstetrics-gynecology GME program
- Teach normal, physiologic birth
- Supervise and educate midwifery students, nursing students, medical students, and interns from multiple specialties during their obstetrics-gynecology rotation
- Model and enhance a multidisciplinary team approach to obstetrical education and collaborative consultation

Midwifery students, medical students, and residents freely interact with one another, working together in case presentations, learning from each other, and filling in knowledge gaps. Midwifery students learn when and how to consult, and residents learn how to provide appropriate consultation. A hallmark of the service is a maternal–fetal medicine subspecialist who serves as a consultant to the midwifery service on both clinical and interdisciplinary professional issues. Practicing midwives have full participation and responsibility as GME faculty. The midwife faculty role includes:

- Participation in the daily turnover of labor and delivery census with the shift-change between staff and residents (utilizing TeamSTEPPS) using a multidisciplinary report with prioritized needs
- Evaluation of medical student and resident competencies by a designated midwife member of the Clinical Competency Committee
- Participation in medical student interviews for placement and matching for the obstetrics-gynecology GME program
- Assessment of residents for possible competency needs, performance plans, and program awards

Through collaborative assessment of the resident program, midwife and physician faculty became aware that residents desired improved continuity with obstetrical patients and increased satisfaction in prenatal interactions. The residents also expressed a sense of inadequacy in provision of routine obstetrical care. The faculty assessed that these concerns were related to indirect supervision of routine obstetrical care during the first year of residency as well as the faculty assumption that 4th-year medical students possessed baseline skills. Previous adjustments to staff supervision of medical students and 1st-year residents did not result in significant improvements in the residents' knowledge and skills.

The faculty decided to try the established CenteringPregnancy program as a vehicle for resident education and direct supervision of prenatal care as well as assessment of the residency curriculum in relation to meeting ACGME core competencies. CenteringPregnancy is an evidence-based method of group health care delivery that promotes safety, efficacy, timeliness, and culturally appropriate, equitable care (Centering Healthcare Institute, 2015). The essential elements of CenteringPregnancy overlap with the ACGME core competencies. CenteringPregnancy incorporates on-going self-assessment of learning by patients and providers, an exceptional fit with ACGME core competencies. The model for this program was presented by the faculty team at the Council on Resident Education in Obstetrics and Gynecology (Figure 26.1).

The CenteringPregnancy program, as a method of supervision and teaching, included the midwifery "listen to women" philosophy of care (Kathryn, 1993). The program aimed to help the residents understand the patients' experiences in learning, to improve collaborative team work, and to promote engagement in ongoing quality improvement and patient-safety programs. At this facility, midwife and physician faculty and residents are formally trained in the CenteringPregnancy model. The training includes leading the group as a facilitator and promoting effective listening skills with both verbal and behavioral cues. Residents are assigned a midwife or physician faculty mentor and a prenatal care group. The residents are required to participate in each session for their group. Each intern is matched with a midwife CenteringPregnancy mentor to focus on physiologic pregnancy and birth. The Centering groups consist of a mixture of patients who have chosen either midwife or physician care. To maximize continuity of care, patients' due dates are coordinated with the residents' rotation schedules in the hope that they may attend as many individual births from their group as possible.

After each session, debriefing between the resident and faculty mentor includes a review of clinical performance; identifying individual patient needs, that is, ordering laboratory work or consults; and developing short-term goals for the next session (both for the resident and for the patients). Midway through the Centering group's progression (session #5 or #6), the mentor and resident review patient and resident satisfaction, the resident's clinical and knowledge competency, and the resident's level of ease with the group model. Scheduling CenteringPregnancy group care for residents demands particular attention to

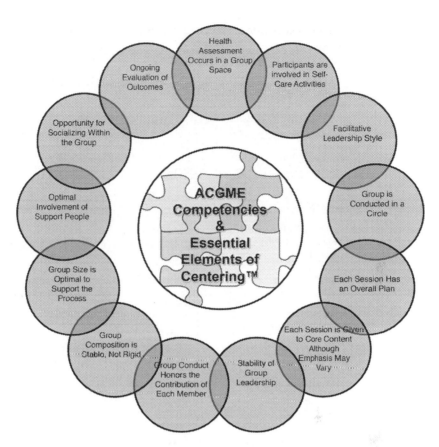

**Figure 26.1**   ACGME core competencies compared to CenteringPregnancy®
essential elements.

ACGME, Accreditation Council for Graduate Medical Education.

*Source:* Foglia, Chinn, Munroe, and Backman (2013). Poster reprinted with permission from Madigan Army Hospital team presentation to Council on Resident Education in Obstetrics and Gynecology.

GME requirements as well as subspecialty rotation requirements. The following objectives are incorporated within the 4-year residency program. In the first year, residents perform all physical assessments with the midwifery faculty mentor directly observing, validating, and teaching. During the group sessions, interns are in an observer role and are encouraged to participate and facilitate discussions as their clinical skills and knowledge levels allow. In the second and third years, residents perform all physical assessments under direct observation of the midwife or obstetrician mentor with increased emphasis on identification of issues recommended for subspecialty consultation or referrals. During the group sessions, the resident is encouraged to be more proactive in planning activities for each session, and to participate more as the facilitator with the mentor acting in a cofacilitator role. Finally, in year 4, residents may choose to lead another CenteringPregnancy group as an elective, functioning independently in the presence of an experienced cofacilitator.

The faculty has observed improvement in knowledge; skills; teamwork; quality improvement; and faculty, staff, and patient satisfaction. Outcomes identified are as follows:

- Improved knowledge areas, including lactation knowledge and management of complications, parenting skills and social support of a new family, and comfort positions in the second stage of labor
- Improved skills areas, including time management and skill performance with Doptone, fundal height, Leopold's maneuvers, blood pressure, and weight gain assessment, including when to consult a subspecialist
- Full participation in the interprofessional teams, facilitating quality improvement and patient safety
- Elevated resident and patient satisfaction, assessed via surveys and direct feedback, as compared to individual patient appointments
- Less frustration among residents who appreciated a relaxed atmosphere, a sense of continuity, knowing patients when they attend their births, having the staff readily available, and learning how to listen
- Increased confidence in routine assessment and skills as the residents moved to caring for more complicated patients
- Faculty satisfaction with their role and with the continuity of care with their patients and their resident

This collaborative model for GME has proven to be highly satisfying for all participants as it improves competency, compliance, patient safety, and interdisciplinary communication. This model demonstrates collaboration between the midwife and the resident. Some patient comments included, "You all really seem to enjoy working together . . . even when you disagree" and "This is not what I thought the relationship was like between doctors and midwives!"

## CONCLUSION

There are many excellent examples of IPE occurring in academic institutions and medical centers throughout the United States, each offering ideas on building collaborative relationships among midwives, physicians, and other health care providers. Successful collaboration begins with knowledge, skills, and attitudes that foster trust and respect and builds on role clarity, common goals, and effective communication. These skills can and should be taught as basic competencies in education programs for health professionals. Health care educators should address and modify existing programs to include IPE competencies. An IPE agenda for midwifery and obstetric education needs to:

- Align core competencies between midwifery students and obstetric residencies, including clinical and teamwork competencies
- Coordinate elements of simulation, didactic, and clinical instruction

- Address the structural differences among the education programs, that is, academic calendars for midwifery and medical education and consider the progression of midwifery education versus rotations of medical residency
- Seek funding streams for IPE as medical and midwifery education funding models are disparate
- Promote clinical sites for midwifery students in residency programs
- Analyze process and outcome data for IPE initiatives

IPE and collaborative practice have the capability to improve patient safety and experience significantly and to shape midwifery practice in the future.

## ACKNOWLEDGMENT

The opinions or assertions contained herein are the private views of the authors and are not to be construed as official or as reflecting the views of the U.S. Department of Defense.

## REFERENCES

Abu-Rish, E., Kim, S., Choe, L., Varpio, L., Malik, E., White, A. A., . . . Zierler, B. (2012). Current trends in interprofessional education of health sciences students: A literature review. *Journal of Interprofessional Care, 26*(6), 444–451. doi:10.3109/13561820.2012.715604

Accreditation Council for Graduate Medical Education (ACGME). (2013). ACGME program requirements for graduate medical education in obstetrics and gynecology. Retrieved from https://www.acgme.org/acgmeweb/Portals/0/pfassets/programrequirements/220_obstet rics_and_gynecology_07012015.pdf

Agency for Healthcare Research and Quality (AHRQ). (2015). TeamSTEPPS®: Strategies and tools to enhance performance and patient safety. Retrieved from http://www.ahrq.gov/pro fessionals/education/curriculum-tools/teamstepps/index.html

American Board of Obstetrics and Gynecology (ABOG). (2015). Certification process. Retrieved from https://www.abog.org/new/information.aspx?cat=Certification_Process&id=1

American College of Nurse-Midwives (ACNM). (2015a). Accreditation Commission for Midwifery Education (ACME). Retrieved from http://www.midwife.org/Accreditation

American College of Nurse-Midwives (ACNM). (2015b). Certification. Retrieved from http://www.midwife.org/Certification

American College of Obstetricians and Gynecologists (ACOG). (2015). Council on resident education in obstetrics and gynecology (CREOG). Retrieved from http://www.acog.org/About-ACOG/ACOG-Departments/CREOG

Angelini, D. J., O'Brien, B., Singer, J., & Coustan, D. R. (2012). Midwifery and obstetrics: Twenty years of collaborative academic practice. *Obstetrics and Gynecology Clinics of North America, 39*(3), 335–346. doi:10.1016/j.ogc.2012.05.002

Armstrong, J. (2015). Women's health in the age of patient protection and the Affordable Care Act. *Clinical Obstetrics and Gynecology, 58*(2), 323–335. doi:10.1097/GRF.0000000000000096

Barr, H., Freeth, D., Hammick, M., Koppel, I., & Reeves, S. (2000). Evaluations of interprofessional education: A United Kingdom review for health and social care. Retrieved from http://caipe.org.uk/silo/files/evaluations-of-interprofessional-education.pdf

Barr, H., & Low, H. (2011). Principles of interprofessional education. Retrieved from http://caipe.org.uk/resources/principles-of-interprofessional-education

Berwick, D. M., Nolan, T. W., & Whittington, J. (2008). The triple aim: Care, health, and cost. *Health Affairs, 27*(3), 759–769. doi:10.1377/hlthaff.27.3.759

Blanchard, M. H., & Kriebs, J. M. (2012). A successful model of collaborative practice in a university-based maternity care setting. *Obstetrics and Gynecology Clinics of North America, 39*(3), 367–372. doi:10.1016/j.ogc.2012.05.005

Brandt, B., Lutfiyya, M. N., King, J. A., & Chioreso, C. (2014). A scoping review of interprofessional collaborative practice and education using the lens of the Triple Aim. *Journal of Interprofessional Care, 28*(5), 393–399. doi:10.3109/13561820.2014.906391

Centre for Advancement of Interprofessional Education (CAIPE). (2015). Defining interprofessional education. Retrieved from http://caipe.org.uk/resources/defining-ipe

Centering Healthcare Institute. (2015). Essential elements. Retrieved from http://centering-healthcare.org/pages/centering-model/elements.php

Cooper, E. M. (2009). Innovative midwifery teaching for medical students and residents. *Journal of Midwifery and Women's Health, 54*(4), 301–305. doi:10.1016/j.jmwh.2009.04.001

D'Amour, D., & Oandasan, I. (2005). Interprofessionality as the field of interprofessional practice and interprofessional education: An emerging concept. *Journal of Interprofessional Care, 19*(Suppl. 1), 8–20. doi:10.1080/13561820500081604

DeJoy, S., Burkman, R. T., Graves, B. W., Grow, D., Sankey, H. Z., Delk, C., . . . Less, A. (2011). Making it work: Successful collaborative practice. *Obstetrics & Gynecology, 118*(3), 683–686. doi:10.1097/AOG.0b013e318229e0bf

Foglia, L., Chinn, M., Munroe, M., & Backman, M. (2013, February). *Effectively meeting the core competencies with group prenatal care.* Poster session presented at the meeting of the Council on Resident Education in Obstetrics and Gynecology (CREOG) and Association of Professors of Gynecology and Obstetrics (APGO), Phoenix, AZ.

Himmelstein, D. U., Jun, M., Busse, R., Chevreul, K., Geissler, A., Jeurissen, P . . . Woolhandler, S. (2014). A comparison of hospital administrative costs in eight nations: US costs exceed all others by far. *Health Affairs, 33*(9), 1586–1594. doi:10.1377/hlthaff.2013.1327

Hutchison, M. S., Ennis, L., Shaw-Battista, J., Delgado, A., Myers, K., Cragin, L., & Jackson, R. A. (2011). Great minds don't think alike: Collaborative maternity care at San Francisco General Hospital. *Obstetrics & Gynecology, 118*(3), 678–682. doi:10.1097/AOG.0b013e3182297d2d

Institute of Medicine (IOM). (2003). *Health professions education: A bridge to quality.* Washington, DC: National Academies Press. Retrieved from http://iom.nationalacademies.org/Reports/2003/Health-Professions-Education-A-Bridge-to-Quality.aspx

Interprofessional Education Collaborative Expert Panel. (2011). *Competencies for interprofessional collaborative practice: Report of an expert panel.* Washington, DC: Interprofessional Education Collaborative. Retrieved from http://www.aacn.nche.edu/education-resources/ipecreport.pdf

Kathryn, E. L. (1993). Listen to women. The ACNM's vision. *Journal of Midwifery and Women's Health, 38*(5), 285–287. doi:10.1016/0091-2182(93)90108-S

Kozhimannil, K. B., Abraham, J. M., & Virnig, B. A. (2012). National trends in health insurance coverage of pregnant and reproductive-age women, 2000 to 2009. *Women's Health Issues, 22*(2), e135–e141. doi:10.1016/j.whi.2011.12.002

Lasser, K. E., Himmelstein, D. U., & Woolhandler, S. (2008). Access to care, health status, and health disparities in the United States and Canada: Results of a cross-national population-based survey. In C. Harrington & C. Estes (Eds.), *Health policy: Crisis and reform in the U.S. health care delivery system* (5th ed., pp. 379–383). Sudbury, MA: Jones & Bartlett.

Marshall, N., Egan, S., Flores, C., Kirsch, A., Mankoff, R., & Resnick, M. (2012). Working toward a common goal: A collaborative obstetrics and gynecology practice. *Obstetrics and Gynecology Clinics of North America, 39*(3), 373–382.

McConaughey, E., & Howard, E. (2009). Midwives as educators of medical students and residents: Results of a national survey. *Journal of Midwifery and Women's Health, 54*(4), 268–274. doi:10.1016/j.jmwh.2009.03.016

Mitchell, P., Wynia, M., Golden, R., Mcnellis, B., Okun, S., Webb, C. E., . . . Von Kohorn, I. (2012). *Core principles and values of effective team-based health care* [Discussion paper]. Washington, DC: Institute of Medicine of the National Academies of Health. Retrieved from https://www.nationalahec.org/pdfs/VSRT-Team-Based-Care-Principles-Values.pdf

Nielsen, P. E., Munroe, M., Foglia, L., Piecek, R. I., Backman, M. P., Cyplier, R., & Smith, D. C. (2012). Collaborative practice model: Madigan Army Medical Center. *Obstetrics and Gynecology Clinics of North America, 39*(3), 399–410. doi:10.1016/j.ogc.2012.05.008

Radoff, K., Natch, A., McConaughey, E., Salstrom, J., Schelling, K., & Seger, S. (2015). Midwives in medical student and resident education and the development of the Medical Education Caucus Toolkit. *Journal of Midwifery and Women's Health, 60*(3), 304–312. doi:10.1111/jmwh.12329

Reeves, S., Lewin, S., Espin, S., & Zwarenstein, M. (2010). *Interprofessional teamwork for health and social care.* Oxford, UK: Wiley Blackwell

Reeves, S., Perrier, L., Goldman, J., Freeth, D., & Zwarenstein, M. (2013). Interprofessional education: Effects on professional practice and healthcare outcomes (update). *Cochrane Database of Systematic Reviews, 2013*(2). doi:10.1002/14651858.CD002213

Smith, D. C. (2015). Midwife–physician collaboration: A conceptual framework for interprofessional collaborative practice. *Journal of Midwifery and Women's Health, 60*(2), 128–139. doi:10.1111/jmwh.12204

Steinhardt, L. (2015). Workshop for new leaders: Innovative midwifery teaching for obstetrics and gynecology residents. *Journal of Midwifery and Women's Health, 60*(3), 313–317. doi:10.1111/jmwh.12292

Taleff, J., Salstrom, J., & Newton, E. R. (2009). Pioneering a universal curriculum: A look at six disciplines involved in women's health care. *Journal of Midwifery and Women's Health, 54*(4), 306–313. doi:10.1016/j.jmwh.2009.03.012

VanderWielen, L. M., Do, E. K., Diallo, H. I., LaCoe, K. N., Nguyen, N. L., Parikh, S. A., . . . Dow, A. W. (2014). Interprofessional collaboration led by health professional students: A case study of the inter health professionals alliance at Virginia Commonwealth University. *Journal of Research in Interprofessional Practice and Education, 3*(3), 1–13.

Wood, D. J. (1991). Toward a comprehensive theory of collaboration. *Journal of Applied Behavioral Science, 27*(2), 139–162. doi:10.1177/0021886391272001

World Health Organization (WHO). (2010). *Framework for action on interprofessional education and collaborative practice.* Health Professions Network Nursing and Midwifery Office. Geneva, Switzerland. Retrieved from http://apps. Interprofessional Education Collaborative .int/iris/bitstream/10665/70185/1/WHO_HRH_HPN_10.3_eng.pdf

# CHAPTER TWENTY-SEVEN

# CREATING A COLLABORATIVE WORKING ENVIRONMENT

Ginger K. Breedlove and John C. Jennings

Collaboration is a process that has shared norms and benefits to participants, based upon informal and formal negotiation. It is based upon rules that structures relationships and decision making (Akaike, 1987). The World Health Organization (WHO) states that collaborative practice occurs when multiple health workers from different professional backgrounds work together with patients, families, and communities to deliver the highest quality of care (WHO Study Group on Interprofessional Education and Collaborative Practice, 2010). The collaborative approach has become essential for the achievement of better health care outcomes and improvements in the delivery of health care services (Nielsen, Jennings & the Presidential Task Force on Collaborative Practice, 2016).

Prior to the passage of the Affordable Care Act (ACA) in 2010, the Institute of Medicine (IOM) proposed six aims for improvement as a road map to a value-based high-performance health care system in the United States (IOM, 2011). The IOM series *Crossing the Quality Chasm* proposed core expectations for safety, effectiveness, efficiency, and equitability for patient-centered care (IOM, 2001). Changes, such as the development of evidence-based care, the advances and availability of technology, and the advent of electronic health records, are supportive of improvements in interpersonal connections and inter-disciplinary collaborative practice. With the increasing complexity of our health care system, collaborative practice models of patient care are arguably best equipped to accomplish the six IOM aims (Nielsen et al., 2016).

The American College of Obstetricians and Gynecologists (ACOG) and the American College of Nurse-Midwives (ACNM) have moved ahead of many sub-specialty interest groups by forming interdisciplinary organizational partnerships to forge a productive working relationship with the intent of championing improvements in collaborative practice in women's health. The two organizations have cooperated in development of quality and safety initiatives, redesign of the well-women visit, maternal health initiatives, leadership of team-based care, the framework for implementation of collaborative team-based care, and legislative advocacy. In July 2015, the authors, the presidential officers of ACOG and ACNM, made a historic visit to Capitol Hill in Washington to advocate jointly for solutions to shortages in maternal health care. On December 9, 2015, during the 114th Congress, Breedlove testified on behalf of House Resolution 1209—The Maternity Care Provider Shortage Act of 2015. This bill, drafted by the ACNM and fully supported by ACOG, amends the Public Service Act to require the Health Resources and Services Administration (HRSA) to designate maternity care health professional shortage areas, review these designations annually, collect and publish data on shortage areas so the right providers can be placed in their professional category with highest need, and defines areas to include assessment of hospital or birth centers. Advocacy for improvements in health care and, particularly the championing of collaborative care, require national, state, and local cooperation among health care organizations and individual providers.

This chapter addresses components essential to the establishment and sustainability of collaborative physician and advanced practice registered nurse (APRN) partnerships in health care. Although many examples will focus on midwifery and women's health care, as this is the principal focus of the authors in this chapter, the concepts and recommendations apply to multiple areas of collaborative care.

## THE CHALLENGES OF THE HEALTH CARE ENVIRONMENT

The need for a strong and affordable health care infrastructure has been the primary impetus for health care reform. The rising health care costs in the United States are unsustainable and the numbers of uninsured persons have been intolerable. According to the IOM (2011), the country has been spending approximately 18% of its gross national product (exceeding $2.6 trillion per year) on health care. The U.S. population is aging, with Medicare enrollment expected to grow on the average of 1.6 million persons per year. Chronic conditions, such as pulmonary disease, heart disease, and diabetes, are present in nearly one half of the U.S. population. The anticipated increase in the number of births and changes in population demographics present workforce challenges for the care of reproductive-aged and postmenopausal women. In many respects, the fragmentation of the health care delivery system has contributed to compromised patient safety and medical errors. A strong, flexible, and collaborative health workforce is one of the best ways to confront these highly complex challenges (IOM, 2011).

Workforce issues in women's health are a significant concern. It is estimated that the United States will have a shortage of 8,000 obstetricians and gynecologists by 2020. There has been no significant increase in the numbers of residency training positions for obstetrics and gynecology. In addition, the numbers of graduates of midwifery programs have only minimally increased and the number of programs training women's health nurse practitioners (NPs) has deceased. There is also a geographic maldistribution of providers of women's health care with most new graduates preferring not to practice in areas where the need is greatest. The United States has a large and diverse population extending from rural settings with minimal resources to urban areas with an abundance of health providers and facilities. Through collaboration among health professionals, it is possible to maintain a level of evidence-based care across sparsely populated areas and among underserved populations in densely populated areas (American Congress of Obstetricians and Gynecologists, 2013; Jennings, 2015; Rayburn, 2011).

Improving the availability and functionality of regionalized systems based on maternal and neonatal levels of care can significantly elevate the accessibility of quality care for mothers and newborns (ACOG & Society for Maternal-Fetal Medicine, 2015). Both international and domestic policy agencies have urged fundamental reform of the health care workforce by increasing interprofessional competencies (Boyce, Moran, Nissen, Chenery, & Brooks, 2009). Variations of collaborative practice models within regionalized systems have the ability to extend access to care and improve efficiency of the workforce. Midwives need to contribute fully in this conversation (Lang, 1974).

The health care marketplace in the United States is evolving from a predominant fee-for-service system to a value- and quality-based reimbursement system while still maintaining some elements of traditional third-party payment. Large numbers of physicians and other health care providers are being employed by integrated health systems as the demand for cost control and quality accountability increases. Patient-centered health care models and accountable care organizations are proliferating, along with an explosion of software designed to identify evidence-based practice options. The changes in the health care are systematic, bold, far reaching, and provide fertile ground for the implementation of collaborative practice (Jennings, 2014; Lockwood, 2012).

## ADVANTAGES OF COLLABORATIVE PRACTICE

Policy makers and health care leaders are looking for innovative strategies that can help develop policy, programs, and practice models to increase the efficiency of potential shortages in the health care workforce (Lockwood, 2012). Collaborative practice strengthens and improves health outcomes. It can also improve access and coordination of health services by the appropriate use of specialist clinical resources with resultant improvements in outcomes for both acute and chronic diseases. The shared responsibility of a collaborative team leverages patient and health care professionals' expertise and provides a mechanism for more efficient delivery and better outcomes of care (Nielsen et al., 2016).

Teams in health care take many forms, ranging from large and broad in scope to small and focused on a particular patient need or clinical process (Nielsen et al., 2016). A clinical care team for a given patient can be composed of various health providers, including physicians, APRNs, midwives, registered nurses, physician assistants, clinical pharmacists, and others. All of these disciplines require training and skills to provide high-quality care coordinated specifically to the patient's clinical needs and circumstances (Siassakos et al., 2011). A key concept and clear advantage of collaborative practice is the ability of each team member to contribute to his or her fullest capability in terms of education, training, and experience (Nielsen et al., 2016). The pursuit of excellence within the teamwork climate leads to a culture of safety, problem solving, and high job satisfaction for the participating providers (Clark, Meyers, Frye, & Perlin, 2011).

Human and financial resources are most efficiently used when collaborative care is built on the strengths of all of the providers on the team (Lockwood, 2014). In many circumstances, solutions to certain clinical problems can only be addressed through the optimized strengths of the collaborative care process. For example, sustainable reductions in cesarean delivery rates cannot be approached directly, but are best approached by the collective efforts of a committed, patient-centered team process (Clark et al., 2011).

Collaborative practice models can provide distinct advantages for all stakeholders involved. For patients, there is increased coordination of care, integration of care, empowerment in decision making, efficient use of time and resources, and the availability to respond to diverse cultural backgrounds. Educators and student participants learn multiple approaches to solving problems, to appreciate and understand other disciplines, and learn to challenge the norms and values of each discipline. Health care professionals have increased job satisfaction, acquire new skills and approaches, focus on their individual expertise, have opportunity to innovate, and learn emphasis on preventive care. The delivery system profits from efficiency, optimization of resources and facilities, decreased burden on acute care facilities, and overall improved quality (Nandiwada & Dang-Vu, 2010).

## PRINCIPLES OF COLLABORATION

Sustainable health care involves receiving the right care at the right time, in the right place by the right people, with coordination and accountability (McDermott, 2011). An essential imperative of collaborative care is that the patient is at the center of decision making and participation in care. Patients should experience "individualization, recognition, respect, dignity and choice in all matters without exception related to themselves, their circumstances, and their relationships in health care" (Berwick, 2009, p. w560). The foundations of collaborative practice are built on a process of education, skill-building, and continuous evaluation.

The guiding principles to establish and maintain a collaborative practice are both distinct and integrated (Nielsen et al., 2016). High-performing teams are "an essential tool for constructing a more patient-centered, coordinated, and effective health care delivery system" (Mitchell et al., 2012, p. 3). Humility and honesty are important values connected to team accountability. This means high-functioning teams rely on team members to recognize practice patterns that compromise quality of care and then take advantage of opportunities to correct failures before they occur (Nielsen et al., 2016).

Certain behaviors have been consistently recognized as facilitators of collaborative practice. These core behaviors include:

- Trust among all parties
- Knowledge and education on the part of all team members
- Shared responsibility and decision making
- Mutual respect among team members for individual expertise
- Nonhierarchic communication between members
- Promotion of each other's skills
- Optimism about the effectiveness and quality of care rendered by the collaborative practice (Mitchell & Crittenden, 2000; Mitchell et al., 2012)

An important cornerstone to the success of a collaborative practice is an operating agreement clarifying the guiding principles and relationships among the providers; including the philosophy, scope of practice (SOP), functions, and organizational structure of clinical services (Dejoy et al., 2011). The division of tasks among members of the team may be based more on the individual patient's problem and needs than on the traditional professional role definitions (Nandiwada & Dang-Vu, 2010).

It is important to define clear expectations for team members and to create well-structured channels of communication (Darlington, McBroom, & Warwick, 2011). It is integral to the success of collaborative practice that an agreement expresses the shared vision and conveys respect and value for the different roles of team members (Nielsen et al., 2016). High-functioning collaborative practices do not necessarily have the same thinking processes and approaches, but their differences can create a positive additive effect (Hutchison et al., 2011).

## TEAM LEADERSHIP

Leadership for interprofessional practices involves emphasis on disease-preventive services, health-promotion counseling, and coordination of team activities. Expected roles in patient-centered care through collaborative practice require education and the development of specific skills. Collaboration and effective team practice are not intrinsic skills, but rather learned practices refined over time. Administrative team leadership, dependent on diverse practice settings and individual preferences, may encompass a broad foundation of organizational, executive, and financial skills. A team leader must have the opportunity to learn the principles and competencies of effective leadership, and to have practice experience needed to build effective team skills (Boyce et al., 2009; Nielsen et al., 2016).

Core leadership competencies required for administration of collaborative practices include competency in clinical practice, respect for other disciplines, knowledge of complexities of strategies for cost savings, and care effectiveness. In addition, team administration requires skills in communication, negotiation, time management, and assessment of group dynamics. Effective administration of a collaborative practice involves a broad understanding of other determinants of health, including housing, social and economic issues, and an understanding of community links that may be essential to providing integrated services (Berwick, 2009; Mitchell & Crittenden, 2000).

Team leadership in the current health care environment can be both situational and dynamic, implying an approach to team leadership that best meets the patient's needs and goals for care. As a consequence, the team leader for an individual patient may be synonymous with the term *lead provider* (Nielsen et al., 2016; Smith, 2015). All health care providers on the clinical team should agree on the most appropriate person to lead the care, based on patient needs. Changes in leadership should occur based on unified agreement concerning the best path of care for the patient at any time. Roles and responsibilities of team members must be clearly defined, but flexibility in roles and team leadership is critical in responding to patient care needs (Mitchell et al., 2012; Nielsen et al., 2016). At a higher level of leadership, there is a need for a systemic organization to build and sustain collaborative teams. Champions for collaborative practice at an institutional level have the ability to enable external support for team practices, desensitize negative effects of imbedded professional culture, and facilitate the logistics of implementation (Barker, Boscoe, & Oandasan, 2005).

## SCOPE OF PRACTICE

With few exceptions, SOP statutes are established via state laws and encompass the legal framework, including regulations, by which individual health professionals practice. Because of the ACA and the rise in health care demand, the health care workforce is being stretched to its limits. As a result, state legislatures are redefining some of the parameters of scope and standards of practice for a variety of health care professionals in order to meet the demand. However, not all states are responding to rapidly changing SOP statutes and regulations for APRNs. The statutes affecting SOP for APRNs have both direct and indirect influence on the practice of midwifery.

Twenty states allow NPs full practice authority (VanVleet & Paradise, 2015). Nineteen states require NPs to have a formal, written collaborative agreement with a physician in order to provide care, and these states restrict NP practice in at least one domain such as treatment, prescribing, or surgical care. In the remaining 12 states, NP practice is even more restricted. These states require physician supervision or delegation for NPs to provide care. In some states NPs have *full practice authority*, which means that practice and licensure law provides for NPs' SOP protection to evaluate patients, diagnose, order and interpret diagnostic tests, initiate and manage treatments—including prescribe medications—under the exclusive licensure authority of the state board of nursing. This is the model recommended by the IOM and National Council of State Boards of Nursing (American Association of Nurse Practitioners, 2015).

More recent, Gilman, and Koslov (2014) cited the findings of several expert bodies stating that APRNs "are safe and effective as independent providers of many health-care services within the scope of their training, licensure, certification, and current practice. Therefore, new or extended layers of mandatory physician supervision may not be justified" (p. 2). The National Governors Association has also encouraged full practice authority for APRNs and SOP changes to increase efficiencies in the current primary care workforce (NGA Center for Best Practices, 2012).

In 2013, in order to facilitate SOP expansion for NPs throughout the United States, the Robert Wood Johnson Foundation (RWJF) convened leaders from nursing and medicine to draft a consensus document. This document built upon findings from the IOM (2010) *Future of Nursing* report (RWJF, 2013). However, the convening group abruptly ended when the draft was leaked to an interim meeting of the House of Delegates of the American Medical Association, leading to many physician groups withdrawing their participation. Remaining participants moved forward, advocating for the following principles:

● The patient must be at the center of interprofessional collaboration
● Interprofessional collaboration is already happening and the problem of achieving consensus to advance SOP is at the organizational level
● The two distinct professions of nursing and medicine have overlapped and approach patient care differently (RWJF, 2013)

"Transition to practice" language is an emerging trend designed to achieve compromise in legislative language when active opposition to expanded SOP statues or regulations is being debated. This legislative language would require a transition period before APRNs can practice independently. Of the 17 states and the District of Columbia that have full practice authority for NPs, four states—Colorado, Maine, Nevada, and Vermont—currently require a transition period before independent practice or prescriptive authority. The transition period, detailed in contact hours or years, designates a period of physician supervision or experienced APRN oversight subsequent to completion of an accredited graduate education program and passing a national certification board examination in the specialty. Many argue the issue is comparing time in education and clinical hours between APRNs (2 years of graduate education) to physician residencies that typically range 3 to 5 years. However, there is no evidence that requiring postgraduate supervision for APRNs will improve patient safety and quality care. The American Nurses Association cautions that requiring additional clinical hours for APRNs after graduation would likely create new, costly bottlenecks for building the provider workforce with no evidence of improved care (Brassard, 2014).

The most comprehensive study of APRN full-practice authority was conducted by the RAND Corporation in the state of Ohio, asking the following key questions:

● What effect do SOP laws for APRNs have on health care access, quality, and cost?
● What effect might relaxing SOP laws have on health care access, quality, and costs, specifically in the state of Ohio? (Brassard, 2014)

The findings suggest that access to care would be enhanced, there would be fewer emergency room visits, patient satisfaction would be higher, and health care costs in the state of Ohio would be reduced (Martsolf, Auerbach, & Arifkanova, 2015).

## EFFECTIVE COMMUNICATION

The authors propose that a leading cause of preventable medical errors is communication failure. Effective communication must be prioritized within all highly functioning, interprofessional, team-based health care teams. The team must continuously refine communication skills based upon mutual trust and respect, allowing for clear and candid channels of communication, accessible across all settings. Technology advancements now facilitate rapid information sharing through electronic health records and telecommunication modalities. With the digital age, however, there is less opportunity for in-person communication exchange.

Team training can improve processes, including communication, coordination, and cooperation. In an evidence-based report, the Agency for Healthcare Research and Quality (AHRQ, 2013) states that settings implementing teamtraining programs have been associated with improvements in patient safety outcomes including reductions in adverse events and reduced mortality. These programs can range from interdisciplinary simulation events scheduled on routine basis to 3-day training sessions utilizing formal curriculum. Teachable communication skills include ensuring that every member of a highly performing team is prepared to be honest, clear, and professional; and can deliver information in a safe environment. Team members should demonstrate capacity to be deep listeners and learn from one another. An equal voice in a room of multidisciplinary team members can be challenging at best, and recognizing signs of tension and disagreement must be addressed (AHRQ, 2013).

In addition to assessing individual attributes of effective communication, organizational barriers can provide a challenge as well. Organizational structures can be designed with high levels of interface or can reinforce silos within systems of care. A team-based approach calls for organizations to embrace relational structures. Setting aside ample time for consultation, patient hand-off, and team processes have all been highlighted as complex activities, often short-circuited due to pressures of high-demand practice settings. Incorporating secure digital portals, electronic records, and personal electronic devices can facilitate continuous and seamless communication among team members. However, not all team members may be skilled in using e-communication tools. Improving health care through interprofessional practice is grounded in effective provider—provider relationships; relational coordination of care; and communication that is frequent, timely, accurate, and focused on problem solving (Gittell, Godfrey, & Thistlethwaite, 2013).

## USE OF INFORMATION TECHNOLOGY

Effective use of information technology (IT) in health care practices (health IT) can help providers improve their ability to deliver high-quality care. Health IT can support quality initiatives that include benchmarking, quality-improvement projects, educational resources for preventive services, decision support tools, and monitoring outcomes of care over time. The ACA emphasized the role of quality improvement (QI) and measurement, and emphasized the role of IT in reducing medical error, improving patient safety, and engaging patients in care (AHRQ, 2014). In the primary care setting, factors that promote QI and a practice culture of health IT include access to health IT tools, knowledge, skills, and processes as well as work flow and a receptive setting. One challenge is the clinician's workload that impedes time to invest in QI projects since attending patients is revenue generating. One solution may be to design a collaborative model of QI projects where all team providers are engaged, recognizing a variety of skill sets that can reduce the workload of one or two individuals (Higgins et al., 2015).

Another factor that may encourage teams to engage in use of health IT is concern for patient safety. Some topics for team attention could be using health IT to make care safer, ensuring the safety of IT, and using health IT safely. When collaborating among multiple providers, the risk for error and patient safety must be considered. As the use of health IT has grown, hardware and software can malfunction, and data can be lost or corrupted during transmission. Deploying complex technologies in an intricate organizational environment among a variety of providers, in and out of hospital settings, can introduce new hazards and safety risks for data accuracy and patient privacy.

Because of the lack of current information on health IT safety, the U.S. Office of Health Information Technology worked with the RAND Corporation to study safety risks and improvement strategies. The project had the following goals:

- Explore the challenges organizations face in deciding whether to participate in health IT safety risk identification and mitigation
- Test a simple diagnostic approach that participating organizations could use to identify health IT safety risks
- Assist organizations in developing and carrying out short-term projects intended to identify and reduce health IT safety risks
- Evaluate the results of the projects
- Evaluate the governance and management approaches used by organizations to manage health IT safety risks
- Identify barriers and facilitators to health IT risk identification and mitigation in hospitals and ambulatory practices (Schneider et al., 2014)

Findings included the importance of fostering collaboration among departments and disciplines and recognizing the contribution of each discipline in terms of perspective and knowledge in detection of IT safety risks. Examples of collaboration included ensuring abnormal laboratory tests are communicated in a timely fashion, core health IT safety measures are in place, and preparing office settings for IT systems. Incorporating principles of safety within the rapidly emerging world of health IT is crucial to improving patients' health, particularly in a collaborative model of team-based care (Schneider et al., 2014).

## ROLE OF INTERPROFESSIONAL EDUCATION

Over the past few years, a growing body of work has shown that interprofessional education (IPE) can improve learners' perceptions of interprofessional practice, and thus lead toward enhanced interdisciplinary collaboration (IOM, 2001). A Cochrane Review published in 2013 included 15 studies measuring the effectiveness of IPE interventions compared to no educational intervention. The studies demonstrating positive outcomes included the interprofessionalism model, which led to increased patient satisfaction, reduction of error rates, and collaborative team behavior (Reeves, Perrier, Goldman, Feeth, & Zwarenstein, 2013). However, more studies are needed to allow conclusions about the variables associated with the effectiveness of IPE, as well as to inform IPE policy development. Study gaps include

- Assessing the effectiveness of IPE interventions compared to separate, profession-specific interventions
- Randomized controlled trials with qualitative strands examining processes relating to the IPE and practice changes
- Cost–benefit analyses (Reeves et al., 2013)

Although robust research will take time, IPE models, encouraged by grant makers at the national level and private donors, are emerging across the health care disciplines. An excellent resource is the National Center for Interprofessional Practice and Education at the University of Minnesota. This center provides a robust variety of IPE resources, educational offerings, access to current grant-funded research projects, and connection to community members. The center is supported by a Health Resources and Services Administration Cooperative agreement, the Josiah Macy Jr. Foundation, the RWJF, the Gordon and Betty Moore Foundation, and the University of Minnesota (National Center for Interprofessional Practice and Education, 2015).

## CHALLENGES AND BEST PRACTICES IN COLLABORATIVE CARE

Barriers to effective collaborative models remain, particularly in terms of the emerging value-based payment structures. As the payment systems evolve for care providers, allocation of patient care services between primary care physicians and other providers will need to be determined to articulate quality and cost variables among a variety of provider types. APRN work schedules often reflect fewer hours and fewer patients than physician counterparts. In order to improve salary adjusted to productivity and quality performance, comparative information must emerge in order to modify and maximize of all providers types (Buerhaus, DesRoches, Dittus, & Donelan, 2014). These issues must be evaluated in an equitable model that defines SOP and types of provision of services.

Barriers to full SOP, based upon education and licensure, is another challenge for APRNs (including midwives). Many practice settings are unwilling to address licensure and local regulations (i.e., hospital bylaws) that restrict APRN admission and clinical privileges for patients needing hospital-based care. This is particularly an issue for full-scope midwifery practice.

All health care providers are required to obtain a National Provider Identifier (NPI) number, assigned by the Centers for Medicare & Medicaid Services. All APRNs who provide medical or health services must have an NPI number. In addition to federal billing guidelines, each state has licensing authority for APRNs, which can differ depending upon the state in which the APRN practices (Wound, Ostomy and Continence Nurses Society, 2012). Hence, many APRNs work in collaborative environments where the APRNs' direct services are not independently billed under their NPIs, but rather are billed "incident to" the physician. This mode of "incident to" billing places the APRN in a dependent role, employed by the physician and making APRN services and revenue generation untraceable (Weiland, 2008). This practice leads to complexity in accurately measuring value-based care by provider type.

Although these barriers are encountered across the country, there are examples of collaborative practice demonstrating best practices. In 2012, *Obstetrics and Gynecology Clinics of North America* dedicated an issue to highlighting successful collaborative practice models between obstetrician/gynecologists and midwives (Kennedy & Waldman, 2012). All 13 articles were coauthored by both categories of providers identified previously and included diverse models of collaborative care in academic practice, private practice, birth centers, Indian Health Services, and army medical centers. The journal highlighted successful interprofessional practice characteristics, describing lessons learned as well as potential challenges and pitfalls. Thematic to the journal series are characteristics of best practice models with established, effective team-based services, providing sustainable health care for women from wellness to acute illness and disease.

## LIABILITY CONCERNS

A variety of collaborative practice physician/APRN models exist throughout the United States, adding complexity in clearly delineating levels of responsibility and risk/liability associated with direct patient care. APRNs may be sole owners of a business, coemployees of a corporate enterprise, employees of a corporation/business or, in some states, formal business partners with physicians. *Vicarious liability* is a legal term discussed in health care that presupposes additional risk borne by physicians who oversee APRN practice. Vicarious liability is a common-law doctrine that suggests that employers or entities have financial responsibility for mistakes made by their employees (Booth, 2007).

In midwifery, where collaborative practice agreements are required, agreements typically include discussion that defines the midwife as independently practicing as long as the patient's health status is normal. If complications arise, the midwife would notify the physician via a consult and then collaboratively manage or refer the patient to medical care. Instead of a direct supervisory role of the physician, the collaborative practice agreement provides for a transition of responsibilities among different health care providers with differing scopes of practice. Nothing in this sort of agreement creates an agency relationship or an employer/employee relationship. Therefore, a collaborative practice arrangement would serve to articulate the nonexistence of the type of relationship necessary to establish vicarious liability. A review of the case law found no reported cases that would support a theory of vicarious liability by virtue of a collaborative practice agreement being in effect (Booth, 2007).

The most extensive study to date on APRN liability demonstrates concern regarding vicarious liability expressed by physicians. However, 17 years of observation demonstrate that APRNs may actually decrease liability, increase patient safety, and decrease costs (Hooker, Nicholson, & Le, 2009). To minimize risk in collaborative relationships, three best practices are as follows:

- A clearly documented articulation of the relationship in employment contracts
- Collaborative practice agreements as required by state
- Clarity in SOP based upon hospital bylaws and privileges (Hooker, Nicholson, & Le, 2009)

The presence of a collaborative practice agreement establishes the duty for a physician to intervene only to the extent that the agreement dictates. In states in which APRNs have been granted authority to practice autonomously, implications of vicarious liability of physicians related to supervisory authority over the APRN is not likely to incur.

## CONCLUSION

Creating a collaborative working environment in the health care setting requires intent to work together toward a defined mission and vision of shared care. The rapid growth of persons seeking health care and the looming crisis of provider shortage across primary care and women's health disciplines demands all health professionals practice at the full scope of their education, certification, and licensure. Talking openly about collaboration and the challenges, opportunities, and principles for success will break through the silos and boundaries. Successful models of collaboration require old organizational models of power and structure to shift and be replaced by models that are satisfying, not forced.

## REFERENCES

Agency for Healthcare Research and Quality (AHRQ). (2013). Making health care safer II: An updated critical analysis of the evidence for patient safety practices. Retrieved from http://www.ahrq.gov/research/findings/evidence-based-reports/ptsafetyuptp.html

Agency for Healthcare Research and Quality (AHRQ). (2014). National healthcare quality report, 2013. Retrieved from http://www.ahrq.gov/research/findings/nhqrdr/nhqr13/index .html

Akaike, H. (1987). Factor analysis and AIC. *Psychometrika, 52*(3), 317–332. doi:10.1007/BF02294359

American Association of Nurse Practitioners. (2015). State practice environment. Retrieved from https://www.aanp.org/legislation-regulation/state-legislation/state-practice-environment

American Congress of Obstetricians and Gynecologists (ACOG). (2013). *The Ob-Gyn distribution atlas.* Washington, DC: Author. Retrieved from http://www.acog.org/Resources-And-Publications/The-Ob-Gyn-Workforce

American College of Obstetricians and Gynecologists (ACOG), & The Society for Maternal-Fetal Medicine. (2015). Obstetrical care consensus. Retrieved from http://www.acog.org/Resources-And-Publications/Obstetric-Care-Consensus-Series/Levels-of-Maternal-Care

Barker, K. K., Bosco, C., & Oandasan, I. F. (2005). Factors in implementing interprofessional education and collaborative practice initiatives: Findings from key informant interviews. *Journal of Interprofessional Care, 19*(Suppl. 1), 166–176. doi:10.1080/13561820500082974

Berwick, D. M. (2009). What "patient-centered" should mean: Confessions of an extremist. *Health Affairs, 28*(4), w555—w565. doi:10.1377/hlthaff.28.4.w555

Booth, J. W. (2007). An update on vicarious liability for certified nurse-midwives/certified midwives. *Journal of Midwifery and Women's Health, 52*(2), 153–157. doi:10.1016/j.jmwh.2006.11.004

Boyce, R. A., Moran, M. C., Nissen, L. M., Chenery, H. J., & Brooks, P. M. (2009). Interprofessional education in health sciences: The University of Queensland health care team challenge. *Medical Journal of Australia, 190*(8), 433–436.

Brassard, A. (2014). *Transition to full practice authority for APRNs.* Retrieved from http://www.theamericannurse.org/index.php/2014/09/02/transition-to-full-practice-authority-for-aprns

Buerhaus, P. I., DesRoches, C. M., Dittus, R., & Donelan, K. (2014). Practice characteristics of primary care nurse practitioners and physicians. *Nursing Outlook, 63*(2), 144–153. doi:10.1016/j.outlook.2014.08.008

Clark, S. L., Meyers, J. A., Frye, D. K., & Perlin, J. C. (2011). Patient safety in obstetrics—The Hospital Corporation of America experience. *American Journal of Obstetrics and Gynecology, 204*(4), 283–287. doi:10.1016/j.ajog.2010.12.034

Darlington, A., McBroom, K., & Warwick, S. (2011). A northwest collaborative practice model. *Obstetrics & Gynecology, 118*(3), 673–677. doi:10.1097/AOG.0b013e31822ac37f

Dejoy, S., Burkman, R. T., Graves, B. W., Grow, D., Sankey, H. Z., Delk, C., . . . Hallisey, J. (2011). Making it work: Successful collaborative practice. *Obstetrics & Gynecology, 118*(3), 683–686. doi:10.1097/AOG.0b013e318229e0bf

Gilman, D. J., & Koslov, T. I. (2014). *Policy perspectives: Competition and the regulation of advanced practice nurses,* Washington, DC: Federal Trade Commission. Retrieved from https://www.ftc.gov/system/files/documents/reports/policy-perspectives-competition-regulation-advanced-practice-nurses/140307aprnpolicypaper.pdf

Gittell, J. H., Godfrey, M., & Thistlethwaite, J. (2013). Interprofessional collaborative practice and relational coordination: Improving healthcare through relationships. *Journal of Interprofessional Care, 27*(3), 210–213. doi:10.3109/13561820.2012.730564

Higgins, T. C., Crosson, J., Peikes, D., McNellis, R., Genevro, J., & Meyers, D. (2015). Using health information technology to support quality improvement in primary care [White paper]. (Agency for Healthcare Research and Quality Publication No. 15-0031-EF). Retrieved from https://pcmh.ahrq.gov/sites/default/files/attachments/Using%20Health%20IT%20 Technology%20to%20Support%20QI.pdf

Hooker, R. S., Nicholson, J. G., & Le, T.. (2009). Does the employment of physician assistants and nurse practitioners increase liability? *Journal of Medical Licensure and Discipline, 95*(2), 6–16.

Hutchison, M. S., Ennis, L., Shaw-Battista, J., Delgado, A., Myers, K., Cragin, L., & Jackson, R. A. (2011). Great minds don't think alike: Collaborative maternity care at San Francisco General Hospital. *Obstetrics & Gynecology, 118*(3), 678–682. doi:10.1097/AOG.0b013 e3182297d2d

Institute of Medicine (IOM). (2001). *Crossing the quality chasm: A new health system for the 21st century.* Washington, DC: National Academies Press. Retrieved from http://iom .nationalacademies.org/Global/News%20Announcements/Crossing-the-Quality-Chasm -The-IOM-Health-Care-Quality-Initi

Institute of Medicine (IOM). (2010). *The future of nursing: Leading change, advancing health.* Washington, DC: National Academies Press. Retrieved from http://iom.nationalacademies .org/Reports/2010/The-Future-of-Nursing-Leading-Change-Advancing-Health.aspx

Institute of Medicine (IOM). (2011). *The healthcare imperative: Lowering costs and improving outcomes—Workshop series summaries.* Washington, DC: National Academies Press. Retrieved from http://iom.nationalacademies.org/Reports/2011/The-Healthcare-Imperative -Lowering-Costs-and-Improving-Outcomes.aspx

Jennings, J. C. (2014). Optimizing women's health care resources. *Obstetrics & Gynecology, 124*(1), 1–4. doi:10.1097/AOG.0000000000000323

Jennings, J. C. (2015). Women's healthcare: Initiatives and challenges. *Women's Health, 11*(6), 801–804. doi:10.2217/whe.15.36

Kennedy, H. P., & Waldman, R. (Eds.). (2012). Collaborative practice in obstetrics and gynecology [Special issue]. *Obstetrics and Gynecology Clinics of North America, 39*(3), 323–452.

Lang, D. M. (1974). The professional midwife on the perinatal team: Proceedings of the VIII World Congress of Gynecology and Obstetrics. *Excerpta Medica International Congress Series, 412,* 392–397.

Lockwood, C. J. (2012). A crystal ball view of healthcare in 2016. Retrieved from http:// contemporaryobgyn.modernmedicine.com/contemporary-obgyn/news/modernmedicine/ modern-medicine-feature-articles/crystal-ball-view-healthcare

Martsolf, G. R., Auerbach, D. I., & Arifkanova, A. (2015). *The impact of full practice authority for nurse practitioners and other advanced practice registered nurses in Ohio.* Santa Monica, CA: RAND Corporation. Retrieved from http://www.rand.org/pubs/research_reports/ RR848.html

McDermott, J. (2011). Harnessing our opportunity to make primary care sustainable. *New England Journal of Medicine, 364*(5), 395–397. doi:10.1056/NEJMp1014256

Mitchell, P., Wynia, R., Golden, R., McNellis, B., Okun, S., Webb, C. E., . . . Von Kohorn, I. (2012). Core principles &;; values of effective team-based health care [Discussion paper].

Washington, DC: Institute of Medicine. Retrieved from https://www.nationalahec.org/pdfs/vsrt-team-based-care-principles-values.pdf

Mitchell, P. H., & Crittenden, R. A. (2000). Interdisciplinary collaboration: Old ideas with new urgency. *Washington Public Health*, *17*, 51–53.

Nandiwada, D. R., & Dang-Vu, C. (2010). Transdisciplinary health care education: Training team players. *Journal of Health Care for the Poor and Underserved*, *21*(1), 26–34. doi:10.1353/hpu.0.0233

National Center for Interprofessional Practice and Education. (2015). Homepage. Retrieved from https://nexusipe.org

NGA Center for Best Practices. (2012). The role of nurse practitioners in meeting increased demands for primary care. Retrieved from http://www.nga.org/cms/home/nga-center-for-best-practices/center-publications/page-health-publications/col2-content/main-content-list/the-role-of-nurse-practitioners.html

Nielsen, P., Jennings, J. C., & the Presidential Task Force on Collaborative Practice. (2016). *Collaboration in practice: Implementing team-based care*. Washington, DC: American College of Obstetricians and Gynecologists.

Rayburn, W. F. (2011). *The obstetrician and gynecologist workforce in the United States: Facts, figures, and implications 2011*. Washington, DC: American Congress of Obstetricians and Gynecologists. Retrieved from http://www.acog.org/Resources-And-Publications/The-Ob-Gyn-Workforce

Reeves, S., Perrier, L., Goldman, J., Freeth, D., & Zwarenstein, M. (2013). Interprofessional education: Effects on professional practice and healthcare outcomes (update). *Cochrane Database of Systematic Reviews*, *2013*(3). doi:10.1002/14651858.CD002213.pub3

Robert Wood Johnson Foundation (RWJF). (2013). How to foster interprofessional collaboration between physicians and nurses: Incorporating lessons learned in pursuing a consensus. Retrieved from http://www.rwjf.org/content/dam/farm/reports/program_results_reports/2013/rwjf403637

Schneider, E. C., Ridgely, M. S., Meeker, D., Hunter, L. E., Khodyakov, D., & Rudin, R. (2014). *Promoting patient safety through effective health information technology risk management* [Research report]. Office of the National Coordinator for Health Information Technology, U.S. Department of Health and Human Services. Washington, DC: RAND.

Siassakos, D., Fox, R., Hunt, L., Farey, J., Laxton, C., Winter, C., & Draycott, T. (2011). Attitudes toward safety and teamwork in a maternity unit with embedded team training. *American Journal of Medical Quality*, *26*(2), 132–137. doi:10.1177/1062860610373379

Smith, D. C. (2015). Midwife–physician collaboration: A conceptual framework for interprofessional collaborative practice. *Journal of Midwifery and Women's Health*, *60*(2), 128–139. doi:10.1111/jmwh.12204

VanVleet, A., & Paradise, J. (2015, January). Tapping nurse practitioners to meet rising demand for primary care. *The Henry J. Kaiser Family Foundation Issue Brief*. Retrieved from http://files.kff.org/attachment/issue-brief tapping-nurse-practitioners-to-meet-rising-demand-for-primary-care

Weiland, S. A. (2008). Reflections on independence in nurse practitioner practice. *Journal of the American Academy of Nurse Practitioners*, *20*(7), 345–352. doi:10.1111/j.1745-7599.2008.00330.x

WHO Study Group on Interprofessional Education and Collaborative Practice. (2010). Framework for action on interprofessional education and collaborative practice. Retrieved from http://www.who.int/hrh/resources/framework_action/en

Wound, Ostomy and Continence Nurses Society. (2012). National Public Policy Committee/ APRN Workgroup: Reimbursement of advanced practice registered nurse services—A fact sheet. *Journal of Wound Ostomy Continence Nurses, 39*(Suppl. 2), S7–S16. doi:10.1097/ WON.0b013e3182478df0

# CONCLUSION: POLICY AND ADVOCACY— FOSTERING BEST PRACTICES IN A DYNAMIC HEALTH CARE ENVIRONMENT

Lisa Summers

Since the 1920s, when Mary Breckinridge rode her horse to visit the mountain women in their cabins in rural Appalachia, midwives have gathered evidence to document and support best practices (Cockerham & Keeling, 2012; Cunningham et al., 2010). Yet the evolution of health care in the United States reflects many trends that hindered rather than supported midwifery practice; for example, the move from home to hospital birth, a workforce built on increased training of specialists, and a growing acceptance of intervention in the physiologic birth process. It is clear that evidence does not always drive practice. Indeed, the very foundation of this book is to explore whether contemporary practices are based on scientific evidence.

Many factors beyond the scientific evidence influence midwives and midwifery practice. This book has integrated the role of policy and advocacy in an evolving health care system. It addresses the complex health care environment and provides a foundation for examining midwifery practice through a lens of policy and advocacy. Policy questions arise around implementing best practices, that is, what policy levers have been and can be used to support out-of-hospital birth? How have policy makers changed the clinical approach to elective induction? How do we advocate building a stronger and more diverse workforce?

*Health policy*, as defined by the World Health Organization (WHO), refers to "decisions, plans, and actions that are undertaken to achieve specific health care goals within a society" (para. 1) and "defines a vision for the future which in turn helps to establish targets and points of reference for the short and medium term" (WHO, 2016, para. 1). Although the policy is largely driven by individuals whose full-time job is to develop and analyze plans and actions, all midwives have an important role to play in defining the vision for women's health care and influencing those decisions, plans, and actions. Everywhere in the world it is critical that midwives achieve and maintain a degree of "literacy" in understanding the system in which they work. What are the policies that can facilitate or hinder the abilities to practice evidence-based midwifery?

Until recently, it was difficult to engage policy makers in women's health, particularly maternity care. In the United States, the limited attention paid to the health care system focused on chronic care and the impact that aging baby boomers would have on Medicare. That situation has changed dramatically in the past several years. The national debate on reforming the U.S. health care system and several other key developments has created a perfect storm (Howell, Palmer, Benatar, & Garrett, 2014). It has never been more critical for midwives to understand and engage in policy and advocacy.

Although the Patient Protection and Affordable Care Act (ACA) was not the sweeping reform sought by some advocates, it did usher in an era of insurance reforms that have had a significant impact on women's health (U.S. Department of Health & Human Services [DHHS], 2014) that provide opportunities for midwifery. This includes the elimination of denial of coverage for preexisting conditions, thereby increasing access to pregnancy-related care; key preventive services provided cost-free by midwives mandated for many Americans; and outreach and enrollment efforts that increase access to care for vulnerable populations of women.

Midwives need to understand how the move toward value-based purchasing, with less emphasis on payment for procedures and more emphasis on primary and preventive care, provides opportunities for describing midwifery care and empowering midwives as primary care providers. The ACA established the Center for Medicare and Medicaid Innovation (CMMI or "The Innovation Center") within the Centers for Medicare & Medicaid Services (CMS) to test payment and service delivery models. Strong Start is a CMMI initiative that is raising awareness of the value of two midwife-led innovations: centering and birth centers.

A key component of the ACA is the establishment of essential health benefits (EHBs), a set of comprehensive health care service categories that certain health plans were required to cover beginning in 2014. States expanding Medicaid coverage must provide these benefits to people eligible for Medicaid, and insurance policies must cover these benefits in order to be offered in the health insurance marketplaces. The EHBs include maternity and newborn care, but how that care is being defined is still a question (National Partnership for Women & Families, Childbirth Connection, 2012). Does it include midwifery? Birth centers? This is an example of the need to attend to the details and the need for strong advocacy (American College of Nurse-Midwives [ACNM], 2013).

Opposition to the ACA has taken many forms, but perhaps most significant in terms of implementation was the legal challenge to increase coverage through Medicaid expansion. With Medicaid as the source of payment for about half of all births in the country (Medicaid and CHIP [Children's Health Insurance Program] Payment and Access Commission [MACPAC], 2013), this is a particularly important issue for midwives. The ACA expands Medicaid for most low-income adults up to 138% of the federal poverty level, but the June 2012 Supreme Court decision left Medicaid expansion decisions to the states (Kaiser Family Foundation, 2012). The status of state action on Medicaid expansion is constantly changing, highlighting the need for midwives to be aware of trusted nonpartisan resources for finding current information, such as the Henry J. Kaiser Family Foundation (Kaiser Family Foundation, 2015).

Despite partisan challenges, there is agreement that the U.S. health care system is unsustainable. There is a growing understanding of the need to pursue *the triple aim*: improving the individual experience of care, improving the health of populations, and reducing the cost of care (Berwick, Nolan, & Whittington, 2008). Midwives need to be fluent in this language to communicate the value of midwifery care. There is a growing realization among policy makers of the importance of maternal–child health (MCH) care and the lifelong costs that result when good care is not provided at the beginning of life.

Within the government, the Maternal and Child Health Bureau (MCHB) has long administered programs designed to improve MCH care, including the Title V Maternal and Child Health Block Grant Program and Healthy Start. In 2012, MCHB launched the Collaborative Improvement & Innovation Network (CoIIN), a public–private partnership that aims to leverage this growing awareness. These efforts are gaining traction in part because of a growing understanding of the "the life course perspective," an approach to examining racial and ethnic disparities in birth outcomes first proposed by Lu and Halfon (2003). Thought leaders in MCH policy are proposing an agenda for MCH policy and programs that integrates the life course perspective (Fine, Kotelchuck, Adess, & Pies, 2009). We need to address determinants of both health and spending (Halfon, 2009).

Some circumstances that have created this perfect storm might seem marginally relevant to midwifery, but should not be underestimated. The Consensus Model was a critical document released at an opportune time and provides opportunities for midwives to influence policy (ACNM, 2008). Likewise, the Robert Wood Johnson Foundation (RWJF) and Institute of Medicine (IOM) report, *The Future of Nursing: Leading Change, Advancing Health* (IOM, 2010), contains recommendations and key messages that present a valuable opportunity for midwives as well as the strong coalitions of diverse stakeholders that are convening in a Campaign for Action led by AARP (RWJF & AARP, 2015). Midwives can leverage these opportunities to build alliances with key partners in business and consumer organizations, lifting barriers to midwifery practice.

An understanding of evidence and best practices is absolutely necessary, but often not sufficient. Midwives must understand the potential for policy decisions to influence the growth of midwifery and the midwifery model. For example, the National Quality Strategy proposes nine *levers* or approaches that stakeholders can use to strengthen programs, and it is not difficult to recognize how those policy levers can influence the scale and spread of midwifery: public reporting of quality measures driving women to look at maternity care differently, payment reform that rewards and incentivizes providers, and midwifery framed as an innovation in health care quality improvement (Alliman, Jolles, & Summers, 2015). These levers can facilitate rapid adoption within and across organizations and communities (Alliman et al., 2015). Policy makers' eyes may glaze over (or they may squirm in their chairs) with the discussion of epigenetics, nitrous oxide, or birth tubs, but they will be alert to improved quality, engaged consumers, and cost savings.

## FINAL THOUGHTS

### There Is Power in Numbers

Midwifery has grown both nationally and internationally, and birth is becoming safer in large part as a result of effective advocacy. Individuals can be eloquent advocates for a cause, but it is often difficult for an individual midwife or even a group of midwives to know where and how to give voice to an issue. Professional associations make it their business to understand and find those opportunities, but that important business requires resources. Millennials are less inclined to join professional associations, diminishing the capacity of associations to influence policy, but the need for strong membership in professional associations has not diminished. Membership in professional associations provides midwives the ability to combine individual advocacy with organizational capacity, and each member contributes to the strength of the collective voice.

### It's All About Relationships

This text has explored the importance of working collaboratively with nursing, medicine, consumer advocates, and the business community. Formal coalitions are not always the right strategy, but going at it alone rarely works without significant resources (TCC Group for The California Endowment, 2011). Midwives must be aware of and ready to partner with organizations waking up to MCH, from the National Governors Association to the Catalyst for Payment Reform.

### The Time Is Now

The vision of the ACNM, "A midwife for every woman" (ACNM, 2015), has never been more achievable.

## REFERENCES

Alliman, J., Jolles, D., & Summers, L. (2105). The innovation imperative: Scaling freestanding birth centers, CenteringPregnancy, and midwifery-led maternity health homes. *Journal of Midwifery and Women's Health, 60*(3), 244–249. doi:10.1111/jmwh.12320

American College of Nurse-Midwives (ACNM). (2008). Consensus model for APRN regulation: Licensure, accreditation, certification and education. Retrieved from http://www.midwife .org/Consensus-Model-for-APRN-Regulation-Licensure-Accreditation-Certification -Education

American College of Nurse-Midwives (ACNM). (2013). Coverage for birth center and midwifery services under Medicaid and the health insurance marketplaces: Discussion of key questions. Retrieved from www.midwife.org/acnm/files/ccLibraryFiles/Filename/ 000000003595/CoverageforBirthCenterandMidwiferyServices-10-5-13.pdf

American College of Nurse-Midwives (ACNM). (2015). Forging our future: ACNM 2015–2020 strategic plan. Retrieved from www.midwife.org/ACNM/files/ccLibraryFiles/FILENAME/ 000000005401/2015-20-strategicplanexecsummary-final-070915.pdf

Berwick, D. M., Nolan, T. W., & Whittington, J. (2008). The triple aim: Care, health, and cost. *Health Affairs*, 27(3), 759–769. doi:10.1377/hlthaff.27.3.759

Cockerham, A. Z., & Keeling, A. W. (2012). *Rooted in the mountains, reaching to the world: Stories of nursing and midwifery at Kentucky's Frontier School, 1939–1989.* Louisville, KY: Butler Books.

Cunningham, F. G., Bangdiwala, S. I., Brown, S. S., Dean, T. M., Fredericksen, M., Rowland Hogue, C. J., . . . Zimmet, S. C. (2010). NIH consensus development conference draft statement on vaginal birth after cesarean: New insights. *NIH Consensus and State-of-the-Science Statements*, 27(3), 1–42.

Fine, A., Kotelchuck, M., Adess, N., & Pies, C. (2009). A new agenda for MCH policy and programs: Integrating a life course perspective [Policy brief]. Retrieved from http://cchealth .org/lifecourse/pdf/2009_10_policy_brief.pdf

Halfon, N. (2009). Life course health development: A new approach for addressing upstream determinants of health and spending. Washington, DC: National Institute for Healthcare Management. Retrieved from http://www.nihcm.org/pdf/ExpertVoices_Halfon_FINAL.pdf

Howell, E., Palmer, A., Benatar, S., & Garrett, B., (2014). Potential Medicaid cost savings from maternity care based at a freestanding birth center. *Medicare and Medicaid Research Review*, 4(3), 1–13. doi:10.5600/mmrr.004.03.a06

Institute of Medicine (IOM). (2010). The future of nursing: Leading change, advancing health. Retrieved from http://iom.nationalacademies.org/Reports/2010/The-Future-of-Nursing -Leading-Change-Advancing-Health.aspx

Kaiser Family Foundation. (2012). Focus on health reform. A guide to the Supreme Court's decision on the ACA's Medicaid expansion. Retrieved from https://kaiserfamilyfoundation .files.wordpress.com/2013/01/8347.pdf

Kaiser Family Foundation. (2015). Status of state action on the Medicaid expansion decision. Retrieved from http://kff.org/health-reform/state-indicator/state-activity-around-expanding -medicaid-under-the-affordable-care-act

Lu, M. C., & Halfon, N. (2003). Racial and ethnic disparities in birth outcomes: A life-course perspective. *Maternal and Child Health Journal*, 7(1), 13–30. doi:10.1023/A:1022537516969

Medicaid and CHIP Payment and Access Commission (MACPAC). (2013). *Maternity services: Examining eligibility and coverage in Medicaid and CHIP.* June 2013 Report to the Congress on Medicaid and CHIP. Retrieved from https://www.macpac.gov/publication/report-to -the-congress-on-medicaid-and-chip-613

National Partnership for Women & Families, Childbirth Connection. (2012). Guidelines for states on maternity care in the essential health benefits package [Fact sheet]. Retrieved from http://transform.childbirthconnection.org/wp-content/uploads/2012/08/REPRO -Guidelines-for-States-on-Maternity-Care7-30–12.pdf

Robert Wood Johnson Foundation (RWJF), & AARP. (2015). Future of nursing: Campaign for action at the Center to Champion Nursing in America. Retrieved from http://campaign foraction.org

TCC Group for The California Endowment. (2011). What makes an effective coalition? Evidence based indicators of success. Retrieved from www.tccgrp.com/pdfs/index.php?pub=What_Makes_an_Effective_Coalition.pdf

U. S. Department of Health & Human Services (DHHS). (2014). Key features of the Affordable Care Act. Retrieved from http://www.hhs.gov/healthcare/facts-and-features/key-features-of-aca/index.html

World Health Organization (WHO). (2016). Health policy. Retrieved from http://www.who.int/topics/health_policy/en

# INDEX

39092 09653970 7

Printed in the United States
By Bookmasters